COOPER AND GUNN'S

Tutorial Pharmacy

Edited by

S. J. CARTER B Pharm, FPS

Deputy Head of the School of Pharmacy
City of Leicester Polytechnic

With contributions by

Present and past members of the
staff of the above school

Sixth Edition

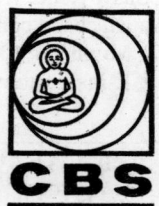

CBS Publishers & Distributors Pvt. Ltd.

New Delhi • Bengaluru • Chennai • Kochi • Kolkata • Mumbai
Hyderabad • Nagpur • Patna • Pune • Vijayawada

ISBN: 81-239-0904-7

First Indian Edition: 1986
Reprint: 1999, 2000, 2004, 2005

This edition has been published in India by arrangement with
M/s Pitman, London

Published by **Satish Kumar Jain** and produced by **Varun Jain** for
CBS Publishers & Distributors Pvt. Ltd.,
4819/XI Prahlad Street, 24 Ansari Road, Daryaganj, New Delhi - 110002
delhi@cbspd.com, cbspubs@airtelmail.in • www.cbspd.com
Ph.: 23289259, 23266861, 23266867 • Fax: 011-23243014

Corporate Office: 204 FIE, Industrial Area, Patparganj, Delhi - 110 092
Ph: 49344934 • Fax: 011-49344935
E-mail: publishing@cbspd.com • publicity@cbspd.com

Branches:
- *Bengaluru:* 2975, 17th Cross, K.R. Road, Bansankari 2nd Stage,
  Bengaluru - 70 • Ph: +91-80-26771678/79 • Fax: +91-80-26771680
  E-mail: cbsbng@gmail.com, bangalore@cbspd.com
- *Chennai:* No. 7, Subbaraya Street, Shenoy Nagar, Chennai - 600030
  Ph: +91-44-26681266, 26680620 • Fax: +91-44-42032115
  E-mail: chennai@cbspd.com
- *Kochi:* Ashana House, 39/1904, A.M. Thomas Road, Valanjambalam,
  Ernakulum, Kochi • Ph: +91-484-4059061-65
  Fax: +91-484-4059065 • E-mail: cochin@cbspd.com
- *Kolkata:* 6-B, Ground Floor, Rameshwar Shaw Road, Kolkata - 700014
  Ph: +91-33-22891126/7/8 • E-mail: kolkata@cbspd.com
- *Mumbai:* 83-C, Dr. E. Moses Road, Worli, Mumbai - 400018
  Ph: +91-9833017933, 022-24902340/41 • E-mail: mumbai@cbspd.com

Representatives:

• Hyderabad: 0-9885175004	• Nagpur: 0-9021734563
• Patna: 0-9334159340	• Pune: 0-9623451994
• Jharkhand: 0-9811541605	• Uttarakhand: 0-9716462459

Printed at NeekunjPrintProcess,Sonipat,Haryana

Tutorial Pharmacy

Contents

Acknowledgements

The use of material contained in the *British Pharmacopoeia* is by permission received from the General Medical Council.

The use of material contained in the *British Pharmaceutical Codex* is by permission received from the Pharmaceutical Society of Great Britain.

Material from British Standards and the booklet, *The Use of SI Units*, is reproduced by permission of the British Standards Institution, 2 Park Street, London W1Y 4AA, from whom copies of the complete Standards and the booklet may be purchased.

We are indebted also to Messrs Glaxo Laboratories Limited for providing Figure 27.13, to Mrs Rosina Faulkner who prepared many of the figures in Chapter 19, to Mrs Cynthia Palmer, Mrs Maureen Richards, and Mrs Valerie Travers for their painstaking typing of parts of the text and, particularly, to Mrs Joan Carter who prepared a number of illustrations, critically read some of the manuscript, checked references and illustrations, assisted with the assembly of the index, and, in innumerable other ways, gave invaluable help.

Contributors

J. A. Box B PHARM, FPS *Senior Lecturer in Pharmaceutical Microbiology, City of Leicester Polytechnic* Part 3, Chapters 26 to 32 inclusive.

S. J. Carter B PHARM, FPS Part 3, Chapters 33 and 34 and the sections on rickettsiae and viruses in Chapter 27.

H. W. Fowler B PHARM, C ENG, AMI CHEM E, FPS, M INST PKG *Lecturer in Chemical Engineering, University College of Swansea* Part 1, Chapter 1, and Part 2, excluding Chapter 19.

C. Gunn B PHARM, FPS *Former Head of the School of Pharmacy, City of Leicester Polytechnic* Part 4.

C. H. R. Palmer B PHARM, PhD, MPS, DBA *Senior Lecturer in Radiopharmacy, City of Leicester Polytechnic* Part 5.

J. H. Richards B PHARM, PhD, MPS *Reader in Physical Pharmaceutics, City of Leicester Polytechnic* Part 1, excluding Chapter 1, and Appendix.

D. N. Travers B PHARM, MSc, MPS, Graduate Member of Institute of Chemical Engineers. *Senior Lecturer in Pharmaceutical Engineering, City of Leicester Polytechnic* Chapter 19.

Preface

During the preparation of this edition, Mr Colin Gunn retired from the editor-ship but, happily, the experience of this outstanding teacher of pharmaceutics has been available to us during the revision. It was he who, wisely, decided that it was no longer possible for one author to prepare a general textbook of pharmaceutics, and who invited me and several other colleagues from the Leicester School of Pharmacy to help with the work. Our contributions are listed on page v.

A major feature of this revision is the greater depth to which many of the fundamental aspects of pharmaceutics have been treated. This has necessitated deletions elsewhere: including the section on the history of pharmacy, because several textbooks on this subject are available; the chapter on surgical dressings, because much of the information that was included previously is more appro-priately taught in pharmacognosy; the detailed descriptions of the preparation of products from vegetable sources, because, today, these have little relevance in most fields of pharmaceutical practice; and the discussion of endocrine glands and hormones, a large part of which is covered in physiology courses.

Further thought has been given to the distribution of material between this book and the companion volume *Dispensing for Pharmaceutical Students*. Future editions of the latter will continue to concentrate on the practical aspects of pharmaceutics that are of particular relevance to the retail and hospital pharmacist, and will include more information on the applications of the principles of formulation and packaging. For reference, a list of the contents of the eleventh edition is included at the back of this volume.

Certain topics, formerly in *Dispensing for Pharmaceutical Students*, have been transferred to this book; for example, the preparation of tablets, which is more appropriately considered under the unit operation of compaction, and the subjects of disinfection and disinfectants, because their theoretical background is large. Radioactive isotopes has been included as a new topic because of the increasing use of radiopharmaceuticals in medicine.

A further important change is the introduction of the International System of Units (SI units). This has presented a number of difficulties (*see* Chapter 1) and was further complicated by the fact that even experienced supporters of the scheme do not always agree on the interpretation of some of the recommendations. In consequence, one or two of our decisions may appear debatable; nevertheless, there is no doubt that, as the system has been adopted throughout most of the world, pharmacy students should be using it now.

School of Pharmacy
City of Leicester Polytechnic

S. J. Carter

PART ONE

Physical Pharmaceutics

1

Units

THE metric system has been a part of pharmaceutical practice for many years; indeed, as long ago as 1867, the first edition of the *British Pharmacopoeia* used metric quantities for volumetric analysis. This was extended in the 1898 edition to gravimetric analysis, and quantities for preparations were stated in parallel, using the metric and the Imperial systems. In the 1914 *Pharmacopoeia*, the quantities for preparations were expressed in metric only, although doses still used Imperial weights and measures, with an approximate metric equivalent. This continued until 1963, when doses were stated in the metric system only, so that all official standards became entirely metric. The metrication of pharmacy was completed on 1st March 1969, when all dispensing under the National Health Service was transferred to this system.

The use of metric weights and measures is, however, only part of a much greater change in which a rationalised system of metric units is coming into international use. Known as the *Système International d'Unités*, with *SI* as the accepted abbreviation, the objective is to derive almost all the quantities needed from a few base units, and to provide rules for the use of SI units to reduce errors and avoid ambiguities.

This book uses SI units, with recommended multiples and sub-multiples, and follows the recommendations of the International Organisation for Standardisation (ISO) and the British Standards Institution (BSI) with a few exceptions that are finding general acceptance where other permitted units are more convenient in practice than the recommended SI units.

In addition, it will be found that non-recommended units are used in certain cases where quotation is made from sources such as the *British Pharmacopoeia* which, at the time of writing, uses metric units, but does not yet follow SI recommendations.

The system of SI units has two important features:

1. All relationships are decimal.
2. It is a coherent system of units and in this respect it differs from metric systems previously in use. A coherent system is one in which the product or quotient of any two unit quantities is the unit of the resultant quantity. Thus, unit velocity results when unit length is divided by unit time, unit acceleration when unit velocity is divided by unit time, and unit force when unit mass is multiplied by unit acceleration. As well as providing straightforward relationships, this eliminates a number of special units and avoids former problems, such as the confusion between mass, force, and weight.

SI BASE UNITS

Six base units are used in the SI system (Table 1.1).

Table 1.1

Quantity	Unit	Symbol
length	metre	m
mass	kilogramme	kg
time	second	s
electric current	ampere	A
thermodynamic temperature	kelvin	K
luminous intensity	candela	cd

SUPPLEMENTARY SI UNITS

Certain additional supplementary units are used, including the radian (rad) for plane angles.

DERIVED SI UNITS

Further SI units are derived from the base units and are stated in terms of these units. Some of the derived units, which are used in this book and which have special names, are listed in Table 1.2. The remainder are included in the list of all symbols and units given in Table 1.4.

MULTIPLES AND SUB-MULTIPLES

As far as possible, numerical values should be kept between 0·1 and 1000, so that multiples and

Table 1.2
Derived SI Units with Special Names

Quantity	Name of SI unit	Symbol	Expressed in terms of SI base units or derived units
frequency	hertz	Hz	$1 \text{ Hz} = 1/s$
force	newton	N	$1 \text{ N} = 1 \text{ kg m/s}^2$
work, energy, quantity of heat	joule	J	$1 \text{ J} = 1 \text{ N m}$
power	watt	W	$1 \text{ W} = 1 \text{ J/s}$

submultiples are recommended for use, based on the decimal range given in Table 1.3.

Thus, kilogramme represents 10^3 g and microgramme represents 10^{-6} g.

Table 1.3
Decimal Multiples and Sub-multiples

Factor by which unit is multiplied	Prefix	Symbol
10^{12}	tera	T
10^9	giga	G
* 10^6	mega	M
* 10^3	kilo	k
10^2	hecto	h
10	deca	da
10^{-1}	deci	d
10^{-2}	centi	c
* 10^{-3}	milli	m
* 10^{-6}	micro	μ
10^{-9}	nano	n
10^{-12}	pico	p
10^{-15}	femto	f
10^{-18}	atto	a

To minimise the number of multiples and submultiples and to reduce the risk of error, only prefixes that represent 10 to a power that is a multiple of 3 are recommended. Those in use in this book are marked in Table 1.3 with an asterisk (*).

To avoid confusion, all calculations are performed in SI units themselves and not in decimal multiples or sub-multiples. In addition, only one prefix is applied to a unit at one time; for example, the term micrometre is used for one millionth of a metre, and not the term milli-millimetre.

EXCEPTIONS TO THE USE OF PREFERRED SI UNITS

Volume

The SI unit for volume is the cubic metre, with the cubic millimetre as the recommended sub-multiple. In practice, it is useful to have a unit of intermediate size and the litre is in common use. This name has been adopted as a synonym for the cubic decimetre and is used for general statement of volumes, with the millilitre as sub-multiple.

Pressure

The SI unit of force is the *newton*, defined as that force which when applied to a mass of 1 kilogramme gives it an acceleration of 1 metre per second per second. The newton per square metre is the SI unit for pressure, but for many purposes the unit is too small. For convenience, a unit known as the *bar* has been suggested, where 1 bar = 10^5 N/m^2. The advantage of the bar is that, for all practical purposes, 1 bar = 1 atmosphere pressure, so that pressures from 0 to 1 bar refer to pressures below atmospheric, while pressures from 1 bar upwards are above atmospheric. For high vacuum work, the unit N/m^2 is retained.

Temperature

The SI unit for temperature is the base unit of thermodynamic temperature, namely the kelvin (K), which is used in all calculations, and generally for physicochemical purposes.

As a 'customary' or practical unit, the degree Celsius (°C) is retained. This is identical to the former degree Centigrade, the change in name being due to the fact that the 'grade', and hence the 'centigrade', has another meaning in some countries.

The degree Celsius and the kelvin are identical units of temperature interval, but since 0°C = 273·15 K, then T°C = T + 273·15 K. It follows, therefore, that temperature intervals or temperature differences are the same in both cases, and these are stated in calculations as K. Hence, if water at 20°C is to be heated by a steam jacket at 100°C, the temperature difference is 80 K. To illustrate these various points:

The unit K is used in the Arrhenius equation, Eqn (6.35), which indicates the effect of temperature on the rate constant of a chemical reaction.

The coefficient of thermal conductivity is used in calculations in Chapter 12 and refers to a temperature interval, so that the units are W/mK.

The reference to the saturation temperature of steam at a pressure of two bars, made in Chapter 12,

Table 1.4
List of SI Units and Decimal Multiples and Sub-multiples

Quantity	SI unit	Multiple or sub-multiple units	Other permitted units
Part I: Space and time			
plane angle	rad (radian)		
length	m	mm	
	(metre)	μm	
area	m²	mm²	
volume	m³	mm³	litre and ml
			(1 litre = 1 dm³)
time	s	ks	minute, hour, day
	(second)	ms	
velocity	m/s		
Part II: Periodic and related phenomena			
frequency	Hz (hertz)		
rotational frequency	1/s		
Part III: Mechanics			
mass	kg	Mg	
	(kilogramme)	g	
		mg	
		μg	
density (mass density)	kg/m³		
force	N (newton)		
pressure	N/m²	kN/m²	bar
		MN/m²	(1 bar = 10⁵ N/m²)
viscosity (dynamic)	N s/m²		
kinematic viscosity	m²/s		
surface tension	N/m		
energy, work	J (joule)	kJ	
power	W (watt)		
Part IV: Heat			
thermodynamic temperature	K (kelvin)		
Celsius temperature			[°C] (degree Celsius)
temperature interval	K		
heat, quantity of heat	J	kJ	
heat flow rate	W	kW	
density of heat flow rate	W/m²		
thermal conductivity	W/mK		
coefficient of heat transfer	W/m²K		
heat capacity	J/K	kJ/K	
specific energy	J/kg	kJ/kg	
specific latent heat	J/kg	kJ/kg	

is a customary temperature, so that it is given as 120·2°C.

Similarly, Chapter 24 gives data on equilibrium moisture contents for various materials at 20°C.

Amount of Substance (Symbol: n)

An additional unit, the mole, corresponding to the quantity 'amount of substance', has been recommended but it is not as yet approved by the international body concerned with the metric system.

The mole is the amount of substance that contains as many elementary units as there are atoms in 0·012 kg of carbon-12. The elementary unit must be specified and may be an atom, an ion, a molecule, etc. or a specified group of such species. For example—

1 mole of K_2SO_4 has a mass equal to 0·174 16 kg
1 mole of K^+ has a mass equal to 0·039 10 kg
1 mole of K_2^{++} has a mass equal to 0·078 20 kg
1 mole of SO_4^{--} has a mass equal to 0·095 96 kg
1 mole of $\frac{1}{2}SO_4^{-}$ has a mass equal to 0·047 88 kg

Units such as the gramme-molecule, gramme-equivalent, equivalent or gramme-ion will, therefore, become obsolete.

PRESENTATION OF NUMERICAL VALUES

In many countries, the comma is used as the decimal point, whereas it has been practice in the UK to use the comma to separate the digits of large numbers into groups of three.

To avoid confusion, this book follows present British practice whereby the decimal point is a full point placed above the line (·) and digits are separated by a small space between groups of three when five or more digits are used, except when data are expressed in tabular form; thus 1000 and 10 000.

BIBLIOGRAPHY

ANDERTON, P. and BIGG, P. M. (1967) *Changing to the Metric System.* London, H.M. Stationery Office.
British Standards Institution (1969) PD 5686, 1969 *The Use of SI Units.* London, The British Standards Institution.
MCGLASHAN, M. L. (1968) *Physico-chemical Quantities and Units.* London, Royal Institute of Chemistry.

2
Solutions

AN understanding of the properties of solutions, and the factors that affect solubility, is essential to pharmacists because of the importance of solutions in so many areas of pharmaceutical interest.

A true solution may be defined as a mixture of two or more components that form a homogeneous molecular dispersion; i.e. a system in which one component is dispersed as small molecules or ions throughout the other component. This definition differentiates true solutions from homogeneous colloidal dispersions, in which the particles of the dispersed component are larger than those in true solutions. (*See* Chapter 5 for a classification of disperse systems.)

In a solution composed of only two components (a binary system), that component which is dispersed throughout the other is termed the solute, and the component in which the dispersion occurs is termed the solvent. In general, the solvent is present in the greater amount, but several exceptions occur. For example, syrup contains about 65 per cent of sucrose in aqueous solution. In addition, it is often difficult to classify the components of mixtures of miscible liquids, such as alcohol and water, as solutes or solvents because either component may be regarded as the solvent depending on the composition of the mixture.

The Process of Dissolution

The transference of a molecule of a solute into solution in a solvent involves a change in the environments of both solute and solvent. The solute is separated from other similar molecules and becomes surrounded by solvent molecules. In addition, the solvent molecules are separated sufficiently from other similar molecules to create space for the accommodation of the solute molecule. Thus, dissolution will occur only if the solute and the solvent are mutually attracted to a degree that is sufficient to overcome the solute-solute and solvent-solvent intermolecular attractive forces.

Similar types of intermolecular force may contribute to solute-solvent, solute-solute, and solvent-solvent interactions. However, the strengths of these various contributing forces differ considerably. The Appendix shows that the attractive forces exerted between polar molecules are much stronger than those that exist between polar and non-polar molecules or between non-polar molecules themselves.

Thus, in a polar solute, where the intermolecular interaction is appreciable, transference of solute molecules into solution will occur only if the solute-solvent association is even stronger. Such strong solute-solvent interaction will result only if the solvent is also a polar substance (e.g. water), since a non-polar solvent (e.g. benzene) will be unable to exert sufficient attraction on a molecule to cause it to separate from other solute molecules.

Conversely, the dissolution of a non-polar substance such as paraffin wax, the intermolecular attractions of which are relatively weak, will occur only if the solute-solvent interaction is stronger than the solvent-solvent interaction. A marked intermolecular association between solvent molecules, such as that which exists between the molecules of a polar solvent (e.g. water) will therefore tend to prevent dissolution of a non-polar solute, so that solvents for this type of solute tend to be restricted to non-polar liquids (e.g. benzene).

The above considerations are often expressed in the very general manner that 'like dissolves like'; i.e. a polar substance will dissolve in a polar solvent and a non-polar substance will dissolve in a non-polar solvent. However, such a generalisation should be treated with caution, since the intermolecular attractions involved in the process of dissolution are influenced by factors that are not obvious from a consideration of the overall polarity of a molecule. For example, the possibility of hydrogen-bond formation (*see* Appendix) between solute and solvent may be more significant than polarity.

Methods of Expressing the Concentration of Solutions

It is assumed that the student is familiar with concentration terms such as normality and molarity.

Although such expressions are included in many existing reference books for pharmacists, the introduction of the SI system of units has either made them obsolete or will eventually lead to their abandonment.

The methods recommended by McGlashan (1968) for expressing the amount of substance in a given solution include—

(a) the molality of solute, which is defined as the number of moles of solute divided by the mass of the solvent, and its SI units are mole kg^{-1}. (The term molality was used in the cgs scale and, although the name is likely to be retained as the name of an SI quantity, the use of the abbreviation 'molal' is not recognised as a unit symbol by the General Conference on Weights and Measures, and the abbreviation 'm' for molality is to be discouraged because this letter is used as a symbol for metre.)

(b) the concentration of solute, which is defined as the number of moles of solute divided by the volume of the solution, and its SI units are mole m^{-3}.

In addition, it is also possible to express concentration of a solution in terms of the mass or volume of a solute contained in a given mass or volume of solution. It should be remembered that the basic SI units for mass and volume are the kilogramme and cubic metre, respectively. These units may be unwieldy in certain instances, and appropriate prefixes to indicate decimal fractions or multiples should therefore be used. The previous use of the litre as a common unit of volume will probably lead to the use of the cubic decimetre (dm^3) as a common unit of volume. It is unfortunate that the term kilogramme and its symbol kg suggest a multiple of a basic unit, and make difficult construction of decimal fractions of this unit by the addition of prefixes. A new name and symbol will probably be introduced in the future.

PERCENTAGE EXPRESSIONS

The concentration of a solution may be expressed as a percentage; i.e.

$$\text{concentration} = \frac{\text{mass or volume of solute}}{\text{mass or volume of solution}} \times 100$$

Percentage weight in volume (% w/v), percentage weight in weight (% w/w), percentage volume in weight (% v/w) and percentage volume in volume (% v/v) are often used in pharmaceutical practice. For example, the strengths of Pharmacopoeial preparations may be defined as percentages; e.g. Belladonna Tincture (BP 1968) contains 0·03 % w/v of the alkaloids of Belladonna Herb.

Solubility

The solubility of a substance in a solvent at a given temperature and pressure, is the amount of substance that has passed into solution when equilibrium is attained between the solution and excess, i.e. undissolved, substance. The solution that is obtained under these conditions is termed a saturated solution. It is possible to obtain solutions that are supersaturated. However, they are unstable, and scratching the side of the container, the presence of dust, or the addition of undissolved solute will provide nuclei that readily lead to precipitation of the excess solute.

METHODS OF EXPRESSING SOLUBILITY

Solubilities may be expressed quantitatively by the same methods as are used for stating concentration. The *British Pharmacopoeia* (1968) expresses solubilities as the number of parts by volume of solvent required to dissolve one part by weight of a solid or one part by volume of a liquid. Unless otherwise specified, these solubilities apply at room temperature. Figures given under the side heading 'Solubility' in the Pharmacopoeial monographs, are only approximate and are not intended to be official requirements. However, statements under side headings such as 'Solubility in Alcohol' are exact and are intended as part of the official requirements for that substance.

TYPES OF SOLUTION

Solutions may be classified on the basis of the physical states of the components. Since there are three states of matter, i.e. solid, liquid, and gas, nine different types of solution with two components are possible, as shown in Table 2.1.

Solutions of solids in liquids are the most important in pharmacy, and only this type of system is

Table 2.1
Types of Solution

Solute	Solvent
Gas	Gas
Liquid	Gas
Solid	Gas
Gas	Liquid
Liquid	Liquid
Solid	Liquid
Gas	Solid
Liquid	Solid
Solid	Solid

discussed in the present chapter. Further information on most of the systems shown in Table 2.1 that are involved in pharmaceutical processes or products is given in the following chapter.

DETERMINATION OF THE SOLUBILITY OF SOLIDS IN LIQUIDS

The following points should be observed in all solubility determinations.

(a) The solvent and solute must be pure.
(b) A saturated solution must be obtained before any solution is removed for analysis.
(c) The method of separating a sample of saturated solution from undissolved solute must be satisfactory.
(d) The method of analysing the solution must be reliable.
(e) Temperature must be adequately controlled.

A saturated solution is obtained either by stirring excess powdered solute with solvent for several hours at the required temperature until equilibrium has been attained, or by warming the solvent with an excess of the solute and allowing the mixture to cool to the required temperature. It is essential that some undissolved solid should be present at the completion of this stage in order to ensure that the solution is saturated.

A sample of the saturated solution is obtained for analysis by separating the solution from the undissolved solid. Filtration is usually used, but precautions should be taken to ensure that: (a) it is carried out at the temperature of the solubility determination, in order to prevent any change in the equilibrium between dissolved and undissolved solute; and (b) loss of a volatile component does not occur.

Different methods of analysis may be applied to the saturated solution depending on the type of system involved. For example, if one of the components is volatile and one is non-volatile, the amount of the latter can be determined by heating to constant weight. Alternatively, the solute may be converted to an insoluble compound by chemical reaction, and the weight of this may be obtained after filtration and drying. Volumetric analysis may be used, especially for those compounds that exhibit the reactions of acids, alkalis, chlorides, etc. which are readily determined by this means. Physical measurements offer a further means of analysis. For example, electrical conductivity measurements are suitable for sparingly soluble electrolytes, optical rotation may be used for optically active compounds, or a radioactive indicator method may be employed. This latter method

involves the preparation of the test material in such a way that it contains a known proportion of a radioactive indicator. A saturated solution is made and its level of radioactivity may be used to determine the concentration of solute.

FACTORS AFFECTING THE SOLUBILITY OF SOLIDS IN LIQUIDS

1. *Temperature*

In most cases the dissolution of a solid in a liquid involves the absorption of heat; i.e. it is an endothermic process with a positive heat of solution. If this type of system is heated, it will tend to react in a way that will nullify the constraint imposed upon it; i.e. the rise in temperature. This tendency is an example of Le Chatelier's principle. Thus, a rise in temperature will lead to an increase in the solubility of a solid with a positive heat of solution. Conversely, if the dissolution of a solid involves the liberation of heat; i.e. it is an exothermic process with a negative heat of solution, then an increase in temperature will lead to a decrease in the solubility.

Solubility curves are often used to indicate the effect of temperature on the solubility of a given substance. Some of these are shown in Fig. 2.1. It can be seen that potassium nitrate shows a marked increase in solubility with rise in temperature, while calcium acetate shows a small decrease. These

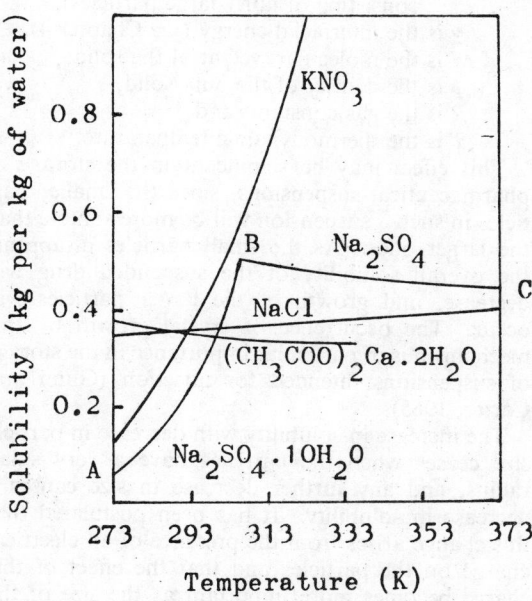

Fig. 2.1 Solubility curves for various substances in water

compounds are therefore examples of substances with positive and negative heats of solution, respectively. The dissolution of sodium chloride involves little absorption of heat, as indicated by the approximately horizontal solubility curve for this compound.

The majority of solubility curves are continuous curves, but abrupt changes in slope may sometimes be observed if the nature of the solid phase in contact with the solution alters. For example, sodium sulphate exists as the decahydrate $Na_2SO_4.10 H_2O$ up to a temperature of $305·55$ K, and its dissolution in water is an endothermic process. Above this temperature the solid is converted into the anhydrous form, Na_2SO_4, and the dissolution of this compound is an exothermic process. The solubility curve therefore exhibits a break at $305·55$ K, which is known as a transition point, and AB and BC in Fig. 2.1 represent the solubility curves for the decahydrate and the anhydrous form of sodium sulphate, respectively.

2. Particle Size of the Solid

The changes in interfacial free energy (see p. 33) that accompany the dissolution of particles of varying sizes cause the solubility of a substance to increase with decreasing particle size, as indicated by Eqn (2.1),

$$\log \frac{s}{s_0} = \frac{2\gamma M}{2·303 RT \rho r} \qquad (2.1)$$

where s is the solubility of small particles of radius r,
s_0 is the normal solubility (i.e. of a solid consisting of fairly large particles),
γ is the interfacial energy (see Chapter 4),
M is the molecular weight of the solid,
ρ is the density of the bulk solid,
R is the gas constant, and
T is the thermodynamic temperature.

This effect may be significant in the storage of pharmaceutical suspensions, since the smaller particles in such a suspension will be more soluble than the larger ones. As the small particles disappear, the overall solubility of the suspended drug will decrease, and growth of the larger particles will occur. The occurrence of crystal growth by this mechanism is of particular importance in the storage of suspensions intended for injection (Gunn and Carter, 1965).

The increase in solubility with decrease in particle size ceases when the particles have a very small radius, and any further decrease in size causes a decrease in solubility. It has been postulated that this change arises from the presence of an electrical charge on the particles and that the effect of this charge becomes more important as the size of the particles decreases (Buckley, 1951).

3. Solvent

It will be appreciated from the discussion of the mechanism of solution that the solubility of a solid depends on the nature of the solvent. The solubilities of a particular solid in a variety of liquids will, therefore, differ. In addition, changes in the properties of a solvent caused by the addition of other substances, may affect the solubility of a solid in the system (p. 12).

Water is the most common solvent encountered in pharmaceutical practice, especially for preparations intended for internal use. Ethanol, usually in various mixtures with water, is also popular. Simple organic liquids such as ether, chloroform, acetone, and various glycols and oils, may be used in addition to water and alcohol in preparations intended for external use. (See Gunn and Carter, 1965, for solvents used in parenteral products.)

4. pH

Many drugs behave as weak acids or bases and their solubility is therefore affected by the pH of an aqueous solvent. For example, a weakly acidic drug such as acetylsalicylic acid (aspirin) will be more soluble in alkaline solution, since it will be converted to the more soluble salt. Conversely, the drug will be precipitated from aqueous solution if the pH is lowered by the addition of a strong acid Similarly, a weakly basic drug will be more soluble in solutions of low pH and will precipitate if the pH is raised by the addition of an alkali.

5. Additional Substances

(a) Common Ion Effect. The solubility of a sparingly soluble electrolyte is decreased by the addition of a second electrolyte that possesses a similar ion to the first. This is known as the common ion effect.

In a saturated solution in contact with undissolved solid, the equilibrium may be represented as follows for a compound AB:

$$AB_{(s)} \rightleftharpoons AB \rightleftharpoons A^+ + B^-$$

undissolved   undissociated   ions
solid   molecule

$\underbrace{\qquad\qquad\qquad}$
species in solution

If the salt is sparingly soluble, then the concentration of solute is sufficiently small to assume complete dissociation into ions. The overall equilibrium may then be represented by

$$AB_{(s)} \rightleftharpoons A^+ + B^- \qquad (2.2)$$

From the Law of Mass Action, the equilibrium constant (K) for this reversible reaction is given by

$$K = \frac{[A^+][B^-]}{[AB]_{(s)}}$$

where the square brackets indicate concentration of the respective components. Furthermore, the concentration of a solid may be regarded as being constant

$$\therefore \quad K = \frac{[A^+][B^-]}{\text{constant}}$$

$$\therefore \quad K_s' = [A^+][B^-] \qquad (2.3)$$

where K_s' is a constant and is known as the solubility product of compound AB.

If each molecule of the salt contains more than one ion of each type, e.g. A_xB_y, then in the definition of the solubility product the concentration of each ion is expressed to the appropriate power; i.e.

$$K_s' = [A^+]^x[B^-]^y$$

These equations for the solubility product are only applicable to solutions of sparingly soluble salts.

If K_s' is exceeded by the product of the concentration of the ions, i.e. $[A^+][B^-]$, then the equilibrium shown above, Eqn (2.2), moves towards the left in order to restore the equilibrium, and solid AB is precipitated. The product $[A^+][B^-]$ will be increased by the addition of more A^+ ions produced by the dissociation of another compound, e.g. $AX \rightarrow A^+ + X^-$, where A^+ is the common ion. Solid AB will be precipitated and the solubility of this compound is therefore decreased. This is known as the common ion effect. The addition of common B^- ions would have the same effect.

The precipitating effect of common ions is, in fact, less than that predicted from Eqn (2.3). The reason for this is explained in the following section.

(b) *Effect of Indifferent Electrolytes.* The solubility of a sparingly soluble electrolyte may be increased by the addition of a second electrolyte that does not possess ions common to the first; i.e. an indifferent electrolyte.

The definition of the solubility product of a sparingly soluble electrolyte in terms of the concentration of ions produced at equilibrium, as indicated by Eqn (2.3), is only an approximation from the more exact thermodynamic relationship expressed by Eqn (2.4),

$$K_s = a_{A^+} \cdot a_{B^-} \qquad (2.4)$$

where K_s is the solubility product of compound AB and a_{A^+} and a_{B^-} are known as the activities of the respective ions. The activity of a particular ion may be regarded as its 'effective concentration'. In general, this has a lower value than the actual concentration, because some ions produced by dissociation of the electrolyte are strongly associated with oppositely charged ions and do not contribute so effectively as completely unassociated ions to the properties of the system. At infinite dilution, the wide separation of ions prevents any interionic association, and the molar concentration (c_{A^+}) and activity (a_{A^+}) of a given ion (A^+) are then equal; i.e.

$$a_{A^+} = c_{A^+}, \quad \text{or} \quad \frac{a_{A^+}}{c_{A^+}} = 1$$

As the concentration increases, the effects of interionic association are no longer negligible, and the ratio of activity to molar concentration becomes less than unity; i.e.

$$\frac{a_{A^+}}{c_{A^+}} = f_{A^+}$$

or

$$a_{A^+} = c_{A^+} \cdot f_{A^+}$$

where f_{A^+} is known as the activity coefficient of A^+. If concentrations and activity coefficients are used instead of activities in Eqn (2.4) then

$$K_s = (c_{A^+} \cdot c_{B^-})(f_{A^+} \cdot f_{B^-})$$

The product of the concentrations, i.e. ($c_{A^+} \cdot c_{B^-}$), will be a constant (K_s') as shown by Eqn (2.3), and ($f_{A^+} \cdot f_{B^-}$) may be equated to $f_{A^+B^-}^2$, where $f_{A^+B^-}$ is the mean activity coefficient of the salt AB, i.e.

$$K_s = K_s' f_{A^+B^-}^2 \qquad (2.5)$$

Since $f_{A^+B^-}$ varies with the overall concentration of ions present in solution (the ionic strength), and since K_s is a constant, it follows that K_s' must also vary with the ionic strength of the solution in an inverse manner to the variation of $f_{A^+B^-}$. Thus, in a system containing a sparingly soluble electrolyte without a common ion, the ionic strength will have an appreciable value and the mean activity coefficient $f_{A^+B^-}$ will be less than one.

From Eqn (2.5) it will be seen that K_s' will, therefore, be greater than K_s. In fact, the concentration solubility product K_s' will become larger and larger as the ionic strength of the solution increases. The solubility of AB will therefore increase as the concentration of added electrolyte increases.

This argument also accounts for the fact that if no allowance is made for the variation in activity with ionic strength of the medium, the precipitating effect of common ions is less than that predicted from the Law of Mass Action.

(c) *Effect of Non-electrolytes on the Solubility of Electrolytes.* The solubility of electrolytes depends on the dissociation of dissolved molecules into ions. The ease of this dissociation is affected by the dielectric constant of the solvent, which is a measure of the polar nature of the solvent. Liquids with a high dielectric constant (e.g. water and formic acid) are able to reduce the attractive forces that operate between oppositely charged ions produced by dissociation of an electrolyte.

If a water-soluble non-electrolyte such as alcohol is added to an aqueous solution of a sparingly soluble electrolyte, the solubility of the latter is decreased because the alcohol lowers the dielectric constant of the solvent and ionic dissociation of the electrolyte becomes more difficult.

(d) *Effect of Electrolytes on the Solubility of Non-electrolytes.* Non-electrolytes do not dissociate into ions in aqueous solution, and in dilute solution the dissolved species therefore consists of single molecules. Their solubility in water depends on the formation of weak intermolecular bonds (hydrogen bonds) between their molecules and those of water. The presence of a very soluble electrolyte (e.g. ammonium sulphate), the ions of which have a marked affinity for water, will reduce the solubility of a non-electrolyte by competing for the aqueous solvent and breaking the intermolecular bonds between the non-electrolyte and water. This effect is important in the precipitation of proteins (p. 60).

(e) *Effect of Complex Formation.* The apparent solubility of a solute in a particular liquid may be increased or decreased by the addition of a third substance which forms an intermolecular complex with the solute. The solubility of the complex will determine the apparent change in the solubility of the original solute. For example, the formation of the complexes between 3-aminobenzoic acid and various dicarboxylic acids has been shown to increase the apparent water solubility of the former compound (Wurster and Kilsig, 1965), and Kostenbauder and Higuchi (1956) have shown that soluble and insoluble complexes may be obtained by interactions between various amides and 4-hydroxybenzoic acid, salicylic acid, chloramphenicol, and phenol. Use is also made of complex formation as an aid to solubility in the preparation of solution of mercuric iodide (HgI_2). The latter is not very soluble in water but it is soluble in aqueous solutions of potassium iodide because of the formation of a water-soluble complex, $K_2(HgI_4)$.

(f) *Effect of Surface Active Agents.* These compounds are capable of forming large aggregates at certain concentrations in aqueous solutions. Organic compounds with low water solubilities are taken into the interior of these aggregates, and the apparent water solubilities of the organic compounds are increased. The phenomenon is termed solubilisation, and more information is given in Chapter 5.

Dissolution Rates

The dissolution of a solid in a liquid involves the transfer of mass from a solid to a liquid phase. The overall transfer process may be regarded as being composed of two consecutive stages. The first of these, which is an interfacial reaction that results in the liberation of solute molecules from the solid phase, is followed by the transport of solute away from the interfacial boundary under the influence of diffusion or convection. Like any complex reaction that involves consecutive stages, the overall rate of mass transfer in dissolution will be determined by the rate of the slowest stage. If the rates of the two consecutive stages are comparable in magnitude, then both stages will influence the overall rate of transfer.

The Noyes-Whitney Eqn (2.6) indicates that the rate of dissolution (dc/dt) is proportional to the surface area, S, of the solid and the concentration gradient ($C_s - C$), where C_s is the concentration of the substance in a thin saturated liquid film (boundary layer) adjacent to the solid surface, and C is the concentration in the surrounding bulk medium. K is a proportionality constant that is known as the dissolution rate constant.

$$\frac{dc}{dt} = KS(C_s - C) \qquad (2.6)$$

This equation assumes that the rate of mass transfer depends on the rate at which the solute diffuses from the thin boundary layer into the bulk solution. Therefore, K will depend on the diffusion coefficient of the solute and the thickness of the diffusion pathway, and it will be influenced by factors that influence the diffusion coefficient and the film thickness.

FACTORS THAT AFFECT DISSOLUTION RATES

1. *Factors Affecting the Complete System*

(a) *Temperature.* It has been shown previously that Le Chatelier's principle will apply to the process of dissolution. An increase in temperature will increase the solubility of a solid with a positive heat of solution. The solid will therefore dissolve at a more rapid rate on heating the system. When complete dissolution has been achieved the system can be cooled to the required temperature, and the substance will remain in solution provided its maximum solubility at the lower temperature is not exceeded. Care should be taken when using this means of increasing the rate of dissolution to ensure that precipitation of the solute does not occur on cooling.

Conversely, a decrease in temperature may be used to increase the dissolution rate of a substance with a negative heat of solution; e.g. paraldehyde.

(b) *Agitation.* The rate of transfer of solute from the boundary layer to the surrounding solute will depend on the concentration gradient between these two regions, as indicated by Eqn (2.6), and on the thickness of the diffusion pathway. This latter factor is included in the value of K in Eqn (2.6). Agitation will help to increase a dissolution rate by reducing the thickness of the diffusion pathway and by bringing fresh solvent into contact with the boundary layer, so producing a high value for $(C_s - C)$. The rate of dissolution may therefore be markedly affected by agitation or stirring, and particular care should be paid to this factor in the measurement of these rates. However, it should be borne in mind that the overall rate of mass transfer by dissolution will be independent of agitation if the interfacial reaction that involves the liberation of molecules from the solid phase into the solution is the rate determining stage.

An increase in dissolution rate may also be achieved by proper positioning of the solid in order to take advantage of the difference in densities of the solution and solvent. A solution is usually denser than its solvent, so that if the solid is supported by some means in the upper part of the liquid the denser solution will fall and be replaced by fresh solvent. This process is less efficient than continuous stirring but it is made use of in the extraction of soluble materials from crude drugs.

2. *Changes in the Characteristics of the Solid*

(a) *Surface Area.* The Noyes-Whitney Eqn (2.6) shows that the dissolution rate is increased by an increase in the surface area of the solid. Reduction in particle size is effective in creating an increase in surface area, as indicated by Eqn (2.7)—

$$S = \frac{6m}{d\rho} \qquad (2.7)$$

where, d is the mean diameter of the particles, m is the mass of the particles, and ρ is the density of the particles. If a unit mass of powder with a density

of 1 is considered, then

$$S = \frac{6}{d}$$

and a ten-fold reduction in the mean particle diameter will provide a similar increase in the surface area.

The porosity of the solid particles will also influence the area of contact between the solid and liquid phases. The rate of dissolution of material from the solid surfaces inside pores is less than that from a plane surface because the pathway for diffusion is longer in the former case. The effect of porosity ceases to be of importance when the pores are of molecular dimensions and become too small to allow access of solvent molecules.

(b) *Polymorphism.* A substance is said to exhibit polymorphism if it can exist in more than one type of structure, which may be stable or metastable. Polymorphism in solids gives rise to a difference in crystalline form between polymorphs of the same substance. This difference may produce a change in the dissolution rates of the polymorphs. For example, Wurster and Taylor (1965b) have shown that three crystalline forms of prednisolone exhibit different dissolution behaviours, and Tawashi (1968) has reported a marked difference in the dissolution rates of two polymorphic forms of aspirin. The pharmaceutical applications of polymorphism have been reviewed by Haleblian and McCrone (1969).

3. *Changes in the Characteristics of the Solvent*

(a) *Viscosity.* An increase in viscosity of the liquid phase will reduce the rate of diffusion of solutes. It is therefore to be expected that dissolution rates dependent on diffusion will be decreased by an increase in viscosity of the solvent, whereas those that are controlled by reactions at the interface will be little affected by changes in viscosity.

(b) *Surface Activity.* It has been postulated that increased dissolution rates obtained in the presence of surface active agents may be caused by a lower interfacial tension, which allows better wetting and penetration by the solvent (Taylor and Wurster, 1965). In addition, changes in the extent of etching of crystal surfaces caused by the presence of surface active agents may lead to increased dissolution rates (Westwood *et al.*, 1962).

The whole subject of dissolution rates has been reviewed by Wurster and Taylor (1965a).

Solubility of Solids in Mixtures of Miscible Liquids

The effect of the addition of a miscible liquid to a solution is of importance in certain pharmaceutical processes and systems. For example, resins are soluble in ethanol but not in water. The former solvent is, therefore, often used in the extraction of resins from crude drugs. The alcoholic solution is then concentrated by evaporation, and the resin is precipitated by pouring into an excess of water. The precipitate can then be collected and washed free from water-soluble impurities. Alcoholic solutions (tinctures) of resins are often used in dispensing practice. If these solutions are diluted with water then the resin is precipitated as a sticky mass. This type of precipitate should be avoided by slowly pouring the resinous tincture into an aqueous dispersion of a protective colloid (p. 61). The mixture should be continuously stirred during this process. The resin should then be precipitated as finely divided particles that are readily dispersible in the aqueous vehicle.

The Distribution of Solutes between Immiscible Liquids

If a substance, which is soluble in both components of a mixture of immiscible liquids, is dissolved in such a mixture, then, when equilibrium is attained at constant temperature, it is found that the solute is distributed between the two liquids in such a way that the ratio of the activities of the substance in each liquid is a constant. This is known as the Nernst distribution law, which can be expressed by Eqn (2.8)—

$$\frac{a_A}{a_B} = \text{constant} \qquad (2.8)$$

where a_A and a_B are the activities of the solute in solvents A and B, respectively. When the solutions are dilute or when the solute behaves ideally, the activities may be replaced by concentrations (c_A and c_B),

$$\frac{c_A}{c_B} = K \qquad (2.9)$$

where the constant K is known as the distribution or partition coefficient. In the case of sparingly soluble substances, K is approximately equal to the ratio of the solubilities (s_A and s_B) of the solute in each liquid; i.e.

$$\frac{s_A}{s_B} = K \qquad (2.10)$$

In most other systems, however, deviation from ideal behaviour invalidates Eqn (2.10).

Association or dissociation of the solute molecules in either solvent should be taken into account, since Eqn (2.9) applies only to an equilibrium between solute molecules in the same state in both liquids. For example, if the solute exists as monomers in solvent A and as dimers in solvent B, the distribution coefficient is given by Eqn (2.11), in which the square root of the concentration of the dimeric form is used:

$$K = \frac{c_A}{\sqrt{c_B}} \qquad (2.11)$$

If the dissociation into ions occurs in the aqueous layer, B, of a mixture of immiscible liquids, then the degree of dissociation (α) should be taken into account as indicated by Eqn (2.12)

$$K = \frac{c_A}{c_B(1 - \alpha)} \qquad (2.12)$$

The solvents, in which the concentrations of the solute—numerators and denominators of Eqns (2.9), (2.11), and (2.12)—are expressed, should be indicated when partition coefficients are quoted. For example, a partition coefficient of 2 for a solute distributed between oil and water may also be expressed as a partition coefficient between water and oil of 0·5.

APPLICATIONS OF THE DISTRIBUTION LAW

1. *Extraction.* Extraction of substances from one phase into another is often used in analytical and organic chemistry and in the removal of active principles from crude drugs. Application of the distribution law to the process of extraction shows that it is more efficient to divide the extracting solvent into a number of smaller volumes that are used in successive extractions rather than to use the total amount of solvent in one single process. (*See* Chapter 22 for more information on extraction, and an example of the method of increasing extraction efficiency.)

2. *Partition Chromatography.* This is a technique used for the separation of components in a mixture. It depends on the difference in the distribution coefficients of the components between two immiscible liquids or between a liquid and a vapour phase. One liquid is maintained stationary by adsorption on to an inert solid support, which may be a powdered solid or strips of a porous material such as filter paper. If a powder is used, then the separation is carried out in a column packed with the powder and its adsorbed liquid phase. The other liquid or vapour is allowed to pass through the column and,

therefore, constitutes a mobile phase. Components of a mixture introduced into the system will become distributed between the mobile and stationary phases in accordance with their partition coefficients, and, provided there is a difference between these coefficients, the components will move at different rates along the column and will eventually become separated.

In paper chromatography, where a filter paper is used to support the stationary liquid phase, the flow of a mobile liquid phase may be made to occur in a vertical or horizontal direction through a strip of paper, or in a radial direction through a paper disc. Whatever the direction of flow the basic principles of the separation technique remain the same as those explained above. More information on the theories and techniques of chromatography is given by Heftmann (1961).

3. *Release of Drugs from Certain Dosage Forms.* Some common dosage forms such as suppositories and ointments are often formulated in water-immiscible bases. The rate of release of medicaments from these dosage forms into aqueous body fluids or secretions will depend on several factors. One of the most important of these is the partition coefficient of the medicament between the base and the body fluid. The effect of partition between water immiscible bases and body fluids is also made use of in the formulation of products intended to provide a prolonged release of drug.

4. *Passage of Drugs through Living Membranes.* The cell membrane is considered to behave as a lipoidal barrier surrounding the cells. One of the main routes of penetration of drugs into cells therefore involves the partition of the substances between these lipoidal layers and the aqueous body fluids with which they are in contact. The partition coefficient of the drug is therefore important in all processes that involve the transport and distribution of drugs throughout the body; e.g. the absorption of drugs from the gastro-intestinal tract, distribution of drugs between various tissues, and penetration of drugs to the sites where they can exert their pharmacological activity (*see* Chapter 6 for more information).

The uptake of preservatives and other substances by micro-organisms is also influenced by the partition coefficient of the compound between the cells and the surrounding aqueous phase (*see* Chapter 31).

5. *Preservation of Emulsions and Creams.* Emulsions and creams are systems comprised of two immiscible phases, one of which is dispersed as globules throughout the other. Micro-organisms usually multiply in the aqueous phase of this type of system, and preservatives must therefore be capable of exerting their activity in this phase. However, most preservatives are usually soluble in both oil and water and will be distributed between these two phases in an emulsion and cream. This distribution will affect the concentration of the substance in the aqueous phase and should be taken into account when deciding the overall concentration of preservative to be used in these systems (*see* Chapter 31).

6. *The Formulation of Solubilised Systems.* Use is often made of compounds known as solubilising agents as a means of increasing the apparent water solubility of organic compounds in the formulation of pharmaceutical preparations. The process is known as solubilisation and it may be regarded as a partition of the organic compound between the interior of the colloidal aggregates (micelles p. 64) formed by the solubilising agents and the surrounding aqueous phase. The activity of the solubilised compound is related to its concentration in the aqueous phase, and a knowledge of the partitioning effect therefore becomes necessary for the proper formulation of such preparations.

7. *Determination of Equilibrium Constants for the Formation of Intermolecular Complexes.* If an intermolecular complex is formed in one phase of an immiscible liquid mixture between a solute A that is only soluble in that phase and a second solute B that is soluble in both phases, then the partition coefficient of the latter will differ from the value that is observed in the absence of A. This change in partition coefficient may be used to determine the equilibrium constant for the formation of the intermolecular complex. This method has been used by Higuchi and his co-workers (1969) to determine the equilibrium constants for a variety of complexes involving compounds of pharmaceutical interest.

Colligative Properties of Solutions

These are the physical properties of a solution that depend on the proportion of dispersed solute particles that are present in the solution. The colligative properties arise from the attractive forces that are exerted by the solute on the solvent. For example, such attractive forces reduce the tendency of the solvent to escape from the liquid as a vapour, and the vapour pressure of the solvent is therefore reduced by the presence of a solute.

The other colligative properties are: (*a*) the elevation of boiling point, (*b*) the depression of freezing point, and (*c*) the osmotic properties. The last of these properties is the most important from a pharmaceutical point of view and the implications of this effect are given by Gunn and Carter (1965).

BIBLIOGRAPHY

BARROW, G. M. (1966) *Physical Chemistry.* 2nd ed. McGraw-Hill, London.

GUCKER, F. T. and SEIFERT, R. L. (1967) *Physical Chemistry.* English Universities Press, London.

HILDEBRAND, J. H. and SCOTT, R. L. (1962) *Regular Solutions.* Prentice Hall Inc., New Jersey.

HOOVER, J. E. (Ed.) (1970) *Remington's Pharmaceutical Sciences.* 14th ed. Chapter 19, Mack Publishing Co., Pennsylvania.

MARON, S. H. and PRUTTON, C. F. (1958) *Principles of Physical Chemistry.* 3rd ed. Macmillan, New York.

MARTIN, A. N., SWARBRICK, J. and CAMMARATA, A. (1969) *Physical Pharmacy.* 2nd ed. Henry Kimpton, London.

ROSE, J. (1961) *Dynamic Physical Chemistry.* Pitman, London.

REFERENCES

BUCKLEY, H. E. (1951) *Crystal Growth.* pp. 29–31. Wiley, New York.

GUNN, C. and CARTER, S. J. (1965) *Dispensing for Pharmaceutical Students.* 11th ed. Pitman Medical, London.

HALEBLIAN, J. and MCCRONE, W. (1969) Pharmaceutical applications of polymorphism. *J. pharm. Sci.,* **58,** 911–929.

HEFTMANN, E. (1961) *Chromatography.* Reinhold, New York.

HIGUCHI, T., RICHARDS, J. H., DAVIS, S. S., KAMADA, A., HOU, J. P., NAKANO, M., NAKANO, N. I., and PITMAN, I. H. (1969) Solvency and hydrogen bonding interactions in non-aqueous systems. *J. pharm. Sci.,* **58,** 661–671.

KOSTENBAUDER, H. B. and HIGUCHI, T. (1956) Formation of molecular complexes by some water soluble amides. I. Interaction of several amides with *p*-hydroxybenzoic acid, salicylic acid, chloramphenicol, and phenol. II. Effect of decreasing water solubility on degree of complex formation. *J. pharm. Sci.,* **45,** 518–522 and 810–813.

MCGLASHAN, M. L. (1968) *Physico-chemical Quantities and Units.* Monographs for teachers, No. 15, Royal Institute of Chemistry, London.

TAWASHI, R. (1968) Aspirin: Dissolution rates of two polymorphic forms. *Science,* **160,** 76.

TAYLOR, JR., P. W. and WURSTER, D. E. (1965) Dissolution kinetics of certain crystalline forms of prednisolone. II. Influence of low concentrations of sodium lauryl sulphate. *J. pharm. Sci.,* **54,** 1654–1658.

WESTWOOD, A. R. C., OPPERHAUSER JR., H., and GOLDHEIM, D. L. (1962) Anomalous solution and etching phenomena. *J. appl. Phys.,* **33,** 1764–1766.

WURSTER, D. E. and KILSIG, D. O. (1965) Effect of complex formation on dissolution kinetics of *m*-aminobenzoic acid. *J. pharm. Sci.,* **54,** 1491–1494.

WURSTER, D. E. and TAYLOR JR., P. W. (1965a) Dissolution rates. *J. pharm. Sci.,* **54,** 169–175.

WURSTER, D. E. and TAYLOR JR., P. W. (1965b) Dissolution kinetics of certain crystalline forms of prednisolone. *J. pharm. Sci.,* **54,** 670–676.

3

Phase Equilibria

A PROPER understanding of certain systems and processes that are encountered in pharmaceutical practice necessitates a knowledge of the principles that govern the equilibria between solid, liquid, and gaseous phases.*

The Phase Rule

The conditions relating to physical equilibria between various states of matter are conveniently expressed by the Phase Rule, which was derived by J. Willard Gibbs in 1876. In order to understand this rule it is first necessary to explain what is meant by the terms 'phase', 'number of components', and 'degrees of freedom'.

PHASE

A phase is defined as any homogeneous and physically distinct part of a system that is separated from other parts of the system by definite boundaries. For example, ice, water, and water vapour are three separate phases; each is physically distinct and there are definite boundaries between them. Pure liquids or solutions constitute homogeneous phases, but two immiscible liquids (or solutions) constitute two phases since there is a definite boundary between them. A mixture of gases always constitutes one phase because the mixture is homogeneous and there are no bounding surfaces between the different gases in the mixture.

NUMBER OF COMPONENTS

The number of components of a system is the smallest number of independent chemical constituents necessary to express the concentration of all phases present in the system. For example, in the three-phase system ice, water, and water vapour, the number of components is one, since each phase can be expressed in terms of H_2O. A mixture of salt

---

* It is assumed that the student is familiar with the kinetic theory of matter and the properties of solids, liquids, and gases.

and water is a two component system since both chemical species are independent.

DEGREES OF FREEDOM

The number of degrees of freedom is the number of variable conditions such as temperature, pressure, and concentration that it is necessary to state in order that the condition of the system at equilibrium may be completely defined. The significance of the number of degrees of freedom of a system will be better understood after considering the specific equilibria that are discussed in the succeeding sections on phase equilibria.

The relationship between the number of phases, P, components, C, and degrees of freedom, F, for equilibria that are influenced only by temperature, pressure, and concentration is given by Eqn (3.1) which is a quantitative expression of the Phase Rule.

$$F = C - P + 2 \qquad (3.1)$$

The application of Eqn (3.1) to various systems of pharmaceutical interest will obviously depend on the number of components present in individual systems. For the convenience of discussing these systems, it is therefore better first to consider those with one component only, and then to move on to those with two components. The succeeding sections are therefore based on such a division, and in each case an attempt will be made to discuss a range of pharmaceutical systems that are examples of each category.

In these discussions the effects of temperature, pressure and composition on the phase equilibria will be indicated by graphs called phase diagrams, which show the variation of a transition temperature such as a boiling point or a melting point with pressure or composition. Representation of the simultaneous effect of three variables would require three axes. This can be achieved with three-dimensional models but if one variable is fixed the resulting planar diagram can be regarded as a section through such a model. The difficulties associated with the representation of three variables do not arise in systems containing one component because no variation in the compositions of these systems can occur. It is therefore sufficient to consider only the effects of variation in temperature and pressure.

SYSTEMS OF ONE COMPONENT

The phase diagram for the ice–water–water vapour system (Fig. 3.1) may be used to illustrate the interpretation of these diagrams for one-component systems. This particular diagram is also of importance in the understanding of the process of freeze drying.

In a diagram such as Fig. 3.1, the areas each correspond to a single phase. The number of degrees of freedom is therefore given from Eqn (3.1) as

$$F = 1 - 1 + 2 = 2$$

This means that temperature and pressure can be varied independently within these areas. For example, by varying the temperature and pressure, a mass of water under conditions corresponding to point w_1 in Fig. 3.1 may be converted to a mass at higher temperature and pressure at point w_2; i.e. this independent variation of temperature and pressure has not altered the number of phases in the system. However, if the conditions are such that the system corresponds to a point that lies on one of the lines AO, BO, or CO, then two phases now exist in equilibrium with each other, since these lines form the boundaries between different phases. The number of degrees of freedom is reduced, because, from Eqn (3.1) $F = 1 - 2 + 2 = 1$. This means that a single variable exists when equilibrium is established between two phases, and if the pressure is altered the temperature will assume a particular value or, conversely, if the temperature is altered the pressure will have a definite value.

Melting Points

The boundary BO represents the coexistence of liquid water and solid ice at various temperatures and pressures. BO therefore indicates the effect of pressure on the melting point of ice, and the negative slope of this line shows that the melting point decreases as the pressure increases. If at any point on this line the pressure is increased while the temperature is maintained constant, then all the ice will be converted to liquid water; i.e. only one phase will remain instead of the two original phases that were in equilibrium at the point on BO. Thus, in order to maintain equilibrium conditions between the two phases, the temperature and pressure must not be varied independently of each other.

Boiling Points

The boundary CO, which is known as the vapour pressure curve, represents the coexistence of liquid water and water vapour under various conditions.

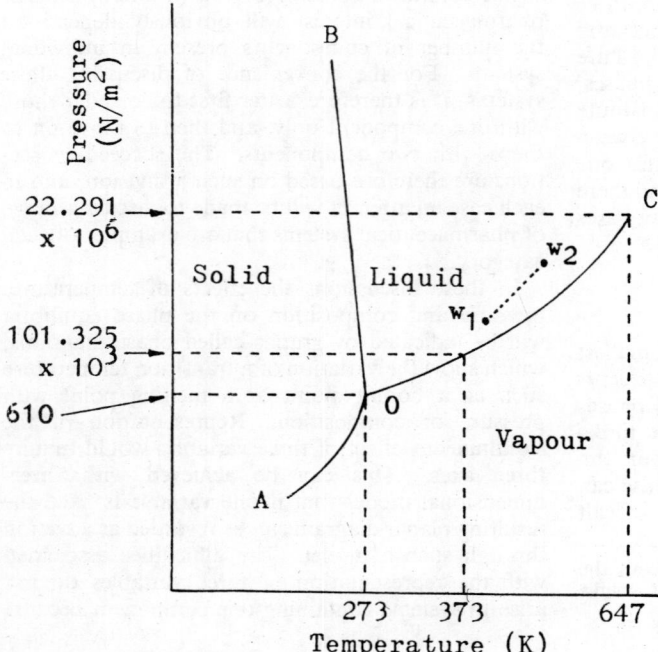

Fig. 3.1 Phase diagram for water at moderate temperatures and pressures (not drawn to scale)

The temperature and pressure again cannot be varied independently otherwise a change from a two-phase system to a single-phase system will occur. For example, if the pressure is kept constant at any point along CO while the temperature is increased, then all the water will be converted to vapour and only one phase will remain. CO therefore represents the effect of pressure on the boiling point of water and it has an upper limit at the critical temperature of water (647 K*). This is the temperature above which it is impossible to liquefy water vapour.

Equilibria that involve vapours are affected appreciably by variation in pressure. Tabulated boiling points should therefore be quoted at a definite pressure (usually atmospheric pressure, i.e. $1 \cdot 013\ 25 \times 10^5$ N/m²), and experimentally obtained values should be converted to values at the appropriate pressure for the purposes of comparison with previously reported ones. Changes in the boiling point of a compound may be calculated from Eqn (3.2), which is known as the Clapeyron equation. (The derivation of this is given in most textbooks of physical chemistry—see Bibliography.)

$$\frac{dT}{dp} = \frac{T(V^G - V^L)}{L_V} \qquad (3.2)$$

In Eqn (3.2), V^G and V^L are the volumes occupied by one mole of the gas and liquid, respectively, L_V is the latent heat of vaporisation of the liquid, T is the thermodynamic temperature, and dT/dp is the change in boiling point with pressure.

A similar Eqn (3.3) can be used to calculate the effect of pressure on melting points, and in this equation V^S is the volume occupied by one mole of the solid, L_f is the latent heat of fusion of the solid, dT/dp is the change in melting point with pressure, and the remaining terms are defined as before:

$$\frac{dT}{dp} = \frac{T(V^L - V^S)}{L_f} \qquad (3.3)$$

Since the equilibrium at a melting point does not involve vapour, then the effect of pressure is very small compared with the effect on boiling points.

Triple Points

In Fig. 3.1 the boundary lines meet at O, which is the only point in the diagram where three phases may coexist in equilibrium and it is therefore termed a triple point. The application of the Phase Rule

equation to the system at O shows that

$$F = 1 - 3 + 2 = 0$$

The system is therefore invariant; i.e. any change in pressure or temperature will result in an alteration of the number of phases that are present.

The triple point for water occurs at a temperature of 273·159 8 K and a pressure of 610 N/m². Thus, the triple point temperature is 0·009 8°C above the usual freezing point of water at $1 \cdot 013\ 25 \times 10^5$ N/m². However, application of Eqn (3.3) will show that a change in pressure from 610 N/m² to $1 \cdot 013\ 25 \times 10^5$ N/m² will produce a decrease in the freezing point of water of only 0·007 5°C. The difference between this calculated value and the observed value is caused by the common presence of air dissolved in water.

Sublimation and Sublimation (Freeze) Drying

The boundary AO, which is known as the sublimation pressure curve for ice, indicates the conditions for the coexistence of vapour and solid phases in equilibrium. A mass of ice may be converted directly into water vapour by heating, provided that the pressure is kept below the triple point pressure. This transition is particularly valuable in drying compounds that are sensitive to the higher temperatures usually associated with drying techniques. Removal of water by means of sublimation is termed sublimation or freeze drying and the importance of the triple point in this process should be appreciated at this stage. Further information on the actual drying process is given in Chapter 24.

Polymorphism

Some substances can exist in more than one type of crystal structure. This ability is known as polymorphism and the different structures are termed polymorphs. If the substance is an element then the phenomenon is called allotropy instead of polymorphism.

A reversible change from one polymorph to another frequently occurs at a definite temperature, and both structures can therefore exist in equilibrium at this temperature. Crystalline forms that exhibit this type of behaviour are said to be enantiotropic. For example, the rhombic crystal structure, which is the stable form of sulphur at ordinary temperatures, is converted to the monoclinic structure at 368·5 K, and the transition is reversed at this point on cooling from a higher temperature. Since each enantiomorph represents a separate phase, the number of degrees of freedom that exist when equilibrium is established between them is restricted

---

* The freezing point of water on the thermodynamic temperature scale is equal to 273·15°C. This value has been approximated to 273°C in this chapter unless stated otherwise.

to one, and the transition temperature is therefore affected by pressure. Thus, in a system containing a solid that is able to exist as two polymorphs, an additional line is required in the phase diagram to represent the boundary between the two solid forms. The inclusion of an extra boundary increases the number of triple points in a phase diagram. The sulphur phase diagram is the classical example of such a system and the Bibliography should be consulted for an explanation of this diagram. The phase diagram of water at very high pressures could, in fact, be used to illustrate the phenomenon of polymorphism, because ice may exist in several different forms. However, this would not be very satisfactory as a simple illustration owing to the rather complicated nature of the phase diagram of water under these conditions.

In some cases the change from one polymorphic form to another occurs in one direction only and reversion is not possible in a direct manner. Substances that exhibit this type of polymorphism are termed monotropic. For example, diamond can be converted directly into graphite but the reverse process is not directly possible.

The polymorphic changes between the crystalline forms of fatty acids and glycerides are nearly always monotropic. Theobroma oil, which is used in the preparation of suppositories, is a polymorphous, natural substance. It consists mainly of a single glyceride and usually melts over a narrow temperature range (34 to 36°C), which is just below normal body temperature. The four polymorphic forms of this substance are shown in Table 3.1 together with

Table 3.1
The Polymorphic Forms of
Theobroma Oil

Polymorph	m.p. (°C)
Metastable γ form	18
Metastable α form	22
Metastable β' form	24
Stable β form	34·5

their melting points. If, during the course of preparation of suppositories, theobroma oil is heated to about 35°C or above and completely liquefied, then the resulting suppositories are too soft for proper administration and tend to melt at ordinary room temperatures. It has been pointed out (Riegelman, 1955) that the excessive heating will cause complete destruction of the nuclei of the stable β form. Consequently, the mass tends to supercool to about 15°C before crystallisation reoccurs in the form of the metastable α, β', and γ forms with a melting

point of 22 to 24°C. If the initial heating is limited to about 33°C the mass is sufficiently fluid for pouring, but the nuclei of the stable β form are preserved and cause the separation of β crystals with a melting point of 34·5°C on cooling.

Polymorphism may also be exhibited by liquids. For example, cholesteryl acetate melts to produce a turbid liquid which becomes clear at a higher transition temperature. The turbid and clear forms of polymorphic liquids have different optical properties and the turbid forms have been referred to as liquid crystals, although the terms anisotropic or mesomorphic liquids are preferable. The transition temperature for the change from mesomorphic liquid to clear liquid is pressure dependent.

The different crystal structures of polymorphic forms of the same substance will cause a difference in the thermodynamic activities of the polymorphs (Higuchi and co-workers, 1963). This is of importance in pharmacy, since many drugs exhibit polymorphism and their activities will govern their stabilities and their rates of solution. Thus, one polymorph may be more stable than others. In addition, one may show a greater rate of solution and may therefore be absorbed from the gastrointestinal tract at a greater rate than other forms, and so produce a higher plasma concentration. For example, the effect of polymorphism on the availability of methylprednisolone and sulphathiazole has been investigated by Higuchi and his co-workers (1963, 1967), and Aguiar and his co-workers (1967) have shown that the polymorphic state of chloramphenicol palmitate has a significant influence on the blood levels of chloramphenicol in humans. If the existence of polymorphism is unrecognised, then the possibility of variation in the availability of a given drug from successive doses may arise. The pharmaceutical applications of polymorphism have been reviewed by Haleblian and McCrone (1969).

SYSTEMS OF TWO COMPONENTS

Table 3.2 shows the effect of the number of phases on the degrees of freedom in a two-component system. When one phase only is present there are

Table 3.2
The Degrees of Freedom in
Two-component Systems

P	F
1	3
2	2
3	1
4	0

three degrees of freedom; i.e. temperature, pressure, and composition. Thus, the behaviour of a two component system may be represented completely only by a three-dimensional diagram showing the relations between the three variables. However, it is more convenient to use separate two-dimensional diagrams which show the relation between two of the variables while the third is kept constant; e.g. diagrams showing the variation of pressure with composition at constant temperature, or the variation of composition with temperature at constant pressure.

Solid-Vapour Systems of Two Components

The conversion of an anhydrous salt to a hydrated form, the transition of one hydrated form to a higher hydrate, and the phenomena of deliquescence, hygroscopicity, efflorescence, and exsiccation are examples of the equilibria in systems containing a solid and water vapour.

HYDRATION AND DEHYDRATION OF SALTS

Each hydrated form of a salt exerts a definite vapour pressure at a given temperature. The relation between this value and that of the vapour pressure of water vapour in the atmosphere surrounding the salt is of importance in deciding the type of hydrate formed under various conditions.

EFFLORESCENCE AND EXSICCATION

If the vapour pressure of a hydrated salt is greater than the pressure exerted by the water vapour in the surrounding atmosphere then the salt will attempt to attain equilibrium with its surroundings, and therefore tend to lose water to form a lower hydrate or an anhydrous salt. This phenomenon is known as efflorescence.

The pressure of water vapour in the atmosphere is about 13.33×10^2 N/m^2 at 293 K, and therefore hydrates with vapour pressures greater than this will tend to exhibit efflorescence and be unstable, provided that the lower hydrate that is formed still exerts a vapour pressure greater than the surrounding atmosphere. If this is not so, then water will be taken up from the atmosphere by the lower hydrate as fast as it is formed and the final equilibrium will depend on the rates at which water is lost or taken up by the two hydrates. For example, the behaviour of the various forms of sodium carbonate may be represented by the following scheme—

$Na_2CO_3.10\,H_2O$　　v.p. $= 32 \times 10^2$ N/m^2 at 293 K

　　↓ spontaneous dehydration;
　　　i.e. efflorescence.

$Na_2CO_3.H_2O$　　v.p. $= 16 \times 10^2$ N/m^2 at 293 K

　　↑↓ efflorescence not observable
　　　because anhydrous salt is
　　　rapidly hydrated.

Na_2CO_3 (anhyd.)　　v.p. $= 0$

Since the vapour pressure exerted by the decahydrate is much greater than that of normal atmosphere it loses water by the process of efflorescence and is converted to the monohydrate. The vapour pressure of the latter is still above that of the atmosphere, but further apparent loss of water does not occur since the anhydrous salt is rehydrated at a faster rate than dehydration of the monohydrate.

The vapour pressure of hydrated salts, and therefore the rate of efflorescence, increases with rise in temperature. The process of accelerating the rate of efflorescence by increasing the temperature in order to remove water of crystallisation from a hydrated salt is known as exsiccation, although this term is also used where water is not normally lost by efflorescence. For example, the pentahydrate of copper sulphate may be converted to the trihydrate by heating to 303 K. Two further molecules of water are removed at 373 K to yield the monohydrate, and the remaining molecule of water is removed at 473 K to yield the anhydrous salt.

Since the instability that arises from efflorescence is caused by the loss of water vapour, the common method of minimising such deterioration involves the use of containers that prevent the loss of water vapour. The additional precautions of using well-filled containers with a minimum amount of atmosphere above the efflorescent material and storage in a cool place are also advisable.

DELIQUESCENCE AND HYGROSCOPICITY

Both of these terms are used to indicate that a material takes up water vapour from the atmosphere and is converted to a more hydrated form. In the case of a hygroscopic substance the more hydrated state is still a solid but deliquescence implies the eventual formation of a liquid phase; i.e. a solution. In both phenomena, however, the final more hydrated state must still exert a lower vapour pressure than that of the water vapour in the surrounding atmosphere. If this is not so then the newly formed hydrated state will immediately lose water by efflorescence and revert to the initial state.

Thus, for a liquid phase to be produced by deliquescence, it is necessary that the vapour pressure exerted by a saturated solution of the deliquescent material should be less than 13.33×10^2 N/m². The following scheme showing the behaviour of sodium hydroxide may be used as an example of deliquescence.

NaOH.H$_2$O   v.p. is very low at 293 K

| Deliquescence

↓

Saturated
solution   v.p. $= 1.33 \times 10^2$ N/m² at 293 K
of NaOH

| Further deliquescence

↓

Unsaturated
solution   v.p. = v.p. of atmospheric moisture
of NaOH

Other deliquescent materials include potassium hydroxide, sodium lactate and potassium carbonate, while examples of hygroscopic materials include exsiccated sodium sulphate, ammonium chloride, and squill.

Storage precautions for pharmaceutical preparations that are deliquescent or hygroscopic are aimed at the maintenance of a moisture-free atmosphere inside the container. The closures of the latter should therefore prevent the access of water vapour, and official monographs usually direct that such substances should be stored in 'well-closed' containers. In addition, a well-filled container limits the volume of atmosphere in the container and, therefore, further reduces the uptake of moisture by the product. In certain cases, where the product is particularly susceptible to moisture, a drying agent may be placed inside the container. The drying agent is usually contained in small packets, made from a material that is pervious to water vapour, in order to prevent contact between the agent and the product. Silica gel is often used in this way and it may contain an indicator to show when its drying properties are no longer satisfactory. Anhydrous cobaltous chloride, which is blue, may be used as an indicator, since it is converted to a pink hydrate when the silica gel has adsorbed its maximum amount of water vapour.

Liquid-Liquid Systems of Two Components; Solutions of Liquids in Liquids

The degree of miscibility of two liquids may be used as a basis for the classification of these systems into

the following types:

1. Completely miscible liquids.
2. Partially miscible liquids.
3. Immiscible liquids.

1. COMPLETELY MISCIBLE LIQUIDS

A solution of one liquid in another in contact with vapour from the liquid mixture constitutes a two-phase system of two components. The Phase Rule therefore indicates that such a system will possess two degrees of freedom; i.e.

$$F = 2 - 2 + 2 = 2.$$

Thus, the system will be completely defined by two variables. For example, if the temperature and composition are fixed, the vapour pressure must have a definite value, or if the pressure and composition are fixed then the equilibrium will only be maintained at a particular temperature.

In diagrams involving vapour pressures exerted by solutions of liquids in liquids it is necessary to consider the application of Raoult's law. This states that the partial vapour pressure exerted by each component is proportional to its molar concentration in the solution. The law may be expressed by Eqn (3.4):

$$p = p_A + p_B = p_A^0 x_A + p_B^0 x_B \qquad (3.4)$$

where p is the total vapour pressure above a liquid mixture containing x_A and x_B mole fractions of components A and B, respectively, p_A^0 and p_B^0 are the vapour pressures exerted by the pure components, and p_A and p_B are the partial vapour pressures exerted by the components in the liquid mixture.

Ideal Solutions. Raoult's law is obeyed by only a few solutions of liquids in liquids. However, it is convenient to consider an ideal solution, to which this law applies, and to discuss real solutions in terms of the deviations in their behaviour from that of an ideal solution.

A graph showing the variation in the partial pressure of each component in an ideal solution, with the composition of the solution at constant temperature, should produce a straight line which passes through the origin, since $p_A = p_A^0 x_A$ and $p_B = p_B^0 x_B$. The line for each component can be represented on the same diagram as shown in Fig. 3.2, where $O_A p_A^0$ and $O_B p_B^0$ indicate the variations in partial pressures exerted by components A and B, respectively, with the composition of the mixture. From Eqn (3.4), and by applying simple geometry, it can be shown that the line $p_A^0 p_B^0$ will indicate the variation in the total vapour pressure with composition.

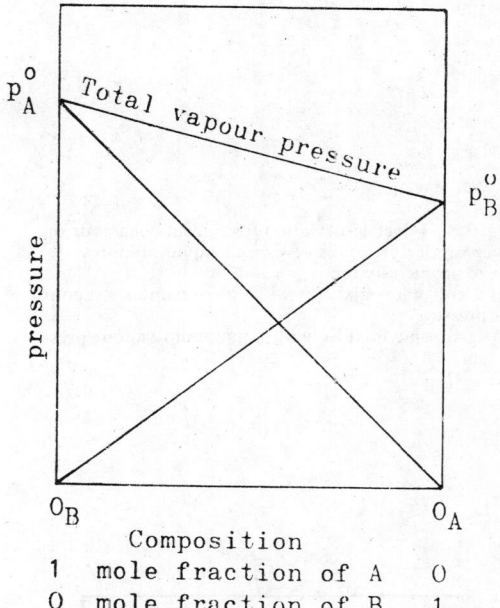

Composition

1   mole fraction of A   0

0   mole fraction of B   1

Fig. 3.2   Vapour-composition diagram for an ideal solution

Real Solutions.   As previously stated, only a few actual solutions show ideal behaviour. The components of these ideal solutions have a similar chemical structure; e.g. benzene and toluene, *n*-hexane and *n*-heptane, ethyl bromide and ethyl iodide.

Most systems show varying degrees of deviation from Raoult's law, depending on the nature of the liquids and on the temperature. When interactions such as hydrogen bonding, salt formation, or hydration occur between the components of a solution, then the vapour pressure of each component is lowered with respect to the behaviour of an ideal solution and the system is said to exhibit a negative deviation from Raoult's law; e.g. chloroform and acetone, pyridine and acetic acid, water and nitric acid.

In most systems, the vapour pressures are greater than those of an ideal solution and positive deviations from Raoult's law are therefore exhibited. This type of behaviour occurs when the components differ in their polarity, length of hydrocarbon chain, and degree of association; e.g. carbon tetrachloride and cyclohexane, benzene and ethanol, water and ethanol. The degree of deviation from Raoult's law decreases as the temperature increases, since the effects of the differences in the natures of the components are reduced at higher temperatures.

Conversely, a decrease in temperature may lead to a decrease in miscibility of the two components and phase separation may occur.

The occurrence of deviations from ideal behaviour allows the classification of solutions of liquids in liquids into three types.

(*a*) Systems where the total vapour pressure is always intermediate between those of the pure components; i.e. there is neither a maximum nor minimum in the vapour pressure-composition diagram as shown in Fig. 3.3(*a*). These systems are known as zeotropic mixtures and examples include carbon tetrachloride and cyclohexane, and water and methanol.

(*b*) Systems that exhibit a maximum value in the vapour pressure-composition diagrams as shown in Fig. 3.3(*b*). These are known as azeotropic mixtures with a maximum vapour pressure or minimum boiling point and examples include benzene and ethanol, and water and ethanol.

(*c*) Systems that exhibit a minimum value in the vapour pressure-composition diagrams as shown in Fig. 3.3(*c*). These are known as azeotropic mixtures with a minimum vapour pressure or maximum boiling point. and examples include chloroform and acetone, pyridine and acetic acid, and water and nitric acid.

The effects of these different types of behaviour on the results of distillation of liquid mixtures is of importance in various pharmaceutical fields. However, before these distillations can be considered, it is necessary to take into account the composition of the vapour that is in equilibrium with the liquid mixtures of different compositions. The previous vapour pressure diagrams show only the relation between vapour pressure and composition of the liquid phase. If these diagrams are drawn to show the variation in vapour pressure with both vapour and liquid compositions, the results may be represented by Fig. 3.4(*a*), (*b*), and (*c*), respectively.

The upper curves in these figures represent the variation in total vapour pressure with composition of the liquid phase, and the lower curves represent the variation in total vapour pressure with composition of the vapour phase. The different areas correspond to the existence of liquid, vapour, or liquid plus vapour, as shown in the diagrams.

When equilibrium is established between liquid and vapour phases the vapour pressure must be constant. It can therefore be seen that the compositions of the vapours (v_1 to v_5) that are in equilibrium with liquids of compositions given by l_1 to l_5 are obtained by drawing horizontal tie-lines through the points on the liquid composition curves that correspond to l_1 to l_5. The points at which these lines intersect the vapour curves provide the compositions

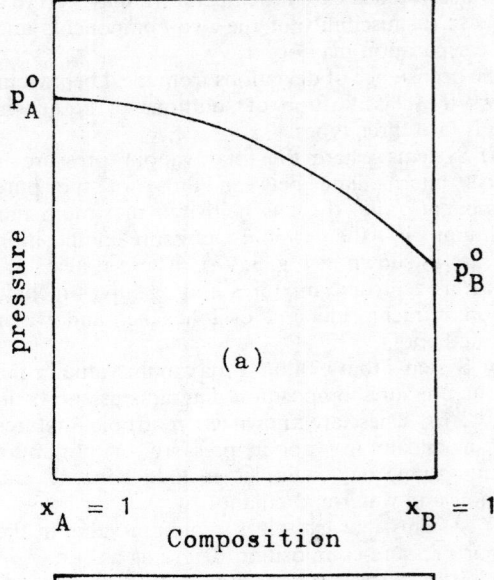

Fig. 3.3   Effect of deviation from ideal behaviour on total vapour pressures of various liquid mixtures
(a) zeotropic mixture
(b) azeotropic mixture with a maximum vapour pressure
(c) azeotropic mixture with a minimum vapour pressure

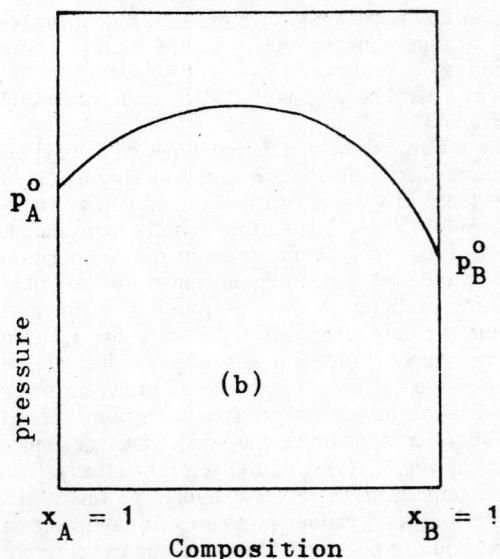

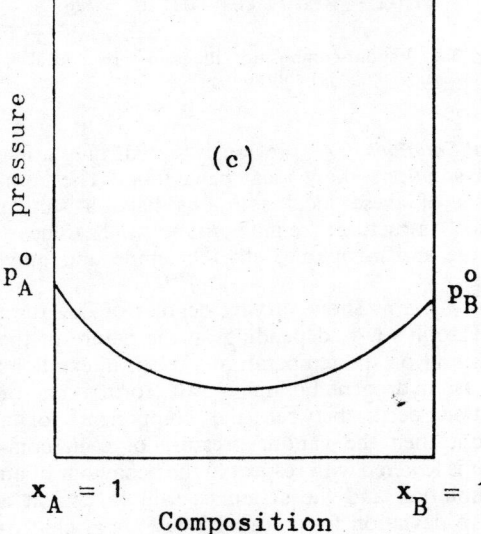

v_1 to v_5. It can be seen from Fig. 3.4(a) that the vapour phase in equilibrium with a particular liquid composition is richer in the more volatile component A; i.e. the component with the higher vapour pressure. This is known as Konowaloff's Rule.

The point M in Fig. 3.4(b) and (c) corresponds to the formation of an azeotrope, which is a mixture with a lower or higher vapour pressure than is exerted by any other composition in the system. It will be observed that the liquid and vapour have identical compositions at this point.

Distillation of Solutions of Liquids in Liquids

(a) Zeotropic Mixtures. For the purpose of explaining the effects of distillation it is more convenient to use a phase diagram (Fig. 3.5) that shows the variation in boiling point with composition of the liquid and vapour phases at constant pressure. It should be observed that the upper and lower curves in Fig. 3.5 represent the vapour composition and the liquid composition, respectively, and that the areas corresponding to liquid and vapour phases are

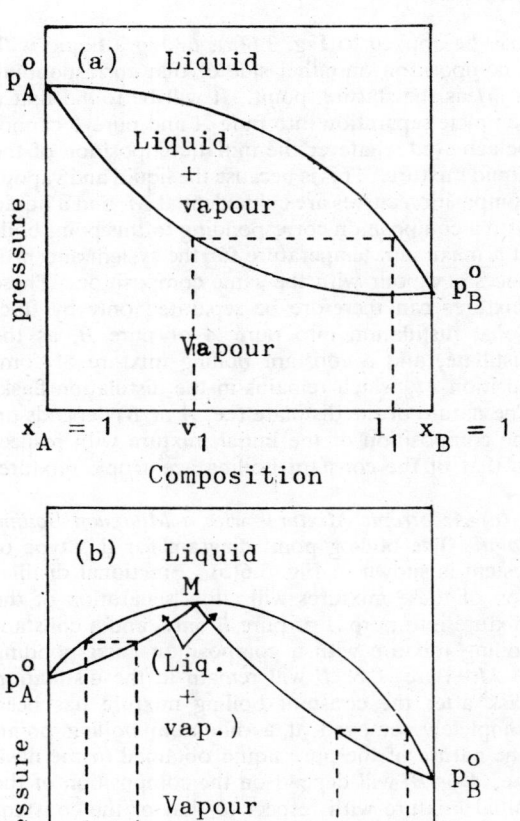

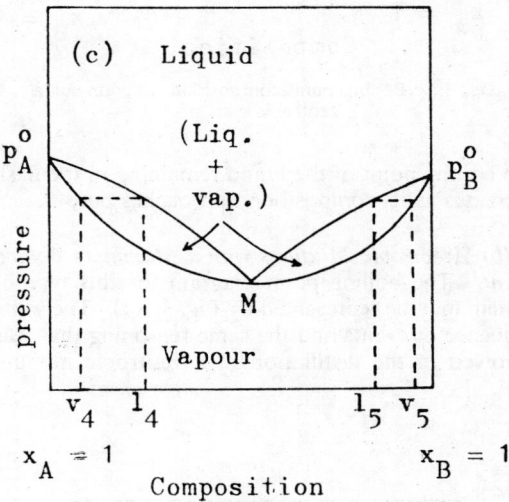

Fig. 3.4 Vapour pressure diagrams showing liquid and vapour composition curves for various liquid mixtures
(*a*) zeotropic mixture
(*b*) azeotropic mixture with a maximum vapour pressure
(*c*) azeotropic mixture with a minimum vapour pressure

transposed when compared with the vapour pressure diagrams shown in Fig. 3.4(*a*). Konowaloff's Rule can still be seen to apply in the boiling point diagram, since a liquid with a composition corresponding to l_1 will boil at temperature T_1 and be in equilibrium with vapour of composition l_2. This vapour is therefore richer in component A, which has the lower boiling point (T_A) and is therefore the more volatile component of the liquid mixture.

It can also be seen from Fig. 3.5 that if the vapour of composition l_2 is removed and condensed it will give a liquid of composition l_2. If this liquid is subsequently heated it will boil at temperature T_2 to provide a vapour of composition l_3 that is even richer in component A; i.e. the composition of the distillate will approach closer to pure A as more stages of heating and condensation are involved. Conversely, as vapour that is richer in A is removed

from the distillation flask the composition of the liquid remaining in the flask gradually approaches pure B. Thus, the components of a zeotropic mixture may be separated completely by the process of fractional distillation, which involves the occurrence of many individual stages of vaporisation and condensation in a distillation column. (*See* Chapter 23 for more information on distillation as a unit operation.)

If the Phase Rule is applied to the two-component system in the distillation flask where two phases (i.e. liquid and vapour) are present, it can be shown that two degrees of freedom exist:

$$F = 2 - 2 + 2 = 2$$

Since the pressure is kept constant, the temperature will therefore change as the composition varies in order to maintain the same number of phases; i.e.

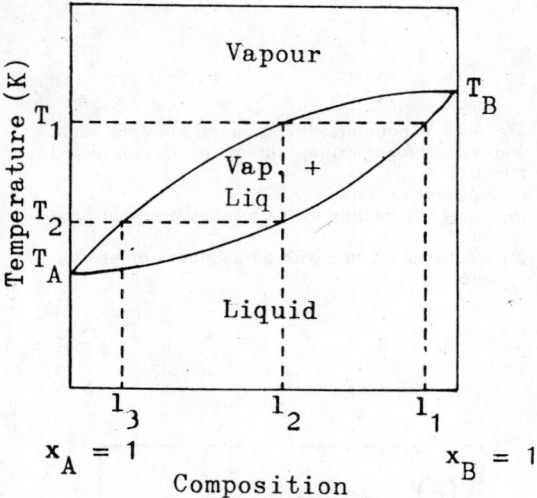

Fig. 3.5 Boiling point-composition diagram for a zeotropic system

may be applied to Fig. 3.6(a), taking a liquid with a composition on either side of that corresponding to M as the starting point. It will be found that a complete separation into pure A and pure B cannot be achieved whatever the initial composition of the liquid mixture. This is because the liquid and vapour composition curves are coincident at M, and a liquid with a composition corresponding to this point boils at a maximum temperature for the system and produces a vapour with the same composition. These mixtures can therefore be separated only by fractional distillation into pure A or pure B, as the distillate, and a constant boiling mixture of composition M, which remains in the distillation flask. The nature of the distillate (i.e. A or B) depends on the composition of the initial mixture with respect to that of the constant boiling azeotropic mixture.

(c) *Azeotropic Mixtures with a Minimum Boiling Point.* The boiling point diagram for this type of system is shown in Fig. 3.6(b). Fractional distillation of these mixtures will allow separation of the mixture into pure A or pure B only, and a constant boiling mixture with a composition corresponding to M. Pure A or B will remain in the distillation flask after the constant boiling mixture has been completely removed at a minimum boiling point. The nature of the pure liquid obtained in the flask (i.e. A or B) will depend on the composition of the initial mixture with respect to that of the constant boiling azeotrope.

the boiling point of the liquid remaining in the flask increases as its composition approaches pure B.

(b) *Azeotropic Mixtures with a Maximum Boiling Point.* The boiling point diagram for this type of system may be represented by Fig. 3.6(a). The same sequence of events and the same reasoning that was involved in the distillation of a zeotropic mixture

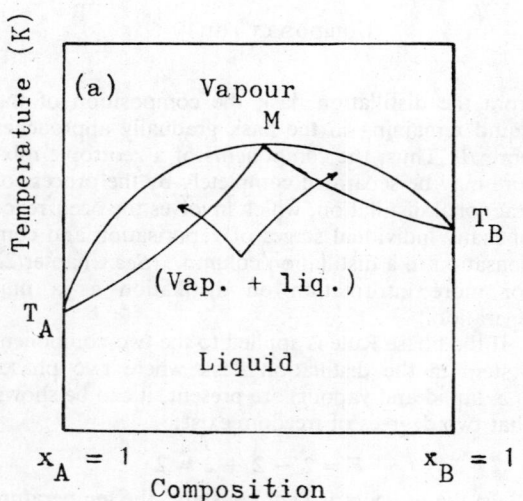

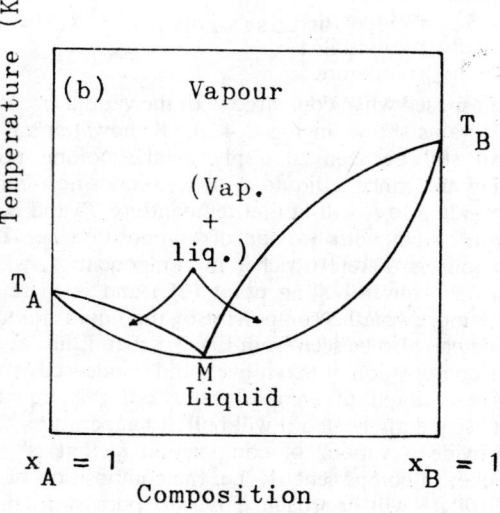

Fig. 3.6 Boiling point-composition diagrams for azeotropic mixtures
(a) maximum boiling point azeotrope   (b) minimum boiling point azeotrope

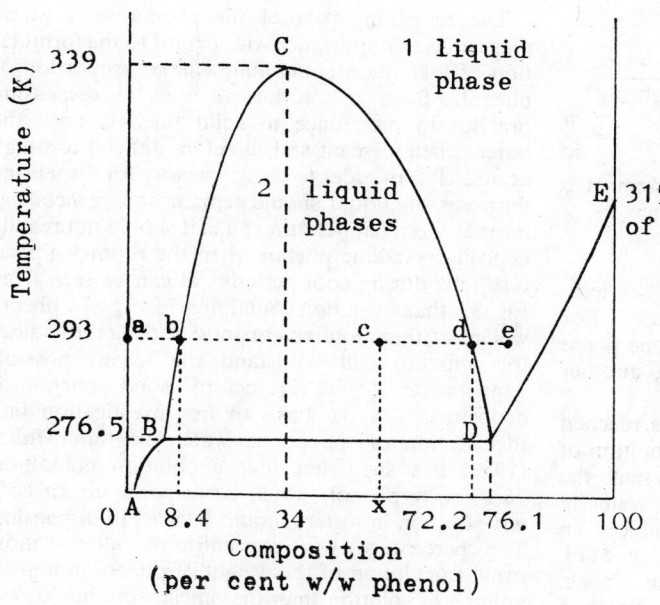

Fig. 3.7 Temperature-composition diagram for the phenol-water system (at 101 325 N/m²)

2. PARTIALLY MISCIBLE LIQUIDS

These systems may be divided into the following types for the convenience of discussion.

(*a*) *Systems Showing an Increase in Miscibility with Rise in Temperature.* A positive deviation from Raoult's law arises from a difference in the cohesive forces that exist between the molecules of each component in a liquid mixture. This difference becomes more marked as the temperature decreases and the positive deviation may then result in a decrease in miscibility sufficient to cause the separation of the mixture into two phases. Each phase consists of a saturated solution of one component in the other liquid. Such mutually saturated solutions are known as conjugate solutions.

The equilibria that occur in mixtures of partially miscible liquids may be followed either by shaking the two liquids together at constant temperature and analysing samples from each phase after equilibrium has been attained, or by observing the temperature at which known proportions of the two liquids, contained in sealed glass ampoules, become miscible, as shown by the disappearance of turbidity.

Phenol-Water System. The temperature-composition diagram of phenol and water at constant pressure (Fig. 3.7) is convenient to use in the explanation of the effects of partial miscibility in systems that show an increase in miscibility with rise in temperature.

The areas shown in Fig. 3.7 each correspond to the existence of various phases as shown in the diagram. The most important part of the diagram, for the purpose of the present discussion, is that indicated by the line *BCD*, which separates a single-phase system of one liquid from a two-phase system of two mutually saturated liquids. If gradually increasing amounts of phenol are added to water at 293 K, the composition moves along the line *abcde*. Between *a* and *b* there is only one liquid phase, and application of the Phase Rule shows that there are three degrees of freedom:

$$F = 2 - 1 + 2 = 3$$

This means that temperature and composition must be specified in order to define the system completely at constant pressure. The aqueous solution is eventually saturated at a composition corresponding to *b* (containing 8·4 per cent phenol). The line *BC* therefore represents the effect of temperature on the solubility of phenol in water. If more phenol is added, then a second layer separates. This is a saturated solution of water in liquid phenol. Thus, at a total composition corresponding to point *c* (i.e. containing *x* per cent phenol) two conjugate solutions will exist as separate phases. The compositions of these phases will correspond to points *b* and *d* respectively (i.e. one solution contains 8·4 per cent phenol in water and the other contains 27·8 per cent water in phenol). The relative amounts of these solutions at 293 K are given by

Amount of saturated solution of phenol in water
Amount of saturated solution of water in phenol
$$= \frac{cd}{bc}$$

Application of the Phase Rule to the system at c shows that there are two degrees of freedom:

$$F = 2 - 2 + 2 = 2$$

Thus, the system is completely defined if the temperature is specified at constant pressure. For example, at 293 K the system consists of one phase with a composition corresponding to b and another with a composition corresponding to d.

If more phenol is added, the point d is reached where the system consists of a saturated solution of phenol in water. Thus, the line DC represents the effect of temperature on the solubility of water in phenol. Further addition of phenol produces an unsaturated solution of water in phenol (i.e. at e).

It can be seen that BC and DC meet at C; i.e. above C only one liquid phase can exist. The two components are therefore miscible in all proportions above C, which is known as the upper critical temperature (upper CST). The composition at C corresponds to a mixture containing 34 per cent phenol and such a mixture will remain separated into two layers up to a higher temperature than any other. Application of the Phase Rule to the system at C shows that this point is invariant; i.e. the upper CST is fixed at 339 K for the phenol-water system at atmospheric pressure (101 325 N/m²).

The remaining part of the phenol-water phase diagram is of importance with regard to the formulation of a solution containing a large proportion of phenol. Such a solution is used in dispensing practice in preference to solid phenol, since the latter is deliquescent and therefore difficult to weigh accurately. In order to be satisfactory for dispensing purposes the liquid should remain homogeneous at normal room temperatures; i.e. it should not readily deposit crystalline phenol when the room temperature falls during cool periods. It can be seen from Fig. 3.7 that a solution containing 76·1 % w/w phenol will meet this requirement most satisfactorily since this mixture will withstand the lowest possible temperature (276·5 K) before solid phenol is deposited. On the basis of his investigation into this section of the phenol-water diagram Mulley (1959) has suggested that a solution containing 76·1 % w/w phenol, which corresponds to an 80 % w/v solution in water, should be used in dispensing. The percentage w/v concentration allows more rapid calculation of the weight of phenol in a given volume of solution than the official solution known as Liquefied Phenol BP 1968, which contains 80 % w/w phenol in water. In addition, the official formulation deposits phenol at a higher temperature (about 283 K).

(b) *Systems Showing a Decrease in Miscibility with Rise in Temperature.* A few mixtures, which probably involve compound formation, exhibit a lower critical solution temperature (lower CST), e.g. triethylamine plus water, paraldehyde plus

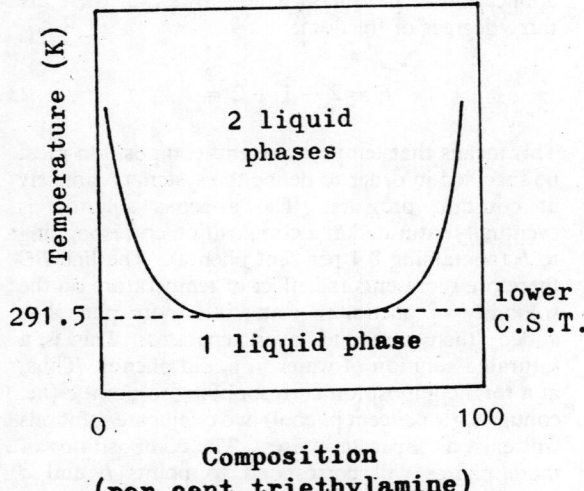

Fig. 3.8 Temperature-composition diagram for the triethylamine-water system (at 101 325 N/m²)

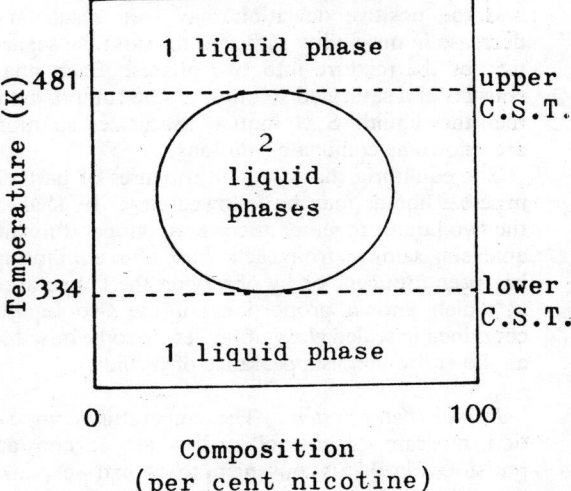

Fig. 3.9 Temperature-composition diagram for the nicotine-water system (at 101 325 N/m²)

water. The formation of a compound produces a negative deviation from Raoult's law, and miscibility therefore increases as the temperature falls, as shown in Fig. 3.8.

The effect of temperature on miscibility is of use in the preparation of paraldehyde enemas, which usually consist of a solution of paraldehyde in normal saline. Cooling the mixture during preparation allows more rapid solution, and storage of the enema in a cool place is recommended. (N.B. Enemas should be warmed to body temperature before use.)

(c) Systems Showing Upper and Lower CSTs. The decrease in miscibility with increase in temperature in systems having a lower CST is not indefinite. Above a certain temperature, positive deviations from Raoult's law become important and miscibility starts to increase again with further rise in temperature. This behaviour produces a closed-phase diagram as shown in Fig. 3.9, which represents the nicotine-water system.

In some mixtures where an upper and lower CST are expected, these points are not, in fact, observed since a phase change by one of the components occurs before the relevant CST is reached. For example, the ether-water system is expected to exhibit a lower CST, but water freezes before the temperature is reached.

The Effects of Added Substances on Critical Solution Temperatures

It has already been stated that a CST is an invariant point at constant pressure. These temperatures are very sensitive to impurities or added substances. In general, the effects of additives may be summarised by Table 3.3.

The increase in miscibility of two liquids caused by the addition of a third substance is referred to as blending. This is made use of in the formulation of Solution of Cresol with Soap BP 1968, which contains 50 per cent cresol. Cresol is only partially miscible with water but the soap in this preparation decreases the upper CST and produces complete miscibility at ordinary temperatures.

3. IMMISCIBLE LIQUIDS

In a mixture containing two immiscible liquids each liquid exerts its own vapour pressure independently of the other. The total vapour pressure, p, is therefore equal to the sum of the separate vapour pressures of the pure compounds (p_A^0 and p_B^0, respectively), i.e.

$$p = p_A^0 + p_B^0$$

Table 3.3
The Effects of Additives on CST

Type of CST	Solubility of additive in each component	Effect on CST	Effect on miscibility
Upper	Approx. equally soluble in both components	Lowered	Increased
Upper	Readily soluble in one component but not in other	Raised	Decreased
Lower	Approx. equally soluble in both components	Raised	Increased
Lower	Readily soluble in one component but not in other	Lowered	Decreased

The application of the Phase Rule to the distillation of such a system, which involves two liquids in equilibrium with a vapour, shows that only one degree of freedom exists,

$$F = 2 - 3 + 2 = 1$$

i.e. the boiling point is constant at constant pressure and is independent of the composition. Since the liquid mixture will boil when its total vapour pressure is equal to atmospheric pressure, it follows that the boiling point is lower than that of either pure component, even the one with the lowest boiling point. After one of the components has been completely removed by distillation the boiling point will rise to that of the remaining component.

The constant boiling mixture will produce a vapour in which the number of molecules of each component (n_A and n_B, respectively) is proportional to its vapour pressure if ideal behaviour occurs, i.e.

$$\frac{n_A}{n_B} = \frac{p_A^0}{p_B^0} \tag{3.5}$$

But

$$n_A = \frac{m_A}{M_A} \quad \text{and} \quad n_B = \frac{m_B}{M_B} \tag{3.6}$$

where m_A and m_B are the masses of each component in the vapour and M_A and M_B are their molecular weights, and from Eqns (3.5) and (3.6)

$$\frac{m_A}{M_A} \times \frac{M_B}{m_B} = \frac{p_A^0}{p_B^0}$$

$$\frac{m_A}{m_B} = \frac{p_A^0 M_A}{p_B^0 M_B} \tag{3.7}$$

Equation (3.7) indicates that the ratio of A to B by weight in the distillate is proportional to the ratios of their partial pressures and their molecular weights. Thus, if an immiscible mixture of water and an organic compound is distilled, a high proportion of the distillate will be comprised of the organic compound, since water has a low molecular weight. This process is known as steam distillation and it is often used in pharmaceutical chemistry as a means of purifying organic compounds that do not react and are immiscible with water. In practice, the process may also be applied to liquids that are partially miscible with water (e.g. aniline). It is especially useful in the purification of liquids with high boiling points, e.g. essential oil of almond, and in the extraction of volatile oils, e.g. clove and eucalyptus oils, which are obtained at the lower distillation temperature without decomposition or loss of aroma.

Liquid-Gas Systems of Two Components; Solutions of Gases in Liquids

A saturated solution of a gas in a liquid is produced when equilibrium is attained between the dissolved gas and that which remains undissolved above the liquid. The amount of gas that will dissolve depends on the temperature and the pressure of the gas, provided that no reaction occurs between the gas and the liquid.

The effect of pressure is indicated by Henry's law, which states that 'at constant temperature, the solubility of a gas in a liquid is directly proportional to the pressure of the gas above the liquid'. The law may be expressed by Eqn (3.8)

$$x = kp \qquad (3.8)$$

where, x is the mole fraction of the dissolved gas, p is the partial pressure of the gas above the solution, and the proportionality constant k is known as Henry's law constant.

The effect of gas pressure is made use of in preparing effervescent solutions containing carbon dioxide, which is maintained in solution by increasing the pressure of carbon dioxide in the atmosphere above the liquid in the container. It should be borne in mind that the solubility of carbon dioxide does not follow Henry's law, because a reaction occurs (i.e. $CO_2 + H_2O \rightleftharpoons H_2CO_3$). However, the equilibrium of this reaction will be influenced by the solubility of CO_2, which will, in turn, be influenced by the pressure.

Equation (3.8) also applies to the solubility of each gas in a solution of several gases in the same liquid, provided that x and p represent the mole fraction and partial pressure, respectively, of a particular gas. Henry's law is most applicable at high temperatures and low pressures. As the pressure rises the value of k may vary.

The solubility of most gases in liquids decreases as the temperature rises. This provides a means of removing dissolved gases. For example, carbon dioxide-free Water for Injections may be prepared by boiling Water for Injections and preventing the access of atmosphere during cooling. The presence of electrolytes may also decrease the solubility of a gas in water by a 'salting out' process, which is caused by the marked attraction exerted between the electrolyte and water.

Solid-Solid Systems of Two Components; Solutions of Solids in Solids

When two solids are melted together and the resultant liquid is cooled, then the components may be deposited either independently or as a single homogeneous phase, which is known as a solid solution. Both components participate in the lattice structure of the solid solution.

Solid solutions may be classified in a similar manner to solutions of liquids in liquids, into completely and partially miscible mixtures and immiscible mixtures. The Bibliography should be consulted for phase diagrams of these systems.

The production of alloys often involves the formation of solid solutions; e.g. gold/silver, gold/platinum. However, Goldberg and his co-workers (1965, 1966a, b, and c) have investigated the usefulness of solid solutions of urea and slowly soluble drugs such as griseofulvin and chloramphenicol. They suggest that when in contact with water, urea is dissolved rapidly from these systems and the remaining drug is in a molecular state of subdivision and therefore dissolves more rapidly than the original compound.

Solid-Liquid Systems of Two Components; Solutions of Solids in Liquids

The effect of pressure on a solid–liquid system is small. The 'reduced Phase Rule' is therefore often used in connection with these systems and this is expressed by Eqn (3.9),

$$P + F' = C + 1 \qquad (3.9)$$

where, P and C are defined as before, and F' is the number of degrees of freedom in addition to pressure. Any system in which a vapour phase is not taken into account is known as a condensed system. Equilibria in these systems are therefore represented by temperature-composition diagrams at constant pressure, and the greatest value of F' is two.

The behaviour of two component solid–liquid systems can be classified into three types.

1. Systems that show the formation of a eutectic mixture.
2. Systems that show the formation of a compound with a congruent melting point (i.e. the compound, which consists of one component solvated by the other, yields a liquid with the same composition as the compound on melting).
3. Systems that show the formation of a compound with an incongruent melting point (i.e. the compound undergoes fusion on heating to a certain temperature and produces a liquid and a new solid phase, the composition of which is different from that of the original compound).

Systems of the first type, which involve the formation of a eutectic mixture, have found certain applications of pharmaceutical interest. The other types are of less importance. No further comment will be made regarding these, and the Bibliography should be consulted if more information is required.

Formation of Eutectic Mixtures

The ice-potassium chloride system, whose behaviour is represented by the phase diagram shown in Fig. 3.10, may be used as an example of the type of system that involves the formation of a eutectic.

In Fig. 3.10, A and B represent the melting points of ice and KCl, respectively. If KCl is added to water, the freezing point of the latter is reduced as indicated by AC, which therefore represents the

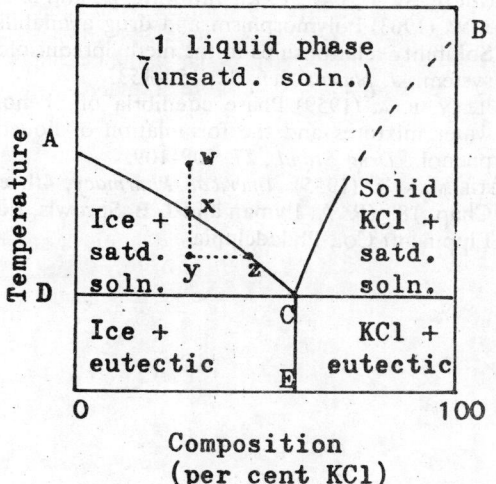

Fig. 3.10 Temperature-composition diagram for the KCl-water system

effect of composition on the temperature at which ice separates from the system. Similarly, if water is added to KCl the melting point of the latter is lowered, and BC therefore represents the effect of composition on the temperature at which solid KCl separates from the system.

At C, both solid components can exist in equilibrium with a liquid of definite composition. Application of the 'reduced Phase Rule' shows that the system is invariant at this point since there are no degrees of freedom.

$$F' = 2 + 1 - 3 = 0$$

This means that the mixture will freeze completely at a constant temperature D, which is lower than the freezing points of either pure component.

Further understanding of the phase diagram may be obtained by considering the effects of cooling a solution of KCl in water represented by point w in Fig. 3.10. If the solution is cooled to point x on the freezing curve AC, then some ice will separate out. Further cooling to y will produce more ice and the remaining solution will become more concentrated since it will contain all the original KCl. The composition of this remaining solution will correspond to point z. Therefore, as the temperature falls, the composition of the remaining liquid moves along AC. A limit is reached when the remaining solution is saturated with KCl, and, on cooling this solution, ice and KCl separate out in the same ratio in which they exist in the saturated solution, and the temperature remains constant at D until all the saturated solution has solidified. The mixture, which separates at this temperature, is termed a eutectic (or a cryohydrate, if one of the components is water) and its composition is given by E. Although the eutectic has a definite melting point, the following evidence suggests that it is an intimate mechanical mixture and not a compound.

(a) The components can be separated mechanically.
(b) The addition of each component raises the melting point of the eutectic. The melting point of a compound would be lowered on admixture with another substance.
(c) A heterogeneous structure can be seen under a microscope.
(d) X-ray analysis reveals the existence of two phases.

As shown in Fig. 3.10, the areas in the phase diagram each correspond to the existence of various phases or mixtures of phases.

The phase diagram for the water-KCl system may be used to explain the principle of freezing mixtures prepared from ice and salt. If salt is added to ice and a little water, some of the salt will dissolve in the water to produce a system comprised of ice, salt, and solution. Such a system is in stable equilibrium at the eutectic point only. The system will therefore tend to move towards this point and ice will melt and salt will continue to dissolve in the resultant water. Both of these processes are accompanied by absorption of heat and the temperature therefore falls until one of the solid components has been used up completely. If the initial proportions of ice and salt are chosen satisfactorily the eutectic temperature will be reached.

It has been suggested that eutectic mixtures may be useful as a means of increasing the rates of solution of slowly soluble drugs in aqueous body fluids (Goldberg, Gibaldi and Kanig, 1965). It was thought that the rapid solution of the second component (e.g. urea) in eutectic mixtures with these drugs would present the drug in a very fine crystalline form that would be more rapidly soluble than the usual forms of the drug. However, subsequent studies have suggested that the increased dissolution rates of the drugs in the presence of urea is likely to be caused by the formation of solid solutions of these drugs with urea and not by eutectic formation (Goldberg and co-workers, 1966c).

BIBLIOGRAPHY

BARROW, G. M. (1966) *Physical Chemistry*. 2nd ed. McGraw-Hill, London.

GUCKER, F. T. and SEIFERT, R. L. (1967) *Physical Chemistry*. English Universities Press, London.

MARON, S. H. and PRUTTON, C. F. (1958) *Principles of Physical Chemistry*. 3rd ed. Macmillan, New York.

MARTIN, A. N., SWARBRICK, J. and CAMMARATA, A. (1969) *Physical Pharmacy*. 2nd ed. Henry Kimpton, London.

ROSE, J. (1961) *Dynamic Physical Chemistry*. Pitman, London.

WILLIAMS, V. R. and WILLIAMS, H. B. (1967) *Basic Physical Chemistry for the Life Sciences*. Freeman and Co., San Francisco.

REFERENCES

AGUIAR, A. J., KRC JR., J., KINKEL, A. W., and SAMYN, J. C. (1967) Effect of polymorphism on the absorption of chloramphenicol palmitate. *J. pharm. Sci.*, **56**, 847–853.

GOLDBERG, A. H., GIBALDI, M., and KANIG, J. L. (1965) Increasing dissolution rates and gastrointestinal absorption of drugs via solid solutions and eutectic mixtures. I. Theoretical considerations and discussion of the literature. *J. pharm. Sci.*, **54**, 1145–1148.

GOLDBERG, A. H., GIBALDI, M., and KANIG, J. L. (1966a) II. Experimental evaluation of a eutectic mixture: Urea—acetaminophen system. *J. pharm. Sci.*, **55**, 482–487.

GOLDBERG, A. H., GIBALDI, M., and KANIG, J. L. (1966b) III. Experimental evaluation of griseofulvin—succinic acid solid solution. *J. pharm. Sci.*, **55**, 487–492.

GOLDBERG, A. H., GIBALDI, M., KANIG, J. L., and MAYERSOHN, M. (1966c) IV. Chloramphenicol—urea system. *J. pharm. Sci.*, **55**, 581–583.

HALEBLIAN, J. and MCCRONE, W. (1969) Pharmaceutical applications of polymorphism. *J. pharm. Sci.*, **58**, 911–929.

HIGUCHI, W. I., BERNARDO, D. P., and MEHTA, S. C. (1967) Polymorphism and drug availability. II. Dissolution rate behaviour of the polymorphic forms of sulphathiazole and methylprednisolone. *J. pharm. Sci.*, **56**, 200–207.

HIGUCHI, W. I., LAU, P. K., HIGUCHI, T., and SHELL, J. W. (1963) Polymorphism and drug availability. Solubility relationships in the methylprednisolone system. *J. pharm. Sci.*, **52**, 150–153.

MULLEY, B. A. (1959) Phase equilibria of phenol—water mixtures and the formulation of liquefied phenol. *Drug Stand.*, **27**, 108–109.

RIEGELMAN, S. (1955) *American Pharmacy*, 4th ed., Chap. 18. (R. A. Lyman and J. B. Sprowls, Eds). Lippincott Co., Philadelphia.

4

Surface and Interfacial Phenomena

AN INTERFACE is a boundary between two phases, while a surface is strictly a boundary between a solid or liquid phase and a vacuum. However, the latter term is often used to describe the interfaces between a gas and a solid or a gas and a liquid. Surfaces and interfaces can be conveniently classified according to the types of phase they separate; i.e. solid–liquid, solid–solid, and liquid–liquid interfaces and solid-gas and liquid-gas surfaces.

The Role of Surface Molecules of Solids and Liquids in Interfacial Phenomena

The kinetic theory of matter indicates that appreciable forces of attraction exist between molecules in liquids and in solids.* However, the surface molecules of a solid or liquid differ in state from those molecules within the bulk of that phase. This difference will be appreciated from a consideration of Fig. 4.1. The points A and B represent molecules

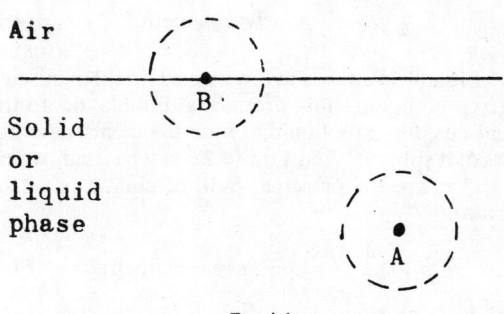

Air

Solid
or
liquid
phase

Fig. 4.1

in the bulk and surface, respectively, of a solid or liquid phase at a given instant, while the circles represent the zones in which molecular attractions between A and B and their surrounding molecules are significant. Since the zone around A contains, on average in any given direction, equal numbers of

* It is assumed that the student is familiar with the basic concepts of the kinetic theory of matter: *see* Bibliography.

molecules all exerting similar forces, then the resultant attraction experienced by A will be zero. In a liquid surface, part of the sphere of molecular attraction around B, i.e. that part that projects above the surface, is occupied by a relatively small number of gas or vapour molecules. In addition to their low numbers, the attractive forces exerted by these molecules are relatively weak. Consequently, the attractions that exist between B and the underlying bulk molecules are not counterbalanced. The surface molecules, therefore, experience a resultant inward attraction and the transference of molecules from the bulk to the surface layer involves the expenditure of energy in order to overcome this inward attraction. It is known from the First Law of Thermodynamics that energy cannot be created or destroyed but can only be converted from one form to another. In this particular example the expended energy is converted into the so-called surface free energy of the system.

In solids it is easier to explain the existence of surface free energy in terms of the unsatisfied forces that project from the surface than on the basis of an inward attraction exerted on the surface molecules. This is because the molecules in a solid are not mobile with respect to each other, as they are in a liquid. If we consider a solid suspended in a vacuum, it is readily appreciated that the projecting attractive forces associated with B are unsatisfied. The surface molecules therefore possess a greater amount of free energy than those in the bulk, and the transference of a molecule from the bulk to the surface of a solid again involves the expenditure of energy, some of which is converted to extra surface free energy.

If a solid block or a bulk liquid is subdivided into many small particles or drops by grinding or spraying, respectively, then the total surface area of the solid or liquid is increased tremendously; i.e. much greater proportions of the molecules are now in the surfaces of the solid or liquid and the total surface free energy of each of these systems is therefore increased. This extra energy is supplied by the work expended in the processes of grinding and spraying. In fact, surface free energy is defined as the work required to extend a surface by unit area. The unit in the SI system is joule/metre^2.

Similar arguments may be applied to the solid–liquid, solid–solid, and liquid–liquid interfaces, and interfacial free energy is defined in a similar manner.

A consideration of thermodynamics also indicates that all systems will tend to react spontaneously in order to reach the state with the lowest total free energy. The existence of surface free energy and the methods by which systems react in order to decrease their total free energies to a minimum give rise to the various surface and interfacial phenomena that are discussed in the following sections of this chapter.

Surface and Interfacial Tension

It has been established above that surfaces possess free energy, and that systems will react spontaneously in order to reach a state with the lowest total free energy.

Since the total surface free energy is directly proportional to the surface area of a solid or a liquid, then one of the methods by which a system can reduce its surface free energy is by contracting the surface area of any solid or liquid within the system to a minimum. This is particularly obvious in liquids in which the molecules are mobile with respect to each other. This mobility is responsible for the tendency of liquid drops suspended in a gas or in an immiscible liquid to assume the minimum ratio of surface area to volume, i.e. a spherical shape, in the absence of other influences such as gravity. The tendency of mobile surfaces to contract can be readily explained by the fact that the surface molecules are continually moving into the bulk at a faster rate than other molecules can move outwards to replace them because of the resultant inward attraction experienced by surface molecules. The number of molecules in a newly formed surface therefore decreases until the surface area reaches a minimum; i.e. until the surface free energy is reduced as much as possible by this means.

Since the liquid surface shows this tendency to contract, it is usual to consider a surface tension, which is defined as the contractile force in newtons, operating in the plane of the surface normal to a line one metre in length. Surface tension is, in fact, the mathematical equivalent of surface free energy and has the same dimensions and magnitude; i.e. surface free energy (joule/metre^2) is equal to surface tension (newton/metre). Although surface free energy is the fundamental property, surface tension is more widely used in liquids since it is usually more convenient to consider problems in terms of a directional surface tension rather than the energy expended per unit increase in surface area.

Pressures Across Curved Liquid Menisci

One of the consequences of surface tension is that an excess pressure (p) is exerted on the concave side of a curved liquid meniscus compared with that exerted on the convex side. Consider a spherical bubble of radius r m divided by an imaginary line into two hemispheres. Surface forces will act around the circumference of the bubble and tend to pull the two hemispheres together. For the bubble to exist, this inward attractive force, which is equal to $2\pi r\gamma$ newtons (where γ N/m is the surface tension of the liquid) must be counteracted by a force that tends to push the hemispheres apart; i.e. the pressure on the inside concave surface of the bubble must be greater than that on the outer convex surface. If this excess pressure is denoted by p newtons/metre^2, then the total force pushing the hemispheres apart is given by $\pi r^2 p$ newtons since the area over which the pressure is exerted is that which separates the two hemispheres. Thus, at equilibrium—

$$\pi r^2 p = 2\pi r\gamma \quad \text{newtons}$$

and, therefore, by rearrangement—

$$p = \frac{2\gamma}{r} \quad \text{newtons/metre}^2 \qquad (4.1)$$

Equation (4.1) applies to any curved liquid meniscus; e.g. to a liquid film around a bubble or to the meniscus of a bulk liquid. Often the meniscus is not part of a sphere; then Eqn (4.2) may be used, where r_1 and r_2 are the principal radii of curvature of the surface.

$$p = \left(\frac{1}{r_1} + \frac{1}{r_2}\right)\gamma \quad \text{newtons/metre}^2 \qquad (4.2)$$

The Shape of Liquid Surfaces and the Wetting of Solids by Liquids

Liquid drops in contact with solid surfaces can assume different shapes, as shown in Fig. 4.2.

The degree of wetting of a solid by a liquid can be conveniently expressed in terms of the contact angle (θ), since a decrease in the value of θ results in a greater contact between the solid and the liquid. The particular value of θ depends on the relative values of the tensions associated with the liquid–solid interface (γ^{LS}) and the gas–solid and gas–liquid surfaces (γ^{GS} and γ^{GL}, respectively) as shown

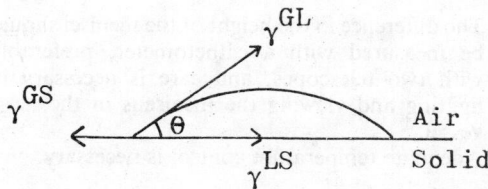

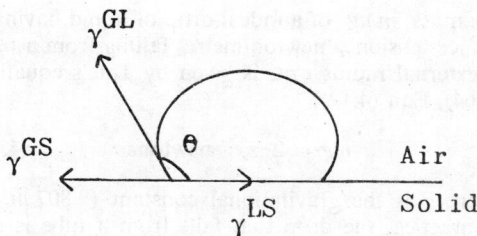

Fig. 4.2 Examples of the shapes of liquid drops in contact with solids

by Eqn (4.3).

$$\gamma^{GS} = \gamma^{LS} + \gamma^{GL} \cos \theta \qquad (4.3)$$

This equation is obtained by using the cosine rule to equate the opposing horizontal components of the tensions shown in Fig. 4.2; i.e. the component acting towards the left-hand side of a horizontal line drawn in the plane of the paper is $\gamma^{GS} \cos 0 \, (= \gamma^{GS})$ and the components acting towards the right-hand side are $\gamma^{LS} \cos 0 + \gamma^{GL} \cos \theta \, (= \gamma^{LS} + \gamma^{GL} \cos \theta)$. From Eqn (4.3) it follows that if γ^{GS} is greater than γ^{LS} then $\cos \theta$ must be positive, i.e. $\theta < \pi/2$ radians, and conversely, if γ^{GS} is less than γ^{LS} then θ must lie between $\pi/2$ and π radians.

Marked variation between the values of contact angles in different systems can be observed from visual examination of the shapes of liquid menisci in glass tubes. For example, in the case of liquids, such as water, that wet glass the meniscus is concave upwards (i.e. θ is very small) whereas liquids, such as mercury, that do not wet glass exhibit a meniscus that is concave downwards (i.e. θ is large).

The Mechanism of Capillary Rise

Consider a capillary tube placed vertically in a liquid that wets the walls of the tube and that is held in a large container so that the liquid surface in this container is flat. The initial state of the system may be represented by Fig. 4.3(a). However, Eqn (4.1) indicates that there is an excess pressure on the concave side of the liquid meniscus in the capillary tube. This means that the pressure, p_A, at a point A

immediately below the meniscus is less than the pressure, p_B, at a point B immediately above the meniscus by an amount equal to $2\gamma/r$; i.e.

$$p_B - p_A = \frac{2\gamma}{r} \quad \text{newtons/metre}^2 \qquad (4.4)$$

This difference in pressure will be appreciable since r, the radius of curvature of the meniscus inside the tube, is small. The difference in pressure, p_C and p_D, at points C and D, which are above and below the meniscus in the large container, respectively, is equal to $2\gamma/r_0$. However, in this case the pressure difference is negligible since the radius of curvature, r_0, at this point is so large, i.e.

$$p_C = p_D \quad \text{newtons/metre}^2 \qquad (4.5)$$

In addition, the pressures at B and C are both equal to the atmospheric pressure,

$$\therefore \quad p_B = p_C \quad \text{newtons/metre}^2 \qquad (4.6)$$

Thus, from Eqns (4.5) and (4.6)

$$p_B = p_D \quad \text{newtons/metre}^2 \qquad (4.7)$$

and from Eqns (4.4) and (4.7)

$$p_D - p_A = 2\gamma/r \quad \text{newtons/metre}^2 \qquad (4.8)$$

The difference in pressures within the liquid, as indicated by Eqn (4.8), produces a driving force which causes the liquid to rise up the capillary tube. Equilibrium is reached when the hydrostatic pressure of the column of liquid is equal to $2\gamma/r$. If at equilibrium the height of the column is h m, as shown in Fig. 4.3(b) then

$$2\gamma/r = h\rho g \quad \text{newtons/metre}^2 \qquad (4.9)$$

where ρ is the density of the liquid in kg/m^3 and g is the gravitational constant (9·807 m/s^2).

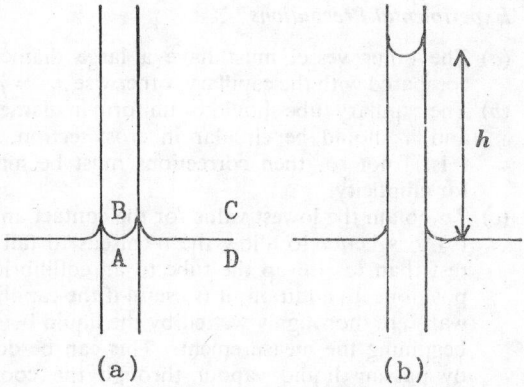

Fig. 4.3 Stages in the rise of a liquid up a capillary tube

Measurement of Surface Tension

Three of the most common methods of measuring surface tension are described below, together with the relevant correction factors and practical precautions that must be taken into account to obtain accurate results. Details of other methods are given in the references cited in the Bibliography.

1. THE CAPILLARY RISE METHOD

This is one of the most accurate methods and is based on the measurement of the height to which a liquid rises in a capillary tube. Equation (4.10), which is a rearranged form of Eqn (4.9) can be used for approximate determinations.

$$\gamma = \frac{h \rho g r}{2} \quad \text{newtons/metre} \quad (4.10)$$

For more accurate results certain modifications of this equation should be taken into account to allow for—

(a) a change in the value of the contact angle (θ) between the liquid and the walls of the tube from the zero value assumed in Eqn (4.10) to a finite value,

(b) the hydrostatic pressure exerted by the small volume of liquid contained in the meniscus above the point from which the height h is usually measured, and

(c) the difference in the density of the liquid (ρ^L) inside the capillary tube and that of the vapour (ρ^V) outside the tube.

The corrected equation is—

$$\gamma = \frac{\left(h + \frac{r}{3}\right)(\rho^L - \rho^V)gr}{2 \cos \theta} \quad \text{newtons/metre} \quad (4.11)$$

Experimental Precautions

(a) The outer vessel must have a large diameter compared with the capillary, otherwise $p_C \neq p_D$.

(b) The capillary tube should be uniform in diameter and it should be circular in cross-section. If this is not so, then corrections must be made for ellipticity.

(c) To obtain the lowest value for the contact angle (θ) it is better to allow the meniscus to fall to rest than to rise up the tube to an equilibrium position. In addition, it is useful if the capillary walls are thoroughly wetted by the liquid before beginning the measurement. This can be done by passing liquid vapour through the cooled capillary, or by evacuating the capillary just before filling.

(d) The difference in the height of the menisci should be measured with a cathetometer, preferably with two telescopes, and care is necessary in lighting and viewing the meniscus in the large vessel.

(e) Adequate temperature control is necessary.

2. THE DROP WEIGHT METHOD

The mass, m kg, of an ideal drop of liquid having a surface tension γ newton/metre, falling from a tube of external radius r m, is given by Tate's equation (1864), Eqn (4.12),

$$mg = 2\pi r \gamma \quad \text{newtons} \quad (4.12)$$

where g is the gravitational constant (9·807 m/s²). In practice, the drop that falls from a tube is not ideal since the drop is constricted at the point where the break occurs to a diameter less than that of the tip of the tube. In addition, only part of the liquid protruding from the tip actually breaks away, and this falls in the form of more than one drop.

Harkins and Brown (1919) introduced a correction factor which takes the shape of the drop into account, and Eqn (4.13) then becomes

$$mg = 2\pi r \gamma \cdot f\left(\frac{r}{V^{-3}}\right) \quad \text{newtons} \quad (4.13)$$

The correction factor $f(r/V^{-3})$ is a function of the radius of the tip r and the cube root of the volume, V, of the drop. It is, in fact, the fraction of an ideal drop that actually falls, and Harkins and Brown give tables and graphs showing the value of their correction factor for various values of the actual ratio r/V^{-3}

An error is often introduced by attempting to obtain 'relative' values of surface tension by comparing drop weights of two different liquids. The results can be used in this way only if the surface tensions and densities of the two liquids and the tips of the tubes are chosen so that the values of r/V^{-3} are within the narrow limits where the correction curve is approximately horizontal.

Experimental Precautions

(a) The tip should be sharply ground with no imperfections in the outer circumference.

(b) The drops should be allowed to form slowly, especially in the later stages, otherwise the weight of the drop is greater than expected due to the effects of liquid streaming into the drop during the final, relatively slow stages of detachment.

(c) Adequate temperature control is necessary.

(d) It is normal practice to collect 20 to 30 drops in a determination, and calculate the average weight of one drop. Since the time of formation and collection of a single drop may take several minutes, it is necessary to prevent loss in weight of the collected sample brought about by evaporation.

The degree of attention paid to the above practical precautions has led to the development of various types of apparatus. These range from the simple type of stalagmometer shown in Fig. 4.4 to the more sophisticated apparatus used by Harkins and Brown (1919).

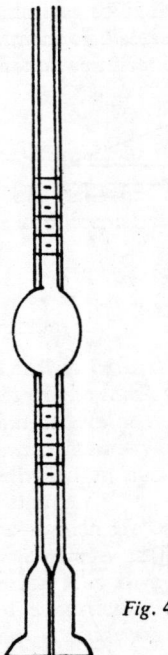

Fig. 4.4 Simple stalagmometer

3. DU NOUY TENSIOMETER

This instrument (Fig. 4.5) measures the force required to detach a platinum wire ring from the surface of a liquid. This force is applied by means of a torsion wire attached to a scale calibrated directly in units of surface tension. This calibration takes into account the fact that the surface tension forces act along the inner and outer circumferences of the wire ring but it is only suitable for approximate readings since it is based on the following Eqn (4.14),

$$P = 4\pi R\gamma \quad \text{newtons} \qquad (4.14)$$

where, P is the maximum pull on the whole ring, R is the radius of the ring (from the centre of the ring to the centre of the wire) in metres, and γ is the surface tension of the liquid in newtons/metre.

For more accurate results it is necessary to multiply the scale reading observed on the tensiometer by a correction factor (F) which was introduced by Harkins and Jordan (1930) and depends on R^3/V and also on the ratio R/r, where V is the volume of liquid raised above the surface and r is the radius of the wire. Harkins and Jordan give tables of F for various values of R^3/V and R/r. The value of V may be calculated by initial determination of the scale deflections necessary to return the boom to its zero position when known weights are placed on the ring in air. The constant ratio of weight:scale reading may then be used to determine the weight of liquid raised by the ring for any scale reading. The corresponding volume can then be obtained from a knowledge of the density of the liquid.

Experimental Precautions

(a) The wire of the ring should be in the horizontal plane.
(b) The vessel containing the liquid should be large enough for the curvature of the surface not to affect the shape of the liquid drop raised by the ring.
(c) The surface of the liquid should be free from wave motion.
(d) There should be no motion of the ring except for a very slow upward movement.
(e) Temperature control should be adequate, and there should be no evaporation with consequent cooling of the surface.

Effect of Temperature on Surface Tension

When a liquid in equilibrium with its vapour is heated, the interface between the two phases disappears at the critical temperature; i.e. there is no surface tension at this temperature. Thus, there is a general tendency for the surface tension of liquids to decrease as the temperature rises, provided no changes in molecular composition occur. This decrease arises from thermal expansion of the liquid in so far as this reduces the number of molecules that lie within the zone of molecular attraction (*see* Fig. 4.1).

The relationship between temperature and surface tension is expressed by Eqn (4.15),

$$\gamma = \gamma_0\left(1 - \frac{T}{T_c}\right)^{1.2} \quad \text{newtons/metre} \qquad (4.15)$$

where γ is the surface tension at temperature T, γ_0 is the surface tension at thermodynamic zero, and

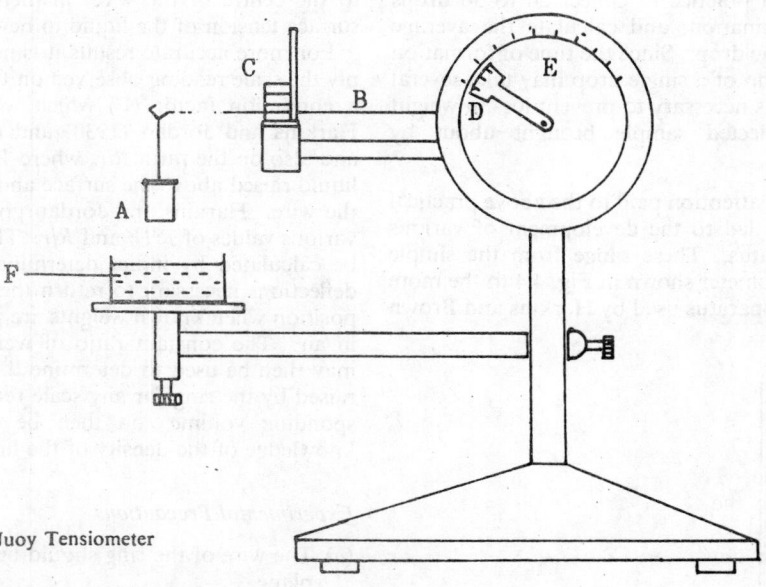

Side view

*Fig.*4.5   The Du Nuoy Tensiometer
A. Platinum loop
B. Light boom
C. Mirror for aiding zero adjustment of boom
D. Vernier
E. Scale calibrated in units of surface tension
F. Liquid under test
G. Torsion wire
H. Screw for adjusting torsion in wire when
     bringing boom to zero
J. Screw for increasing torsion in wire
K. Dash-pot for damping oscillations of boom

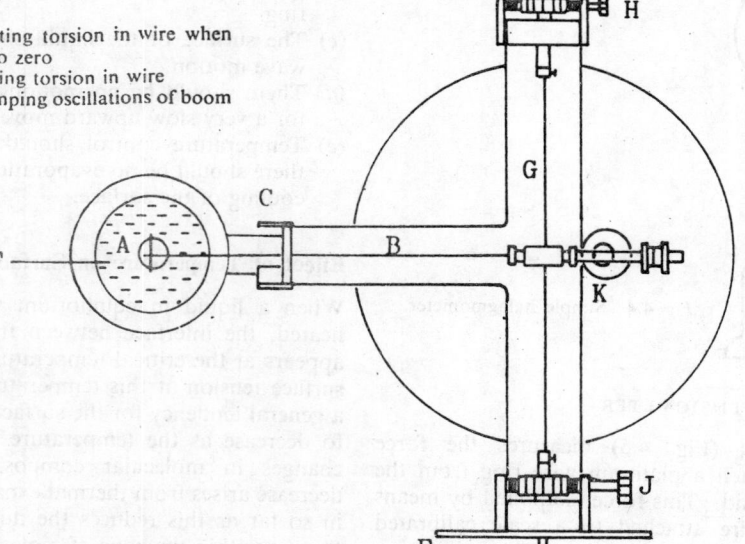

Plan view

T_c is the critical temperature of the liquid; i.e. the temperature at which the interface between the liquid and its saturated vapour disappears.

Orientation of Molecules of Pure Liquids at Surfaces and Interfaces

The inward attraction experienced by the surface molecules of a liquid will tend to result in a particular orientation of these molecules with respect to the plane of the surface. This orientation arises from the difference in the strengths of attraction between the various groups in the surface molecules and the underlying molecules. Consequently, those groups with the strongest associated attractive forces will tend to be directed inwards, and those with the weakest associated fields will tend to project from the surface. This orientation offers a further means by which the total surface free energy of a system is reduced to a minimum; i.e. in addition to the tendency for the surface to assume a minimum area for a given volume.

The tendency towards a definite orientation will be disrupted by thermal effects so that the surface and

underlying layers of a liquid long-chain alcohol or carboxylic acid, for example, may be represented by Fig. 4.6(a). The rod-like ends of the diagrammatic molecules represent groups with relatively low attractive forces (e.g. hydrocarbon chains) whereas the globular ends represent more polar groups (e.g. —OH and —COOH groups) with greater associated forces.

The type of orientation of the surface molecules of a given liquid is markedly influenced by the nature of the other phase with which it is in contact. For example, if either the alcohol or carboxylic acid shown in Fig. 4.6(a) is in contact with a more polar phase such as water or glass, which will exert a relatively strong attractive force, then the interfacial molecules of the organic liquid will tend to become orientated with their polar groups directed outwards as shown in Fig. 4.6(b).

Effects of Solutes on the Surface Tension of Liquids

The composition of a newly formed surface of a solution is the same as that of the bulk phase. However,

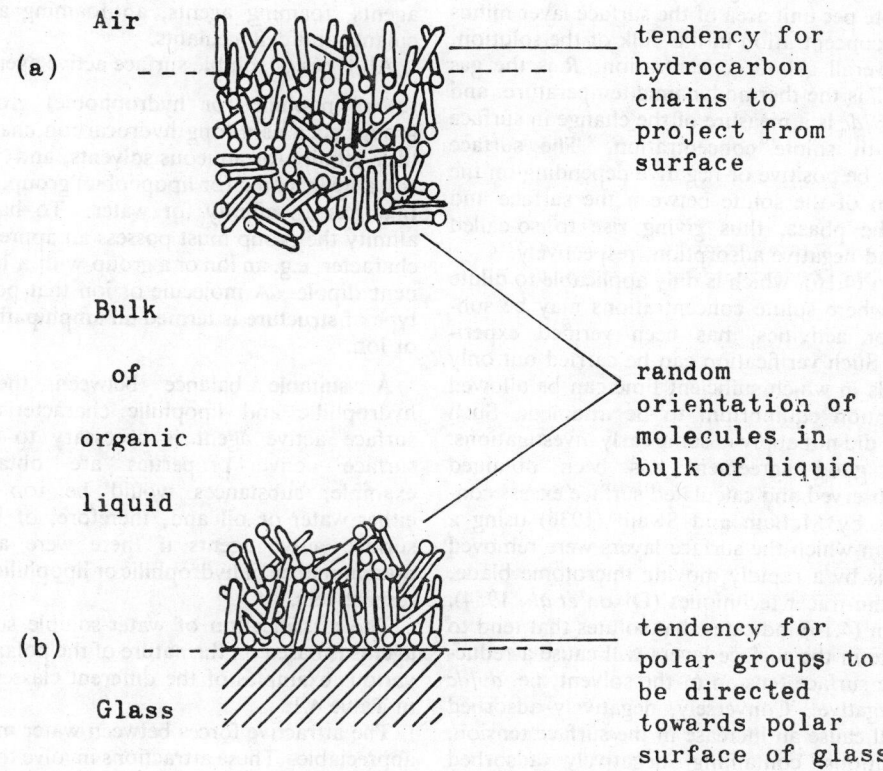

(a) Air — tendency for hydrocarbon chains to project from surface

Bulk of organic liquid — random orientation of molecules in bulk of liquid

(b) Glass — tendency for polar groups to be directed towards polar surface of glass

Fig. 4.6   The orientation of molecules at surfaces and interfaces

the unequal forces that exist between the underlying molecules and the solute and solvent molecules in the fresh surface will eventually produce a surface layer with a different composition from that of the bulk solution, since those surface molecules that are attracted most strongly by the underlying liquid will be removed most rapidly from the surface and replaced by other molecules. The rate at which an equilibrium is established depends on the nature of the solute and solvent and may vary between values of the order of 0·1 s for small molecules or ions in aqueous solution to several days for some colloidal solutions.

The surface properties of the solution, including the surface tension, will depend on the composition of the surface layer and will therefore be affected by the distribution of the solute between this layer and the bulk solution. The quantitative relationship between solute distribution and surface tension is expressed by Gibbs adsorption isotherm Eqn (4.16)

$$\Gamma = \frac{-c}{RT} \cdot \frac{d\gamma}{dc} \qquad (4.16)$$

where Γ is the surface excess concentration of the solute, which may be regarded as the concentration of the solute per unit area of the surface layer minus the solute concentration in the bulk of the solution, c is the overall solute concentration, R is the gas constant, T is the thermodynamic temperature, and the term $d\gamma/dc$ is a measure of the change in surface tension with solute concentration. The surface excess may be positive or negative depending on the distribution of the solute between the surface and bulk of the phase, thus giving rise to so-called positive and negative adsorption, respectively.

Equation (4.16), which is only applicable to dilute solutions where solute concentrations may be substituted for activities, has been verified experimentally. Such verification can be carried out only by methods in which sufficient time can be allowed for adsorption equilibrium to be attained. Such conditions did not apply in some early investigations. However, good agreement has been obtained between observed and calculated surface excess concentrations by McBain and Swain (1936) using a trough from which the surface layers were removed for analysis by a rapidly moving microtome blade, and by radio-tracer techniques (Dixòn et al., 1954).

Equation (4.16) indicates that solutes that tend to concentrate in the surface layers will cause a reduction in the surface tension of the solvent, i.e. $d\gamma/dc$ will be negative. Conversely, negatively adsorbed solutes will cause an increase in the surface tension.

In solutions containing negatively adsorbed solutes there is little change in the composition of the surface layer when compared with that of the pure solvent. Consequently, only small increases in surface tension are observed in·these cases.

In solutions containing positively adsorbed solutes, the composition of the surface layer may change markedly from that of the pure solvent, depending on the nature of the solute and solvent and the concentration of the solution. For example, there may be a slight lowering of surface tension with increase in concentration as in the case of many mixtures of organic liquids, since the surface tensions of the majority of organic liquids are fairly similar ($< 35 \times 10^{-3}$ newtons/metre). However, the greater difference between the surface tension of water (about 72×10^{-3} newtons/metre) and organic liquids leads to a considerable decrease in the surface tension of aqueous solutions of organic compounds even at low concentrations.

Surface Active Agents

Solutes that cause a marked decrease in the surface tension of the solvent are termed surface active agents or surfactants. These substances are of importance in a wide variety of fields as emulsifying agents, detergents, solubilising agents, wetting agents, foaming agents, antifoaming agents, flocculants and deflocculants.

All types of soluble surface active agent contain—

(a) a lipophilic (or hydrophobic) group; i.e. a group, such as a long hydrocarbon chain, that has little affinity for aqueous solvents, and
(b) a hydrophilic (or lipophobic) group, i.e. a group that has an affinity for water. To have such an affinity the group must possess an appreciable polar character, e.g. an ion or a group with a large permanent dipole. A molecule or ion that possesses this type of structure is termed an amphipathic molecule or ion.

A suitable balance between the opposing hydrophilic and lipophilic characteristics of the surface active agent is necessary to ensure that surface active properties are obtained. For example, substances would be too soluble in either water or oil and, therefore, of little use as surface active agents if there were an excessive predominance of hydrophilic or lipophilic properties, respectively.

The classification of water-soluble surface-active agents is based on the nature of the polar group, and various examples of the different classes are shown in Table 4.1.

The attractive forces between water molecules are appreciable. These attractions involve the formation of hydrogen bonds between adjacent molecules that

Table 4.1

The Classification of Synthetic Surface Active Agents

Class	Surface active agent	Chemical formula (in aqueous solution)		Surface inactive ion
		Lipophilic group	Hydrophilic group	
1. Anionic				
(a) Alkali soaps	Potassium stearate	$C_{17}H_{35}$ ————————	———————— COO^-	K^+
(b) Organic sulphates	Sodium lauryl sulphate (sodium dodecyl sulphate)	$C_{12}H_{25}$ ————————	———————— OSO_3^-	Na^+
(c) Organic sulphonates	Sodium cetyl sulphonate (sodium hexadecane sulphonate)	$C_{16}H_{33}$ ————————	———————— SO_3^-	Na^+
2. Cationic				
(a) Quaternary ammonium compounds	Cetyl trimethyl ammonium bromide or cetrimide (hexadecyl trimethyl ammonium bromide)	$C_{16}H_{33}$ ————————	———————— $\overset{+}{N}(CH_3)_3$	Br^-
(b) Pyridinium compounds	Dodecyl pyridinium chloride	$C_{12}H_{25}$ ————————	———————— $\overset{+}{N}C_5H_5$	Cl^-
3. Ampholytic Amino-acids	N-dodecyl -alanine		(i) in alkaline solution (e.g. NaOH)—anionic	
		$C_{12}H_{25}$ ————————	———————— $NH-CH_2-CH_2-COO^-$	Na^+
			(ii) in acid solution (e.g. HCl)—cationic	
		$C_{12}H_{25}$ ————————	———————— $\overset{+}{N}H_2-CH_2-CH_2-COOH$	Cl^-
			(iii) at iso-electric point—zwitterion	
		$C_{12}H_{25}$ ————————	———————— $\overset{+}{N}H_2-CH_2-CH_2-COO^-$	none
4. Non-ionic				
(a) Alcohol-polyethylene glycol ethers	Polyethylene glycol 1000 monocetyl ether (cetomacrogol 1000)	$CH_3-(CH_2)_n$ ———————— $n = 15$ or 17	———————— $(O-CH_2-CH_2)_m-OH$ $m = 20-24$	none
(b) Fatty acid-polyethylene glycol esters	Polyethylene glycol 40 monostearate	$CH_3-(CH_2)_{16}$ ————————	———————— $CO-(O-CH_2-CH_2)_{40}-OH$	none
(c) Fatty acid-polyhydric alcohol esters	Sorbitan mono-oleate	$C_{17}H_{33}$ ————————	———————— $COO-CH_2$ —	none
	Polyoxyethylene sorbitan mono-oleate	$C_{17}H_{33}$ ————————	———————— $COO-CH_2$ —	none

A more detailed classification of surface active agents is given by Schwartz and Perry (1949) and Moilliet *et al.* (1961). In addition, Lower (1962) gives a list of the chemical structures and trade names of surface active agents produced in the UK in 1961.

tend to become arranged in a particular manner. Water may therefore be said to possess a relatively high degree of structure. The presence of a solute will cause the replacement of some intermolecular water bonds by attractive forces between the solute and water. If these latter forces are appreciable, then the solute will remain in solution. However, in a surface active agent, although the forces of attraction between the hydrophilic groups and water are appreciable, those between the hydrocarbon chains and water are much weaker than the hydrogen bonds between water molecules. The system therefore tends to react in order to limit the degree of contact between water and the hydrophobic groups by the following methods—

(a) The hydrocarbon chains of molecules or ions in true solution tend to assume a coiled configuration, thus reducing the area of contact that would exist if these chains were extended.

(b) Although some molecules of the surface active agent are in true solution the majority are adsorbed at the surface, the hydrophilic groups remaining in contact with water, while the hydrocarbon chains tend to project from the surface. This type of adsorption is, of course, responsible for the marked effect of surface active agents on the surface properties of water.

Traube's rule (1891) states that in a homologous series the concentration required to produce an equal lowering of surface tension decreases by a factor of three for every CH_2 group added to the hydrocarbon chain. Thus, the differences in the free energies of adsorption of a homologous series of surface active agents are approximately equal. This fact has been interpreted as evidence for suggesting that the adsorbed molecules lie with their hydrocarbon chains parallel to the surface since in this orientation each CH_2 group has a similar position with respect to the surface. However, this orientation has been criticised, and alternative suggestions involving either a coiled hydrocarbon chain in the adsorbed molecules (Ward, 1946), or an orientation in which the hydrocarbon chains project from the surface and show a random hindered rotation around the C—C bonds (Aronow and Witten, 1958), have been made, together with explanations of the significance of the factor of three observed by Traube.

In addition to their marked effect on the surface properties of the solvent, surface active agents also show unusual changes in their physical properties at reasonably well-defined concentrations. These changes are attributed to the association of the amphipathic molecules or ions into aggregates of colloidal dimensions, which are known as micelles.

The formation of these aggregates and the properties of the colloidal solutions are dealt with in more detail in Chapter 5.

ADSORPTION AT SOLID–GAS AND SOLID–LIQUID INTERFACES

The irregular shapes of solid particles indicate the absence of a surface tension similar to that operating in liquids. In addition, it is impossible to extend the surface of a solid without upsetting the lattice structure of the component crystals. The changes in energy that result when the crystal lattices are altered make the estimation of changes in true surface free energy difficult and are also responsible for the difference in the ways in which the surface energies of solids and liquids are manifested. In general, the phenomena that do not involve the disruption of crystal lattices, e.g. adsorption and wetting, are thought to depend solely on the existence of surface free energy in solids.

If a solid comes into contact with a gas or a liquid there is an accumulation of gas or liquid molecules at the interface; i.e. the densities of the gas or liquid at the interface are greater than their bulk densities. This phenomenon is known as adsorption. (Since adsorption is a surface phenomenon it should be distinguished from absorption, which involves penetration of the absorbing material by the molecules of the absorbed substance.) The occurrence of adsorption at the solid–gas interface is easy to perceive since it causes a decrease in the pressure of the gas. However, the effects of adsorption at the solid–liquid interface are less obvious because the concentration of molecules in the bulk of a liquid is relatively great so that the detection of this type of adsorption is more difficult. In adsorption at the interface between a solid and liquid that contains two components (e.g. a solution or a mixture of miscible liquids), then the effects of adsorption are again readily demonstrable because the different degrees of adsorption of the two components result in a concentration change in the bulk of the solution.

It has already been pointed out that adsorption is one of the phenomena that occur at interfaces as a result of the tendency of a system to attain the lowest state of free energy. The surface (or interfacial) free energy that arises from the residual attractive forces on the surface molecules is reduced by the interaction of these forces with those of the adsorbed molecules. The irregular shapes of, solid particles and the roughness of solid surfaces introduces a further factor which complicates any quantitative treatment of phenomena that occur at solid surfaces. This factor is the variation in the activity of different sites on the solid surface; e.g. the activity of a site on a plain surface will be different from that of a similar site at the bottom of a crack in the surface. Thus, the attractive forces exerted by the solid surface will be heterogenous, the adsorbed molecules will first be attracted to those sites with the highest activity, and subsequent adsorption will occur at the sites of decreasing activities.

In the majority of its practical applications the process of adsorption involves, in fact, the displacement of previously adsorbed molecules by others. For example, the adsorption of gases often involves the displacement of air by another gas, and adsorption from solution often involves the displacement of solvent molecules by a more strongly adsorbed solute. However, a system that contains two components only, i.e. the adsorbing material (the adsorbent) and the substance that is adsorbed (the adsorbate), is more simple to consider from a theoretical point of view. For this reason the adsorption of gases by evacuated solids will first be discussed, followed by an account of adsorption at the solid–liquid interface.

Adsorption at the Solid–Gas Interface

The interactions between the solid adsorbent and the adsorbed gas or vapour molecules may range from a surface reaction, which is similar to a normal chemical reaction, to weak attractions similar to those responsible for the condensation of gases and vapours. It is therefore convenient to classify adsorption systems into chemisorption and physical adsorption on the basis of the interactions that are involved. The characteristic properties of these types of adsorption are listed in Table 4.2 in order to allow comparisons to be made.

Table 4.2
The Characteristics of Physical Adsorption and Chemisorption

	Physical adsorption	*Chemisorption*
1. Adsorption forces	Weak physical forces (van der Waals forces)* Heat of adsorption is usually <50 kJ/mole. May be regarded as a surface condensation	Involves transfer or sharing of electrons between adsorbent and adsorbed molecules. Heat of adsorption is usually about 60 to 420 kJ/mole. May be regarded as a surface reaction.
2. Specificity	Non-specific; i.e. will occur to some degree in any system.	Specific; i.e. only occurs when reaction is possible between adsorbent and adsorbate.
3. Reversibility	Reversible; i.e. adsorbate can be removed easily from surface in an unchanged form.	Often irreversible; i.e. adsorbate is removed with difficulty usually in a changed form: e.g. oxygen adsorbed by carbon is removed as carbon dioxide.
4. Effect of temperature	Process is exothermic; i.e. amount of adsorption decreases with rise in temperature.†	Surface reaction only proceeds above a certain temperature.‡ Reaction is usually exothermic.¶
5. Number of adsorbed layers	Monomolecular layer formed at low pressures followed by additional layers as pressure increases. Condensation of vapour in capillaries of porous solids may occur.	Restricted to formation of a monolayer.
6. Rate of adsorption	Usually rapid at all temperatures.	Usually proceeds at a finite rate which increases rapidly with rise in temperature.

* The appendix gives information on the various forces involved in physical adsorption.

† The exothermic nature of the process is indicated by the thermodynamic equation $\Delta G = \Delta H - T\Delta S$, where ΔG, ΔH, and ΔS are the changes in free energy, heat content, and entropy, respectively, that occur during a physicochemical process. For a spontaneous process such as adsorption ΔG must be negative; i.e. the process must lead to a decrease in the free energy of the system. In addition, the adsorbed molecules will have less freedom than those in the gaseous state; i.e. there is a decrease in the disorderly orientations of the gas molecules on adsorption and ΔS will be negative. Consequently, the term $-T\Delta S$, where T is the thermodynamic temperature, will be positive, and, therefore, from the above equation, H must be negative and the process is exothermic.

‡ Physical adsorption at low temperatures may give way to chemisorption at higher temperatures.

¶ It is often stated that all adsorptions are exothermic. However, some chemisorptions may be endothermic (Thomas, 1961).

ADSORPTION ISOTHERMS

It is normal practice to express the results of an adsorption process in the form of a graph showing the variation in the amount of gas or vapour adsorbed, x, by a given mass, m, of the adsorbent, with the equilibrium pressure, p, of the gas at constant temperature. These graphs are known as adsorption isotherms. In vapour adsorption it is more common to use the relative vapour pressure, p/p_0, where p_0 is the saturated vapour pressure, instead of simply the equilibrium pressure.

The majority of isotherms for the adsorption of gases or vapours by solids may be classified on the basis of their shapes into Types I–V as shown by Fig. 4.7.

Many attempts have been made to obtain a relationship between the amount of adsorption and the pressure of gas in the system. Since these relationships are quantitative expressions of the shapes of graphs given in Fig. 4.7, the equations themselves are also referred to as adsorption isotherms. The most common are those suggested by Freundlich, Langmuir, and by Brunauer, Emmett, and Teller.

The Freundlich adsorption isotherm, which is expressed by Eqn (4.17), was the earliest of these adsorption isotherms and it was deduced empirically from its agreement with a large number of experimental results.

$$\frac{x}{m} = kp^{1/n} \qquad (4.17)$$

In Eqn (4.17), x and m are defined as before, and n and k are constants for a particular system at constant temperature. The power of p is usually written in the form of a fraction ($1/n$, where $n > 1$) to indicate that the increase in the amount of adsorption at the low pressures, where this equation is usually valid, is less rapid than the increase in the pressure itself. In fact, the value of $1/n$ is often between 0·3 and 0·5.

The agreement of experimental data with Eqn (4.17) may be checked by plotting $\log x/m$ against $\log p$. A straight line with a slope of $1/n$ and an intercept of $\log k$ should be obtained if the equation is applicable.

Langmuir (1916) attempted to explain adsorption in terms of a dynamic equilibrium determined by

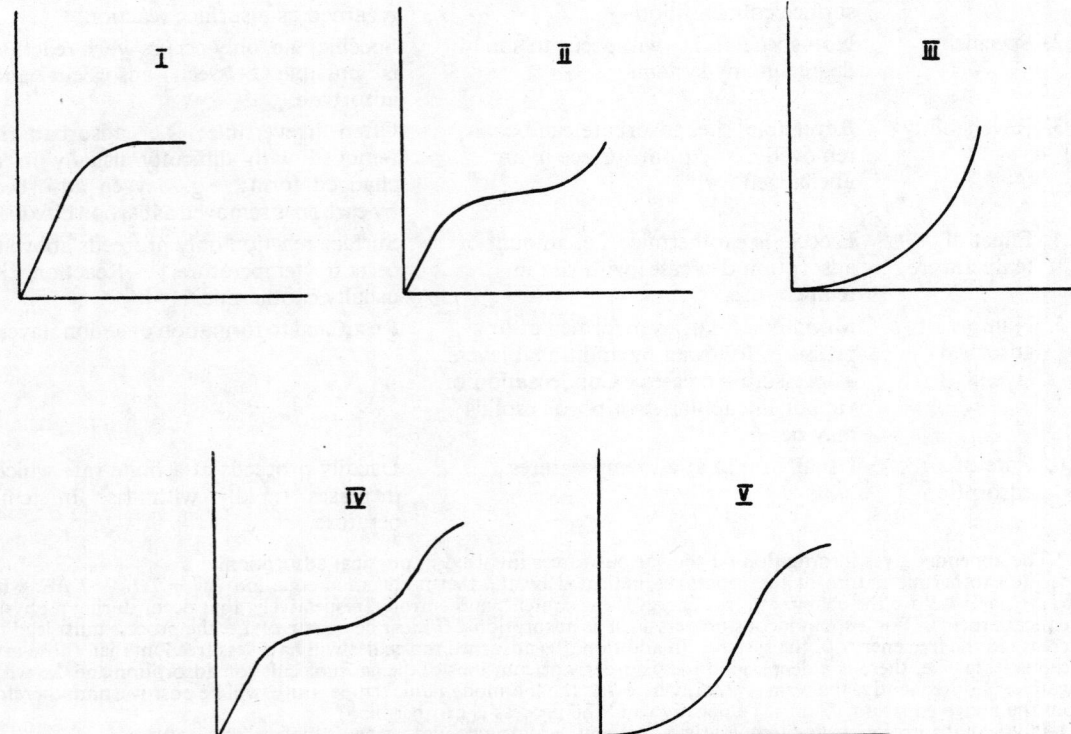

Fig. 4.7 Classification of isotherms for the adsorption of vapours by solids according to Brunauer *et al.* (1940)
Ordinates, x/m Abscissae, p/p_0

the rates at which gas molecules were adsorbed and desorbed. The rate of adsorption at any instant was considered to be proportional to the amount of 'free' surface available at that instant and to the pressure of the gas in the system. The rate of desorption was considered to be proportional to the fraction of the surface onto which the gas was already adsorbed. In addition, it was assumed that the interaction between adsorbed molecules and the adsorbent involved forces similar to short-ranged chemical bonds, so that the adsorption of only a monolayer was envisaged.

This approach resulted in the Langmuir adsorption isotherm which is expressed by Eqn (4.18), where x, m, and p are defined as before, and a and b are constants for a given system at constant temperature.

$$\frac{x}{m} = \frac{abp}{1 + ap} \qquad (4.18)$$

In the original derivation of Eqn (4.18), the constant a is the ratio of the rate constants for the adsorption and desorption processes, and the constant b is the amount of gas required to produce an adsorbed monolayer over the whole surface of the adsorbent. However, the Langmuir adsorption isotherm is often successfully applied to systems where the assumptions made by Langmuir are obviously invalid. In these cases, the constants a and b can no longer be defined as above and are arbitrary constants only.

The applicability of the Langmuir adsorption isotherm to experimental data may be checked by rearranging Eqn (4.18) to the form shown in Eqn (4.19).

$$p \cdot \frac{m}{x} = \frac{1}{b} \cdot p + \frac{1}{ab} \qquad (4.19)$$

It can be seen from Eqn (4.19) that a graph of pm/x against p should give a straight line with a slope of $1/b$ and an intercept of $1/ab$ if the equation is obeyed.

The Langmuir adsorption isotherm is capable of application only to isotherms represented by Type I in Fig. 4.7. Many attempts have been made to derive an equation that is applicable to all the different types of adsorption isotherm. One of the more successful approaches is due to Brunauer et al. (1938). These workers considered that multilayers of gas were adsorbed and assumed that the forces involved in physical adsorption are the same as those responsible for the condensation of gases. Since these forces have a very short range the effect of the solid was considered to be appreciable only on the first layer of adsorbed molecules. The possibility of multilayer formation depended, therefore, on the degree of interaction between the gas molecules. Equation (4.20), which is the result of this

approach, is known as the BET adsorption isotherm.

$$\frac{p}{x(p_0 - p)} = \frac{1}{x_m h} + \frac{h - 1}{x_m h} \cdot \frac{p}{p_0} \qquad (4.20)$$

where x = the amount of gas adsorbed per unit weight of adsorbent at the equilibrium pressure p, x_m = the amount of gas adsorbed per unit weight of adsorbent when the surface of the latter is covered with a monolayer of adsorbed molecules, p_0 = the saturated vapour pressure of the gas, and h = a constant, which is a function of the difference between the heat of adsorption of the gas in the first layer (E_a) and the heat of condensation of the gas (E_c) as shown by Eqn (4.21).

$$h = e^{-E_a - E_c/RT} \qquad (4.21)$$

The agreement of experimental data with Eqn (4.20) may be verified by plotting $p/x(p_0 - p)$ against p/p_0. A straight line with a slope of $h - 1/x_m h$ and an intercept of $1/x_m h$ is obtained if the equation is applicable.

The derivation of Eqn (4.20) neglects the existence of lateral interactions between molecules adsorbed in any layer and assumes that the energy of adsorption is independent of the amount already adsorbed in that layer. In addition, it is assumed that the energy of interaction between two adjacent layers of adsorbed molecules is the same, irrespective of their positions relative to the solid surface.

Since Eqn (4.20) reduces to the Langmuir equation for systems in which adsorption is restricted to monolayer formation, it is therefore applicable to isotherms of Type I in Fig. 4.7. In addition, the BET equation can be applied to isotherms of Type II, in which the further rise after the first plateau is attributed to the adsorption of layers beyond the monolayer level. However, the agreement of Eqn (4.20) with the experimental results for this type of isotherm is satisfactory only when the relative pressure (p/p_0) is within the range of 0·05 to 0·35.

It has been suggested that the failure of Eqn (4.20) below a relative pressure of 0·05 arises from the non-uniformity of the surface sites, which results in a variation in the value of E_a for different parts of the surface, and which cannot be accounted for satisfactorily in a quantitative manner. Furthermore, the poor agreement above a relative pressure of 0·35 has been ascribed to the effect of the walls of narrow pores in the solid on the thickness of the adsorbed films. This effect can be taken into account by rather complicated modifications of Eqn (4.20) (Gregg, 1965).

Except for Type IV isotherms at low pressures, where they resemble Type II isotherms, the BET equation appears to be of little use in describing quantitatively the isotherms of Types III to V. However, modifications of the equation are available which allow a reasonable agreement with a Type IV isotherm (Gregg, 1965).

THE CAPILLARY CONDENSATION THEORY

In adsorption of vapours by porous solids, it is considered that much of the adsorption at high relative pressures is caused by condensation of the vapour in the fine capillaries of the solid. The occurrence of condensation at pressures lower than normal saturated vapour pressures follows from a consideration of the Kelvin equation, which indicates the relationship between the equilibrium vapour pressure, p, in a capillary of radius r and the normal saturated vapour pressure, p_0. This relationship is represented by Eqn (4.22) in which γ is the surface tension of the liquid, V is its molecular volume, R is the gas constant, and T is the thermodynamic temperature.

$$\ln \frac{p}{p_0} = \frac{-2\gamma V}{rRT} \qquad (4.22)$$

Equation (4.22) indicates that condensation of a vapour will occur at pressure p in all those capillaries with a radius less than r in a porous solid. This theory is supported by the fact that at pressures equal to or just below the saturated vapour pressure the amounts of adsorbed vapours for different substances calculated as liquid volumes are the same for a given adsorbent (Gurvich, 1915). Thus, the efficiency of a porous solid in adsorbing vapour at high relative pressures is determined mainly by the total volume of the pores that are accessible to the vapour.

Adsorption at the Solid–Liquid Interface

The adsorption of solutes from solution at the solid–liquid interface has been studied to a lesser extent than gas adsorption, although the phenomenon has been used practically for centuries; e.g. in the clarification of liquids. It is only in more recent years that the theories of adsorption from solution have become more developed, and the importance of the solvent recognised.

The isotherms for adsorption from solution have been classified into four main groups depending on the shape of the initial part of the isotherm (Giles et al., 1960). Each of these groups is then subclassified on the basis of the shape of the isotherm at higher concentrations. The classification is shown in Fig. 4.8.

The initial curvature of the S curves indicates that

adsorption becomes easier as the equilibrium concentration rises. This curve is characteristic of systems in which the solute molecule is monofunctional, i.e. the solute molecule has a single point of strong attachment on to the adsorbent, and there is an appreciable intermolecular interaction within the adsorbed layer. These conditions usually result in the vertical orientation of adsorbed molecules. The S curve may also be indicative of strong competition by the solvent or other species for the adsorbent sites.

The L curve is so-called because it is similar in shape to the Langmuir isotherm, a type of curve most commonly obtained for adsorption from dilute solution. The shape of the curve shows that the amount of adsorbed solute increases as the concentration increases until a limiting 'plateau' value is reached. In systems producing this type of curve the adsorbate molecules are likely to be adsorbed flat on the surface of the adsorbent, or vertically if there is little competition from the solvent for the adsorption sites.

The H or High Affinity curve is characteristic of systems in which there is a strong interaction between the adsorbent and adsorbate, which results in complete removal of solute from solutions of low concentration. Such a system may involve a chemisorption mechanism or the adsorption of micellar aggregates. (See Chapter 5 for information about structure of micelles.)

The C curve represents a constant partition of the solute between the adsorbent and solution. It seems to occur in systems that involve fibrous materials such as wool, where the penetration of the solute increases as the concentration in solution increases.

From a consideration of the above comments it can be seen that the shape of an isotherm for a particular system may provide information about the interaction between the adsorbate and adsorbent, the orientation of the adsorbed molecules, and the competition offered by the solvent.

Although attempts have been made to find a universal equation applicable to all solution isotherms, a suitable one has not been developed due to the wide variety and complexity of systems.* Also, as pointed out by Kipling (1965), 'many equations have proved inadequate because the role of the solvent has been neglected'. Equations analogous to the Freundlich, Langmuir, and BET isotherms (i.e. Eqns 4.17, 4.18, and 4.20) have been used for adsorption from solution by introducing a

---

* The Gibbs Adsorption Isotherm applies to adsorption at all interfaces. However, it involves a further term (interfacial tension) and therefore does not describe adsorption solely in terms of the concentration of the solution.

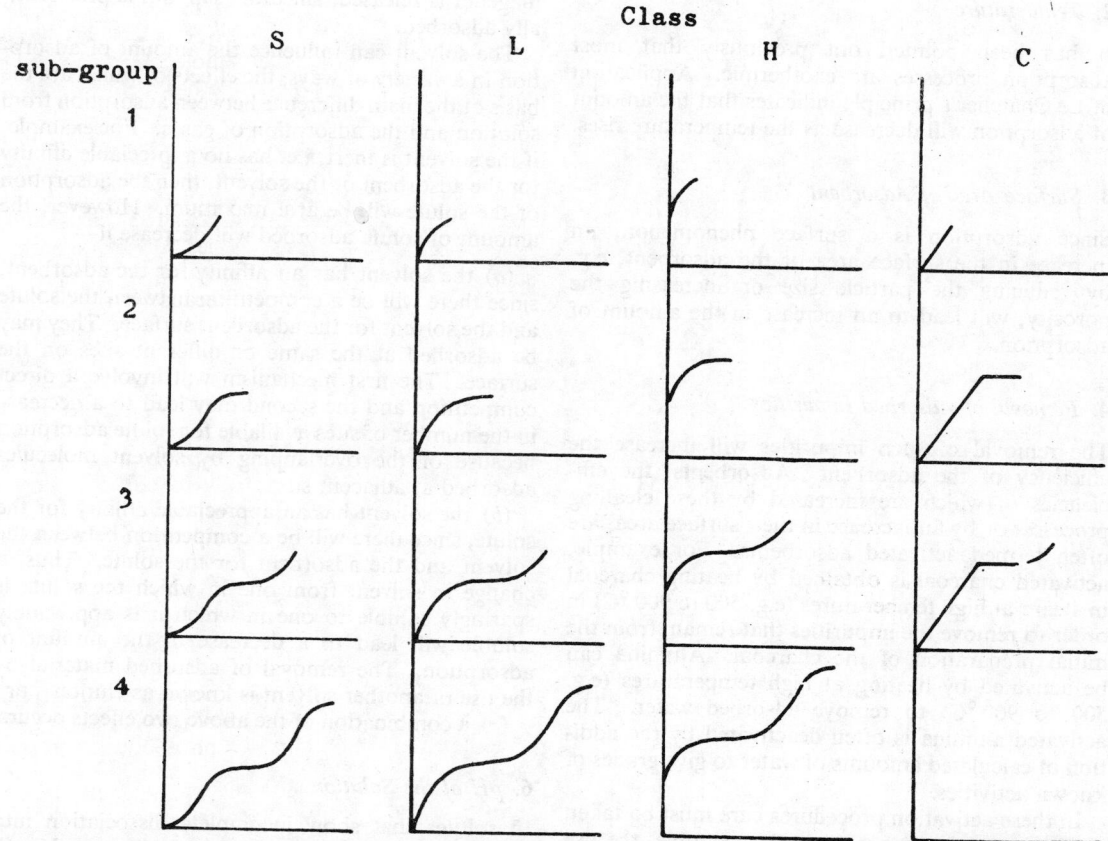

Fig. 4.8 Classification of isotherms for the adsorption of solutes from solution according to Giles and co-workers (1960) Ordinates—amount of solute adsorbed per unit weight of adsorbent   Abscissae—equilibrium concentration of solution

term for solute concentration instead of pressure. For example, the Langmuir isotherm, which has probably found the greatest application to solution data, becomes

$$\frac{x}{m} = \frac{abc}{1 + ac} \qquad (4.23)$$

where, c is the equilibrium concentration of the solute, x is the amount of solute adsorbed by a given mass (m) of adsorbent, and a and b are constants for a given system at constant temperature. Although the use of these equations for adsorption from solution may not be entirely satisfactory from a theoretical point of view, they often fit the isotherm obtained for the adsorption of solutes from dilute solution (Kipling, 1965).

Kipling (1951) and Kipling and Tester (1952) have introduced the concept of a 'composite isotherm'. This takes into account the adsorption of all the components of a system (e.g. the solvent as well as

the solute) by combining the individual isotherms for each component. However, in the case of dilute solutions the 'composite isotherm' is often indistinguishable from the usual solute isotherm and, therefore, there is little advantage to be gained from using it in place of the simpler Langmuir isotherm.

FACTORS AFFECTING ADSORPTION FROM SOLUTION

1. *Solute Concentration*

An increase in the concentration of the solute will cause an increase in the amount of adsorption that occurs at equilibrium until a limiting value is reached. It should be borne in mind that for most adsorptions from solution the *relative* amount of solute removed from solution is greater in dilute solutions.

2. Temperature

It has been pointed out previously that most adsorption processes are exothermic. Application of Le Chatelier's principle indicates that the amount of adsorption will decrease as the temperature rises.

3. Surface Area of Adsorbent

Since adsorption is a surface phenomenon, an increase in the surface area of the adsorbent, e.g. by reducing the particle size or increasing the porosity, will lead to an increase in the amount of adsorption.

4. Removal of Adsorbed Impurities

The removal of such impurities will increase the efficiency of the adsorbent. Adsorbents, the efficiencies of which are increased by these cleaning processes or by an increase in their surface area, are often termed activated adsorbents. For example, activated charcoal is obtained by heating charcoal in steam at high temperatures (e.g. 500 to 900 °C) in order to remove the impurities that remain from the initial preparation of the charcoal. Alumina can be activated by heating at high temperatures (e.g. 500 to 900 °C) to remove adsorbed water. The activated alumina is often deactivated by the addition of calculated amounts of water to give grades of known activities.

In these activation procedures care must be taken to obtain maximum activity. For example, the use of high temperatures in the activation of alumina may result in a decrease in the total surface area by a 'sintering' process. In addition, an inactive form of alumina (α-alumina) is produced at temperatures in excess of 1000 °C.

5. Adsorbent-Solute Interactions and Solvent Competition

The adsorption of a solute from dilute solution involves breaking solute-solvent bonds and adsorbent-solvent bonds and the formation of adsorbent-solute bonds. The strength of the various interactions between the components of a system, i.e. adsorbent, solute and solvent, will depend on their mechanisms, which, in turn, depend on the structures of the components. It is quite possible that an adsorbent will have a strong affinity for a particular type of solute, which will therefore be adsorbed preferentially from a mixed solution. This gives rise to what is known as selective adsorption. For example, charcoal will adsorb the dye magenta from solution. However, if saponin is added to the system the

magenta is released, since the saponin is preferentially adsorbed.

The solvent can influence the amount of adsorption in a variety of ways, the effects of which are the basis of the main difference between adsorption from solution and the adsorption of gases. For example, if the solvent is inert, i.e. has no appreciable affinity for the adsorbent or the solvent, then the adsorption of the solute will be at a maximum. However, the amount of solute adsorbed will decrease if—

(a) the solvent has an affinity for the adsorbent, since there will be a competition between the solute and the solvent for the adsorbent surface. They may be adsorbed at the same or different sites on the surface. The first mechanism will involve a direct competition and the second may lead to a decrease in the number of sites available for solute adsorption because of the overlapping by solvent molecules adsorbed at adjacent sites;

(b) the solvent has an appreciable affinity for the solute, since there will be a competition between the solvent and the adsorbent for the solute. Thus, a change in solvent from one in which the solute is sparingly soluble to one in which it is appreciably soluble will lead to a decrease in the amount of adsorption. The removal of adsorbed material by the use of another solvent is known as elution; or

(c) a combination of the above two effects occurs.

6. pH of the Solution

In solutes that show incomplete dissociation into ions in solution the effect of a change in pH will depend on whether the ionised or unionised species is the most strongly adsorbed.

APPLICATIONS OF ADSORPTION IN PHARMACY AND ALLIED FIELDS

1. Decolorising Agents

The removal of traces of coloured impurity is often achieved by the use of an adsorption process. For example, the decolorisation of a liquid may be effected by shaking or heating with approximately one per cent of activated charcoal. After standing, the charcoal plus adsorbed impurity is removed by filtration. Care must be exercised when carrying out decolorisation processes in order to ensure that active ingredients are not also removed by adsorption. This is particularly likely to happen if alkaloidal solutions are decolorised by the use of activated charcoal.

An attempt is made to standardise the adsorptive capacity of decolorising charcoal in the BP by comparing the amount of bromophenol blue remaining in alcoholic solution after adsorption has occurred. Two tests for the adsorptive capacity of Charcoal BPC are given. One involves the adsorption of chloroform vapour and the other involves adsorption of phenazone from aqueous solution. The results of tests such as these should be treated cautiously, since it does not necessarily follow that the decolorising powers of various samples of charcoal for the removal of other solutes will parallel the results obtained with bromophenol blue or phenazone.

2. Desiccants and Drying Agents

Water is strongly adsorbed by alumina and silica gel. The last traces of water are therefore often removed from organic solvents by passage through a column of alumina or silica gel. These materials are also used as desiccants to maintain a dry atmosphere inside electronic apparatus, and small packets are sometimes included inside the containers of pharmaceutical preparations that may be affected adversely by a high humidity.

3. Adsorption Chromatography

This is a separation technique based on the difference in affinity of an adsorbent for various solutes. The different affinities result in a variation in the partition of the solutes between the liquid/solid interface and the liquid phase. If the latter moves through a stationary column of the adsorbent, then the rates of movement of the solutes will vary; for example, a strongly adsorbed solute will spend more time adsorbed on to the stationary phase than a weakly adsorbed solute and, consequently, the former will move through the column at a slower rate than the latter. Eventually some degree of separation will be obtained.

The applications of chromatography to compounds of pharmaceutical interest are many, since it is a standard method of separation and purification in most laboratories. The student is therefore recommended to read one of the available textbooks on this subject.

4. Surface Area Determination

Many of the properties of a powder are influenced by its surface area; e.g. rate of solution, rate of oxidation, hygroscopicity, sedimentation behaviour, resistance to gas flow, bulk density and associated packing problems.

Measurement of the adsorption of gases or solutes provides one of the commonest means of determining the specific area, S_a, i.e. the surface area per unit weight (or unit volume) of the powder. The majority of the adsorption methods are based on Eqn (4.24) and involve the determination of the following two parameters.

(a) The monolayer capacity, x_m, i.e. the amount of adsorbate required to produce a complete monolayer on the adsorbent surface.

(b) The surface area occupied by each molecule in the monolayer (A_0). This involves a knowledge of the orientation of the adsorbed molecules with respect to the surface.

$$S_a = x_m . N_A . A_0 \qquad (4.24)$$

In Eqn (4.24), x_m is expressed in moles and N_A is Avogadro's constant ($6·023 \times 10^{23}$ mole^{-1}).

The accurate determination of x_0 is difficult in the case of adsorption from solution because adsorbed solvent molecules may prevent close packing of the adsorbed solute in the formation of a monolayer; i.e. the latter may consist of solute and solvent molecules. In addition, the orientation of the adsorbed solute will vary with the type of solvent, and A_0 is difficult to evaluate, especially in complex asymmetric molecules such as dyes. (These compounds are often used in surface area determinations because of the ease of analysis of coloured solutions.) These difficulties are either avoided or are not so marked in the adsorption of small gas molecules, e.g. nitrogen and argon. Absolute values for the specific surface area are therefore more reliable when obtained from gas adsorption measurements, although reasonable agreement has been obtained between such values and those determined by the adsorption of 4-nitrophenol from solution (Giles and Nakhwa, 1962). The common application of adsorption from solution is in the measurement of specific surface areas on a relative basis, e.g. for quality control. This use arises from the experimental simplicity of the method compared with the practical difficulties associated with the measurement of gas adsorption.

5. Medicinal Adsorbents

Kaolin and charcoal are both used as gastrointestinal adsorbents for the removal of toxic materials, and charcoal is also useful as a general antidote for poisoning by compounds such as atropine, strychnine, oxalic acid, and phenolphthalein. It should be borne in mind that these adsorbents may also take up vitamins, drugs, enzymes, and trace materials. Their continued use may therefore lead to unwanted effects such as vitamin and mineral deficiencies, incomplete medication, and interference with digestive processes.

Kaolin is useful in external preparations such as poultices for dressing boils, suppurating wounds and ulcers. Kaolin is also used for its drying properties in dusting powders for application to moist lesions.

6. *Miscellaneous Applications*

(*a*) Activated charcoal has been used for removing pyrogens from injections (Gunn and Carter, 1965).

(*b*) The concentration of penicillin and streptomycin may be effected by adsorption from dilute solution followed by recovery.

(*c*) The pore sizes of some filters are often slightly larger than the normal dimensions of retained particles. However, penetration of filters is prevented by several mechanisms, one of which involves adsorption of the particles onto the walls of the pores.

(*d*) The stability of colloids is often dependent on the adsorption of ions onto their surfaces, and the

mechanism of action of protective colloids is thought to involve the adsorption of hydrophilic material onto hydrophobic particles (*see* Chapter 5).

(*e*) The stability of emulsions depends on the adsorption of the emulsifying agent at the oil/water interface (*see* Chapter 5).

(*f*) Pharmacological activity may involve adsorption of drug molecules at receptor sites in the cell (Ariens and Simonis, 1964).

(*g*) The rheological properties of suspensions are markedly affected by the adsorption of various materials especially surface active agents, at the liquid/solid interface (*see* Chapter 7).

(*h*) The adsorption of drugs by solid excipients included in many pharmaceutical formulations may have an important effect on the rate of drug release from these formulations and on the rate of absorption of the drugs (Wurster and Polli, 1961 and 1964; Sorby, 1965; Sorby *et al.*, 1966).

Electrical Effects at Interfaces

The existence of a difference in electrical potential across a solid–liquid interface is demonstrated by the following phenomena.

(*a*) *Electrophoresis*

This involves the movement of dispersed particles through a liquid medium under the influence of an electrical field.

(*b*) *Electro-osmosis*

This involves the movement of a liquid relative to a fixed solid under the influence of an applied field.

(*c*) *Streaming Potential*

This is the potential difference set up across a fixed porous plug of solid when a liquid is forced through it.

(*d*) *Sedimentation Potential*

This is the potential difference set up between the top and bottom of a suspension of solid particles in a liquid when the particles settle under the influence of gravity.

The above phenomena are termed electrokinetic phenomena since they are concerned with a potential difference associated with the relative movement between two phases separated by an interface.

The difference in electrical potential across an interface indicates that there must be a particular distribution of charges near to the interface. This distribution is referred to as an electrical double layer and its initial structure was proposed by Helmholtz

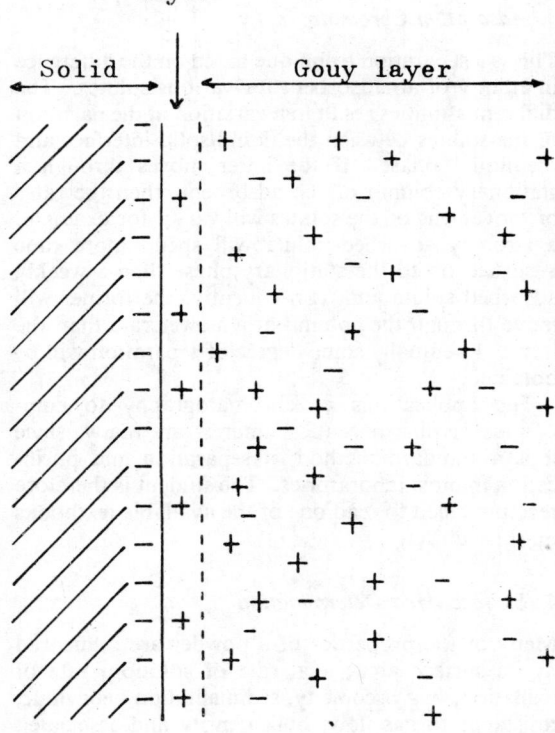

Fig. 4.9   The electrical double layer at a flat negatively charged solid surface

in 1879. Various modifications have been suggested since then, and the present theory is discussed below.

The Electrical Double Layer

Consider a solid surface carrying negative charges in contact with an aqueous solution containing positive and negative ions. The negatively charged solid surface will influence the distribution of ions in the neighbouring layers of the solution. Thus, positive ions will be attracted towards the solid surface and negative ions repelled away from it. However, this distribution will also be affected by thermal agitation which will tend to redisperse the ions in solution. The resulting effect creates a diffuse layer of solution, in which the concentration of positive ions gradually decreases on moving away from the interface, and the concentration of negative ions gradually increases. However, this diffuse layer contains a sufficient excess of positive ions to neutralise the negative charges on the solid surface. This type of distribution of charges is referred to as an electrical double layer. The surface charges form the fixed part of this double layer and the layers of liquid containing the excess oppositely charged ions constitute the diffuse part. The separation of charge in the electrical double layer gives rise to a decrease in potential, ψ, across the double layer from its value at the surface of the solid, ψ_0, to zero at the edge of the diffuse layer where a condition of electro-neutrality is reached.

Sometimes thermal agitation is insufficient to overcome the attractive forces between the solid surface and oppositely charged ions. For example, strong attractions will exist if the ions in solution carry several charges (e.g. multivalent ions) or if additional forces are involved in the adsorption process (e.g. as in the adsorption of surface active agents). Strong adsorption of these types of oppositely charged ions will result, and these are held in the so-called Stern layer. The remaining oppositely charged ions are distributed in a diffuse layer (the Gouy layer) similar to that described previously. The structure of the electrical double layer is shown diagrammatically in Fig. 4.9 in which δ and d

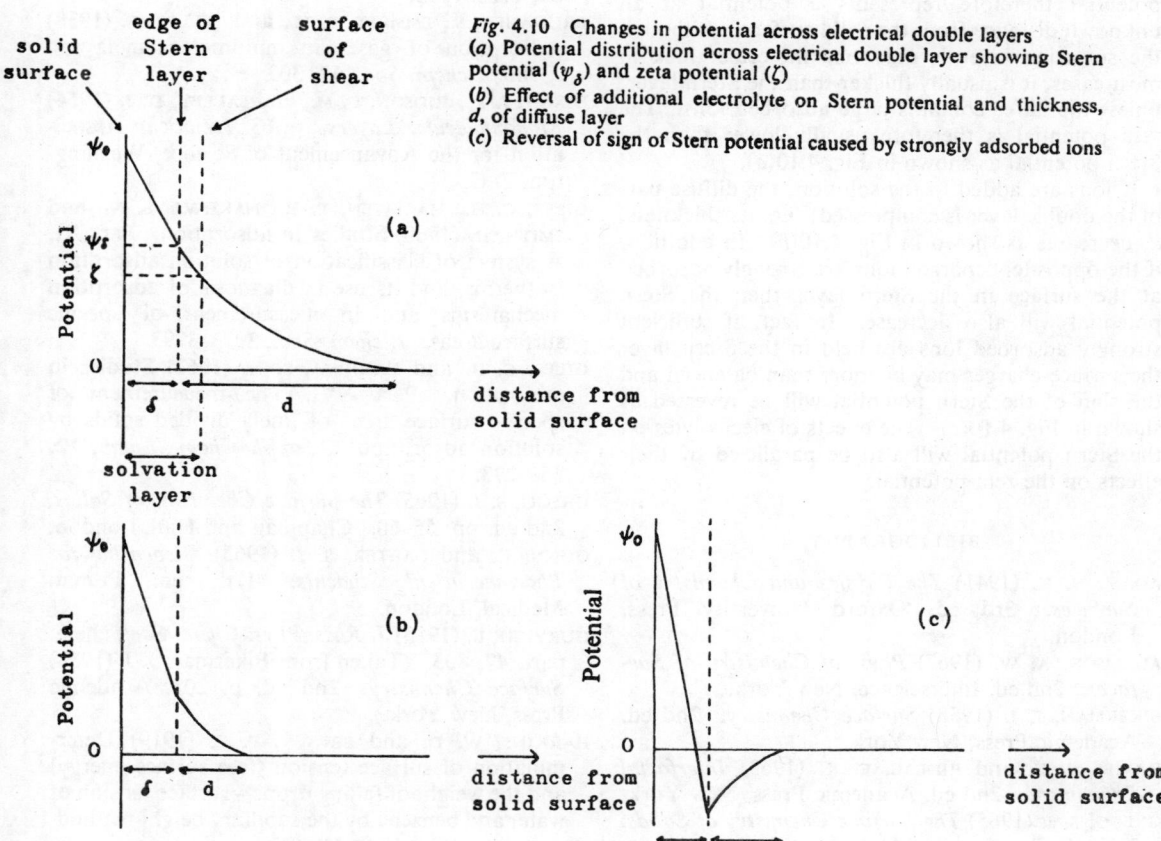

Fig. 4.10 Changes in potential across electrical double layers
(*a*) Potential distribution across electrical double layer showing Stern potential (ψ_δ) and zeta potential (ζ)
(*b*) Effect of additional electrolyte on Stern potential and thickness, *d*, of diffuse layer
(*c*) Reversal of sign of Stern potential caused by strongly adsorbed ions

represent the thicknesses of the Stern and Gouy layers respectively.

The distribution of ions shown in Fig. 4.9 will affect the potential at varying distances from the surface of the solid. This change is illustrated by Fig. 4.10(a). It can be seen that the potential decreases linearly across the Stern layer from the surface potential, ψ_0, to the Stern potential, ψ_δ, which is the value at the boundary between the Stern and Gouy layers, and then falls more and more slowly until it is zero at the edge of the Gouy layer.

A layer of liquid molecules will also be adsorbed on to the solid. This solvating layer is strongly held to the surface and is therefore of importance in electrokinetic phenomena since the outer surface of this layer represents the boundary of relative movement between the solid and the liquid. This surface is therefore termed the surface of shear. The potential at this point is termed the zeta, ζ, or electrokinetic potential, and it may be calculated from measurements of the electrokinetic phenomena mentioned previously. The thickness of the solvating layer of liquid molecules is ill-defined and the zeta potential therefore represents a potential at an unknown distance from the solid surface. Although the solvating layer is only one molecule thick in most cases, it is usually thicker than the Stern layer, unless the latter contains large adsorbed ions. The zeta potential is therefore usually lower than the Stern potential as shown in Fig. 4.10(a).

If ions are added to the solution, the diffuse part of the double layer is compressed; i.e. its thickness, d, decreases as shown in Fig. 4.10(b). In addition, if the oppositely charged ions are strongly adsorbed at the surface in the Stern layer then the Stern potential will also decrease. In fact, if sufficient strongly adsorbed ions are held in the Stern layer the surface charges may be more than balanced and the sign of the Stern potential will be reversed as shown in Fig. 4.10(c). The effects of electrolytes on the Stern potential will also be paralleled by their effects on the zeta potential.

BIBLIOGRAPHY

ADAM, N. K. (1941) *The Physics and Chemistry of Surfaces*. 3rd ed. Oxford University Press, London.

ADAMSON, A. W. (1967) *Physical Chemistry of Surfaces*. 2nd ed. Interscience, New York.

BIKERMAN, J. J. (1958) *Surface Chemistry*. 2nd ed. Academic Press, New York.

DAVIES, J. T. and RIDEAL, E. K. (1963) *Interfacial Phenomena*. 2nd ed. Academic Press, New York.

GREGG, S. J. (1965) *The Surface Chemistry of Solids*. 2nd ed. Chapman and Hall, London.

KIPLING, J. J. (1965) *Adsorption from Solutions of Non-electrolytes*. Academic Press, New York.

MOILLIET, J. L., COLLIE, B., and BLACK, W. (1961) *Surface Activity*. 2nd ed. Spon, London.

TROTMAN-DICKENSON, A. F. and PARFITT, G. D. (1966) *Chemical Kinetics and Surface/Colloid Chemistry*. Pergamon Press, London.

VERWEY, E. J. W. and OVERBEEK, J. TH. G. (1948) *Theory of the Stability of Lyophobic Colloids*. Elsevier, Amsterdam.

REFERENCES

ARIENS, E. J. and SIMONIS, A. M. (1964) A molecular basis for drug action. *J. Pharm. Pharmac.*, **16**, 137–157.

ARONOW, R. H. and WITTEN, L. (1958) Theoretical derivation of Traube's rule. *J. chem. Phys.*, **28**, 405–409.

BRUNAUER, S., DEMING, L. S., DEMING, W. S., and TELLER, E. (1940) On a theory of the van der Waals adsorption of gases. *J. Amer. chem. Soc.*, **62**, 1723–1732.

BRUNAUER, S., EMMETT, P. H., and TELLER, E. (1938) Adsorption of gases in multimolecular layers. *J. Amer. chem. Soc.*, **60**, 309

DIXON, J. K., JUDSON, C. M., and SALLEY, D. J. (1954) *Monomolecular Layers*. p. 63, American Association for the Advancement of Science, Washington, D.C.

GILES, C. H., MACEWEN, T. H., NAKHWA, S. N., and SMITH, D. (1960) Studies in adsorption. **Part XI.** A system of classification of solution adsorption isotherms, and its use in diagnosis of adsorption mechanisms and in measurement of specific surface areas. *J. chem. Soc.*, 3973–3993.

GILES, C. H. and NAKHWA, S. N. (1962) Studies in adsorption. Part XVI. The measurement of specific surface areas of finely divided solids by solution adsorption. *J. appl. Chem., Lond.*, **12**, 266–273.

GREGG, S. J. (1965) *The Surface Chemistry of Solids*. 2nd ed. pp. 55–60. Chapman and Hall, London.

GUNN, C. and CARTER, S. J. (1965) *Dispensing for Pharmaceutical Students*. 11th ed. Pitman Medical, London.

GURVICH, L. (1915) *J. Russ. Phys. Chem. Soc.*, chem. part, **47**, 805. (Taken from Bikerman, J. J. (1958) *Surface Chemistry*. 2nd ed. p. 203. Academic Press, New York.)

HARKINS, W. D. and BROWN, F. E. (1919) Determination of surface tension (free surface energy) and the weight of falling drops—surface tension of water and benzene by the capillary height method. *J. Amer. chem. Soc.*, **41**, 499.

HARKINS, W. D. and JORDAN, H. F. (1930) Determination of surface tension. *J. Amer. chem. Soc.*, **52**, 1751.

KIPLING, J. J. (1951) Adsorption of non-electrolytes from solution. *Q. Rev. chem. Soc.*, **5**, 60–74.

KIPLING, J. J. (1965) *Adsorption from Solutions of Non-electrolytes.* p. 25. Academic Press, London.

KIPLING, J. J. and TESTER, D. A. (1952) Adsorption from binary mixtures: Determination of individual adsorption isotherms. *J. chem. Soc.*, 4123–4133.

LANGMUIR, I. (1916) *J. Amer. chem. Soc.*, **38**, 2219.

LOWER, E. S. (1962) Dictionary of British surface active agents. Parts 1–7 and Additional Entries. *Mfg Chem.*, **33**, 141–144, 181–184, 241–244, 285–288, 333–336, 371–374, 421–424 and 478.

MCBAIN, J. W. and SWAIN, R. S. (1936) Measurements of adsorption at the air-water interface. *Proc. R. Soc.*, **A154**, 608.

MOILLIET, J. L., COLLIE, B., and BLACK, W. (1961) *Surface Activity.* 2nd ed. Spon, London.

SCHWARTZ, A. M. and PERRY, J. W. (1949) *Surface Active Agents. Their chemistry and technology. Vol. 1.* Interscience, New York.

SORBY, D. L. (1965) Effect of adsorbents on drug absorption. I. Modification of promazine absorption by activated attapulgite and activated charcoal. *J. pharm. Sci.*, **54**, 677–683.

SORBY, D. L., PLEIN, E. M., and BENMAMAN, J. D. (1966) Adsorption of phenothiazine derivatives by solid adsorbents. *J. pharm. Sci.*, **55**, 785–794.

TATE, T. (1864) *Phil. Mag.*, **27**, 176.

THOMAS, J. M. (1961) Textbook errors, 29. The existence of endothermic adsorption. *J. chem. Educ.*, **38**, 138–139.

TRAUBE, I. (1891) *Justus Liebigs Annln. Chem.*, **265**, 27.

WARD, A. F. H. (1946) Thermodynamics of monolayers on solutions. I. Theoretical significance of Traube's rule. *Trans. Faraday Soc.*, **42**, 399–407.

WURSTER, D. E. and POLLI, G. P. (1961) Investigation of drug release from solids. IV. Influence of adsorption on the dissolution rate. *J. pharm. Sci.*, **50**, 403–406.

WURSTER, D. E. and POLLI, G. P. (1964) Investigation of drug release from solids. V. Simultaneous influence of adsorption and viscosity on the dissolution rate. *J. pharm. Sci.*, **53**, 311–314.

5

Disperse Systems

A DISPERSE system may be defined as a system in which one substance (the disperse phase) is dispersed as particles throughout another (the dispersion medium or continuous phase). This type of system can be classified on the basis of the physical states of the two substances. Since matter can exist as gas, liquid, or solid, then nine different types of disperse system are possible in the same way that nine different types of solution are possible (*see* Table 2.1, Chapter 2). With the exception of dispersions of gases in gases, these systems can be further classified on the basis of the size of the dispersed particles as shown in Table 5.1. It should be borne in mind that the sub-division given in the table is not rigid and there is no sharp demarcation between the particle sizes in these systems.

Since true solutions have been discussed in Chapters 2 and 3 the present discussion will be restricted to colloidal dispersions and coarse dispersions. Some examples of these systems are given in Table 5.2.

The Stability of Disperse Systems

The dispersion of one phase as small particles throughout another produces a considerable area of contact between the two phases. Any free energy associated with the interface between the phases will be decreased if the particles aggregate or coalesce because of the reduction in interfacial area that accompanies such aggregation. Since any system will tend to react spontaneously to decrease its free energy to a minimum, it follows that disperse systems are often unstable. Thus, if the interfacial free energy has a positive value, then the particles will eventually aggregate rather than remain in contact with the dispersion medium. Dispersions that exhibit this behaviour are termed lyophobic dispersions. In other systems, known as lyophilic dispersions, an affinity exists between the dispersed particles and the dispersion medium, and this contributes to the stability of these systems.

Colloidal dispersions are usually more stable (i.e. will remain as dispersions longer) than coarse dispersions, since the larger particles in the latter settle more rapidly under the influence of gravity and, unlike colloidal systems, the maintenance of their dispersions is not aided by Brownian movement (*see* below). Some types of disperse system are of particular importance in pharmacy. The factors that contribute to their stability will therefore be discussed together with the preparations and properties of the dispersions.

Colloidal Dispersions of Solids in Liquids

The majority of these systems of interest to pharmacists are dispersions in an aqueous medium. Unless otherwise stated, the discussion in the remainder of this section will be restricted to aqueous systems. The specific terms 'hydrophilic' and 'hydrophobic' will therefore be used instead of the general terms 'lyophilic' and 'lyophobic'. A hydrophilic colloid is a system in which the dispersed particles have an affinity for the aqueous dispersion medium, and a hydrophobic colloid is a system in which the particles exhibit little or no such affinity.

Mechanisms of Stabilisation

The affinity of hydrophilic colloidal particles for an aqueous dispersion medium is sufficient to render these dispersions thermodynamically stable. In fact, hydrophilic materials form colloidal dispersions spontaneously on addition to water.

However, spontaneous coalescence of hydrophobic colloids indicates that these systems are unstable and that attractive forces exist between the particles. Thus, if the latter are to remain in a dispersed state for any considerable time then a stabilising mechanism that reduces the rate of coalescence must operate.

The present theory for the stabilisation of lyophobic colloids was developed independently by Derjaguin and Landau (1941) and Verwey and Overbeek (1948), and is therefore referred to as the DLVO theory. It has also been well explained by

Table 5.1
Types of Disperse System

System	Dispersed particles	Particle size	Notes
True solutions	Small molecules or ions	Usually less than 1×10^{-6} mm	Mixtures of gases are restricted to this type of system
Colloidal dispersions	Single large molecules (or ions) or aggregates of small molecules (or ions)	Larger than those in true solution and have an upper size limit of about 1×10^{-3} mm	
Coarse dispersions	Aggregates of molecules	Larger than those in colloidal dispersions	Particle size ranges from about 1×10^{-3} mm to an upper limit, which depends on the system

other authors (Overbeek, 1952; van Olphen, 1963; Sheludko, 1966). To understand this theory it is necessary first to consider the repulsive and attractive forces that operate between approaching particles, and then to examine the combined effects of these opposing forces.

Repulsive Forces between Approaching Particles

The existence of electrical charges on dispersed particles is demonstrated by the process of electro-

Table 5.2
Examples of Disperse Systems
(true solutions omitted)

Dispersed phase	Dispersion medium	Examples Colloidal	Coarse
Liquid	Gas	Fog	Spray
Solid	Gas	Smoke	Dust
Gas	Liquid	Foam	Foam
Liquid	Liquid	Oil globules $<1 \times 10^{-3}$ mm in water	Emulsion
Solid	Liquid	Colloidal gold in water	Suspension of kaolin in water
Gas	Solid	Solid foam	Solid foam
Liquid	Solid	Mineral oil in wax	Solid emulsion
Solid	Solid	Colloidal gold in glass	Solid suspension

phoresis (*see* later). These charges originate either from ionisation of surface groups or from preferential adsorption of specific ions, known as peptising ions, from solution. The former mechanism applies frequently in hydrophilic colloids, and the latter in hydrophobic colloids.

The presence of charges on the dispersed particles influences the distribution of positive and negative ions in the layers of solution that surround each particle. This distribution is also influenced by thermal motions in the solution. The resultant effect is that each particle is surrounded by an electrical double layer with a structure similar to that described in Chapter 4 for plane solid–liquid interfaces.

When two particles approach each other the diffuse parts of their electrical double layers overlap. This leads to a redistribution of the charge in each layer, and a repulsion will be exerted between the particles. Work must therefore be performed in order to overcome this repulsion and bring the particles close together. The amount of work necessary to bring the particles from an infinite distance apart to a given distance of separation may be calculated. This amount of work is equal to the repulsive potential at that given distance of separation. The continuous line in Fig. 5.1 shows the variation in the repulsive potential with distance of separation of the particles.

Attractive Forces between Approaching Particles

The repulsive forces that arise from the overlapping of electrical double layers still operate even when particles aggregate. An attractive force must therefore exist between particles, and this force must be comparable in its magnitude and range of operation to the repulsive force if the latter is to be overcome during an aggregation process. It is considered that the attraction is provided by van der Waals forces. Although the Appendix indicates that between a pair of atoms these forces are weak and only of short range, it should be pointed out that they are also additive. Thus, the total attraction between two particles will be equal to the sum of all the attractive forces between every atom of one particle and all those of the other. This additive effect not only produces an appreciable force but also increases the range over which this force is exerted. The broken line in Fig. 5.1 represents the variation in attractive potential with distance of separation of the particles.

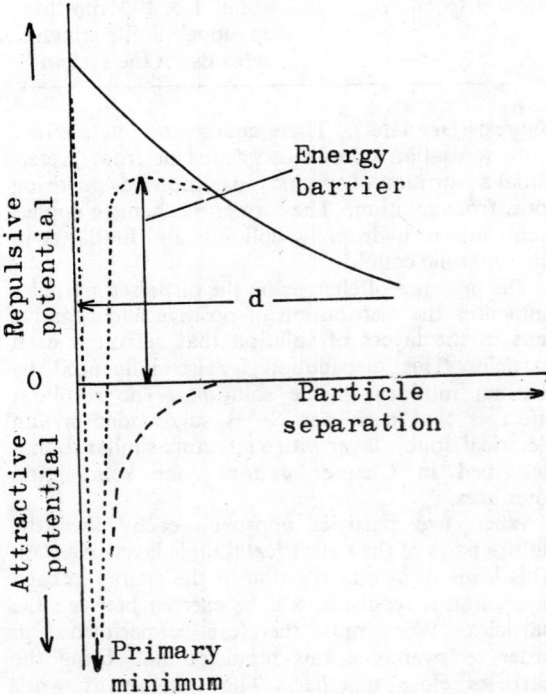

Fig. 5.1 Variation in net potential of interaction (. . . . .) arising from the combined effects of repulsive potential (————) and attractive potential (– – – –) between two approaching particles

Combined Effects of Repulsive and Attractive Forces between Approaching Particles

The dotted line in Fig. 5.1 represents the variation in net potential of interaction with the distance of separation of the particles. This curve is obtained by addition of the repulsive and attractive potentials at each distance, assuming that these separate potentials have opposite signs; e.g. the repulsive potential is regarded as being positive and the attractive potential as negative.

The net interaction curve indicates that as two particles approach each other the repulsive potential

predominates initially, the attractive potential then predominating as the distance between the particles decreases.

The sharp rise of the net interaction curve when the particles are very close is caused by additional short-range repulsive forces that have not been taken into account in the previous discussion. These forces may arise from the contact of points on the irregular surface of the particles (the Born repulsion) and, also, from the presence of strongly adsorbed molecular layers of water on each particle. These layers must be desorbed before the particles can approach to closer distances than the thicknesses of these layers.

Since the repulsive potential predominates at the longer distances of separation, coalescence will occur only if the approaching particles possess sufficient activation energy to overcome this repulsion barrier, and pass into the region where the attractive potential predominates. The height of the energy barrier in Fig. 5.1 will determine its effectiveness in preventing the aggregation of dispersed particles. If this barrier is reduced, then the stability of the colloidal dispersion will decrease.

Effect of Electrolytes

An increase in the concentration of ions in the dispersion medium has the effect of compressing the diffuse part of the electrical double layer; i.e. the thickness, d, of this layer is decreased and the repulsive potential decays more rapidly. Thus, the energy barrier that opposes aggregation, decreases as the concentration of added electrolyte increases, and finally disappears as indicated by Fig. 5.2. When the barrier ceases to exist, rapid coalescence of the particles occurs and large aggregates become visible in the system.

The degree of compression of the double layer depends not only on the concentration of added electrolyte but also on the valency of the ion of opposite charge to the colloidal particle. This is known as the Schulze-Hardy rule. Thus, a negatively charged colloid would be coagulated rapidly by a certain concentration of aluminium chloride in the dispersion medium but a greater concentration of barium chloride would be required, since barium cations are only divalent whereas aluminium cations are trivalent. In fact, calculations show that the flocculation value of an electrolyte should be inversely proportional to the sixth power of the valency of the ion of opposite charge. Experimental results show good agreement with these calculations.

The coagulating effect of electrolytes may be used to assess the original stability of a colloidal dispersion. Thus, the greater the concentration of electrolyte required to produce rapid coagulation, the greater the stability of the original system.

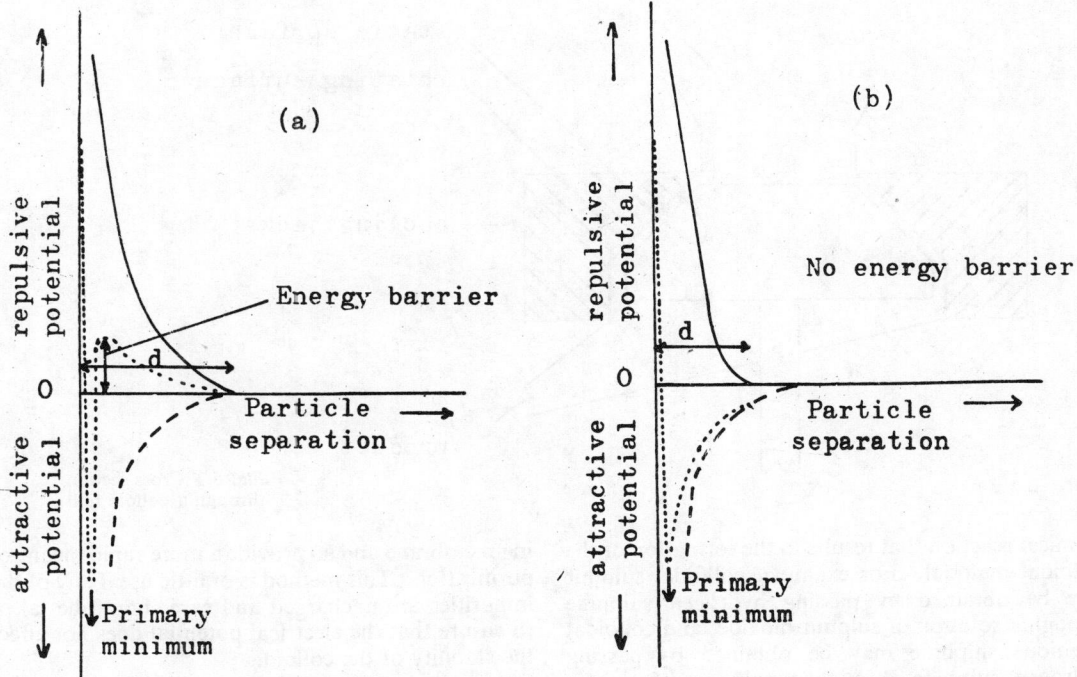

Fig. 5.2 The variation in thickness, *d*, of the electrical double layer and height of energy barrier to coagulation caused by (*a*) intermediate, and (*b*) higher concentrations of electrolyte (*See* Fig. 5.1 for key)

Preparation of Colloids

HYDROPHILIC COLLOIDS

As previously stated, the affinity of hydrophilic colloids for water leads to the spontaneous formation of a colloidal dispersion when the material is placed in contact with water. For example, acacia will readily disperse in water, and gelatin will disperse in hot water. This simple method of dispersion is a general one for the formation of lyophilic colloids.

HYDROPHOBIC COLLOIDS

The preparative methods for hydrophobic colloids may be divided into those methods that involve the breakdown of larger particles into particles of colloidal dimensions (dispersion methods) and those in which the colloidal particles are formed by aggregation of smaller particles such as molecules (condensation methods).

Dispersion Methods

The breakdown of coarse material may be effected by several means.

Colloid Mills. These mills cause the dispersion of coarse material by shearing in a narrow gap between a static cone and a rapidly rotating cone. A diagram of a colloid mill is given in Fig. 5.3.

Electrical Dispersion (Bredig's method). Certain metals may be dispersed by the passage of an electric arc between electrodes made of the metal and immersed in the dispersion medium.

Ultrasonic Irradiation. The passage of ultrasonic waves through a dispersion medium produces alternating regions of cavitation and compression in the medium. The cavities collapse with great force and cause the breakdown of coarse particles dispersed in the liquid.

Peptisation. Because the charges necessary for stabilising colloidal dispersions may originate from the preferential adsorption of specific ions at the surface of the particles, a finely divided solid may be converted into a colloidal dispersion by the addition of such ions to the dispersion medium. This process is known as peptisation.

Condensation Methods

These involve the rapid production of supersaturated solutions of the colloidal material under conditions in which it is deposited in the dispersion medium as colloidal particles and not as a precipitate. The supersaturation is often obtained by means of a

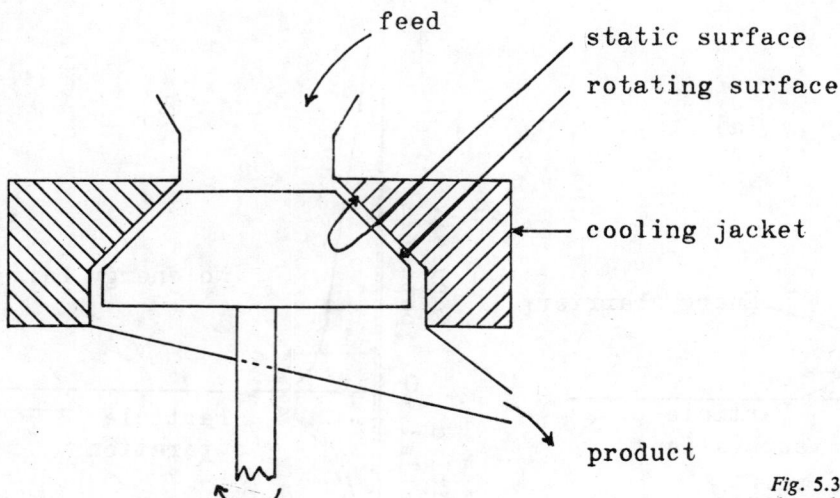

Fig. 5.3 Cross-section through a colloid mill

chemical reaction that results in the formation of the colloidal material. For example, colloidal sulphur may be obtained by passing hydrogen sulphide through a solution of sulphur dioxide, and colloidal arsenious sulphide may be obtained by passing hydrogen sulphide through a solution of arsenic trioxide.

A change in solvent may also cause the production of colloidal particles by condensation methods. If an alcoholic solution of a resin (resinous tincture) is poured slowly into water, a colloidal dispersion of resin particles may be obtained.

Purification of Colloids

DIALYSIS

Colloidal particles are too large to diffuse through the pores of certain membranes such as parchment or cellophane. The smaller particles in true solution are able to pass through these membranes. Use is made of this difference in diffusibility to separate micromolecular impurities from colloidal dispersions. The process is known as dialysis.

A colloidal dispersion may become diluted during dialysis because water will pass through the membrane under the influence of the osmotic pressure of the colloid. Such dilution may be prevented by applying to the colloid a pressure that is equal to or greater than its osmotic pressure. This procedure is referred to as dialysis under pressure.

ELECTRODIALYSIS

An electrical potential may be used to increase the rate of movement of ionic impurities through a dialys-

ing membrane and so provide a more rapid means of purification. This method is of little use if any of the impurities are uncharged and care should be taken to ensure that the electrical potential does not affect the stability of the colloid.

ULTRAFILTRATION

Colloidal particles are too small to be retained by ordinary filter papers. However, filtration through a dialysing membrane may be carried out, but because the rate of flow of the liquid dispersion medium through such membranes is slow it is usual to carry out the filtration process under the influence of either positive pressure or vacuum. Since the sizes of the colloidal particles and the pores in the membrane are so small, the process is referred to as ultrafiltration.

It is possible to manufacture membranes with different degrees of porosity (*see* later). The use of a series of ultrafilters with gradually decreasing pore sizes allows the particle size of a colloid to be determined. Conversely, the pore size of an ultrafilter can be determined by the use of a series of colloidal dispersions of different particle sizes.

The Properties of Colloids

PARTICLE SIZE

The particles in a colloidal dispersion fall within the approximate range of 1×10^{-6} to 1×10^{-3} mm. The actual size may be determined by ultramicroscopic measurements, the use of graded ultrafilters, or the measurement of the rates of sedimentation of the particles in an ultracentrifuge.

ELECTRICAL PROPERTIES

If an electric current is passed through a colloidal dispersion contained in a suitable cell, the particles migrate towards one of the electrodes. This process, which is known as electrophoresis, demonstrates that all the particles in a given system carry a similar charge. In addition, the sign of this charge is indicated by the direction of movement of the particles. Thus, the particles of negatively charged colloids, such as kaolin, sulphur, arsenious sulphide, and metals, will move towards the anode, while the particles of positively charged colloids, such as ferric hydroxide and other metal hydroxides, will move towards the cathode.

Different colloidal materials may possess different electrophoretic mobilities and the process may therefore be used as a method of separating mixtures of colloidal materials. For example, the proteins of blood plasma may be separated by electrophoresis.

The charge carried by colloidal protein molecules, and therefore the direction of movement of these molecules under the influence of an electric current, will depend on the pH of the dispersion medium. This variation in the sign of the charge is explained by the fact that in alkaline solution the carboxylic acid groups of the protein molecules will exist as carboxylate anions, whereas in acid solutions the amino groups of the molecules will be protonated. Thus, proteins are negatively charged in alkaline solutions and positively charged in acid solutions. At an intermediate pH, known as the iso-electric point, the protein exists as a zwitterion, which is electrically neutral, although both groups are ionised. The solubility of the protein is at a minimum at its iso-electric point and therefore precipitation is facilitated at this pH.

OPTICAL PROPERTIES

Colloidal particles are too small to be seen under an ordinary microscope and a colloidal dispersion appears to be perfectly transparent when viewed from the front with a light behind it. However, the colour appears to change if the system is viewed against a dark background at right angles to the incident light, when a turbidity can be seen. Furthermore, if the incident light is restricted to a beam, then a cone of light, known as the Tyndall cone, is observed. These effects arise because the incident light is scattered by the colloidal particles. The progressively greater scattering effect produced as the light passes through the system is responsible for the formation of the Tyndall cone. In addition, the intensity of the scattered light increases with decreasing wavelength. The scattered light therefore has a greater proportion of smaller wavelengths than the incident light, while the transmitted light is deficient in these smaller wavelengths. These changes are responsible for the apparent difference in colour of the system when viewed by scattered or transmitted light. For example, a colloidal dispersion of a white material illuminated by white light will produce a bluish-white scattered light and a yellow-brown transmitted light.

The light-scattering effect is made use of in the design of the ultramicroscope, in which a cell containing the colloid is viewed against a dark background at right angles to an intense beam of incident light. The particles, which exhibit an erratic movement, appear as bright spots against the dark background. The motion of the particles is known as Brownian movement and arises from the bombardment of the particles by the molecules of the dispersion medium. This effect is useful in helping to counteract the effects of sedimentation and in maintaining the dispersion of particles in the continuous medium.

OSMOTIC PROPERTIES

Osmotic pressure is a colligative property (see p. 15) and therefore depends only on the number of particles present in a dispersion. The particles in a colloidal system may consist of aggregates of several molecules, but each of these aggregates acts as a single unit for colligative purposes. The osmotic pressure exerted by such a system will therefore be small. If the colloidal particles consist of single large molecules then the osmotic pressure may be used to calculate the molecular weight of the colloidal material. This method is often used for long-chain polymers, but a correction may be necessary to allow for the Donnan membrane effect, which is discussed later (see p. 73)

Differences in Properties of Hydrophilic and Hydrophobic Colloids

Some of the differences in the properties of the two types of colloid have already been mentioned in the previous sections. These and other differences are summarised in Table 5.3.

It will be observed from Table 5.3 that hydrophilic colloids are much more stable to the presence of added electrolytes than hydrophobic colloids. The instability of the latter type has already been explained in terms of the compression of the diffuse part of the electrical double layer in the presence of additional counter-ions. A similar effect is insufficient to cause the rapid coalescence of hydrophilic colloids since these are also stabilised by the affinity that exists between the colloidal particles and the

Table 5.3
A Comparison of the Properties of Hydrophilic and Hydrophobic Colloids

Property	*Hydrophilic colloids*	*Hydrophobic colloids*
1. Ease of dispersion of material in dispersion medium.	Usually occurs spontaneously.	Special treatment necessary.
2. Stability towards electrolytes.	High concentrations of very soluble electrolytes are necessary to cause precipitation.	Relatively low concentrations of electrolytes will cause precipitation.
3. Stability towards prolonged dialysis.	Stable.	Unstable because ions necessary for stability are removed.
4 Reversibility after precipitation (i.e. colloidal dispersion reforms when precipitated material is added to fresh dispersion medium).	Reversible.	Irreversible.
5. Tyndall effect.	Weak. Particles are not easily detected by ultramicroscope.	Strong. Particles are readily detected by ultramicroscope.
6. Viscosity.*	Usually higher than that of dispersion medium.	Similar to that of dispersion medium.
7. Protective ability (*see* later).	Capable of acting as protective colloids.	Incapable of acting as protective colloids and often require addition of such a material for stability.

* Further information on the viscosity of colloidal dispersions is given in Chapter 7.

dispersion medium. Precipitation of hydrophilic colloids therefore involves a reduction in this affinity as well as the removal of any energy barrier arising from a repulsive potential between the particles. Very soluble electrolytes such as ammonium sulphate will compress the double layer and so remove an energy barrier. In addition, since the ions of such electrolytes are strongly hydrated, high concentrations of such ions will compete so successfully for the molecules of the dispersion medium that the affinity of the latter for the colloidal particles is reduced. These combined effects lead to the precipitation of hydrophilic colloids, and the process is known as 'salting out'. Variation in the stabilities of different hydrophilic colloids affects the concentration of soluble electrolyte required to produce their precipitation. The components of a mixture of hydrophilic colloids can therefore be separated by a process of fractional precipitation, which involves the 'salting out' of the various components at different concentrations of electrolyte. This technique is used in the purification of antitoxins (*see* p. 403).

Effects of Mixing Different Colloids

1. MUTUAL PRECIPITATION

This may occur when two hydrophobic colloids with oppositely charged particles are mixed, due to the attractive forces exerted between the particles.

2. COACERVATE FORMATION

When oppositely charged hydrophilic colloids are mixed, a layer rich in colloidal material may separate. This layer is known as a coacervate.

3. SENSITISATION

In the presence of very small amounts of hydrophilic colloid a hydrophobic colloid may become more susceptible to precipitation by electrolytes. This effect, known as sensitisation, is thought to arise from the adsorption of various parts of each chain-like hydrophilic colloid onto several hydrophobic particles.

4. PROTECTION

The stability of hydrophobic colloids towards the precipitating effects of electrolytes is increased by the presence of hydrophilic colloids in concentrations several times those required for sensitisation. Hydrophilic colloids used in this way are termed protective colloids. Their protective action is considered to arise from their adsorption over the entire surface of each hydrophobic particle, so that the latter acquires some hydrophilic properties and is therefore able to withstand the effects of electrolytes.

The protection afforded to a specific hydrophobic colloid is often used as an indication of the relative abilities of a series of hydrophilic colloids to act as protective colloids. For example, the 'Gold Number', introduced by Zsigmondy, is the number of milligrammes of protective colloid that must be added to 10 cm³ of a standard colloidal suspension of gold to prevent flocculation on the addition of 1 cm³ of a 10 per cent NaCl solution. In the same way the 'Congo Red' number depends on the flocculation of a standard dispersion of congo red by a given amount of KCl. Such methods of comparing the protective abilities of hydrophilic colloids are influenced by the nature of the hydrophobic colloid.

The relative abilities as indicated by Gold or Congo Red numbers may therefore be different for other systems.

Pharmaceutical Applications of Colloids

It has been suggested that the efficiency of certain substances used in pharmaceutical preparations may be increased if colloidal forms are used, since these have large surface areas; for example, the adsorption of toxins from the gastro-intestinal tract by kaolin, and the rate of neutralisation of excess acidity in the stomach by aluminium hydroxide may be increased if these compounds are used in colloidal forms.

The use of colloidal iron and colloidal iodine is said to alter the effects of these compounds, the former being less astringent than crystalloidal iron and the latter less toxic than iodine in aqueous solution.

In the purification of proteins, use is made of the changes in solubility of colloidal materials caused by the presence of electrolytes or changes in pH.

The protective ability of hydrophilic colloids is used to prevent the coagulation of hydrophobic particles in the presence of electrolytes. The increased viscosity of a liquid that results from dispersion of a hydrophilic colloid is used to retard the sedimentation of particles in pharmaceutical suspensions; i.e. the hydrophilic colloids are used as suspending agents.

Blood plasma substitutes are colloidal dispersions in which the particle size is such that they are retained in the blood vessels for an adequate time (e.g. Dextran Injection BP 1968).

Association Colloids

It has already been mentioned (Chapter 4) that surface active agents behave as normal compounds in dilute solutions but at certain reasonably well-defined concentrations relatively sharp changes occur in the physical properties of these solutions. These changes are attributed to the association of the amphipathic molecules or ions into aggregates of colloidal dimensions, that are known as micelles.

Ionic and non-ionic substances that exhibit this type of behaviour are referred to collectively as association colloids. Although the older term 'colloidal electrolyte' is strictly applicable to all ionised colloidal materials it is usually reserved for ionic association colloids. Since the early work in this field was carried out solely on ionic association colloids the term 'colloidal electrolyte' is still sometimes used erroneously as a synonym for 'association colloids'.

Critical Micelle Concentration and Micellar Structure

The minimum concentration at which physical properties of solutions of association colloids show marked changes is known as the critical micelle concentration, which is often written in an abbreviated form as CMC. The formation of micelles was originally suggested by McBain to explain the apparently anomalous changes in osmotic properties and electrical conductivity with concentration in solutions of ionic associated colloids. The conductivity indicated that a considerable degree of electrolytic dissociation was occurring in solution, whereas the osmotic properties indicated that considerable aggregation of ions into single colligative units was also occurring above the CMC. McBain's original suggestion allowed for the existence of two types of micelle. These types were—

(*a*) a small, approximately spherical, charged micelle, which existed in all concentrations, i.e. above and below the CMC, and which was largely responsible for the appreciable electrical conductivity, and

(*b*) a large undissociated lamellar micelle, which only existed above the CMC and was responsible for the low osmotic properties at such concentrations.

Hartley later suggested that the experimental facts could be explained on the basis of a single type of micelle. Hartley's model, shown in Fig. 5.4, consists of a spherical charged micelle with a radius

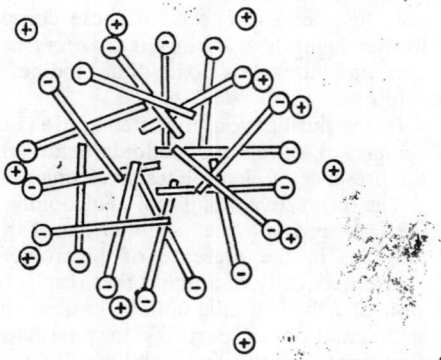

Fig. 5.4   The Hartley spherical micelle

approximately equal to the chain length of the amphipathic ion.

The spherical type of micelle is now accepted as existing in all solutions of association colloids at and just above the CMC. However, in more concentrated solutions physical measurements, e.g. X-ray diffraction, viscosity, light scattering, indicate the existence of large asymmetric micelles. The rearrangement from spherical to larger and more widely separated asymmetric micelles has been ascribed to a reaction of the system in an effort to reduce the intermicellar repulsive forces that arise from the closer and closer approach of spherical micelles as the concentration of amphipathic material increases. Present evidence suggests that different micellar shapes, e.g. rods, lamellae, are formed in different systems.

STABILITY AND SIZE OF SPHERICAL MICELLES

The cohesive force between water molecules is much stronger than either the attraction between the lipophilic parts of the surface active agents or the attraction between water and the lipophilic chains. Therefore, the surface active agent tends to be squeezed out of solution in order to reduce the large degree of separation of water molecules that would be caused by the presence of many monomeric amphipathic molecules. This effect, which tends to cause a phase separation, is counterbalanced to some extent by the hydrophilic nature of the polar groups. In addition, the attractive forces between water molecules decay very rapidly with distance of separation since they are inversely proportional to somewhere between the fourth and seventh power of the distance (*see* Appendix). Thus, the work of separating water molecules by a relatively large distance on the formation of a micelle is little different from that involved in the introduction of an amphipathic monomer.

The electrical repulsion between adjacent similarly charged ions tends to disrupt the micelles of an ionic surface active agent. In such a case, micelle formation is therefore dependent on the balance between this disruptive effect and the constructive 'squeezing out of solution' effect. Since the electrical repulsive effect is absent in non-ionic micelles, various suggestions have been made regarding the existence of a factor that would tend to oppose micelle formation; e.g. cross-sectional area and solvation of the hydrophilic group. However, the precise nature of such a factor is still in doubt. The association of ionic and non-ionic surface active agents is also aided by the 'hydrophobic bonding' between the hydrocarbon chains. This type of bonding involves weak van der Waals forces of attraction, the effect of which is therefore of less significance than those mentioned previously. In addition, an increase in temperature will have a disruptive effect on the formation of micelles since their rate of deaggregation will be increased.

The size of a spherical micelle depends on the structure of the surface active agent. In the Hartley model of a micelle the radius is approximately equal to the length of the hydrocarbon chain. If the diameter were to increase beyond this point then the unlikely structure would either include a space in the centre into which the hydrocarbon chains could not reach, or the presence of some of the ionic groups between the hydrocarbon chains.

Physical Properties of Solutions of Association Colloids

Since micellar structure and shape influence the physical properties of solutions it is convenient to consider separately the properties of dilute solutions (i.e. up to concentrations just above the CMC, where the micelles are spherical and concentrated solutions containing asymmetric micelles.

DILUTE SOLUTIONS; PHYSICAL PROPERTIES AND METHODS OF DETERMINING CMC.

Colligative Properties

The association of monomeric ions or molecules into micelles at the CMC causes a marked decrease in the colligative properties of solutions of association colloids. A typical graph of osmotic pressure against concentration is shown in Fig. 5.5.

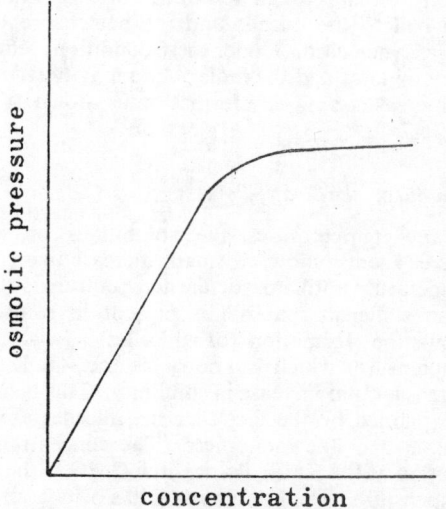

Fig. 5.5 Variation of the osmotic pressure with concentration of a solution of an association colloid

Osmotic pressure, freezing point and vapour pressure measurements have been used to determine CMCs. However, such determinations are not common since these methods are more tedious and more difficult than others, and their accuracy is dependent on the measurement of relatively small changes in physical properties. In addition, the depression of freezing point method is limited by the fact that many surface active agents are too insoluble at the freezing point of the solvent, and even measurements that are possible at these temperatures have little relationship to practical applications.

Surface Properties

The positive adsorption of surface active agents at the surface of water causes a progressive decrease in surface tension with increase in concentration until the CMC is reached. The micelles formed at and beyond this concentration provide an alternative means of removing the lipophilic groups from the aqueous environment, thus causing a decrease in

free energy of the system. In fact, in such systems orientation of further surface active material in the form of micelles is energetically preferable to its orientation in the surface. Thus, additional material is used in the production of more micelles, and the concentrations in the surface layer and in true solution (i.e. as monomeric units) remain approximately constant beyond the CMC; a graph of surface tension against concentration levels out at this point, as shown in Fig. 5.6.

A minimum is frequently observed in the surface tension curves, shown by the dotted line in Fig. 5.6. Such minima are usually caused by the presence of surface active impurities in the system. The difficult and/or tedious purification procedures are usually responsible for the presence of such impurities. The initial adsorption into the surface layers of the surface active agent and impurity results in the lowering of the surface tension to a greater degree than that given by the pure surface active agent. At the CMC the impurity is leached out of the surface and taken up by the micelles so that the surface tension rises to that of the pure surface active agent beyond its CMC.

Surface tension measurements are useful in the determination of CMCs and the accuracy of the determination is little affected by the actual value of the CMC (cf. with other methods where the accuracy decreases as the CMC becomes smaller). Because of the slow attainment of adsorption equilibrium that occurs in some systems, static methods of surface tension measurement (i.e. methods in which the surface is not disturbed during measurement) are

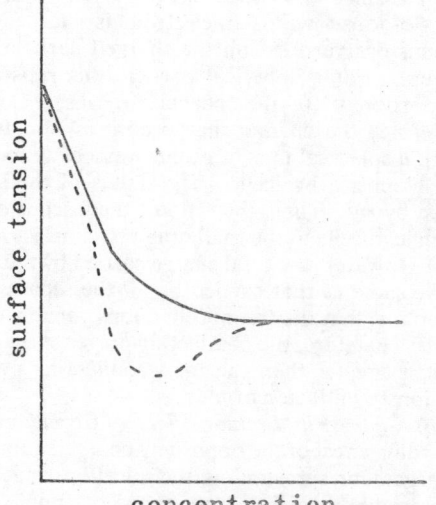

Fig. 5.6 Surface tension–concentration curve for a solution of an association colloid

often more useful, since changes in surface tension with time can be followed.

Electrical Conductivity

The effects of micelle formation on the electrical conductivity of solutions of ionic association colloids are shown in Fig. 5.7(i) and (ii). According to Hartley three factors contribute to these changes.

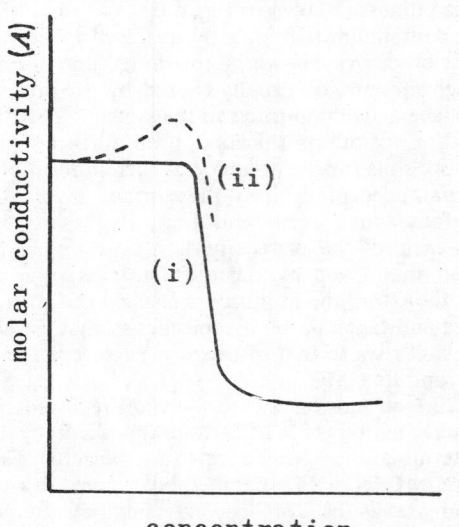

Fig. 5.7 The effect of micelle formation on the molar conductivity (Λ) of a solution at (i) low, and (ii) high field strengths

(a) Change in Viscous Drag Effects. The movement of ions towards an electrode is retarded by the viscous drag exerted on the charged particle by the solvent. For a spherical particle this resistance is proportional to the particle radius. Consider, therefore, the change that occurs in viscous drag when n spherical ions of radius r associate to form a single spherical micelle. The radius of the latter is given by $rn^{\frac{1}{3}}$. Thus, the ratio of the viscous drag on a single micelle to the total drag on n ions is $rn^{\frac{1}{3}}/rn = n^{-\frac{2}{3}}$. However, the total charge carried by the micelle is the same as that carried by all the separate ions, assuming that all the micellar ions remain dissociated. Therefore, the conducting power of the micelle will be greater than the total conducting power of the ions by a factor of $n^{\frac{1}{3}}$.

(b) Changes in 'Braking Effect' of Gegenions. The retarding effect of the oppositely charged atmosphere of gegenions surrounding the micelle is much more appreciable than that experienced by simple ions.

(c) Reduction of Net Charge on Micelle. Since the micellar surface has a high charge density some gegenions adhere to the micelle, thus lowering its net charge.

Under normal conditions the change in electrical conductivity with concentration is represented in Fig. 5.7 (i), since effects (b) and (c) above, which cause a decrease in the molar conductivity (Λ) on micelle formation, outweigh effect (a). However, at high field strengths the micelles move so rapidly that the ionic atmosphere of gegenions cannot reform quickly enough (Wein effect) and the 'braking effect' is therefore reduced. In addition, fewer gegenions are attached to the micelle and the net charge on the latter is increased. Under these conditions, effect (a) predominates and the molar conductivity (Λ) shows an increase on micelle formation as shown at (ii) in Fig. 5.7.

Solubility; the Krafft Point

At low temperatures the solubilities of surface active agents show a small increase with rising temperature until a particular temperature is reached when sufficient material is present in solution to allow the formation of micelles. Beyond this temperature, which is known as the Krafft Point, there is a rapid increase in solubility. This behaviour is explained by the fact that the micelles are more soluble than the monomers. The concentration in solution at the Krafft Point is the CMC at the Krafft temperature. The usefulness of this behaviour in the determination of CMCs is limited by the fact that it is difficult to calculate from the results the CMC at other temperatures.

Light Scattering

The scattering of light by solutions of surface active agents is increased by the aggregation of molecules into micelles. The slopes of graphs of amount of light scattered versus concentration therefore show an abrupt increase at the CMC. In addition to the CMC determination this method allows the aggregation number, i.e. the number of monomers per micelle, to be calculated, and provides information on the shape of the micelle.

Solubilisation

The property of surface active agents to cause an increase in the solubility of organic compounds in aqueous systems is called solubilisation. This property is observed only at and above the CMC, thus indicating that the micelles are involved in the phenomenon. In general, the increased solubility of the solubilised material (solubilisate) can be explained in terms of partition between the aqueous

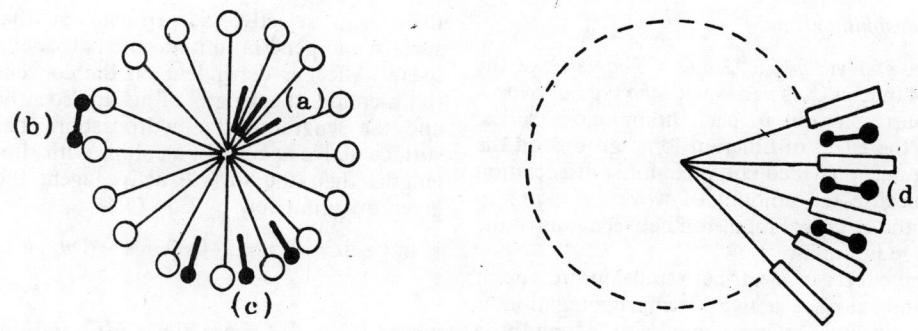

Fig. 5.8   Solubilisation within micelles: (*a*) non-polar hydrocarbon (*b*) polar molecule adsorbed at micelle-water interface (*c*) amphipathic molecules orientated in palisade layer (*d*) polar molecules orientated between polyoxyethylene chains of a non-ionic surface active agent

phase and the hydrocarbon interior of the micelles or by adsorption at the micellar surface. Thus, it is believed that non-polar hydrocarbons are taken into solution in the interior of the micelles, and polar water soluble compounds such as sugar and glycerol are adsorbed at the micelle/water interface, as shown at (*a*) and (*b*) respectively in Fig. 5.8. Compounds with amphipathic character, such as octanol and phenols, are believed to become orientated in the palisade layer in a similar manner to the surface active agent, i.e. with their polar groups directed towards the aqueous phase and their lipophilic groups inside the micelle, as shown at (*c*) in Fig. 5.8. A possible additional mechanism for the effect of non-ionic micelles on the solubility of certain compounds, e.g. phenol, involves inclusion of these compounds between the long hydrophilic polyoxyethylene chains, as shown at (*d*) in Fig. 5.8.

CMCs may be determined by solubilisation measurements preferably using a solid dyestuff that is virtually insoluble in water. The amount of dyestuff in solution remains reasonably constant until the CMC of the surface active agent is reached, and then increases rapidly. Dyes are commonly used in such determinations because of the ease of analysis of the solutions by optical methods. The disadvantages of this method include the long periods of stirring necessary to ensure that equilibrium conditions have been reached, and the fact that the CMCs are affected by the presence of the solubilisate so that the observed values are consequently lower than those obtained by other methods.

Other Methods of Determining CMCs

Refractive index, diffusion rate, viscosity, density, u.v. and i.r. spectrophotometric measurements may also be used in the determination of CMCs. In addition, a method based on the changes in absorption spectra of various compounds on their adsorption by micelles is frequently used (dye absorption method). Pinacoyl chloride and rhodamine G may be used for anionic surface active agents, eosin and fluorescein for cationics, and pinacoyl chloride or iodine for non-ionics. This method suffers from the disadvantage that the CMC may be affected by the presence of the additive.

FACTORS AFFECTING CRITICAL MICELLE CONCENTRATIONS

A. Molecular Structure of the Surface Active Agent

1. *The hydrocarbon chain*

(*a*) *Chain Length.* An increase in the hydrocarbon chain length causes a logarithmic decrease in the CMC at constant temperature as shown by Eqn (5.1)

$$\log C = A - Bm \qquad (5.1)$$

where C is the CMC, m is the number of carbon atoms in the chain, and A and B are constants for a homologous series of compounds.

(*b*) *Branched Hydrocarbon Chains.* Branching of a hydrocarbon chain causes an increase in CMC since the decrease in free energy arising from the aggregation of branched chain molecules is less than that obtained with linear molecules with the same number of carbon atoms.

(*c*) *Unsaturation.* The CMC is increased by about three to four times by the presence of one double bond when compared with the value for the analogous saturated compound.

2. The hydrophilic group

(a) *Type of Hydrophilic Group.* The value of the constant A in Eqn (5.1) varies with the type of hydrophilic group common to each homologous series. However, the effect of different ionic groups on the CMC is small, provided complete ionic dissociation occurs, because the amount of work necessary to overcome the electrical repulsion between ions of the same charge is similar.

Since the effects of electrical repulsion are absent in non-ionic surface active agents aggregation is facilitated and the CMCs are much lower than those of ionic surface active agents.

(b) *Number of Hydrophilic Groups.* The electrical repulsive force between adjacent ions in a micelle increases as the number of ionic groups increases. In addition, an increase in the number of any type of hydrophilic group increases the solubility of the surface active agent. Both these effects will lead to an increase in the CMC.

(c) *Position of Hydrophilic Group.* The CMC tends to increase as the polar group is moved from the terminal position towards the middle of the hydrocarbon chain.

B. Effect of Additives

1. Simple electrolytes

The CMC decreases on addition of salts. The most important factors concerned in the overall effect are the concentration and number of charges on the ions of opposite charge (gegenions) to that carried by the micelle. The effect of these factors is given by Eqn (5.2), where C and C_i are the CMC and

$$\ln C = -K . \ln C_i + \text{constant} \qquad (5.2)$$

total gegenion concentration, respectively, and K is a constant with a value of approximately 0.4 to 0.6. For surface active agents with two ionic groups, Eqn (5.2) becomes

$$\ln C = -2K . \ln C_i + \text{constant} \qquad (5.3)$$

2. Other Surface Active Agents

The CMCs of mixtures of surface active agents appear to vary between the limiting values of the highest and lowest CMCs of the individual components.

3. Alcohols

The CMCs are decreased by the addition of alcohols. The marked effect of alcohols probably arises from their high selective adsorptivity at the micellar surface and penetration into the palisade layer. The overall effect is dependent on the concentration of the alcohol, the length of its hydrocarbon chain, and the length of the hydrocarbon chain of the surface active agent. In alcohols with shorter chain lengths than the surface active agent the effect is given quantitatively by Eqn (5.4)

$$\ln (-dC/dC_a) = -0.69m + 1.1m_a + \text{constant}$$
$$(5.4)$$

where, C and C_a are the CMC and the alcohol concentration, respectively, and m and m_a are the number of carbon atoms in the surface active agent and alcohol respectively.

4. Hydrocarbons

Solubilisation of hydrocarbons causes an increase in micellar size, which results in an increase in the radius of curvature of the micellar surface. This increase in curvature may cause a slight separation of adjacent ions and, therefore, a decrease in the repulsive forces. In addition, the presence of the solubilised hydrocarbon may allow a greater decrease in the surface free energy of the lipophilic part of the surface active agent on micellisation. Consequently, micelle formation is facilitated and the CMC decreases.

Pharmaceutical Applications and Medical Importance of Surface Active Agents

Some of the more general applications of surface active agents, e.g. as emulsifying agents, detergents, wetting agents, etc., have already been mentioned in Chapter 4. The type of application of a particular compound is usually indicated by the balance between its hydrophilic and lipophilic properties. A numerical value (HLB value) can be assigned to this balance from a knowledge of the structural formula of the compound. Thus a detergent and a w/o emulsifying agent would normally possess HLB values of 13–16 and 3–6 respectively. The following list is intended to give more specific examples of the applications and implications of these compounds in pharmacy and related fields.

A. PHYSIOLOGICAL EFFECTS OF SURFACE ACTIVE AGENTS

1. On Micro-organisms

Many surface active agents, especially the quaternary ammonium compounds, have useful antibacterial properties, and preparations containing these compounds are widely used; e.g. disinfectants for instruments and skin, antibacterial creams, and throat lozenges.

This activity of surface active agents is thought to arise from their adsorption at the cell surface, with consequent change in the permeability of the cell membrane and eventual death through loss of essential substances from the cell.

2. On Removal of Bronchial Mucus from the Respiratory Tract

In various acute and chronic infections of the respiratory tract such as bronchitis, asthma and tuberculosis, there is an increase in the amount and viscosity of bronchial mucus. Under certain conditions the mucus tends to dry out and form hard patches which prevent ciliary movement. The inhalation of surface active agents as sprays or mists by aerosol therapy has been shown to be useful in the treatment of these conditions. The action of the surface active agents is probably connected with their ability to promote wetting and, therefore, softening of the hardened mucus, thus facilitating its removal.

3. On Human Skin

It is well known that repeated contact between the skin and certain detergent solutions may cause disorders ranging from mild irritation and 'dry skin' to blisters and pustules. These disorders usually arise from a combination of various effects such as defatting of the skin, change in pH of the skin surface, increased swelling of the skin, and adsorption onto the skin of the surface active agent. These effects may facilitate the onset of infection.

B. THE USE OF SURFACE ACTIVE AGENTS IN PHARMACEUTICAL FORMULATION

4. As Solubilising Agents

(a) Disinfectant Solutions. The apparent water solubility of phenolic compounds such as Cresol BP and Chloroxylenol BP is increased in the presence of an alkali soap. This fact is made use of in the formulation of Lysol BP and Solution of Chloroxylenol BP.

The disinfectant properties of the phenolic compounds are also increased in the presence of these soaps, probably because the surface active agent alters the permeability of the cell membranes of the micro-organisms. However, it must be borne in mind that the presence of an excessive amount of surface active agent may reduce the activity of a given concentration of phenol since there will be a competition for the latter between the micelles and the surface of the micro-organism (see p. 338).

(b) Vitamin Preparations. Many people find that oil-soluble vitamins are unpleasant to take in the form of fish liver oils or as concentrated solutions in oils. This problem may be overcome by the use of oil-in-water emulsions or aqueous solutions of solubilised vitamins. The solubilised systems do not suffer from the instabilities of emulsified preparations. In addition, it has been found that vitamins, such as vitamin A, are more resistant to oxidation in solubilised systems than in emulsions or oily solutions.

(c) Examples of Other Solubilised Systems. Surface active agents have been used to increase the water solubility of phenobarbitone, volatile oils, chloroform, iodine, hormones, dyes, and sulphonamides.

2. As Wetting Agents and Deflocculating Agents

The dispersion of hydrophobic powders in aqueous vehicles is difficult since such powders tend either to float on the water surface or to form large floccules. In the latter case the apparent viscosity of the preparation is increased and homogeneity, even after prolonged shaking, may not be attained. Such properties are often troublesome and may, for example, hinder the pourability of a suspension, the spreading of a lotion, or the withdrawal of the correct dose from an injectable suspension. These problems associated with dispersion may be overcome by the use of a surface active agent which is adsorbed at the solid/liquid interface in such a manner as to increase the affinity of the particles for the surrounding medium and reduce the interparticle attractive forces. These effects are discussed more fully in Chapter 7.

3. As Flocculating Agents

A controlled amount of flocculation is often desirable in the formulation of suspensions in order to obtain the required rheological properties and optimum stability. The aggregation of dispersed particles into floccules may be brought about by the use of a suitable surface active agent. This effect is also discussed more fully in Chapter 7.

4. As Emulsifying Agents

Synthetic and naturally occurring surface active materials are widely used as emulsifying agents. An account of the compounds commonly used, together with the mechanism of their action, is given later in this chapter.

5. As Additives to Ointment and Suppository Bases

The inclusion of surface active agents into the fatty bases used for ointments and suppositories may cause the following effects.

(a) The rate of release of active medicament from these preparations may be accelerated or retarded. The exact mechanisms responsible for these effects have not been clarified. However, contributory effects to an accelerated release rate are thought to include the absorption of water by the base from its aqueous environment and the formation of an emulsion at the base/environment interface. Such emulsification would increase the interfacial area and therefore allow a more rapid exchange of medicament between the two phases. A retardation in a release rate may occur if an increase in the hydrophilic character of a base, brought about by the inclusion of a surface active agent, has an adverse effect on the rate of partition of the medicament between the base and its aqueous surroundings.

(b) The capacity of the base to take up aqueous liquids may be improved. There are three official ointments that will take up appreciable amounts of water to form oil-in-water emulsions; i.e. Emulsifying Ointment BP, Cetomacrogol Emulsifying Ointment BPC, and Cetrimide Emulsifying Ointment BPC. Such water-miscible ointments are useful where either miscibility with skin secretions or subsequent removal of the ointment by washing is required.

Many of the commercially available suppository bases contain varying amounts of surface active agents such as glycerol monostearate plus traces of soaps, so that a range of bases having different emulsifying properties and release rates is available.

Gels

In certain concentrations dispersions of lyophilic colloids form semi-solid masses, particularly when the solubility of the colloidal material is reduced by change in temperature. These semi-solids are known as gels. The setting of solutions of gelatin and agar on cooling are well-known examples of gel formation. Other methods for the production of gels are available and these include: (a) flocculation of lyophilic colloids by salts or precipitating liquids, (b) evaporation of certain colloidal solutions (e.g. collodion, which is a solution of nitrocellulose in alcohol and ether, forms a nitrocellulose gel when the solvents are removed by evaporation), (c) chemical reactions that lead to a change in shape of the lyophilic molecules (e.g. the denaturation of albumen on heating involves some uncoiling of the protein molecules and a gel structure results), and (d) swelling of a dry colloid (xerogel) when placed in contact with a suitable liquid (e.g. starch granules added to water).

The term gel represents a physical state with properties intermediate between those of solids and liquids. However, it is often wrongly used to describe any fluid system that exhibits some degree of rigidity. It is therefore recommended that the term should be restricted to those systems that satisfy the following criteria, which are similar to those suggested by Hermans (1949):

1. they are coherent colloidal systems of at least two components (the gelling agent and a fluid component);
2. they exhibit mechanical properties characteristic of the solid state;
3. each component is continuous throughout the system.

These criteria are fulfilled by gelatin, agar, and bentonite gels, in which the fluid component is aqueous, and by soft paraffin, in which the fluid component is an organic liquid.

Xerogels

Many gels shrink if the fluid component is removed; e.g. by evaporation or freeze-drying. The remaining solid, which will swell and reform the gel on contact with fresh fluid component, is termed a xerogel. Gelatin sheets, acacia tears, tragacanth strips, starch grains, and leather are all xerogels.

The Structure of Gels

The rigidity of a gel arises from the presence of a network formed by the interlinking of particles of the gelling agent. The nature of the particles and the type of force that is responsible for the linkages determines the structure of the network and the properties of the gel.

The individual particles of a hydrophilic colloid may consist of either spherical or anisometric aggregates of small molecules, or single macromolecules. Possible arrangements of such particles in a gel network are shown in Fig. 5.9. In linear macromolecules the network is comprised of entangled molecules, the points of contact between which may either be relatively small or consist of several molecules aligned in a crystalline order, as shown in Fig. 5.9(c) and (d), respectively.

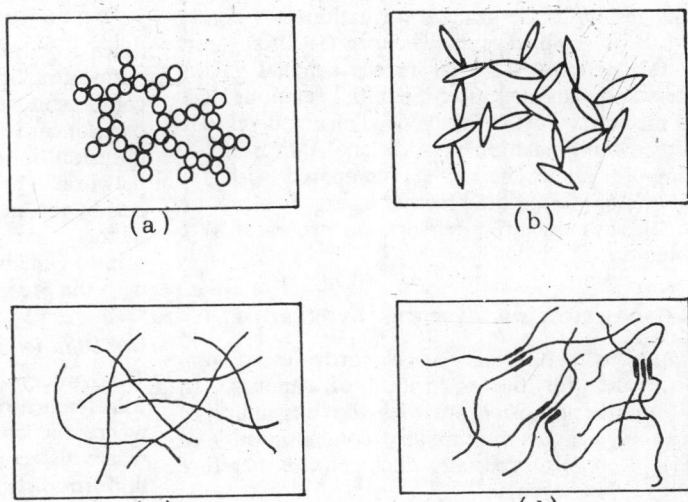

Fig. 5.9 Arrangements of particles in gel structure

The cross-linking of macromolecules by primary valency bonds provides a further mechanism for the formation of a gel network. This behaviour is exhibited by silicic acid gel, which consists of a three-dimensional network of Si—O bonds.

The forces of attraction responsible for the linkages between gelling agent particles may range from strong primary valencies, as in silicic acid gels, to weaker hydrogen bonds and van der Waals forces. The weaker nature of these latter forces is indicated by the fact that a slight increase in temperature often causes liquefaction of a gel. Systems that exhibit this type of transition, such as agar and gelatin gels, are termed thermal gels. In addition, the transition from gel state to a colloidal dispersion may in some cases be brought about by mechanical agitation. Systems, such as bentonite and aluminium hydroxide gels, that exhibit this type of transition are termed thixotropic gels.

The Properties of Gels

1. SWELLING

If a xerogel is placed in contact with a liquid that solvates it then an appreciable amount of the liquid is often taken up and the volume of the xerogel increases. This is referred to as swelling, and the pressure that develops if the xerogel is confined is known as the swelling pressure.

The degree of swelling depends on the number of linkages between individual molecules of the gelling agent and on the strength of these linkages. For example, in a protein xerogel, swelling is at a minimum at the iso-electric point of the protein because the intermolecular linkages are strongest at this point and, therefore, offer more resistance to swelling. In addition, the presence of ions in the swelling liquid influences the degree of swelling of protein xerogels. Sulphate ions, for example, increase the resistance to swelling by forming additional linkages, known as salt bridges, between the protein molecules, whereas the peptising effects of iodide ions produce an increased swelling.

If the gel network consists of primary valency bonds, as in silicic acid gel, the strength of these bonds is sufficient to prevent the occurrence of swelling and only relatively small amounts of liquids are taken up by such systems.

2. SYNERESIS

Gels will often contract spontaneously and exude some of the fluid medium. This effect is known as syneresis and the degree to which it occurs usually decreases as the concentration of gelling agent increases. The occurrence of syneresis indicates that the original gel was thermodynamically unstable. Although syneresis occurs spontaneously it may take place extremely slowly so that the absence of separation of fluid component should not be taken as an indication that the gel is thermodynamically stable.

Blood clot is a common example of a system that exhibits syneresis.

3. AGEING

Colloidal systems usually exhibit slow spontaneous aggregation. This is referred to as ageing. In gels, ageing results in the gradual formation of a denser network of gelling agent. Theimer (1960) suggests that this process is similar to the original gelling process and continues after the initial gelation, since fluid medium is lost from the newly formed gel. He observed the formation of additional thin fibrils in 10-day-old gelatin gels when compared with the fresh gels but found little further change in structure after 21 days since the dehydration processes were slowing down.

4. ADSORPTION OF VAPOURS BY XEROGELS

The porous nature of xerogels provides a large surface area for the adsorption of vapours. In addition, the porosity provides the possibility of uptake of vapour by capillary condensation (*see* p. 46). Xerogels, especially silica gel, are therefore used as drying agents.

The isotherms for adsorption and desorption in a particular system of this type often do not coincide at higher vapour pressures. A hysteresis loop is therefore observed between the curves that represent adsorption and desorption in graphs showing the variation in the amount of vapour taken up at different equilibrium pressures. This behaviour is attributable to the differences that arise when the pores in the xerogel are filled with liquid during adsorption and when they are subsequently emptied during desorption.

5. RHEOLOGICAL PROPERTIES

Gels exhibit the mechanical properties of rigidity, tensile strength, and elasticity that are characteristic of solids. In thixotropic gels these effects are only apparent below the yield value, above which the systems exhibit the flow properties of suspensions.

6. CHEMICAL REACTIONS IN GELS

If the components of a gel are inert towards substances involved in a chemical reaction then the gel forms a suitable medium in which the reaction can be studied since the network provides some protection against disturbances caused by mechanical influences or convection currents. The precipitates produced from such reactions often have a periodic structure; i.e. the precipitate is formed in a rhythmic pattern throughout the gel. Such patterns are often referred to as Leisegang rings. The precipitation of silver chromate that results from the reaction of potassium chromate and silver nitrate in gelatin gel is a common example of this type of behaviour and it is suggested that the layered structure of gallstones offers a further example (Jirgensons, 1958).

7. DIFFUSION IN GELS

Since a gel may be regarded as a random network permeated by pores that are filled with a liquid component, substances that are soluble in the liquid component will tend to permeate through the gel by diffusion in solution through the spaces in the network. The rate of diffusion of substances through gels by this means will therefore be affected by those factors that normally affect simple diffusion in solution and by additional factors that are associated with the presence of the gel network.

(a) Diffusion in Solution

This process may be defined as the spontaneous transference of solute from regions in the solution where the concentration is high to other regions where the concentration is lower, until there is a uniform distribution throughout. The rate of diffusion of a solute is expressed by Fick's first law (Eqn 5.5),

$$\frac{dm}{dt} = -DA\frac{dc}{dx} \qquad (5.5)$$

where dm is the amount of solute diffusing in time dt across an area A under the influence of a concentration gradient dc/dx. D is known as the diffusion coefficient and it has the dimensions of area per unit time. It is not strictly constant but varies with concentration at constant temperature. The value of D obtained from any measurements should therefore be regarded as a mean value for the concentration range that is considered. The negative sign in Eqn (5.5) is necessary because diffusion occurs in the opposite direction to that of increasing concentration (i.e. dc/dx is negative).

The diffusion coefficient for spherical particles that are of colloidal dimensions (i.e. considerably larger than the solvent molecules) is given by Eqn (5.6), which is known as the Sutherland-Einstein equation.

$$D = \frac{RT}{6\eta r N_A} \qquad (5.6)$$

where r is the radius of the spherical particle, η is the viscosity of the liquid medium, R is the gas constant, T is the thermodynamic temperature, and N_A is Avogadro's constant.

Equation (5.6) does not apply to non-spherical particles because the frictional force that opposes their movement will vary with the orientation of the particles.

The rates of diffusion of small molecules and ions are greater than those of colloidal particles. Although the diffusion of the former is impeded by the viscosity of the medium, Eqn (5.6) is not applicable to these systems.

The difference in the rates of diffusion of small and large particles tends to cause the separation of charged colloidal particles from their surrounding atmospheres of gegenions. This effect gives rise to a potential difference that resists further separation and may cause an acceleration or a retardation in the diffusion rate of the colloidal particle depending on the conditions of the experiment. The effect can be suppressed by the addition of sufficient simple electrolyte (e.g. KCl), which provides an excess of gegenions throughout the liquid medium and so prevents the development of potential gradients. However, it is necessary to ensure that the diffusion of this electrolyte does not affect the diffusion of the colloidal material. This is usually achieved by following the diffusion of colloid across a boundary on both sides of which the concentration of simple electrolyte is the same.

(b) The Effects Associated with the Presence of a Gel Network

Sieve Effects. The rates of diffusion of small molecules and ions through gels are virtually the same as their rates of diffusion in simple solution. However, as the size of the diffusing particles becomes comparable with the pore diameter of the gel network diffusion is retarded considerably and ceases when the particles are larger than the widest pores in the gel. This is known as the sieve action of the gel and it may be regarded as a normal filtration process.

The sieve effect of a gel is determined by the average pore diameter. This, in turn, is affected by: (a) the concentration of gelling agent (an increase in this concentration usually results in a decrease in the pore diameter), and (b) by the age of the gel and the conditions under which it has been stored, because an aged gel is usually denser than a freshly prepared one, and the ageing process may be accelerated by conditions that cause loss of the liquid component.

A further consequence of the porous nature of the medium through which diffusion is occurring arises from the fact that the area over which diffusion can take place is not the total surface area of the gel but only the combined surface area of the pores.

Electrical Effects. An electrical double layer, similar to that which surrounds a colloidal particle, will exist at the interface between the walls of the pores in a gel and the liquid that fills these pores. If the capillary walls possess fixed negative charges then the diffuse part of the electrical double layer that is associated with these walls will contain an excess of positive gegenions. However, the diffuse layers extend into the liquid that fills the pores, and

flow of liquid through the gel will tend to displace the gegenions; i.e. the latter are mobile. The effect of gegenion mobility is particularly noticeable when diffusion of an electrolyte through gel occurs. The electrolyte ions that possess a similar charge to the mobile gegenions of the gel are able to enter the pores easily and the mobile gegenions are displaced along the pores. However, the charged framework of the gel will tend to prevent the entry of the other electrolyte ions since they both carry charges with the same sign. This effect gives rise to a selective permeability of the gel for either positive or negative ions. For example, gelatin gel is selectively cation permeable in alkaline media since the gel network then possesses fixed negative charges. Conversely, when the network becomes positively charged as in acid media, the gel is selectively anion permeable.

These effects also apply to the permeability of membranes; further information is given on page 73.

Other Effects. Adsorption of a diffusing solute onto the walls of the pores will retard the rate of diffusion. If a mixture of solutes is passing through the gel then any difference in their affinities for the adsorption sites on the walls may lead to a type of chromatographic separation.

A solute may become distributed between the network phase of a gel and the liquid phase that fills the pores. Diffusion through a gel may therefore proceed by diffusion in solution through the network itself.

Although the viscosity of the medium in which diffusion is occurring will influence the rate of diffusion it should be remembered that in diffusion in gels it is usually the viscosity of the liquid component in the pores that is important in this respect, not the overall viscosity of the gel.

Application of Gels

1. DOSAGE FORMS

Glycogelatin gels are frequently used as a basis for medicated pastilles. They are also used in the formulation of some suppositories, e.g. Glycerin suppositories BP (1968).

Gelatin gels are employed in the preparation of hard and soft capsules that may be used to mask the unpleasant tastes of solids and liquids.

2. MICROBIOLOGICAL MEDIA

Agar and gelatin gels are used as solid media for the culture of micro-organisms (p. 317). The diffusion of antibiotics, antiseptics, vitamins, and enzymes through solid culture media is used in microbiological assays of these materials. Such diffusion produces zones of either retarded or enhanced growth on seeded agar plates depending on the activity of the diffusing substances. The factors involved in this type of assay for antiseptics have been investigated by Cooper and Woodman (1946). These workers determined the diffusion coefficients of crystal violet and penicillin through agar gels by employing an equation, Eqn (5.7) that had been given previously by Eversole and Doughty (1935) for the diffusion of neutral molecules through pure water. If the initial concentration of a solution is m_0 and the concentration at a distance x from the junction of the gel and solution after a time t is m_1 then the diffusion coefficient of the solute is given by

$$4D \, 2 \cdot 303(\log m_0 - \log m_1) = x^2/t \qquad (5.7)$$

A graph of x^2 against t is usually plotted, and the diffusion coefficient is then calculated from Eqn (5.7) by inserting the value of x^2/t obtained from the slope of such a graph. This equation applies to the diffusion of neutral molecules only and must be amended for the diffusion of charged particles to allow for the influence of potential gradients. However, the presence of sufficient simple electrolyte prevents the development of such gradients, and

Eqn (5.7) may then be applied. In addition, Eqn (5.7) was derived for the case of linear diffusion and is not strictly applicable to the radial diffusion that occurs in most cup plate assay techniques. However, the error involved is small if the cups are of large diameter. A consideration of the theoretical aspects of diffusion assays is given by Cooper (1963). Further details of this type of assay are given later in this book (p. 349).

3. GEL FILTRATION

This is a technique for the separation of solutes of different molecular sizes. It is based on the fact that small molecules are able to penetrate into the networks of gels whereas larger molecules are unable to do so. Gels consisting of cross-linked polysaccharide chains are commonly used, e.g. Sephadex (Pharmacia), and chromatographic techniques are employed in the separation process. For example, a solution containing the mixed solutes is passed through a column packed with gel particles and solvent. The largest solute molecules pass between the particles and through the column at a relatively rapid rate, whereas the rate of passage of the smaller solute molecules is reduced by their penetration into the pores of the gel particles.

Dialysing Membranes

The membranes that are used in dialysis and ultra-filtration are usually derivatives of cellulose (e.g. cellulose acetate, nitrocellulose) and may be classed as xerogels. The structure of these materials may be regarded as a microporous network of macromolecules, as indicated by Fig. 5.10, which shows that the molecules are usually aggregated into bundles or micelles by secondary forces such as hydrogen bonding.

Preparation of Membranes

Suitable membranes should prevent the escape of colloidal material but allow rapid diffusion of solvent and small molecules. They are usually prepared by evaporation of layers of a solution of the membrane material in a volatile solvent (e.g. ether, acetone). The solution is cast on to either a rotating thimble-shaped mould or a flat surface. Several layers are applied and each is allowed to evaporate under controlled conditions of humidity and temperature before the next one is added. The membrane is finally hardened by immersion in a liquid in which it is insoluble.

If the original solvent is non-volatile the membrane material may be deposited as a film in a support such as filter paper.

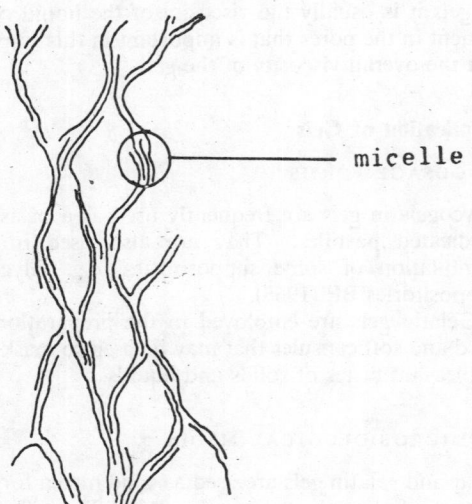

micelle

Fig. 5.10. The structure of dialysing membranes

Permeability of Membranes

The permeability or permeability coefficient (P) of a membrane is given by Eqn (5.8)

$$\frac{Q}{t} = \frac{PA \, \Delta c}{d} \qquad (5.8)$$

where Q is the amount of material that passes through a membrane of area A and thickness d under the influence of a concentration difference Δc in time t.

FACTORS AFFECTING PERMEABILITY

Since the structure of a membrane resembles that of a gel the factors that affect the permeability of membranes are similar to those that affect the rate of diffusion of substances through gels (p. 70).

Pore Size

This is important in determining the contribution of the sieve effect to the permeability of a membrane. The average pore size may be determined by the rate of penetration of water through the membrane, or by the filtration of standardised colloidal particles of varying sizes. For example, colloidal gold particles, the size of which had been previously determined in the electron microscope, were used by Zsigmondy. It is also useful to know the degree of uniformity of pore size. This is often expressed as the ratio of the maximum pore size, which is determined by measuring the minimum pressure required to produce a stream of air bubbles through the membrane, to the average pore diameter, which is determined from the rate of flow of water as indicated previously.

Satisfactory membranes should possess pores that fall within a narrow range of sizes. Preparative methods therefore attempt to produce membranes of different grades with reproducible characteristics. This involves careful control of all factors that may influence pore size during the preparation of membranes. For example, the temperature and humidity under which evaporation of the volatile solvent is carried out are controlled since the final pore size depends on the extent of drying; the shorter the drying time the greater the pore size. In addition, solvent mixtures containing gelifying liquids as well as normal solvents are used to preserve the regularity of a gel during the hardening process. These liquids cause swelling of the gel material as opposed to complete solution. They are not removed by the evaporation but dissolve out of the membrane into the hardening liquid, thus preserving the porosity of the initial gel in the final membrane. If only solvent liquids are used the resulting membranes are very compact and relatively impermeable.

The pore size may also be affected by various treatments after the membranes are formed. For example, stretching by means of hydrostatic pressure, partial digestion by cellulose enzymes or treatment with zinc chloride solution will all increase the permeability of cellophane membranes, while longitudinal stretching or acetylation cause a decrease in permeability (Craig and Konisberg, 1961).

Electrical Effects

(a) *Charges on Membranes.* These will influence the permeability of membranes to anions and cations in the same way as they affect diffusion through gels. Thus, a membrane such as collodion, which possesses fixed anions and mobile cations, will be selectively permeable to cations, since these are able to displace the original cations through the pores, anions being repelled by the negatively charged membrane material. Conversely, a membrane with fixed cations and mobile anions will be selectively permeable to anions. The separation of charge that results from such selectivity produces a difference in electrical potential between the opposite sides of the membrane.

(b) *The Donnan Membrane Effect.* The diffusion of small ions through a membrane will be affected by the presence of a charged macromolecule that is unable to penetrate the membrane because of its size. This is known as the Donnan membrane effect and it may be explained by considering a system consisting of a solution of sodium chloride separated by a membrane from another solution containing a charged macromolecule (R^-) and its gegenion (Na^+). If the initial concentration of sodium chloride is c_1 and that of the macromolecule is c_2 the system may be represented diagrammatically as

Initial concn.
$$\begin{array}{cc|cc} Na^+ + Cl^- & & Na^+ + R^- \\ c_1 \quad\quad c_1 & & c_2 \quad\quad c_2 \end{array}$$

In dilute solutions the product of the concentrations of the diffusible ions (i.e. Na^+ and Cl^-) will be equal on both sides of the membrane when equilibrium is established. The condition of electroneutrality must also apply; i.e. the concentrations of positively and negatively charged ions on each side of the membrane must balance. If the amount of sodium chloride that has diffused through the membrane when equilibrium has been established is x then the system may be represented as

$$Na^+ + Cl^- \mid Na^+ + R^- + Cl^-$$

Equilibrium

concn. $(c_1 - x)$ $(c_1 - x)$ $\mid$ $(c_2 + x)$ c_2 x

$\therefore$ at equilibrium $(c_1 - x)(c_1 - x) = (c_2 + x)x$

$\therefore \qquad\qquad c_1^2 - 2c_1x + x^2 = c_2x + x^2$

$\therefore \qquad\qquad\qquad\qquad c_1^2 = c_2x + 2c_1x$

$$= x(c_2 + 2c_1)$$

$\therefore \qquad\qquad\qquad\qquad x = \dfrac{c_1^2}{(c_2 + 2c_1)}$

$$\therefore \qquad\qquad \frac{x}{c_1} = \frac{c_1}{(c_2 + 2c_1)}$$

$$(5.9)$$

In Eqn (5.9) x/c_1 represents the fraction of sodium chloride that has diffused through the membrane when equilibrium has been established. It can be seen that this fraction is influenced by the concen- tration of the non-diffusible ion R^-. If the unequal distribution of diffusible electrolyte that occurs in the presence of a charged macromolecule is not taken into account then determination of the osmotic pressure exerted by the macromolecule will be incorrect. However, if the concentration of diffusible electrolyte is relatively high then the denominator on the right-hand side of Eqn (5.9) is approximately equal to $2c_1$ (i.e. c_2 may be ignored). The equation then reduces to $x/c_1 = \frac{1}{2}$, indicating that the simple electrolyte is equally distributed on both sides of the membrane and that the Donnan effect is negligible in such cases.

Solubility Effects. Substances may pass through membranes by diffusion in solution through the membrane material itself. This process involves an initial partition of the substance between the original solvent and the membrane material. It may be of importance when an aqueous solution of an organic solute is in contact with a membrane with marked lipoidal properties (*see* Chapter 6).

Aerosols

Aerosols are colloidal dispersions of liquids or solids in gases. In general, mists and fogs possess liquid disperse phases, while smokes, fumes, and dusts are dispersions of solid particles in gases.

Stability

Fogs and smokes appear to be very stable when compared with the aqueous dispersions of colloidal particles discussed in the preceding section. How- ever, the concentration of particles in the latter is usually of the order of 10^{10} mm^{-3}, whereas the concentration of particles in fogs and smokes is much lower (about 10^3 mm^{-3}). Aqueous dispersions of similar low concentrations would be even more stable than the fogs and smokes, since the particles in the latter are not stabilised to any appreciable extent by electrical charges, which may arise from collisions between the particles and naturally occurring ions in air.

Preparation

In common with other colloidal dispersions aerosols may be prepared by either dispersion or condensa- tion methods. The latter type involves the initial production of supersaturated vapour of the material that is to be dispersed. This may be achieved by supercooling the vapour. The supersaturation eventually leads to the formulation of nuclei, which grow into particles of colloidal dimensions.

The preparation of aerosols by dispersion methods is of greater interest in pharmacy and may be achieved by the use of pressurised containers. For example, the pressure inside these containers may be produced by a liquefied gas, which is known as the propellant. If a solution or a suspension of active ingredients is contained in the liquid propellant or in a mixture of this liquid and an additional solvent then when the valve on the container is opened the vapour pressure of the propellant forces the mixture out of the container. The large expansion of the propellant at room temperature and atmospheric pressure produces a dispersion of the active ingredi- ents in air. Although the particles in such dispersions are usually larger than those in colloidal systems, the term aerosols is still generally applied to them.

Various types of product can be obtained by the use of different propellants, valves, and solvents. These products range from aerosols to sprays, which contain larger liquid particles, and to foams and semi-solid products such as toothpaste. A review of the various aspects of pressurised containers used for these different products is given by Sciarra (1970).

Applications and Advantages in Pharmacy

The advantages obtained from the use of pressurised containers, such as those used for the production of aerosols, are common to all the types of product that may be presented in this way; e.g. foams, sprays, and semi-solids. These advantages include—

(a) ease of use,

(b) protection from contamination with foreign materials, since the product is sealed inside the container (this is particularly important in the preservation of sterility),

(c) protection from the effects of air and moisture,

(d) regulation of dosage by the use of a metered valve (although such metering is no more accurate than oral dosage forms it is an advantage when used for topical preparations),

(e) economic usage of dosage form, when, for example, metered valves are used for expensive topical preparations which may otherwise be formulated as ointments, creams or lotions. The usage of these latter dosage forms will

depend on the user's attitude to economy and often involves some loss of the product on an applicator.

The use of aerosols as a dosage form is particularly important in the administration of drugs via the respiratory system or nasal passages. In addition to local effects, systemic effects may be obtained if the drug is absorbed into the bloodstream from the lungs.

Topical preparations are also well suited for presentation as aerosols or sprays. The irritation of a sore wound caused by the rubbing in of an ointment or cream is avoided, and the cooling effect of aerosols containing liquefied gases may be advantageous.

Suspensions

Stability

As previously stated, coarse suspensions are less stable than colloidal dispersions since the larger particles in the former settle more rapidly under the influence of gravity. Nevertheless, it is possible to obtain suspensions of relatively coarse particles that will remain as dispersions for considerable periods.

The factors that determine the rate of sedimentation are indicated by Stokes's law (Eqn 5.10)

$$u = \frac{d^2(\rho_s - \rho_l)g}{18\eta} \qquad (5.10)$$

where, u is the average velocity of sedimentation of the particles, d is the mean diameter of the particles, ρ_s is the density of the solid particles, ρ_l is the density of the fluid phase, η is the viscosity of the fluid phase, and g is the acceleration due to gravity.

Stokes's law was derived for dilute suspensions of rigid uniform spheres settling at a velocity which produced no turbulence in the fluid medium. Under such conditions the particles do not interfere with each other; i.e. free settling occurs.

Equation (5.10) is not applicable to the more concentrated suspensions usually encountered in pharmaceutical practice, since the particles in these suspensions are rarely spherical and their concentrations are high enough to interfere with the sedimentation of individual particles; i.e. hindered settling occurs. However, the factors indicated by Eqn (5.10) are still important, and an increase in the mean particle size or in the difference between the densities of the solid and liquid phases will produce a faster rate of sedimentation, while an increase in the viscosity of the liquid medium will decrease the sedimentation rate.

FLOCCULATED AND DEFLOCCULATED SUSPENSIONS

Aggregation of particles will also lead to a more rapid rate of sedimentation because the size of the sedimenting units is increased. As pointed out previously, the existence of a positive free energy associated with the interface between solid particles and liquid medium will mean that the dispersion is unstable from a thermodynamic point of view. Aggregation of the particles will tend to occur spontaneously in order to reduce this interfacial free energy. However, the rate of coalescence of particles will depend on the combined effects of repulsive and attractive forces that exist between approaching particles in a similar manner to the effects that were discussed in relation to the stability of colloidal dispersions. Thus, the overlapping of electrical double layers that occurs when two particles approach each other gives rise to a repulsive force and the attractive force arises from the van der Waals interactions between all the atoms in one particle and all those of the other.

In coarse suspensions of lyophobic materials the size of the dispersed particles introduces an effect that is not apparent in colloidal dispersions. The van der Waals attractive force falls off with distance more slowly than the repulsive force so that although the latter is greater than the attractive force at some distances of separation, and thus gives rise to a repulsion barrier, the van der Waals forces may again predominate at larger distances and produce a secondary minimum in the net interaction energy curve for the approach of two particles. Since the total attractive force is approximately proportional to the size of the dispersed particles, it follows that the secondary minimum is more pronounced for

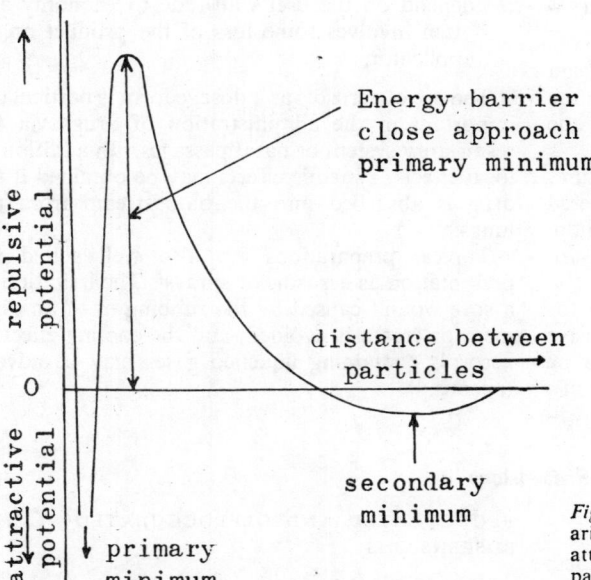

Fig. 5.11 Variation in net potential of interaction arising from the combined effects of repulsive and attractive forces between two approaching coarse particles

coarse particles than for those of colloidal dimensions. This difference between coarse and colloidal dispersions is illustrated by a comparison of Fig. 5.11, which represents the variation in net potential for the approach of coarse particles, with Fig. 5.1, which relates to colloidal systems, when it will be seen that no secondary minimum is evident in the latter figure.

The existence of two minima in the net potential energy curve for the interaction between coarse particles allows two types of coagulation to occur in these systems. If approaching particles possess sufficient energy to overcome the repulsion barrier they will come into very close contact in the deep primary minimum. In order to reseparate they will need to acquire even more energy since the barrier to redispersion is represented by the difference in levels of the primary minimum and the repulsion barrier maximum. Since this barrier to redispersion is relatively great, separation of particles coagulated in this manner does not occur easily.

The second type of coagulation may arise from the trapping of an approaching particle in the secondary minimum. Since this minimum is shallow and the particles remain separated by a thin film of liquid, the resulting coagulation is more reversible and the aggregated particles are easily redispersed by mechanical agitation. Although the DLVO theory (p. 54) predicts that a secondary minimum will exist for all lyophobic dispersions it may be too shallow to have any significant effect, since the influence of gravity on coarse particles may

be greater than the attractive force exerted between particles. In addition, the shape of the particles may be important; for example, as the particles become more elongated the effect of the secondary minimum becomes significant in relation to gravitational forces.

If aggregation of the particles in a suspension does occur then the system is said to be flocculated. The nature of the flocs will be determined by the closeness of contact of the individual particles. Aggregation in the primary minimum will produce rather compact flocs, and an increase in the proportion of aggregations in the secondary minimum will increase the fluffy nature or porosity of the flocs.

If the barrier to repulsion is sufficient to prevent aggregation in the primary minimum and the effect of the secondary minimum is insignificant then the particles will remain as individual units and the system is said to be deflocculated. Solvation effects will also help to maintain the dispersion of individual particles and any lyophilic properties of the surface of the particles, e.g. caused by the adsorption of surface active agents, will tend to produce a deflocculated suspension.

The Sedimentation Behaviour of Flocculated and Deflocculated Suspensions

It has already been pointed out that the formation of aggregates will cause an increase in the rate of sedimentation of particles since the size of the sedimenting units is increased. Thus, a flocculated suspension will show a more rapid sedimentation rate than a deflocculated system. The rate of sedimentation in a flocculated system is often referred to as subsidence and it depends not only on the size of the aggregates or flocs but also on their porosity, since the liquid medium flows through, as well as around, them as they fall.

In addition to their different sedimentation rates there is a difference in the nature of the sediment that is formed by the two types of suspension. In a flocculated suspension the loose structure of the rapidly sedimenting flocs tends to be preserved in the sediment, which therefore contains an appreciable amount of entrapped liquid. The volume of the final sediment is therefore relatively large and the sediment is easily redispersed by agitation. It should be noted that the sedimentation volume of a flocculated suspension may show small decreases on storage due to the compaction of underlying flocs by the material resting upon them in the sediment.

In a deflocculated suspension the repulsive forces between individual particles allow the particles to slip past each other in a sediment. This property, together with the slow rate of sedimentation, which prevents the entrapping of liquid medium, allows the formation of a compact sediment; i.e. one with a small volume. This type of sediment is usually difficult to redisperse by agitation and is often referred to as a cake.

Pharmaceutical suspensions usually contain a reasonable distribution of particle sizes. In such systems the largest particles will sediment first and the smaller ones will fall slowly through the supernatant liquid. This is particularly noticeable in deflocculated suspensions where the particles retain their individual identities and the supernatant liquid often remains cloudy because of the presence of the smallest particles when the majority of the sediment has already formed. However, in a completely flocculated suspension even the smallest particles are involved in floc formation so that they do not remain in the supernatant, which is therefore not cloudy (Michaels and Bolger, 1964).

Figure 5.12 illustrates the difference in appearance of flocculated and deflocculated suspensions after various periods of standing in an undisturbed condition.

Rheological Properties of Suspensions

These properties are discussed in more detail in Chapter 7, where it will be seen that flocculated suspensions tend to exhibit plastic or pseudoplastic behaviour while deflocculated systems tend to be dilatant. This means that the apparent viscosity of flocculated suspensions is relatively high when the applied shearing stress is low but it decreases as the applied stress increases. In fact, if plastic behaviour is exhibited then the system behaves like a solid up to a particular shearing stress, which is known as the yield value, and no flow occurs in the system until this value is exceeded. Conversely, the apparent viscosity of deflocculated suspensions is low at low shearing stresses and increases as the applied stress increases. One of the important consequences of this difference in behaviour is that deflocculated suspensions are easy to pour, whereas flocculated ones are not, since the shearing stresses involved in pouring are relatively low. However, dilatant suspensions are often troublesome, and attention to this type of system should be paid in milling operations because the high speed involved in some of these operations may cause such an increase in viscosity that the mill may sieze up. It should be reiterated that this paragraph gives only a brief indication of the differences in the rheological properties of flocculated and deflocculated suspensions, and Chapter 7 should be consulted for explanations of these and other properties.

Pharmaceutical Applications of Suspensions

A pharmaceutical suspension consists of a dispersion of finely divided insoluble material suspended in a liquid medium. Most suspensions are prepared and stored in their final form until required for use. In other cases, where unwanted effects may be caused by prolonged contact between the solid particles and the liquid dispersion medium, the suspension is prepared immediately before use and is acceptable for only a limited period thereafter. For example, Ampicillin Mixture BPC (1968) is a suspension of ampicillin or ampicillin trihydrate in a suitable flavoured aqueous vehicle. However, the antibiotic is susceptible to hydrolysis and the activity of an aqueous suspension gradually decreases. The BPC therefore directs that the mixture should be freshly prepared by dispersing the dry mixed ingredients in Purified Water, stored in a cool place, and used within one week of preparation.

The major applications of suspensions in pharmacy can be conveniently divided into the following groups.

(a) Preparations for Oral Administration

A suspension provides a convenient means of administering an insoluble nrug, especially where difficulty may be encountered in swallowing solid dosage forms such as tablets or capsules. Solids such as kaolin, magnesium carbonate, calcium

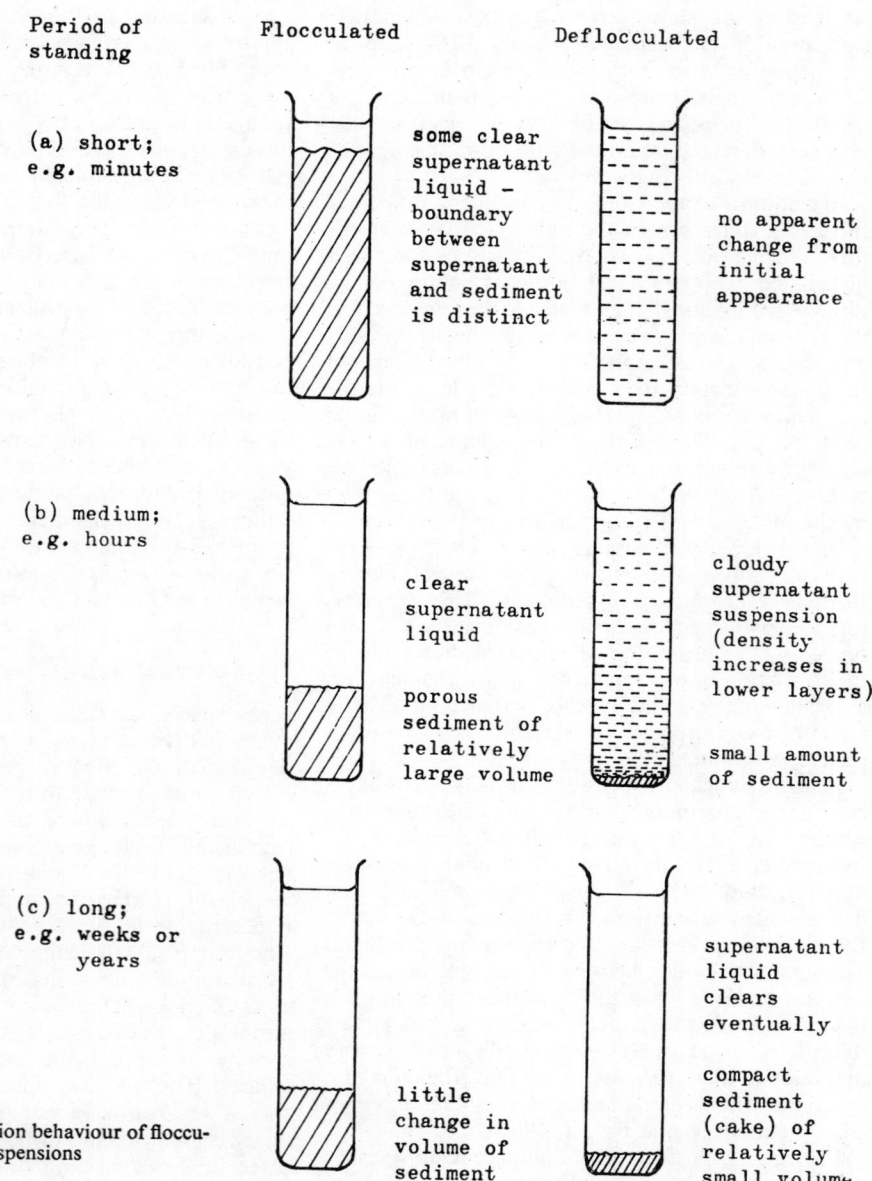

Period of standing	Flocculated		Deflocculated	
(a) short; e.g. minutes		some clear supernatant liquid – boundary between supernatant and sediment is distinct		no apparent change from initial appearance
(b) medium; e.g. hours		clear supernatant liquid porous sediment of relatively large volume		cloudy supernatant suspension (density increases in lower layers) small amount of sediment
(c) long; e.g. weeks or years		little change in volume of sediment		supernatant liquid clears eventually compact sediment (cake) of relatively small volume

Fig. 5.12   The sedimentation behaviour of flocculated and deflocculated suspensions

carbonate, and magnesium trisilicate are often administered for their adsorptive or antacid properties in the treatment of gastric disorders. The effectiveness of these substances is influenced by the surface areas of the solids and administration as fine powders in the form of suspensions allows a large surface area to be available immediately for contact with the gastric contents.

Insoluble derivatives are often used to reduce the unpleasant taste of the active form of drugs and the formulation of these insoluble compounds in suspensions is common. For example, insoluble chloramphenicol palmitate is used in Chloramphenicol Mixture BPC (1968) to reduce the bitter taste of the free base.

(b) Suspensions for Injection

Such preparations are of particular importance in the field of depot therapy. The various types of product and the problems associated with their formulation are discussed by Gunn and Carter (1965).

(c) Suspensions for External Use

Preparations of this type that are pourable are usually referred to as lotions (e.g. calamine lotion) and those that possess semi-solid characteristics are termed pastes (e.g. zinc and salicylic acid paste and magnesium sulphate paste).

The physico-chemical problems associated with the formulation of pharmaceutical suspensions are concerned with the control of sedimentation behaviour and rheological properties, both of which are influenced by the degree of flocculation in a particular system. In addition, the sedimentation behaviour is influenced by the rheological properties of the liquid continuous phase. Because of this interdependence of properties relevant to the formulation of pharmaceutical suspensions, the problems associated with this type of formulation are discussed in the section concerned with the rheology of suspensions (Chapter 7).

Emulsions

An emulsion is a dispersion of a liquid as globules in another liquid that is immiscible with the first. The diameters of the globules usually vary between about 0.1×10^{-3} to 100×10^{-3} mm. One of the liquids is usually water and the other is an oil. Two types of emulsion are possible; i.e. oil-in-water (o/w) and water-in-oil (w/o) and examples of both types are frequently encountered in pharmaceutical and cosmetic preparations. A third component is required to stabilise the emulsion because a simple dispersion of oil in water (or water in oil) obtained by vigorous shaking of the two liquids is unstable and coalescence of the globules and eventual separation into two phases occurs rapidly. This additional component is termed the emulsifying agent, emulgent, or emulsifier.

Emulsifying Agents

Various types of agent are used as indicated by the following list.

1. SYNTHETIC SURFACE ACTIVE AGENTS

A classification of these has already been given in Chapter 4. This type of agent is the most common in modern emulsion technology and many commercial products are available. Surface active agents may be used singly or in combination with other surface active agents for the purpose of stabilising an emulsion. For w/o emulsions the balance between the hydrophilic and lipophilic properties of the emulsifier should be such as to give an HLB value in the range 3 to 6 (see p. 66) and for an o/w emulsion the HLB value of the emulsifier should be in the range 8 to 13. For a particular emulsion the required HLB value of the emulsifier may be calculated more precisely and many surface active agents have been synthesised to satisfy the requirements of specific systems.

2. MACROMOLECULAR EMULSIFYING AGENTS

The majority of these agents produce o/w emulsions. In addition, many of them are obtained from natural sources and therefore may vary in quality.

(a) Gums

Acacia is the most common gum used in pharmaceutical preparations. It is particularly useful for emulsions prepared with a mortar and pestle, provided that the correct proportions of oil, water, and gum are employed in the preparation of a so-called primary emulsion that may then be diluted with more aqueous phase. These proportions depend on the nature of the oil phase and more information on the preparation of emulsions by this means is given by Gunn and Carter (1965).

Tragacanth gum is often included in emulsion formulations but is not a very efficient agent when used alone. It is usually used as an additional agent in emulsions containing acacia as the main emulsifier.

(b) Carbohydrates and Derivatives

Starch is a poor emulsifying agent but is sometimes used in the preparation of enemas containing oils. Cellulose derivatives such as methylcellulose and sodium carboxymethylcellulose, and soluble salts of alginic acid are often used.

(c) Proteins

Certain proteins such as gelatin and casein are occasionally used in pharmaceutical emulsions.

3. FINELY DIVIDED SOLIDS

Solid particles that are wetted by oils and water may be adsorbed around the globules in an emulsion, and provide stability against coalescence. Examples of solid emulsifying agents used in pharmacy include aluminium hydroxide and bentonite, both of which yield o/w emulsions.

Determination of Emulsion Type

Several tests are available to distinguish between o/w and w/o emulsions. The most common of these involve: (a) miscibility tests with oil or water—the emulsion will only be miscible with liquids that are miscible with its continuous phase; (b) conductivity measurements—systems with aqueous continuous phases will readily conduct electricity whereas systems with oily continuous phases will not; and (c) staining tests—the oil is stained by the incorporation of a dye that does not partition into the aqueous phase and facilitates microscopic examination of the emulsion and determination of its type. Details of these tests are given by Gunn and Carter (1965).

Types of Instability in Emulsions

A stable emulsion may be defined as a system in which the globules retain their initial character and remain uniformly distributed throughout the continuous phase. Various types of deviation from this ideal behaviour are common.

1. BREAKING OR CRACKING

This involves coalescence of the dispersed globules and produces eventual separation of the emulsion into two phases. It will occur if the barriers to coalescence are inefficient or if they are weakened by some means. Some of the factors that cause breaking are—

(a) The addition of a substance that is incompatible with the emulsifier may destroy its emulsifying ability, e.g.

  (i) The effect of large anions on cationic emulsifying agents.
 (ii) The effect of magnesium and calcium ions in hard water on the alkali soaps.
(iii) The effect of phenolic substances on cetomacrogol.

It should be noted that a stable emulsion must not be taken as conclusive evidence of the absence of incompatibility between an emulsifying agent and other ingredients. Satisfactory tests on the particular activities of these other ingredients should be carried out on new formulations.

Incompatibilities between an emulsifying agent and another ingredient may produce a compound that stabilises the opposite type of emulsion to the initial emulsifier so that phase reversal or phase inversion occurs. For example, the addition of sufficient calcium chloride to an o/w emulsion stabilised by a sodium soap causes phase inversion, and the resulting w/o emulsion is stabilised by the calcium soap that is formed by reaction between the original emulsifier and the added calcium chloride.

(b) An increase in temperature will increase the number of collisions between globules that are effective in overcoming the barriers to coalescence. This effect is made use of in accelerated tests on the stability of emulsions.

(c) An increase in temperature may coagulate certain types of macromolecular emulsifying agent (e.g. proteins). Such adverse effects of high temperature must be taken into account if temperature is used in accelerated testing as a means of increasing the rate of coalescence.

(d) Freezing of the aqueous phase will produce ice crystals that may exert unusual pressures on the oil globules. In addition, dissolved salts will concentrate in the remaining unfrozen water and may affect electrical barriers to coalescence.

(e) Attempts to incorporate excessive amounts of disperse phase may cause breaking of an emulsion or phase inversion. It can be shown that uniform spheres arranged in the closest packing will occupy 74 per cent of the total volume irrespective of their size. Although it is possible to obtain more concentrated emulsions than this, because of the non-uniform sizes of the globules, there is a critical point at which the emulsion will break.

2. CREAMING

This involves the concentration of dispersed globules in either the upper or lower layers of the emulsion. It is caused by the influence of gravity on the globules, since they usually have a different density from that of the continuous phase. If the globules have a lower density they will tend to concentrate in the upper layers of the system. This is common in dilute o/w emulsions; the cream on milk is a familiar example. Globules will settle to the lower layers if they have a greater density than the continuous phase. This is common in dilute w/o emulsions.

In creaming, the dispersed globules retain their identities and do not coalesce as they do in breaking. Furthermore, a uniform dispersion of globules can be re-obtained by shaking the system. Creaming is not therefore such a serious instability as breaking, since redispersion by shaking cannot be brought about in breaking. However, creaming is undesirable from a pharmaceutical point of view because a creamed emulsion is inelegant in appearance, provides the possibility of inaccurate dosage, and increases the likelihood of coalescence, since the globules are closer together in the cream.

To prevent or delay creaming it is necessary to understand the factors that influence the rate at which it occurs. These factors are similar to those involved in the sedimentation rates of coarse suspensions and are indicated by Stokes' law (Eqn 5.10). A consideration of this equation will show that the rate of creaming will be decreased by (a) a reduction in the mean globule diameter, (b) a decrease in the difference in the densities of the two phases, and (c) an increase in the viscosity of the continuous phase. Conversely, it will be increased by centrifugation which increases the value of g in the equation, and by an increase in temperature, which will decrease the viscosity of the continuous phase.

The main factors utilised in reducing the rate of creaming in pharmaceutical emulsions are—

(a) reduction in mean globule diameter—this is usually achieved by using an efficient homogeniser;
(b) increase in viscosity of the continuous phase by using thickening agents; for example tragacanth and methylcellulose for o/w emulsions and soft paraffin for w/o emulsions;
(c) storage at low temperatures—freezing the aqueous phase should be avoided since this may cause breaking of the emulsion. This method is less attractive to manufacturers as a sole means of ensuring adequate stability because it introduces a stability factor that passes out of their control when the product is sold.

Although creaming is prevented altogether by equalisation of the densities of the two phases this method is little used in pharmaceutical practice since it usually involves the addition of substances that are unacceptable in medicinal preparations.

3. FLOCCULATION OR COAGULATION

This involves globules aggregating into loose masses within the emulsion. The globules do not coalesce and may be redispersed by shaking. Thus, flocculation is less serious than breaking. However, as is emphasised later, flocculation must precede coalescence in the overall process of breaking, and factors that prevent or retard flocculation will therefore increase the stability of emulsions.

Assessment of Stability

Approximate assessments of the relative stabilities of a series of emulsions may be obtained from estimations of the degree of separation of the dis-

perse phase as a distinct layer, or from the degree of creaming. These methods are suitable only for unstable emulsions that exhibit rapid breaking or creaming, and difficulties may arise in measuring the degree of separation accurately.

More precise assessments are obtained from changes in the distribution of globule sizes in an emulsion with time. Microscopy provides the simplest way of determining a globule size distribution but this method is very tedious since large numbers of globules must be measured. Several other methods, which have been reviewed by Sherman (1968), are available.

The single determination of a globule size distribution, such as that shown in Fig. 5.13, is not sufficient for the purposes of assessing stability because stability is not related to the initial globule size in an emulsion. The changes in the shapes of such curves on ageing of the emulsion must be considered. Instability arising from coalescence results in a decrease in the total number of globules and an increase in the size of the remainder, hence the maximum in the distribution curves moves towards the right in Fig. 5.13 and, also, decreases in height. Stability can therefore be assessed in terms of the rate at which such changes occur.

It is possible to observe changes that arise from flocculation, i.e. decrease in the number of single globules, and from coalescence, i.e. the decrease in total number of globules. The kinetics of flocculation and coalescence have been investigated by van den Tempel (1953) and reviews of these and other studies are given by Becher (1965) and Kitchener and Mussellwhite (1968).

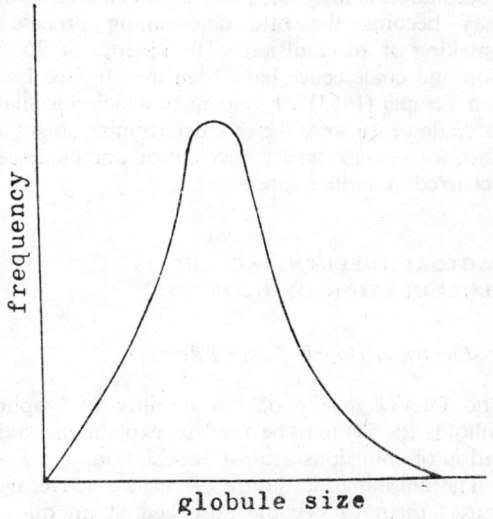

Fig. 5.13 Globule size distribution in an emulsion

Theories of Stability of Emulsions

Several theories attempt to explain the stability of emulsions. Some of the earliest suggestions considered that the reduction in interfacial tension between the oil and water, caused by adsorption of the emulsifying agent at the interface, was the main stabilising factor. However, although a reduction in this interfacial tension will facilitate the formation of a disperse system, if the tension still possesses a finite value, coalescence and breaking will lead to a decrease in the total free energy associated with the oil-water interface. The Bibliography should be consulted for reviews of these and other previous suggestions since the present discussion will be limited to modern theories.

It has already been pointed out that breaking is the most serious instability of emulsions since it is not reversed by shaking. However, it should be noted that the actual coalescence of globules must be preceded by their aggregation or flocculation. In other words, breaking is a two-stage process that involves flocculation followed by coalescence. In any process that involves two consecutive stages, the overall reaction rate is determined by the slower of the two. In breaking emulsions the rate determining stage may therefore be flocculation or coalescence, and whichever is responsible is determined by the properties of the particular emulsion. For example, in a very dilute emulsion the slow rate of flocculation between the low number of globules will tend to be the rate determining stage. In such a case the actual stability of the emulsion will be markedly influenced by those factors that determine the rate of flocculation. In more concentrated emulsions the rate of flocculation is increased, when the coalescence stage may become the rate determining process for breaking of an emulsion. The kinetics of flocculation and coalescence have been investigated by van den Tempel (1953) for systems in which flocculation or coalescence were the rate determining stages and, also, for systems where flocculation and coalescence occurred at similar rates.

FACTORS INFLUENCING THE FLOCCULATION OF GLOBULES

1. Electrical Double Layer Effects

The DLVO theory of the stability of lyophobic colloids (p. 54) may be used to explain the stabilisation of emulsions against flocculation.

The amphipathic nature of surface active agents causes them to become adsorbed at an oil-water interface in a particular manner; i.e. with their hydrophilic groups projecting into the aqueous phase and their lipophilic groups projecting into the oily phase. Such adsorption often increases the density of charges around dispersed globules. This is particularly obvious in the case of ionic surface active agents adsorbed at the interface between an oil globule and a surrounding aqueous phase, as shown by Fig. 5.14.

O/w Emulsions. The presence of charges on the surface of dispersed oil globules will create an electrical double layer around each globule. Overlapping of these double layers gives rise to a repulsion, which opposes the van der Waals force of attraction between approaching globules. The variation in net energy of interaction with distance of separation of the globules is shown in Fig. 5.15. Thus, if the potential energy barrier is high enough, colliding globules will not make contact but will bounce apart, and the emulsion will be stable except for the creaming effects. If the approaching globules are able to overcome the energy barrier they will pass into the primary minimum, where they are held by strong attractive forces. In this position the globules will be separated only by very small distances and their stability will be determined by the resistance to rupture of the interfacial films of adsorbed emulsifying agent.

In o/w emulsions, flocculation may also occur in the secondary minimum shown in Fig. 5.15. The attractive forces in this position are relatively weak and the globules are separated by a layer of continuous phase. These aggregates are easily separated by mechanical agitation.

For the repulsive energy barrier to be efficient in preventing globules from passing into the primary minimum it is necessary for the charge density on each globule to be appreciable. This fact implies that an ionised emulsifying agent should form a relatively close packed film around the globules. Such a film is referred to as a condensed film. However, close packing of similarly charged amphipathic ions in an interfacial film will be hindered by the repulsive forces between the similar charges. Thus, a lipophilic hydrocarbon chain of sufficient length must be present in the molecules of the emulsifying agent to promote their adsorption and produce a condensed film. This effect is illustrated by a comparison of the emulsion stabilising abilities of potassium stearate ($C_{17}H_{35}$ COOK) and potassium laurate ($C_{11}H_{23}$ COOK). The longer hydrocarbon chain in the former soap promotes adsorption at the oil-water interface because of its greater hydrophobic character, and the electrostatic barrier is sufficient to provide a good degree of stability to an emulsion. The adsorption of potassium laurate at the oil-water interface is less than that of the stearate since the hydrocarbon chain is shorter. The amount of

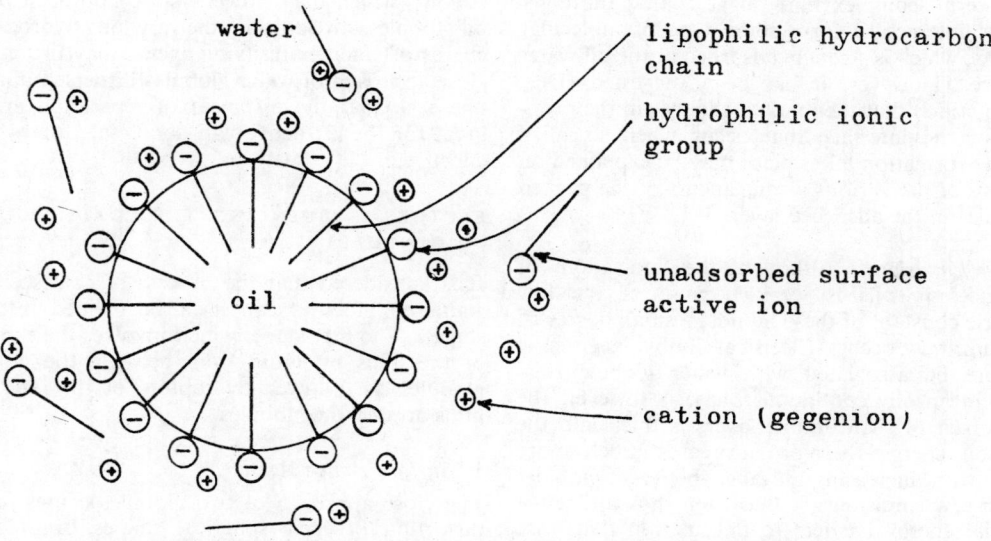

Fig. 5.14   Adsorption of surface active ions on to an oil globule in an o/w emulsion

adsorption is insufficient to provide a satisfactory electrostatic barrier, and poor emulsion stability is obtained with this compound.

The adsorption of a water-soluble amphipathic agent at an oil-water interface is also promoted by the presence of an oil-soluble amphipathic substance in the oil phase. In fact, the effect is mutual and the adsorption of the oil-soluble substance is also increased by the presence of the water-soluble compound. This mutual effect leads to the formation of closely packed films that are referred to as complex condensed films. If the water-soluble agent is ionised, then the electrostatic barrier to flocculation in the primary minimum is increased by complex film formation. Mixtures of water-soluble and oil-

soluble amphipathic agents therefore act as efficient emulsifiers although the individual components are only poor emulsifying agents (Schulman and Cockbain, 1940). Such mixtures form the basis of emulsifying waxes such as

(*a*) Emulsifying Wax BP (1968)
        Sodium lauryl sulphate   1 part
        (anionic and water-soluble)
        Cetostearyl alcohol   9 parts.
        (non-ionic and oil-soluble)

(*b*) Cetrimide Emulsifying Wax BPC (1968)
Cetrimide (cationic and water soluble)   1 part
Cetostearyl alcohol (non-ionic and oil-soluble)
                                                                9 parts

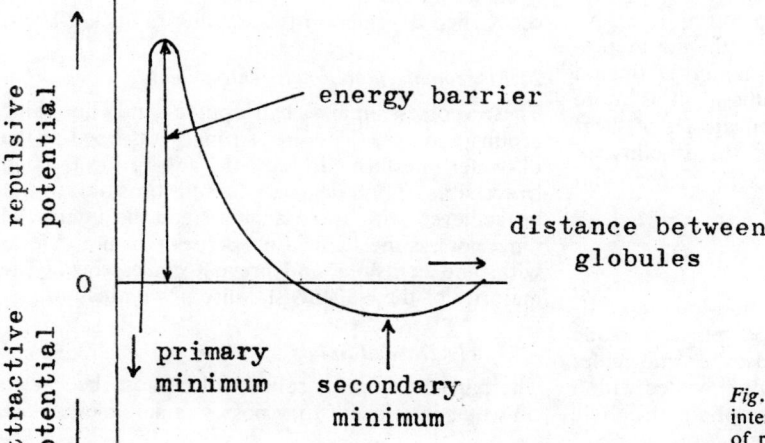

Fig. 5.15   The variation in net potential of interaction arising from combined effects of repulsive and attractive forces between oil globules in an o/w emulsion

The term 'complex film' suggests that the components interact to form some type of molecular complex, which is strongly adsorbed at the oil-water interface. However, it has been suggested (Dervichian, 1958) that the marked changes in the properties of the interface that occur when so-called complex formation takes place may be explained on the basis of the various arrangements of the packed molecules in the adsorbed layer.

W/o Emulsions. Although the ionisation of substances in oils is weak because of the low dielectric constant of these liquids, a small degree of ionisation may occur. Electrical double layers may therefore be associated with water globules dispersed in an oily continuous phase. However, the diffuse part of such double layers is thick and the repulsion energy therefore decreases much more slowly with increasing distance between globules than in o/w emulsions. It has been shown that the potential energy barriers to flocculation that arise from overlapping of electrical double layers are lower in w/o than in o/w emulsions and, furthermore, no secondary minimum is apparent in the net potential energy curves (Sherman, 1963). Flocculation therefore occurs more easily in w/o systems, and flocculated globules are separated only by the small distances associated with primary minima. In addition, the attraction between flocculated globules is strong.

It has been suggested by Schulman and Cockbain (1940) that if the ionic character of an interfacial film is low and its rigidity is high, e.g. unionised solid condensed films, then w/o emulsions will tend to be formed.

2. *Solvation Effects*

It has often been suggested that the effects of hydrophilic groups of adsorbed emulsifier on water molecules in the surrounding aqueous phase give rise to thick solvation sheaths which aid in preventing flocculation. However, although Derjaguin (1964) still advocates this hypothesis, it is more generally believed that solvation effects are of short range and do not contribute to the stability of emulsions against flocculation (Kitchener and Mussellwhite, 1968).

3. *Steric Effects*

The hydrophilic groups of many non-ionic emulsifying agents consist of extended polyethylene oxide chains. Oil globules carrying adsorbed molecules of this type behave as though they are coated with a thick layer of concentrated solution of a hydrophilic

colloid, which may prevent close approach of the oil globules. In addition, the very long hydrocarbon chains of some emulsifying agents may prevent the close approach of water globules dispersed in an oil phase so that the distances of separation are too great for the attractive van der Waals forces to be effective.

FACTORS INFLUENCING THE COALESCENCE OF GLOBULES

It is considered that the process of coalescence of stabilised globules can itself be divided into two stages. The first stage, which involves the drainage of the films of liquid from between the adjacent globules, is followed by rupture of the interfacial films around the globules.

1. *Surface Active Agents*

The close approach of two globules causes mutual distortion of their spherical shapes. In globules stabilised by surface active agents this distortion produces a flattening of the approaching surfaces as the liquid layer that separates them becomes thinner. Since a change from a sphere to any other shape must involve an increase in surface area, it follows that thinning of the liquid lamella between the globules is resisted by surface tension forces. The presence of surface active agent provides additional effects that oppose unequal thinning of the liquid layer. These surface effects delay the drainage time of the liquid from between the globules. When the lamella between the globules reaches a critical dimension, rupture may occur and the globules will coalesce. Mechanical disturbance of the system will increase the likelihood of rupture. If the interfacial films are reasonably stable, drainage may proceed further until the globules are separated by a bimolecular layer of surface active agent containing a small amount of liquid. The resistance to coalescence then depends on the stability of such a layer.

2. *Macromolecular Emulsifying Agents*

These possess many hydrophilic and lipophilic groups and are, therefore, strongly adsorbed at the oil-water interface. In fact, the adsorption is often irreversible. High degrees of emulsion stability can be achieved with these agents since the interfacial films possess mechanical properties that are able to withstand collisions and prevent coalescence. The majority of these agents stabilise o/w emulsions.

3. *Finely Divided Solids*

The particles of such solids will be adsorbed at an oil-water interface if they possess a suitable balance

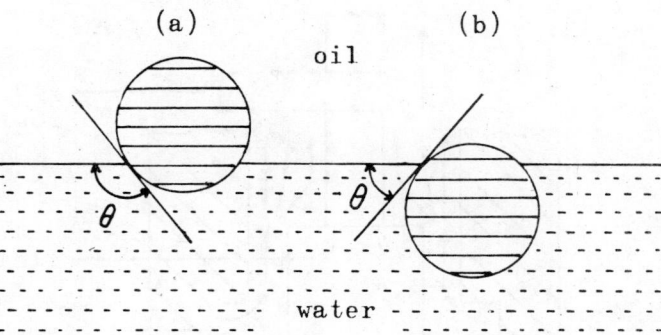

Fig. 5.16 The effect of angle of contact (θ) between solid particles and water on adsorption of particles at the oil-water interface
(a) $\theta > \pi/2$ radians; particle is mainly in the oil phase and will tend to stabilise w/o emulsions
(b) $\theta < \pi/2$ radians; particle is mainly in the aqueous phase and will tend to stabilise o/w emulsions

between their hydrophilic and lipophilic properties. The relative wettabilities of the particles by oil and water will determine their position at the interface, as shown by Fig. 5.16. Since the interfacial area is at a minimum when the bulk of each particle is in the continuous phase, then the type of emulsion that is stabilised is also influenced by the relative hydrophilic and lipophilic properties of the particles.

Although spherical particles are illustrated in Fig. 5.16, anisometric particles are the most efficient emulsion stabilisers. The mechanism of stability is considered to be concerned with the prevention of thinning of liquid lamellae between globules (Kitchener and Mussellwhite, 1968).

The Preparation of Emulsions

The small-scale methods of preparing emulsions are considered by Gunn and Carter (1965). Various types of machine are used for large scale production. These machines may be classified into the following groups.

1. MIXERS, WHISKS OR CHURNS

These involve agitating the ingredients of an emulsion by beaters. The beaters and containing vessel should be designed to provide a continuous movement in all parts of the liquid. In some cases the container may be fitted with a jacket so that heating or cooling effects may be applied.

2. COLLOID MILLS

As the name suggests these mills (see Fig. 5.3) are capable of producing colloidal dispersions. These machines are suitable for preparing emulsions and, unlike the mixers in the previous group, they are capable of continuous production.

3. HOMOGENISERS

These may be operated continuously and are based on the principle that the large globules in a coarse emulsion are broken into smaller globules by passage under pressure through a narrow orifice. Figure 5.17 illustrates the operation of a homogenising valve.

4. ULTRASONIC EMULSIFIERS

If a liquid is subjected to ultrasonic vibrations, alternate regions of compression and rarefaction are produced in it. Cavities are formed in the regions of rarefaction and, later, these collapse with great force which produces emulsification. The required frequency of vibration may be produced electrically, but simple mechanical methods may be used, in which the vibration is produced in a thin metal blade when a jet of the liquid mixture impinges on it. This latter effect is employed in the Rapisonic Homogeniser (Ultrasonics Ltd). Circulation of a coarse emulsion from a reservoir past the vibrating blade into a receiver is involved and further circulation may be applied until an emulsion with the desired globule size distribution is obtained. More information on this machine and its method of use is given by Myers and Goodman (1954).

Pharmaceutical Applications of Emulsions

O/w emulsions are convenient preparations for the oral administration of unpalatable oils or oily solutions of drugs with unpleasant tastes. However, their use in this manner has been decreased by introducing preparations in which the oils are solubilised within micelles, since these systems are not subject to the physical instabilities of emulsions. In addition, the stability of solubilised material is often greater than when it is included in the oil globules of emulsions.

O/w emulsions are also used as a dosage form for the intravenous administration of oils and fats with high calorie contents to patients who cannot ingest food by other means. The globules in these emulsions should be similar in size to chylomicrons.

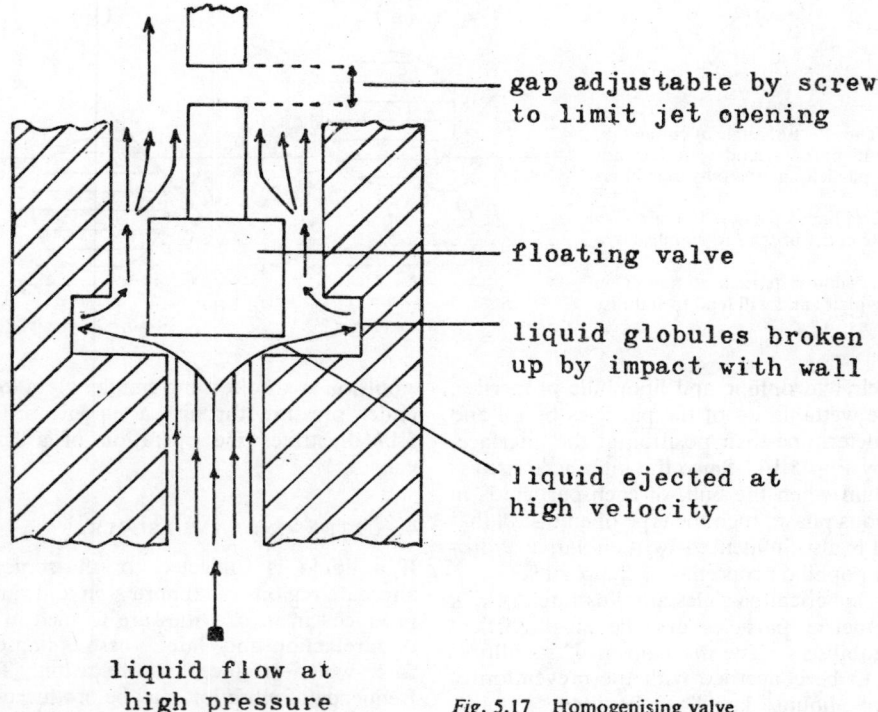

gap adjustable by screw
to limit jet opening

floating valve

liquid globules broken
up by impact with wall

liquid ejected at
high velocity

liquid flow at
high pressure

Fig. 5.17 Homogenising valve

Emulsions of both types (i.e. o/w and w/o) are used extensively in pharmaceutical preparations for external use and in cosmetic preparations. The factors that should be taken into account in formulating these products are considered by Gunn and Carter (1965), Pernarowski (1970), and Becher (1965). The rheological properties of emulsions are a particularly important aspect of the formulation of these systems. The factors that influence these properties are discussed in Chapter 7.

The use of foams in many cosmetic preparations and some pharmaceutical preparations provides an expanding field for the applications of emulsion technology since many of these products are emulsified systems (p. 87).

Foams

A foam is a coarse dispersion of a gas in liquid, which is present as thin sheets or lamellae between the gas bubbles.

Stability of Foams

This is determined by the rate of drainage of the liquid from the foam, which leads to a decrease in the strength of the lamellae. When the lamellae rupture, the liquid contained in them breaks into drops that have a lower total surface than the original film and, consequently, the free energy of the system is decreased. A foam is therefore unstable from a thermodynamic point of view. However, although the lifetimes of foams containing pure liquids and gases are very low, the presence of suitable stabilising agents (foaming agents) can provide almost indefinite stability. Many stabilising agents are available, the most important types of which are the proteins, insoluble powders, and synthetic surface active agents that are adsorbed at the liquid-gas interface.

The drainage rates of liquids from lamellae is reduced by increases in the surface and bulk viscosities of the liquids. In addition, these increases also protect the liquid films against disturbances arising from mechanical and thermal effects. Such changes are particularly important in foam stabilisation, since foaming agents that produce marked increases in the surface viscosity yield foams with high stabilities, whereas those that do not, produce rapidly draining foams of low stability.

The thinning of lamellae is also opposed by the adsorption of ionic foaming agents at the opposite faces of the liquid films. Excessive drainage from such lamellae would bring the similarly charged surfaces closer together. In addition, the increasing concentration of gegenions that builds up in the liquid films tends to oppose drainage by exerting a high osmotic pressure.

The presence of surface active agents also opposes the unequal thinning of liquid films that may, for example, be caused by mechanical shock. This effect arises from the transient change in distribution of the surface active agent that occurs when a film is stretched. It causes the adsorbed monolayer to spread into the extended region of the interface and so prevents an increase in the interfacial free energy.

Foams are often troublesome, and knowledge of the action of substances that cause their destruction (foam breakers or antifoams) is therefore useful. These substances (e.g. ether, n-octanol, silicones) are usually adsorbed at the liquid–gas interface and produce regions of lower surface tension. Extension of the interface in these regions allows further thinning of the lamellae to occur until they eventually rupture.

Preparation of Foams

Foams are usually prepared by shaking the liquid and gas together in the presence of the foaming agent, or by bubbling the gas through a solution of the foaming agent.

The use of pressurised containers for the presentation of foams is of particular interest in pharmacy. The general advantages of this type of container have already been listed (p. 74). Systems used in this type of preparation include:

(a) emulsions containing the liquefied propellant, water, and active ingredients. When the valve on the container is opened the vapour pressure of the propellant forces the emulsion out of the container through a nozzle. At atmospheric pressure and room temperature the emulsified propellant reverts to a vapour and so produces a foam;

(b) emulsified products used in conjunction with soluble compressed gases such as carbon dioxide. This type of system is usually shaken before use in order to disperse some of the gas throughout the liquid concentrate. When the valve is opened, emulsion plus entrapped gas is forced out of the container by the pressure of the compressed gas inside. The liberation of entrapped gas whips the concentrated emulsion into a foam.

Pharmaceutical Applications of Foams

Variation of the ingredients used in the emulsified systems that are presented in pressurised containers allows the formulation of aqueous or non-aqueous foams that are either stable or rapidly breaking. It has been suggested that various types of product would be useful for topical preparations, rectal and vaginal medication and for burn dressings.

A further application of foams is encountered in the preparation of the absorbable haemostats Human Fibrin Foam and Gelatin Sponge (p. 425).

BIBLIOGRAPHY

ADAMSON, A. W. (1967) *Physical Chemistry of Surfaces.* 2nd ed. Interscience, New York.

BECHER, P. (1965) *Emulsions: Theory and Practice.* 2nd ed. Reinhold, New York.

BIKERMAN, J. J. (1958) *Surface Chemistry.* 2nd ed. Academic Press, New York.

DAVIES, J. T. and RIDEAL, E. K. (1963) *Interfacial Phenomena.* 2nd ed. Academic Press, New York.

JIRGENSONS, B. (1958) *Organic Colloids.* Elsevier, Amsterdam.

KRUYT, H. R. (1952 and 1949) *Colloid Science. Vols. I and II.* Elsevier, Amsterdam.

MOILLIET, J. L., COLLIE, B., and BLACK, W. (1961) *Surface Activity.* 2nd ed. Spon, London.

MULLEY, B. A. (1964) *Advances in Pharmaceutical Sciences. Vol. 1.* (H. S. Bean, A. H. Beckett, and J. E. Carless, Eds). Academic Press, London. Chapter 2.

SHERMAN, P. (1968) *Emulsion Science.* Academic Press, London.

SHINODA, K., NAKAGURA, T., TAMAMUSHI, B., and ISEMURA T. (1963) *Colloidal Surfactants.* Academic Press, London.

TROTMAN-DICKENSON, A. F. and PARFITT, G. D. (1966) *Chemical Kinetics and Surface and Colloid Chemistry.* Pergamon, London.

WILLIAMS, V. R. and WILLIAMS, H. B. (1967) *Basic Physical Chemistry for the Life Sciences.* Freeman and Co., San Francisco.

REFERENCES

BECHER, P. (1965) *Emulsions: Theory and Practice.* 2nd ed. Reinhold, New York.

COOPER, K. E. (1963) *Analytical Microbiology.* (F. Kavanagh Ed.) Academic Press, London. Chapter 1.

COOPER, K. E. and WOODMAN, D. (1946) The diffusion of antiseptics through agar gels, with special reference to the agar cup assay method of estimating the activity of penicillin. *J. Path. Bact.* **58,** 75–84.

CRAIG, L. C. and KONISBERG, W. (1961) Dialysis studies III. Modification of pore size and shape in cellophane membranes. *J. phys. Chem., Ithaca* **65**, 166–172.

DERJAGUIN, B. V. and LANDAU, L. D. (1941) Theory of the stability of strongly charged lyophobic sols and the adhesion of strongly charged particles in solutions of electrolytes. *Acta phys.-chim. URSS*, **14**, 633.

DERJAGUIN, B. V. (1964) *Nineteenth Symposium of the Society of Experimental Biology*, Swansea, 55.

DERVICHIAN, D. G. (1958) *Surface Phenomena in Chemistry and Biology*. (J. F. Danielli, K. G. A. Pankhurst, and A. C. Riddiford, Eds) Pergamon, London. Chapter 5.

EVERSOLE, W. G. and DOUGHTY, E. W. (1935) Diffusion coefficients of molecules and ions. *J. phys. Chem. Ithaca*, **34**, 289.

GUNN, C. and CARTER, S. J. (1965) *Dispensing for Pharmaceutical Students*. 11th ed. Pitman Medical, London.

HERMANS, P. H. (1949) *Colloid Science. Vol. II.* (H. R. Kruyt, Ed.) Elsevier, Amsterdam. Chapter 12.

JIRGENSONS, B. (1958) *Organic Colloids*. Elsevier, Amsterdam.

KITCHENER, J. A. and MUSSELLWHITE, P. R. (1968) *Emulsion Science*. (P. Sherman, Ed.). Academic Press, London. Chapter 2.

MICHAELS, A. S. and BOLGER, J. C. (1964) Particle interactions in aqueous kaolinite dispersions. *Ind. Engng. Chem. Fundamentals*, **3**, 14–20.

MYERS, J. A. and GOODMAN, J. E. (1954) Pharmaceutical applications of ultrasonics. *Pharm. J.* **173**, 422–424.

OVERBEEK, J. TH. G. (1952) *Colloid Science. Vol. I.* (H. R. Kruyt, Ed.) Elsevier, Amsterdam. Chapter 2.

PERNAROWSKI, M. (1970) *Remington's Pharmaceutical Sciences*. 14th ed. Mack Publishing Co., Pennsylvania. Chapter 80.

SCHULMAN, J. H. and COCKBAIN, E. G. (1940) Molecular interactions at oil–water interfaces. (I) Molecular complex formation and the stability of oil-in-water emulsions. (II) Phase inversion and the stability of water-in-oil emulsions. *Trans. Faraday Soc.* **36**, 651–660 and 661–668.

SCIARRA, J. J. (1970) *Remington's Pharmaceutical Sciences*. 14th ed. Mack Publishing Co., Pennsylvania. Chapter 90.

SHELUDKO, A. (1966) *Colloid Chemistry*. Elsevier, Amsterdam.

SHERMAN, P. (1963) Changes in the rheological properties of emulsions on ageing, and their dependence on the kinetics of globule coagulation. *J. phys. Chem. Ithaca* **67**, 2531–2537.

SHERMAN, P., Ed. (1968) *Emulsion Science*. Academic Press, London. Chapter 4.

THEIMER, W. (1960) Structure and ageing of gelatin gels. *Z. Naturf.* Pt. 15b, 346–350.

VAN DEN TEMPEL, M. (1953) Stability of oil-in-water emulsions. I The electrical double layer at the oil-water interface. II Mechanism of the coagulation of an emulsion. III Measurement of the rate of coagulation of an oil-in-water emulsion. *Recl. Trav. chim. Pays-Bas Belg.* **72**, 419–432, 433–441 and 442–461.

VAN OLPHEN, H. (1963) *An introduction to Clay Colloid Chemistry*. Interscience, London.

VERWEY, E. J. W. and OVERBEEK, J. TH. G. (1948) *Theory of the Stability of Lyophobic Colloids*. Elsevier, Amsterdam.

6

Kinetics

INVESTIGATIONS on the rates at which changes occur in a particular system and the factors that influence such rates are known as kinetic studies. They are useful in providing information that (a) gives an insight into the mechanism of the change involved, and (b) allows prediction of the degree of change that will occur after a given time has elapsed.

In general, the theories and laws of chemical kinetics are well proven and provide a sound basis for the application of such studies to pharmaceutical problems that involve chemical reactions; e.g. the decomposition of medicinal compounds. However, kinetic studies of the processes involved in the absorption of drugs into, their distribution within, and removal from living organisms are more recent. The theoretical basis of drug kinetics is therefore often less well-founded than that of chemical kinetics. Nevertheless, the application of knowledge derived from these studies allows a more rational approach to be made towards the synthesis of medicinal compounds with particular activities and to the effects of formulation on these activities. In addition, the increasing amount of information that is becoming available will increase the application of these studies in pharmacy.

This chapter attempts to indicate the more important applications of kinetic studies in pharmacy. Those concerned with chemical reactions will be discussed initially and followed by those concerned with the behaviour of drugs in living organisms.

CHEMICAL KINETICS

EXTENT OF REACTION

Consider the formation of a compound B from the reaction between two molecules of a compound A; e.g. a dimerisation. This reaction may be described by Eqn (6.1).

$$2A = B \qquad (6.1)$$

The extent to which this reaction has proceeded may be defined in terms of the change in either the amount of product B or the amount of reactant A.

The change in the amount of B is the difference between the amount of B produced (n_B) and the amount of B present at the starting point ($n_{B,0}$). (The starting point is usually the beginning of the reaction where $n_{B,0} = 0$.) Thus, the extent of reaction (ξ) defined in terms of the change in amount of substance B is given by Eqn (6.2).

$$\xi = n_B - n_{B,0} \qquad (6.2)$$

The change in the amount of A is the difference between the amount present at the starting point ($n_{A,0}$) and the amount that remains (n_A). However, two molecules of A are involved in the balanced Eqn (6.1) and the extent of reaction (ξ) defined in terms of the change in the amount of reactant A is given by Eqn (6.3).

$$\xi = \frac{n_{A,0} - n_A}{2} \qquad (6.3)$$

It is obvious from Eqn (6.1) that Eqns (6.2) and (6.3) will give the same value of ξ. It is therefore convenient to write a general equation for the definition of extent of reaction. This is represented by Eqn (6.4),

$$\xi = \frac{n_X - n_{X,0}}{\nu_X} \qquad (6.4)$$

where n_X and $n_{X,0}$ are the actual and initial amounts of a substance X that is involved in a reaction as a reactant or a product. ν_X is called the stoichiometric number of X and it indicates the number of molecules (or atoms, or radicals, or ions) of X that are involved in the balanced equation, which describes the reaction under consideration. When X is a product the difference ($n_X - n_{X,0}$) is positive because the amount of product increases as the reaction proceeds; (i.e. $n_X > n_{X,0}$). However, if X is a reactant, ($n_X - n_{X,0}$) is negative because the amount of X will decrease as reaction proceeds; (i.e. $n_X < n_{X,0}$). This variation in the sign of ($n_X - n_{X,0}$) is overcome by using the convention that the stoichiometric number v_X is positive for a product and negative for a reactant, so that the right-hand side of Eqn (6.4) is always positive.

It can be seen from Eqn (6.4) that the dimension of extent of reaction, ξ, will be amount of substance and, therefore, the units of ξ will be the same as those of n_X, for which the basic SI unit is the mole.

The change in extent of reaction $(d\xi)$ with increasing change in amount of substance X (dn_X) may be expressed by Eqn (6.5), where v_X is defined as before.

$$dn_X = v_X \, d\xi \qquad (6.5)$$

Rate of Reaction ($\dot{\xi}$)

This may be defined as the rate of increase of the extent of reaction (i.e. $d\xi/dt$) as is shown by Eqn (6.6).

$$\dot{\xi} = d\xi/dt \qquad (6.6)$$

The dimensions of $\dot{\xi}$ will be amount of substance per unit time and its basic SI unit will be moles per second (mol s^{-1}). From Eqns (6.5) and (6.6) it can be seen that

$$\dot{\xi} = \frac{d\xi}{dt} = \frac{1}{v_X}\frac{dn_X}{dt} \qquad (6.7)$$

where dn_X/dt may be called the rate of formation of X if X is a product, or the rate of disappearance of X if X is a reactant.

Equations (6.6) and (6.7) are general ones for the definition of rate of reaction and they are independent of the conditions under which a reaction is carried out. For example, they are valid for reactions in which the volume varies with time or where the reaction occurs in more than one phase.

When discussing chemical kinetics it is convenient to divide reactions into two classes; homogeneous and heterogeneous reactions. The former occur in one phase, e.g. in solution, while the latter occur at the interface between two phases, e.g. at solid–gas or solid–liquid interfaces.

HOMOGENEOUS REACTIONS

These reactions are usually classified on the basis of the effect of the concentration of reactants on the rates of increase in concentration of products or decrease in concentration of reactants. To convert Eqn (6.7) to concentration terms it is necessary to divide by the volume, V, of the homogeneous system, when Eqn (6.8) is obtained.

$$\frac{1}{V}\frac{d\xi}{dt} = \frac{1}{Vv_X}\frac{dn_X}{dt} \qquad (6.8)$$

If the volume, V, of the phase does not vary with

time during the reaction then Eqn (6.8) may be written in the form of Eqn (6.9),

$$\frac{1}{V}\frac{d\xi}{dt} = \frac{1}{v_X}\frac{d(n_X/V)}{dt} \qquad (6.9)$$

However, the term n_X/V represents the concentration of substance X and may be replaced by a single term; e.g. c_X or $[X]$, and Eqn (6.9) may be rewritten as,

$$\frac{1}{V}\frac{d\xi}{dt} = \frac{1}{v_X}\frac{dc_X}{dt} = \frac{1}{v_X}\frac{d[X]}{dt} \qquad (6.10)$$

If X is a product the rate at which its concentration increases is represented by the symbol v_X and is equal to the term dc_X/dt in Eqn (6.10). If X is a reactant, then v_X represents its rate of disappearance, given by $v_X = -dc_X/dt$. The minus sign is necessary in this latter case because the concentration of a reactant decreases with time. Thus, the term $-dc_X/dt$ is positive because dc_X is negative.

Order of Reaction

Experiments show that the rates of change in the concentrations of products or reactants usually depend on the concentrations of the reactants. This dependence is indicated by Eqn (6.11),

$$v \propto [A]^a[B]^b \quad \text{or} \quad v = k[A]^a[B]^b \qquad (6.11)$$

where $[A]$ and $[B]$ are the concentrations of reactants A and B respectively, a and b are some powers of these concentrations, and k is a proportionality constant known as the rate constant of the reaction at a particular temperature.

Classification of reactions may be achieved by division into various orders, where the order of a reaction is given by the sum of the powers of the concentration terms involved in equations, such as that represented by Eqn (6.11). For example, in this particular case the order of reaction is given by $(a + b)$. In fact, this represents the overall order of the reaction. It is also possible to refer to the order of a reaction with respect to a particular reactant. Thus, the above reaction is of order a with respect to A, and of order b with respect to B.

Homogeneous reactions are usually interpreted in terms of simple orders of reaction, which are discussed below.

(a) First Order Reactions

The rate of change in the concentrations of products and reactants in this type of reaction is proportional to the first power of the concentration (c_X) of a single reactant (X) and is independent of the concentration of any other substance that may be present.

The rate of formation of a product Y is therefore given by Eqn (6.12) and the rate of disappearance of reactant X is given by Eqn (6.13)

$$v_Y = \frac{dc_Y}{dt} = kc_X \qquad (6.12)$$

$$v_X = -\frac{dc_X}{dt} = kc_X \qquad (6.13)$$

where k is the rate constant.

If the concentration of reactant X at the beginning of a reaction when time $t = 0$ is denoted by a, and the amount that has reacted after time t is denoted by x, then the amount of X that remains at this time is given by $(a - x)$. Equation (6.13) may therefore be rewritten in the form shown by Eqn (6.14)

$$-\frac{dc_X}{dt} = k(a - x) \quad \text{or} \quad \frac{dc_X}{a - x} = -k\,dt \qquad (6.14)$$

where $-dc_X/dt$ represents the rate of decrease in the concentration of X. Integration of Eqn (6.14) between the time limits of 0 and t gives

$$\int_a^{(a-x)} \frac{dc_X}{a - x} = -k \int_0^t dt$$

$$\therefore \quad \ln(a - x) - \ln a = -kt$$

Converting from natural logarithms gives

$$\log(a - x) - \log a = -\frac{kt}{2\cdot303}$$

or

$$\log(a - x) = \log a - \frac{kt}{2\cdot303} \qquad (6.15)$$

It can be seen that Eqn (6.15) is representative of a linear relation (i.e. $y = c + mx$) and the variables are $(a - x)$ and t. If the first order law is obeyed, then a graph of $\log(a - x)$ versus t will give a straight line with a slope of $-k/2\cdot303$ and an intercept at $t = 0$ of $\log a$.

The rate constant k may therefore be calculated from the slope of such a graph. It may also be obtained by substitution of experimental values into Eqn (6.16) which is a rearranged form of Eqn (6.15).

$$k = \frac{2\cdot303}{t} \log \frac{a}{a - x} \qquad (6.16)$$

It can be seen that the dimension of k for a first order reaction is reciprocal time and the basic SI unit is the reciprocal second (s^{-1}).

(b) Second Order Reactions

The rate of change in the concentrations of products and reactants in this type of reaction is proportional either to the second power of the concentration of a single reactant, or to the first powers of the concentrations of two reactants. These two possibilities are illustrated by the following Eqns (6.17) and (6.18), which refer to the rate of decrease in the concentration of reactant X—

(i) $\qquad v_X = -dc_X/dt = k[X][Y] \qquad (6.17)$

(ii) $\qquad v_X = -dc_X/dt = k[X]^2 \qquad (6.18)$

where the rates of concentration change are dependent on the concentrations of reactants X and Y, or X only. In the first type of second order reaction given above the rate of decrease in concentration of reactant Y will be equal to that of X (i.e. $v_Y = v_X$). If the concentrations of reactants X and Y at time $t = 0$ are given by a and b respectively, and the concentration of each substance that has reacted after time t is equal to x, then the concentrations of X and Y that remain after this time are given by $(a - x)$ and $(b - x)$ respectively. Equation (6.17) may therefore be rewritten as

$$-\frac{dx}{dt} = k(a - x)(b - x) \qquad (6.19)$$

where $-dx/dt$ represents the rate of decrease in the concentration of X (or Y). Integration of Eqn (6.19) yields Eqn (6.20)

$$kt = \frac{2\cdot303}{(a - b)} \log \frac{b(a - x)}{a(b - x)} \qquad (6.20)$$

where k is the rate constant.

Rearrangement of Eqn (6.20) yields

$$\log \frac{a - x}{b - x} = \frac{(a - b)kt}{2\cdot303} + \log \frac{a}{b} \qquad (6.21)$$

and if the second order law is obeyed, then a graph of the left-hand side of Eqn (6.21) against time t should produce a straight line with a slope equal to $(a - b)k/2\cdot303$, and an intercept at $t = 0$ of $\log(a/b)$.

When the initial concentrations of reactants X and Y are equal (i.e. $a = b$) or when the second power of a single reactant determines the rate of concentration change, then the integrated form of the rate equation is given by Eqn (6.22)

$$kt = \frac{x}{a(a - x)} \qquad (6.22)$$

Rearrangement of Eqn (6.22) yields

$$\frac{1}{(a - x)} - \frac{1}{a} = kt \qquad (6.23)$$

and if the second law is obeyed then a graph of $1/(a - x)$ against time should produce a straight line with a slope of k and an intercept of $1/a$ at $t = 0$.

It can be shown from the previous equations that the rate constant for a second order reaction has the dimensions of time^{-1} concentration^{-1} and the SI unit is m^3 mol^{-1} s^{-1}.

(c) Pseudo First Order Reactions

If a large excess of one of the reactants in a second order reaction is present throughout the reaction, then its concentration remains virtually constant and the rate of concentration change follows the first order law. Hydrolysis reactions in dilute aqueous solution are common examples of this type of reaction, which is known as a pseudo first order reaction.

However, it should be borne in mind that a decrease in the concentration of water, e.g. caused by a change in the composition of the solvent, may lead to a reaction that follows second order kinetics.

(d) Reactions of Third and Higher Orders

The rates of change in concentrations in this type of reaction are proportional to three concentration terms. However, such reactions are rare and their analysis is complex. Reactions of even higher orders are unlikely to occur.

(e) Zero Order Reactions

The rates of change in the concentrations of re-actants and products in reactions of this type are dependent on some factor other than the concentration of a reactant. They include photochemical reactions that depend on the absorption of light and heterogeneous reactions that depend on the area of the interface at which reaction occurs (p. 94, 96).

The rate of change in concentration of a reactant X is constant in a zero order reaction as indicated by Eqn (6.24), where k is the rate constant, which has the same dimensions as v_X; i.e. mol s^{-1}.

$$v_X = -\frac{dc_X}{dt} = k \qquad (6.24)$$

If the amount of X that reacts in time t is denoted by x then the integrated form of the equation for a zero order reaction is given by

$$x = kt \qquad (6.25)$$

Half-life ($t_{\frac{1}{2}}$)

The half-life of a reaction is the time required for the concentration of a reactant to decrease to half its original value; i.e. when $x = a/2$ in the previous equations. The expressions of half-life in terms of the rate constant (k) for the disappearance of reactant are shown in Table 6.1 for simple orders of reaction. It can be seen from these expressions that half-life can be defined in terms of Eqn (6.26) for the simple orders given in Table 6.1.

$$t_{\frac{1}{2}} \propto \frac{1}{a^{(n-1)}} \qquad (6.26)$$

The half-life of a reaction provides a convenient means of expressing the rate of concentration change of a reactant and is particularly useful because the time taken for complete reaction is theoretically infinite except in zero order reactions.

Methods of Determining the Order of a Reaction

1. Graphical Method

A straight line is obtained when the data from kinetic experiments are plotted in the form that is relevant to the order of a particular reaction. The

Table 6.1
Summary of Information on Reactions of Simple Orders

Order	Integrated rate equation	Half-life equation	Linear graph			
			Ordinate	Abscissa	Slope	Intercept
Zero	$x = kt$	$t_{\frac{1}{2}} = \dfrac{a}{2k}$	x	t	k	0
First	$\log \dfrac{a}{(a-x)} = \dfrac{kt}{2\cdot303}$	$t_{\frac{1}{2}} = \dfrac{0\cdot693}{k}$	$\log(a-x)$	t	$-\dfrac{k}{2\cdot303}$	$\log a$
Second $(a = b)$	$\dfrac{x}{a(a-x)} = kt$	$t_{\frac{1}{2}} = \dfrac{1}{ak}$	$\dfrac{1}{a-x}$	t	k	$\dfrac{1}{a}$

ordinates and abscissae of graphs for simple orders are summarised in Table 6.1, together with the values of the slopes and intercepts of these graphs.

2. Substitution Method

The order of a reaction is indicated by the particular integrated rate equation that gives a constant value of k for data obtained from a kinetic experiment. The integrated equations are given in Table 6.1 for simple orders of reaction.

3. Half-life Method

Consider a reaction in which the initial concentration of the reactant is a_1 and the concentration at a later time is a_2. These concentrations may be regarded as the starting points of two separate reactions, and the corresponding half-lives may be represented by $t_{\frac{1}{2}(1)}$ and $t_{\frac{1}{2}(2)}$, respectively. From Eqn (6.26) it is possible to write that

$$t_{\frac{1}{2}(1)} \propto \frac{1}{a_1^{(n-1)}}$$

and

$$t_{\frac{1}{2}(2)} \propto \frac{1}{a_2^{(n-1)}}$$

$$\therefore \frac{t_{\frac{1}{2}(1)}}{t_{\frac{1}{2}(2)}} = \frac{a_2^{(n-1)}}{a_1^{(n-1)}}$$

$$\therefore \log \frac{t_{\frac{1}{2}(1)}}{t_{\frac{1}{2}(2)}} = (n-1) \log \frac{a_2}{a_1}$$

$$\therefore n = \frac{\log (t_{\frac{1}{2}(1)}/t_{\frac{1}{2}(2)})}{\log (a_2/a_1)} + 1 \qquad (6.27)$$

COMPLEX REACTIONS

Many reactions involve several stages and the kinetics of the overall reaction cannot be expressed in terms of simple orders of reaction. However, it is often possible to determine the order of the separate stages. The following types of complex reaction are encountered frequently and examples of each type are given by Martin et al. (1969) and Saunders (1966).

1. Simultaneous Reactions

These involve the production of two or more products from the same reactant by different reactions, which proceed at different rates. They may be represented diagrammatically as

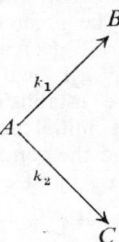

Substitution reactions into aromatic nuclei are examples of this type of complex reaction; e.g. the simultaneous formation of 1- and 4-nitrophenols during the nitration of phenol.

2. Consecutive Reactions

These may be represented diagrammatically as

$$A \xrightarrow{k_1} B \xrightarrow{k_2} C$$

and each stage proceeds at a particular rate. The overall rate will be determined by the rate of the slowest stage.

3. Chain Reactions

These reactions usually proceed at slow rates under normal conditions but these rates are increased, often very markedly, by the presence of substances that are able to produce free radicals. (A free radical is an electrically uncharged atom or group of atoms with an unpaired electron and is highly reactive.) Polymerisation and oxidation of unsaturated organic compounds are important examples of reactions that involve a chain mechanism.

4. Reversible Reactions

These are reactions in which the reaction products react to produce the original reactants. They may be represented diagrammatically as

$$A \underset{k_2}{\overset{k_1}{\rightleftharpoons}} B$$

where the arrows indicate that the opposing reactions are proceeding simultaneously.

The rate of increase in concentration of $A(v_A)$ is given by Eqn (6.28)

$$v_A = \frac{dc_A}{dt} = -k_1 c_A + k_2 c_B \qquad (6.28)$$

where c_A and c_B are the concentrations of substances A and B, and k_1 and k_2 are the rate constants for the forward and reverse reactions, respectively. In the initial stages of reaction the concentration of A will be large while that of B will be small. The product $k_1 c_A$ will therefore be greater than $k_2 c_B$ and the concentration of A will decrease and that of B will increase. Eventually $k_1 c_A$ will equal $k_2 c_B$, and an equilibrium will be established where $dc_A/dt = dc_B/dt = 0$. If the initial concentration of A is denoted by $c_{A.0}$, and the concentrations of A and B at equilibrium are $c_{A.e}$ and $c_{B.e}$ respectively, then

$$c_{B.e} = c_{A.0} - c_{A.e}$$

and

$$\frac{c_{B.e}}{c_{A.e}} = \frac{k_1}{k_2}$$

$$\therefore \quad \frac{c_{A.0} - c_{A.e}}{c_{A.e}} = \frac{k_1}{k_2} = K \qquad (6.29)$$

where K, which is known as the equilibrium constant, is the ratio of the forward reaction rate constant to the reverse reaction rate constant. Its dimensions will depend on the number of concentration terms in the numerator and denominator respectively of Eqn (6.29), and if it is not a dimensionless number, i.e. if the concentration terms do not cancel completely, its units will depend on those in which the remaining terms are expressed.

All chemical reactions probably come to some equilibrium if sufficient time is allowed, provided the products are not removed from the system. However, in many cases reaction may be regarded as being irreversible for practical purposes, since the rate constant for the reverse reaction is very small. The higher the value of K the closer the forward reaction approaches completion.

HETEROGENEOUS REACTIONS

As previously stated these reactions occur at the interface between two phases. Although the rates of these reactions may be defined by the general Eqns (6.6) and (6.7) the interpretation of their kinetics in terms of simple models such as first and second order laws is prevented by the influence of other factors on the rates of concentration change of products and reactants. For example, the area of the interface and the porosity of the solid phase are particularly important in controlling these rates.

Ion Exchange

The exchange of ions between a solid phase and a solution is one of the most important examples of heterogeneous reactions. These reactions involve an exchange between mobile ions associated with a solid and similarly charged ions in a solution and

they may be illustrated by the following equations—

$$RSO_3H + NaCl \rightleftharpoons RSO_3Na + HCl \qquad (6.30)$$

In this equation, RSO_3H represents an insoluble material which produces fixed anions (RSO_3^-) and mobile cations (H^+) on ionisation. The mobile cations are exchangeable with other cations (e.g. Na^+) as shown in the above equation. The insoluble RSO_3H is therefore termed a cation exchanger.

$$RN(CH_3)_3OH + NaCl \rightleftharpoons RN(CH_3)_3Cl + NaOH$$
$$(6.31)$$

This equation represents the exchange of mobile OH^- ions by Cl^- and the insoluble material $RN(CH_3)_3OH$, which contains fixed cations, is termed an anion exchanger.

The materials (RSO_3H and $RN(CH_3)_3OH$) involved in the above reactions are typical examples of organic ion exchange resins, where R represents a resin, which usually consists of polymeric chains of styrene that are cross-linked by divinyl benzene, as shown in Fig. 6.1. An increase in the proportion of divinyl benzene increases the degree of cross-linking and therefore decreases the porosity and increases the rigidity of these resins.

The ion exchange groups (e.g. $-SO_3H$ and $-N(CH_3)_3OH$) are introduced by chemical reaction between the hydrocarbon polymer and suitable reagents. The nature of the ion exchange group that is introduced will determine the type of ions that can be exchanged and provides a means of classifying ion exchange resins into the following groups.

(a) Strong Cation Exchangers

These contain strongly acidic groups such as $-SO_3H$, and the mobile H^+ ions are capable of exchanging with the cations of salts of strong acids. For example, Eqn (6.30) illustrates the exchange of sodium ions from a solution of sodium chloride. The opposing arrows in this equation indicate that the exchange process is reversible and an equilibrium is therefore obtained. The reversibility also indicates that the original acid form of the ion exchange resin (i.e. RSO_3H) can be regenerated from the sodium form by washing with dilute hydrochloric or sulphuric acid.

(b) Strong Anion Exchangers

These contain quaternary ammonium groups attached to the hydrocarbon resin, and the mobile OH^- ions of the hydroxides of these resins are capable of exchanging with the anions of salts of

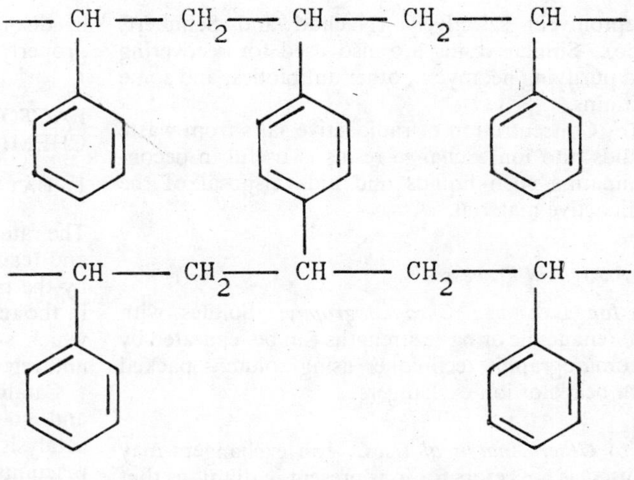

Fig. 6.1 Structure of a styrene–divinyl benzene resin

strong bases. Equation (6.31) illustrates the exchange of chloride ions from a solution of sodium chloride, and the reversibility of this equation indicates that the original ion exchange resin can be regenerated by treatment with dilute NaOH.

(c) Weak Cation Exchangers

These contain weaker acidic groups than the sulphonated strong cation exchangers. For example, carboxylic acid groups may be introduced into the resin structure. This type of resin is only capable of exchanging hydrogen for the cations of weak acids and its efficiency decreases as the pH of the solution decreases because the ionisation of the weakly acidic —COOH groups is depressed at low pH.

(d) Weak Anion Exchangers

These usually contain amine groups and the disappearance of anions from the solution in contact with such exchangers may be explained on the basis of an acid adsorption mechanism, i.e.

$$RNH_2 + HX = RNH_3X$$

or by the following exchange mechanism

$$RNH_2 + H_2O \rightleftharpoons RNH_3^+ + OH^-$$

$$\Updownarrow X^-$$

$$RNH_3X + OH^-$$

APPLICATIONS OF ION EXCHANGERS

1. Demineralisation of Water

This is the most important use of ion exchange. It involves the removal of cations and anions from impurities in water and their replacement by hydrogen and hydroxyl ions respectively. The exchange reactions may be carried out in two separate stages: the first involves passage of the water through a column packed with beads of a cation exchanger; the second involves a similar treatment with an anion exchanger. Each resin can be regenerated easily when necessary. However, it is also possible to carry out the exchange reactions in a single process, which involves the use of a mixed bed of cation and anion exchangers. The different resins must then be separated before regeneration of each can be carried out. Separation is achieved by forcing water into the bottom of the column, when the lighter anion exchanger beads rise above the cation exchanger beads.

This method of water purification is cheaper than distillation and for many purposes the product is superior to distilled water.

Although considerable evidence indicates that certain ion exchange resins will remove pyrogens from water the BP does not allow the use of demineralised water as Water for Injections (Gunn and Carter, 1965).

2. Other Purification Processes

(a) Ionic impurities can be removed from solutions of non-electrolytes such as glycerol, ethanol, and sugars. Similar impurities can also be removed from solutions of macromolecules such as proteins.

(b) The collection and purification of ionic compounds of pharmaceutical importance may be achieved by using ion exchange techniques; for example, streptomycin is a cation and carboxylic acid cation exchange resin may be used in its collection and purification. The efficiency of the process is usually increased by the use of resins that adsorb streptomycin selectively (Nachod and Schubert, 1956). Similar resins are also used for recovering and purifying neomycin, other antibiotics, and some vitamins.

(c) Concentration of radioactive salts from waste liquids into ion exchange resins is useful in decontaminating such liquids and aids disposal of the radioactive material.

3. Analytical Processes

(a) *Ion Exchange Chromatography.* Solutes with different acidic or basic strengths can be separated by chromatographic techniques using columns packed with beads of ion exchangers.

(b) *Other Analytical Uses.* Ion exchangers may be used as collectors for ions present in dilutions that are too low for accurate determination. They may also be used to remove interfering ions before analytical procedures are carried out.

4. Formulation of Prolonged Release Dosage Forms

The exchange of ionic forms of drugs held by resins with ions present in body fluids is a relatively slow process and the rate of exchange can be controlled by variation in the properties of the resin. Such a mechanism is therefore used in formulating dosage forms that are intended to release the drug into the body over a prolonged period.

5. Medical Uses

(a) *As Antacids.* The removal of acid by weak anion exchangers is achieved without causing side effects such as constipation or diarrhoea that often result after treatment with conventional antacids.

(b) *As Laxatives and Anti-obesity Agents.* The marked swelling of weakly crosslinked ion exchange resins allows them to act as bulk laxatives. Such resins are also used as anti-obesity agents because on swelling they create a feeling of fullness in the patient.

(c) *Control of Salt Intake.* A low salt intake by the body is required in the treatment of various oedemas and hypertensive conditions. Cation exchangers allow the use of more salt in the diet of patients suffering from these disorders and the diet can therefore be made more palatable than those that have no or low salt contents.

The potassium level in the blood can also be regulated by cation exchange resins, when necessary, in disorders where the kidneys do not function properly.

FACTORS INFLUENCING RATE OF CHEMICAL REACTIONS

1. CATALYSIS

The rate of change in the concentrations of products and reactants in a chemical reaction may be altered by the presence of a catalyst. The latter takes part in the reaction by forming an intermediate complex which subsequently decomposes into the products and regenerated catalyst.

Catalysts may dissolve in the reaction medium and so result in what is termed homogeneous catalysis, or they may remain as solids, when the reactants are adsorbed on to their surfaces. This latter process is referred to as heterogeneous catalysis.

Homogeneous catalysis includes the effect of pH on the hydrolysis of many compounds. For example, the rate of decrease in concentration of sucrose in acid solution that results from hydrolysis is approximately proportional to the concentration of hydrogen ions. This effect of pH is important in the stabilisation of many pharmaceutical preparations since an optimum pH for maximum stability of an active ingredient often exists. For example, Injection of Ergometrine BP (1968) is adjusted to pH 3 by the addition of maleic acid. In addition, the containers used for many official preparations must comply with a test for the limit of alkalinity (*see* Gunn and Carter, 1965).

Chemisorption is now accepted as being necessary in the process of heterogeneous catalysis. The strong adsorption of reactants at active sites on the surfaces of catalysts produces a local concentration of reactants in a particular orientation. In addition, the bonds within the chemisorbed molecules are weakened. All these factors will affect the rate of reaction. Heterogeneous catalysts are often used in hydrogenation reactions and these catalysts include palladium, platinum, and nickel.

Since heterogeneous catalysis occurs at the surface of a solid catalyst it is influenced by the surface area of the solid and by the presence of other compounds, which may also be adsorbed strongly, and so poison the surface.

Enzymes are usually regarded as heterogeneous catalysts although they are often soluble in water. However, adsorption of the substrate on to the enzyme macromolecules is involved in the catalysed reaction. The first stage of the reaction may be considered to be the formation of a complex, ES, between the enzyme, E, and substrate, S, and this is followed by decomposition of the complex into products plus enzyme. This series of stages may be represented by Eqn (6.32), which shows that the first stage is reversible but the second is not.

$$E + S \underset{k_{-1}}{\overset{k_1}{\rightleftharpoons}} ES \xrightarrow{k_2} E + \text{products} \quad (6.32)$$

The kinetics of such reactions catalysed by enzymes is interpreted by the Michaelis-Menten theory that is named after the original workers in this field. This theory is based on the fact that the second stage in Eqn (6.32) is the rate determining stage, since it is much slower than the first. The changes in concentrations of substrate and products are therefore dependent on the concentration of the complex ES, since this determines the rate of the second stage. However, the concentration of the complex cannot be measured and must therefore be defined in other terms that are measurable. This treatment leads to the Michaelis-Menten Eqn (6.33), which expresses the rate of decomposition of the substrate ($-\mathrm{d}s/\mathrm{d}t$) in terms of the substrate concentration S at any time, a constant, V, which is equal to the maximum rate that is possible (i.e. when all the enzyme is involved in complex formation), and a constant, K_m, that is known as the Michaelis constant. In fact this constant is the ratio of the rate constant for the reverse reaction in the first stage of Eqn (6.32) to the rate constant for the forward reaction in the same stage (i.e. $K_m = k_{-1}/k_1$).

$$v = -\frac{\mathrm{d}s}{\mathrm{d}t} = \frac{K_m V S}{1 + K_m S} \quad (6.33)$$

Equation (6.33) does not permit easy determination of the constants K_m and V, and various forms of it have been suggested to facilitate such determination. For example, the Lineweaver-Burk equation, Eqn (6.34), indicates that a straight line will be obtained if $1/v$ is plotted against $1/S$.

$$\frac{1}{v} = \frac{K_m}{V}\frac{1}{S} + \frac{1}{V} \quad (6.34)$$

The slope of this line is equal to K_m/V and the intercept at $1/S = 0$ is equal to $1/V$ so that these constants can be determined.

2. TEMPERATURE

The effect of temperature on a rate constant, k, is indicated by the Arrhenius equation, Eqn (6.35)

$$k = Z\,e^{-E/RT}$$

or

$$\log k = \log Z - \frac{E}{2\cdot303R}\frac{1}{T} \quad (6\ 35)$$

where Z is a constant that is termed the frequency factor, E is the energy of activation, R is the gas constant, and T is the thermodynamic temperature.

Different interpretations of the constant Z are given by the collision theory and the transition state theory of reaction rates. In addition, there is a slight difference in the interpretation of the constant E, and the student is recommended to read accounts of these theories given in the books listed at the end of this chapter.

It can be seen from Eqn (6.35) that a straight line will be obtained from a graph of $\log k$ against $1/T$ as shown in Fig. 6.2. The constants E and Z may be determined from the slope and intercept of this line, which are equal to $-E/2\cdot303R$ and $\log Z$, respectively. It should be borne in mind that temperature is decreasing when $1/T$ is increasing so that the higher temperatures lie towards the left-hand side of the horizontal axis of the graph.

3. LIGHT

Light energy may be absorbed by certain molecules, which then become sufficiently activated for participation in a reaction. Only frequencies in the visible and ultra-violet regions can provide sufficient energy to cause photochemical reactions. Since the energy for activation is provided by light in these reactions the rates of the latter are independent of temperature. However, it is often difficult to separate photochemical reactions from thermal reactions,

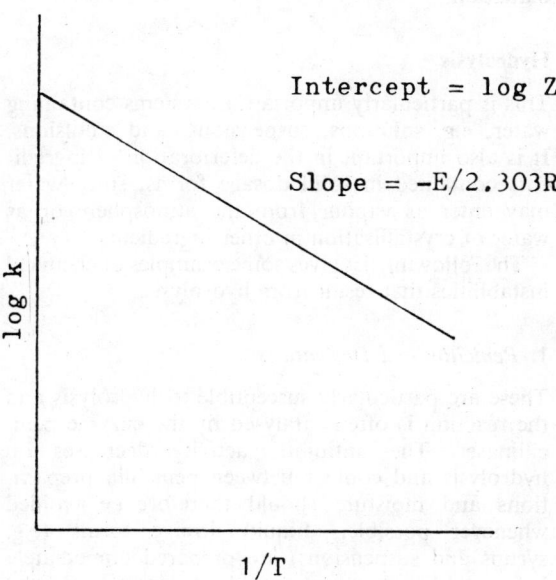

Fig. 6.2 Graph showing plot of the Arrhenius equation

since thermal effects may: (*a*) be involved in the subsequent chain of reactions that often follows a photochemical reaction, or (*b*) arise from the heating effect produced by the increase in kinetic energy of molecules that have collided with others that have absorbed some light energy.

4. SOLVENT

The effects of solvents on the rate constants of chemical reactions are complex. Their influence on the ability of solutes to dissociate into ions is particularly important in reactions that involve these ions.

Stability Testing

Pharmaceutical compounds and preparations often exhibit chemical or physical instabilities. The deterioration that results from such instabilities may lead to:

(*a*) a reduced activity of the compound or preparation,
(*b*) the formation of toxic reaction products, or
(*c*) the formation of an inelegant or unusable product, e.g. a broken emulsion.

In addition, microbial contamination may be unacceptable or lead to deterioration.

Stability testing is therefore carried out to ensure that deterioration does not exceed an acceptable level in order to:

(*a*) ensure the safety of the patient,
(*b*) maintain the activity of the product, and
(*c*) maintain sales, because a deteriorated product is either unusable or a poor advertisement.

The common causes of chemical instability in pharmaceutical materials involve hydrolysis or oxidation.

Hydrolysis

This is particularly important in systems containing water, e.g. solutions, suspensions, and emulsions. It is also important in the deterioration of ingredients contained in solid dosage forms, since water may enter as vapour from the atmosphere or as water of crystallisation in other ingredients.

The following list gives some examples of chemical instabilities that result from hydrolysis.

1. *Penicillin and Derivatives*

These are particularly susceptible to hydrolysis and the reaction is often catalysed by the enzyme penicillinase. The antibiotic activity decreases on hydrolysis and contact between penicillin preparations and moisture should therefore be avoided whenever possible. Liquid dosage forms (e.g. syrups and suspensions) are prepared immediately before use by adding water to the dry ingredients, and unused liquid should be discarded after a relatively short period (e.g. 1 to 2 weeks) if stored at room temperature. Dry preparations may be stored for considerably longer periods; e.g. 2 to 3 years at room temperature for crystalline sodium benzylpenicillin if the moisture content is kept below 0·5 per cent (Johnson, 1967).

2. *Aspirin*

Hydrolysis of this acid to a mixture of acetic and salicylic acids occurs readily and the powdered drug should therefore be protected against atmospheric water vapour. In fact, as Johnson (1967) has pointed out, if aspirin were introduced at the present time as a new drug it would probably be regarded as unsuitable because of its marked instability.

3. *Alkaloids*

Solanaceous alkaloids that contain ester linkages are susceptible to hydrolysis. It is usually assumed that if hydrolysis of the alkaloid occurs in aqueous solution then it is likely to occur in the crude drug if the moisture content increases. Drying the crude drugs excessively may produce a hygroscopic material, which is undesirable, so that an optimum level of drying is usually aimed at.

Other examples of instabilities that arise from hydrolysis are given by Macek (1970), Garrett (1967) and Johnson (1967). In addition, Johnson discusses the physical deterioration that may be caused by moisture.

METHODS OF PROTECTION AGAINST HYDROLYSIS

The obvious method of protection is to prevent contact between the material and water. This method is mainly concerned with protecting the dry material against water vapour and therefore involves control of atmospheric humidity during preparation, purification, and packing, and satisfactory design of the final container so that adequate protection against the entry of water vapour from the atmosphere is provided. Extra protection is also achieved by including porous envelopes containing desiccants in the containers.

Prevention of contact is impossible in liquid dosage forms that contain water. The method of protection is therefore concerned with reducing the rate of hydrolysis in the system. Since many hydrolytic reactions are catalysed by acids and bases, one method of achieving a reduction in the rate of decomposition is by adjusting the pH to an optimum level at which the catalytic effect is at a minimum.

It has also been shown that the formation of molecular complexes between the hydrolysable substance and a second component may inhibit hydrolysis. For example, Higuchi and Lachman (1955) have found that benzocaine is protected against hydrolysis by complexation with caffeine.

Since hydrolysis is a solvolytic reaction the rate at which it causes decomposition is affected by the solubility of the hydrolysable substance. A decrease in solubility caused by a change in pH, or the use of insoluble derivatives, will therefore provide means of reducing the decomposition; for example, insoluble chlorothiazide is stable in neutral aqueous suspension but the soluble sodium salt that is formed in alkaline solution is readily hydrolysed.

Oxidation

Oxidation and reduction involve the loss and gain of electrons, respectively. Many oxidation reactions result from the presence of atmospheric oxygen but the required loss of electrons may sometimes occur even when oxygen is absent; e.g. in reactions between oxidising and reducing agents. However, the decomposition of medicinal compounds usually involves molecular oxygen. Such oxidations are usually termed autoxidations because they occur spontaneously under normal conditions, and often involve free radicals. The latter, which contain one or more unpaired electrons, are particularly reactive and the products of their reactions are often free radicals themselves, hence chain reactions are initiated and proceed until the remaining free radicals are destroyed or rendered less active.

AUTOXIDATION OF UNSATURATED FATS AND OILS

This type of decomposition may be used to illustrate the mechanism of autoxidation and the methods of obtaining protection against its effects. The decomposed products usually develop objectionable odours and tastes and are said to be rancid.

The mechanism of a chain reaction may be considered in terms of the following stages.

(a) Chain Initiation

The presence of unsaturated C=C linkages has an activating effect on adjacent $-CH_2-$ groups in a hydrocarbon chain. The reaction between molecular oxygen and an unsaturated hydrocarbon is considered to involve the abstraction of a hydrogen free radical ($\dot{H}$) from an activated methylene group and results in the formation of a hydrocarbon free radical. This reaction is illustrated by the following equation, in which the free radicals are indicated by a dot over their chemical formulae.

$$-CH=CH-CH_2- \xrightarrow[-\dot{H}]{O_2} -CH=CH-\dot{C}H-$$

Chain initiation may also occur from the ready dissociation of so-called initiators (e.g. benzoyl peroxide) into free radicals or from the effects of heat, light or ionising radiation on some ingredients of an oil, e.g. (i) dissociation of a peroxide (R = hydrocarbon group)

$$R.OOH \rightarrow R\dot{O} + \dot{O}H$$

and (ii) photo-oxidation of a ketone (R and R' = hydrocarbon groups)

$$R.CO.R' \rightarrow R.\dot{C}O + \dot{R}'$$

(b) Chain Propagation

The free radicals produced in the previous stage are involved in further reactions that yield other free radicals. Peroxides are formed as intermediates, but the concentration of these compounds eventually decreases when their rate of decomposition exceeds their rate of production. The use of peroxide values as an indication of the extent of an autoxidation process may therefore be misleading. The reactions involved in the propagation stage can be summarised as follows:

$$\left.\begin{array}{l} \dot{R} + O_2 \rightarrow R\dot{O}_2 \\ R\dot{O}_2 + RH \rightarrow ROOH + \dot{R} \\ \qquad\qquad\qquad \text{hydroperoxide} \end{array}\right\} \begin{array}{l} \text{These reactions} \\ \text{increase the} \\ \text{rate of peroxide} \\ \text{formation} \end{array}$$

$$\left.\begin{array}{l} ROOH \rightarrow R\dot{O} + \dot{O}H \\ 2\,ROOH \rightarrow R\dot{O} + R\dot{O}_2 + H_2O \\ ROOH \rightarrow \text{non-radical products} \end{array}\right\} \begin{array}{l} \text{These reactions} \\ \text{increase the} \\ \text{rate of peroxide} \\ \text{disappearance.} \end{array}$$

(c) Chain Termination

(i) *Self Termination.* This involves reaction between two free radicals and the production of inactive (i.e. non-free radical) products.

(ii) *Chain Breaking Termination* This involves reaction between free radicals and compounds that are known as chain inhibitors and results in the formation of stable and comparatively unreactive free radicals, e.g.

$$\dot{R} + IH \cdot \rightarrow RH + \dot{I}$$

chain inhibitor   stable free radical

Autoxidations may be followed by measuring the amount of oxygen taken up during a reaction. The results of such a measurement are illustrated in Fig. 6.3 which shows that three separate stages may be defined in the reaction. The first of these stages, *AB*, corresponds to an induction period, in which little oxygen is used and the chain initiation reaction occurs. This is followed by propagation, *BC*, where the oxygen uptake increases rapidly until termination begins to occur and the rate of uptake decreases slowly (beyond *C*).

The kinetics of the overall process are affected by the effects of heat and light, both of which increase the rate of autoxidation, by the nature of the fatty material, and by the presence of certain metals and salts, which probably catalyse the decomposition of hydroperoxides.

METHODS OF PROTECTION AGAINST OXIDATION

Reducing agents are often used to provide protection against atmospheric oxygen and oxidising agents. Sodium metabisulphite is commonly used for this purpose in many injections (e.g. Injection of Adrenaline BP).

Antioxidants that are effective against atmospheric oxygen are often used to provide protection against autoxidation. These compounds may influence the chain initiation or propagation stages, or both, and this provides a basis for their classification.

(a) *Chain Initiation Suppressors*

(i) *Ultra-violet Stabilisers.* These absorb ultra-violet radiation and dispose of the energy without forming free radicals. They include phenyl salicylate and 2-hydroxybenzophenone.

(ii) *Hydroperoxide Destroyers.* These react with hydroperoxides to form non-free radical products. They are mainly organic compounds of phosphorus and sulphur and their toxicity precludes any wide use in pharmacy.

(iii) *Metal Deactivators.* These form complexes with metals, which are then unavailable for catalysing peroxide decomposition. They include citric acid, ethylenediamine tetra-acetic acid (EDTA) and 8-hydroxyquinoline. Care must be taken in their use because the metal complex may be even more effective in catalysing peroxide decomposition than the original metal.

(b) *Propagation Suppressors*

These combine with free radicals to produce stable products; i.e. they act as chain terminating agents

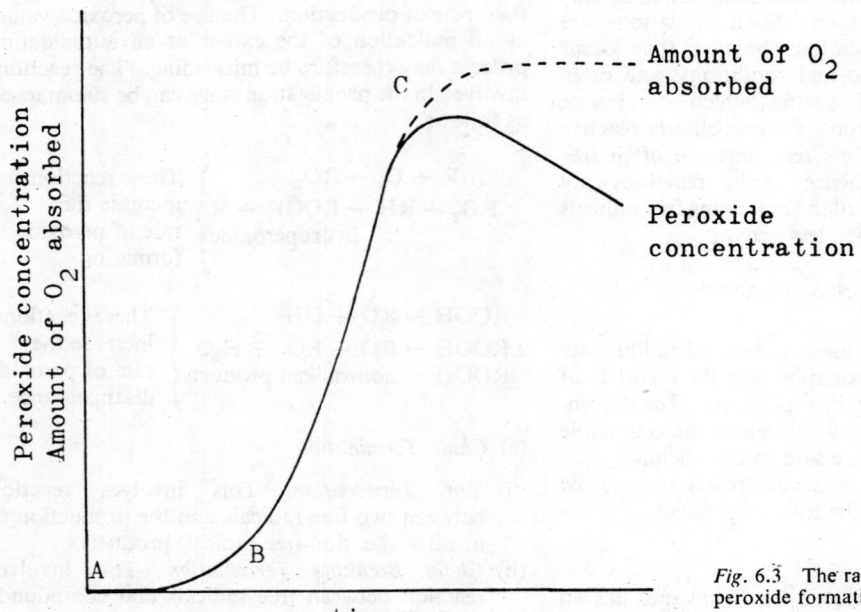

Fig. 6.3 The rates of oxygen absorption and peroxide formation in an autoxidation

They include phenolic and secondary amino compounds, the former type being in common use in pharmaceutical preparations; e.g. butyl hydroxyanisole (BHA), nor-dihydroguaiaretic acid (NDGA), and gallic acid esters such as propyl and n-butyl gallates.

Two or more different antioxidants may be more effective than would be expected on the basis of their individual activities. This is, known as synergism, and in general the best mixtures are those that contain an initiation suppressor and a propagation suppressor. However, the characteristics of the system that requires protection, or its intended storage conditions, may indicate more precise combinations; for example, if prolonged exposure to light is expected then an ultra-violet stabiliser plus a propagation suppressor should be used.

The effectiveness of antioxidants may be determined from their effects on the oxygen uptake of the protected substrate or on the rate of peroxide formation. An increase in the induction period should be obtained with an initiation suppressor and a decrease in the subsequent rate of reaction should be obtained with a propagation suppressor.

Other Types of Chemical Decomposition

Reaction between various ingredients of a formulation may be responsible for a loss in activity or other undesirable change. Examples of incompatibilities that may arise in extemporaneous preparations are given by Gunn and Carter (1965). Reactions occurring in new formulations or arising from the leakage of substances from container materials are less easy to predict.

Isomerisation of a compound to a less active structure may occur, especially in optically active compounds, where the optical activity may be lost during the racemisation which is accompanied by a decrease in pharmacological activity.

Determination of the Cause of Decomposition

The route of a particular decomposition and therefore the factors that cause it may be indicated from a consideration of:

(a) the chemical structure of the decomposing substance,
(b) the chemical structure(s) of the product(s) of decomposition,
(c) the properties of other ingredients, possible impurities and container material,
(d) the storage conditions,
(e) the appearance and odour of the decomposed preparation, and
(f) a knowledge of the behaviour of similar compounds.

More information is obtainable from a series of tests such as that outlined below.

Solution of drug sealed in ampoules

	Series A Contains O_2 above solution in ampoules	Series B Contains N_2 above solution in ampoules
1. Expose to light	A1	B1
2. Heat	A2	B2
3. Store in dark	A3	B3

Results

(a) Decomposition in all cases indicates hydrolysis.
(b) Decomposition in all of series A but not in series B indicates oxidation.
(c) Decomposition in A1 but not A3 indicates a photochemical reaction.
(d) Decomposition in A2 and B2 but not in A1, A3, B1 and B3 indicates a thermal decomposition.

Similar series of tests may be carried out at different pH's to indicate the effect of hydrogen and hydroxyl ion concentrations on decompositions.

Accelerated Stability Testing

Instabilities in modern formulations are often detectable only after considerable storage periods under normal conditions. To reduce the time required to obtain information, various tests that involve storage of the products under conditions that accelerate decomposition have been introduced. The objectives of such accelerated tests may be defined as

1. the rapid detection of deterioration in different initial formulations of the same product—this is of use in selecting the best formulation from a series of possible choices;
2. the prediction of shelf-life, which is the time a product will remain satisfactory when stored under expected or directed storage conditions; and
3. the provision of a rapid means of quality control, which ensures that no unexpected change has occurred in the stored product.

All these objectives are based on obtaining a more rapid rate of decomposition by applying to the product a storage condition that places a higher stress or challenge to it when compared with normal storage conditions. However, the use of this basic method depends on the particular objective required. For example, in the first objective the best formulation from a series of possible choices is the one that exhibits the least amount of decomposition in a given time under the influence of a reasonably high stress. The results of such a test are illustrated in Fig. 6.4(a).

The second objective is achieved by using the results obtained from an accelerated test to predict the amount of decomposition in a product after a longer period of storage under normal conditions. This is illustrated in Fig. 6.4(b) where the amount of decomposition X obtained after the short time t_1 is used to predict the value of Y after time t_2.

The use of accelerated tests in achieving the third objective is illustrated by Fig. 6.4(c) which shows that a single measurement taken after a given time t should fall below an acceptable limit of decomposition for a product subjected to the challenge involved in the test.

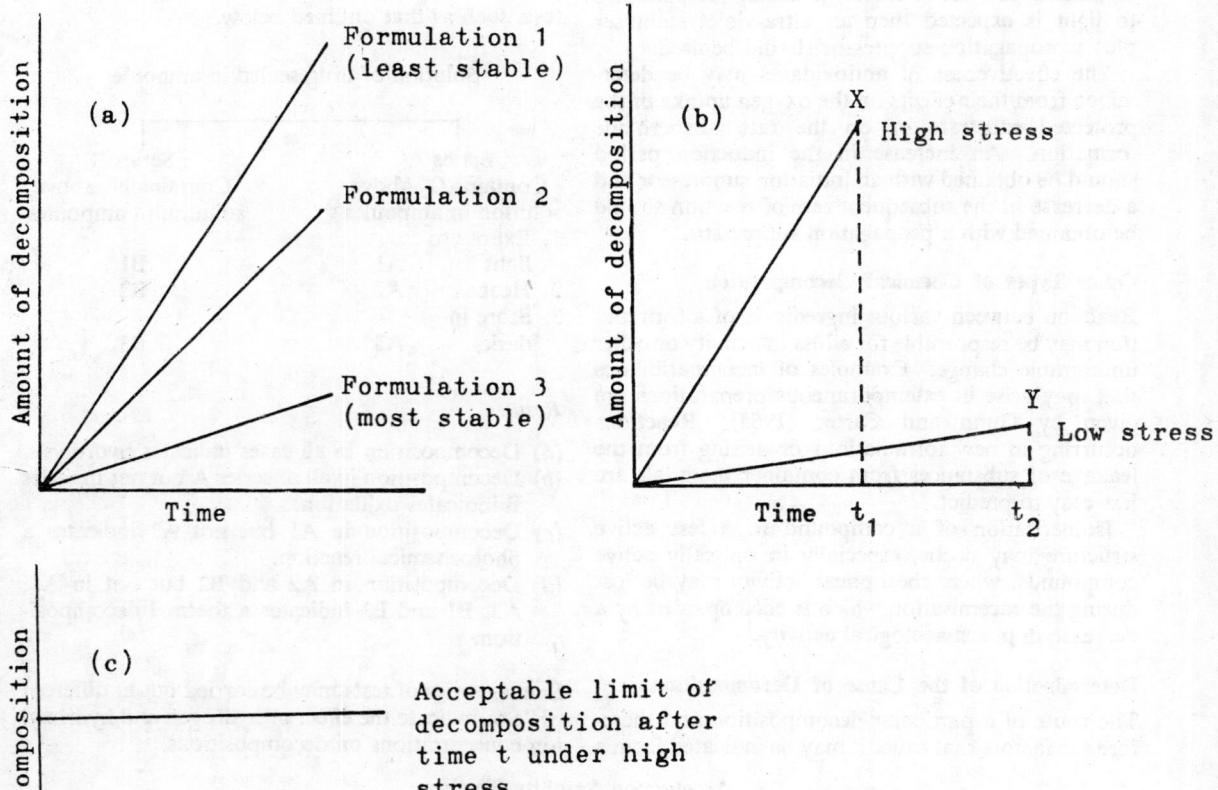

Fig. 6.4 The various aspects of accelerated stability testing

Common High Stresses or Challenges

(a) Temperature

An increase in temperature causes an increase in the rate of chemical reactions. The products are therefore stored at temperatures greater than room temperature. The nature of the product often determines the range covered in the accelerated test. Samples are removed at various time intervals and the extent of decomposition is determined by analysis. Sensitive analytical methods should be used in all stability tests of this nature since small changes may be detected after very short storage periods.

The effects caused by high temperatures should not be confused with those that arise from the effect of low humidity. Such confusion is possible because the relative humidity inside a high temperature storage cabinet will be lower than that in the room. This low humidity causes loss of moisture, which may lead to apparent increases in the concentration of ingredients. If these concentration changes are not allowed for in subsequent analyses decomposition may be unsuspected.

(b) Humidity

Storage of the product in atmospheres of high humidity will accelerate decompositions that result from hydrolysis. Marked acceleration will be obtained if the 'naked' product (i.e. not enclosed in a container) is subjected to these tests, which usually indicate the minimum humidity tolerated by the product without undue decomposition, and are therefore useful in determining the degree of protection that should be afforded by a container.

(c) Light

A source of artificial light is used to accelerate the effects of sunlight or sky light. The source should emit a similar distribution of radiant energy to that in sunlight because photochemical reactions involve the absorption of light of definite wavelengths. Daylight fluorescent lamps provide a satisfactory source, and banks of such lamps may be used to accelerate the effects of light. However, although these lamps do not have a marked heating effect the use of glass plates to reduce such an effect is recommended, otherwise it is difficult to separate the accelerated decomposition caused by light from that caused by increased temperatures.

The Prediction of Shelf-life

This is the second of the objectives that were listed previously and it is based on the application of the Arrhenius equation, Eqn (6.35), which indicates the effect of temperature on the rate constant, k, of a chemical reaction. Figure 6.2 (*see* p. 97) shows that a graph of $\log k$ versus the reciprocal of thermodynamic temperature, $1/T$, is a straight line. If the slope of this line is determined from the results of accelerated tests at high temperatures it is possible to determine the value of the rate constant at other temperatures (e.g. normal room temperature) by extrapolation. Substitution of this value of k into the appropriate order of reaction (i.e. the rate equation that applies to the reaction involved in the particular decomposition) allows the amount of decomposition after a given time to be calculated. As pointed out, this approach involves a knowledge of the order of the reaction involved and preliminary experiments such as those outlined on p. 92 are therefore necessary to determine this order.

Several difficulties and limitations are involved in this aspect of accelerated stability testing. First, as in all accelerated tests, there is the possibility that the application of high stresses may cause reactions that would not take place under the lower stresses associated with normal storage conditions. Secondly, the uncertain conditions defined by the term 'normal storage conditions' introduces a difficulty when attempting to forecast the shelf-life of a product. Unless the storage conditions are defined precisely on the container, then allowance should be made for variations in the conditions likely to be encountered under normal storage. Attempts to allow for such a contingency often involve accepting the shortest shelf-life for the range of conditions likely to be encountered. The climate of the country in which a product is to be marketed is particularly important in defining this range.

Decompositions in formulated products often proceed via a complex reaction series and may involve simultaneous, consecutive, or chain reactions, because the formulated products themselves are complex systems. In addition, the order of a reaction may change after a certain time. Predictions of the extent of decomposition at future times are then impracticable and prolonged tests under normal storage conditions must be carried out.

In spite of these difficulties the application of accelerated testing to pharmaceutical products is often useful, and predicted shelf-lives are sufficiently accurate. Statistical methods of designing such tests have therefore been reported, which allow the selection of the number of replicates, sampling times and other factors involved in the tests to be made on a logical basis for attaining the required degree of accuracy without wasting time on unnecessary experimentation (Tootill, 1961; Jones and Grimshaw, 1963).

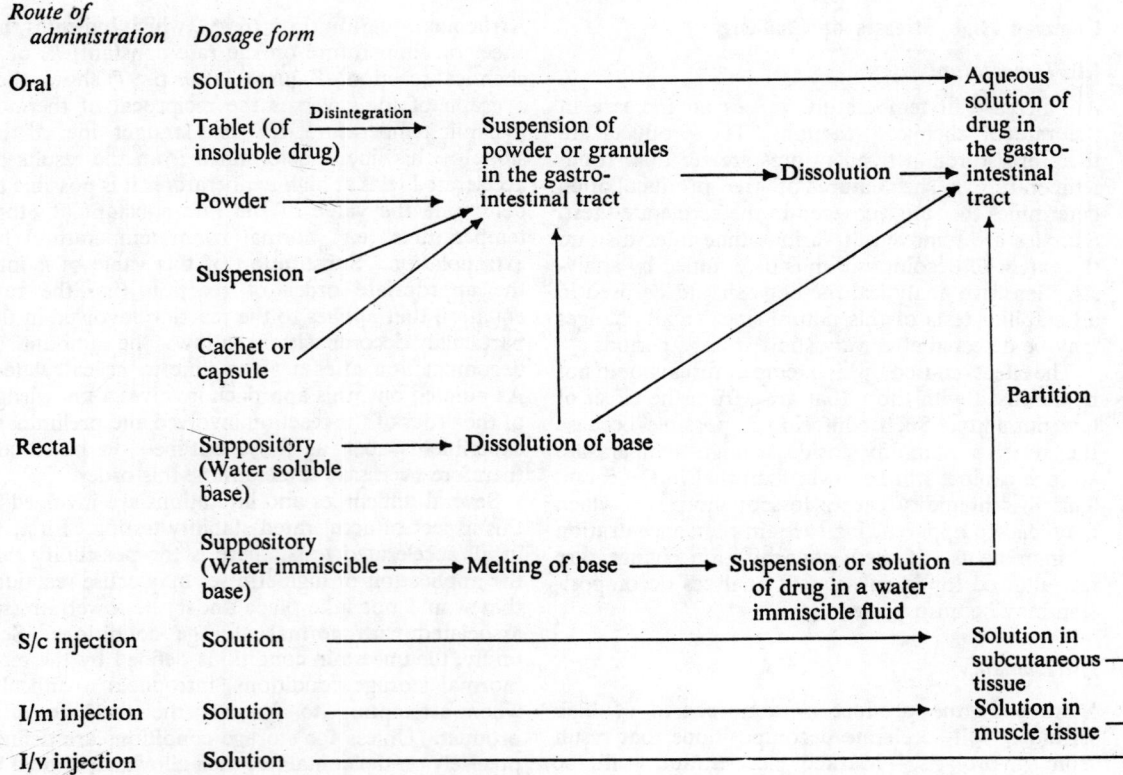

Fig. 6.5 Diagram illustrating some of the factors that influence

KINETICS OF DRUG TRANSPORT *IN VIVO*

The purpose of administering a drug to a patient is to produce a particular response. This response is achieved when enough of the drug is concentrated at a certain site in the body. The number of molecules of the active form of the drug that reach the site where they can exert their effect (locus of action or receptor site) and the rate at which these molecules arrive there depend on several factors. Some of these factors will be generally applicable but others will be determined by the route of administration of the drug and the properties of the dosage form.

Systemically Active Drugs

These are drugs that after absorption into the body are carried to their site of action by the blood. Figure 6.5 illustrates some of the *in vivo* processes that are involved in the transport of such drugs after administration as various dosage forms. It should be realised that all drugs except those injected intravenously must be transported across some type of

body membrane before they can enter the plasma. Transport into other tissues, or excretion, again involves passage through membranes. The various body membranes constitute the major barriers to the movement of drugs *in vivo* and it is therefore necessary to consider the general structure of such membranes and the various mechanisms involved in the transport of substances across them.

STRUCTURE OF THE CELL MEMBRANE

Although a variety of membranes exist in the body (e.g. cytoplasmic membrane surrounding a single cell, sheets of tissue several cells in thickness around certain organs) the same transport mechanisms are involved in all cases. It is therefore useful to consider the structure of a cell membrane and show how this structure is penetrated by different substances.

A cell membrane is regarded as having two layers of lipid molecules orientated with their polar groups

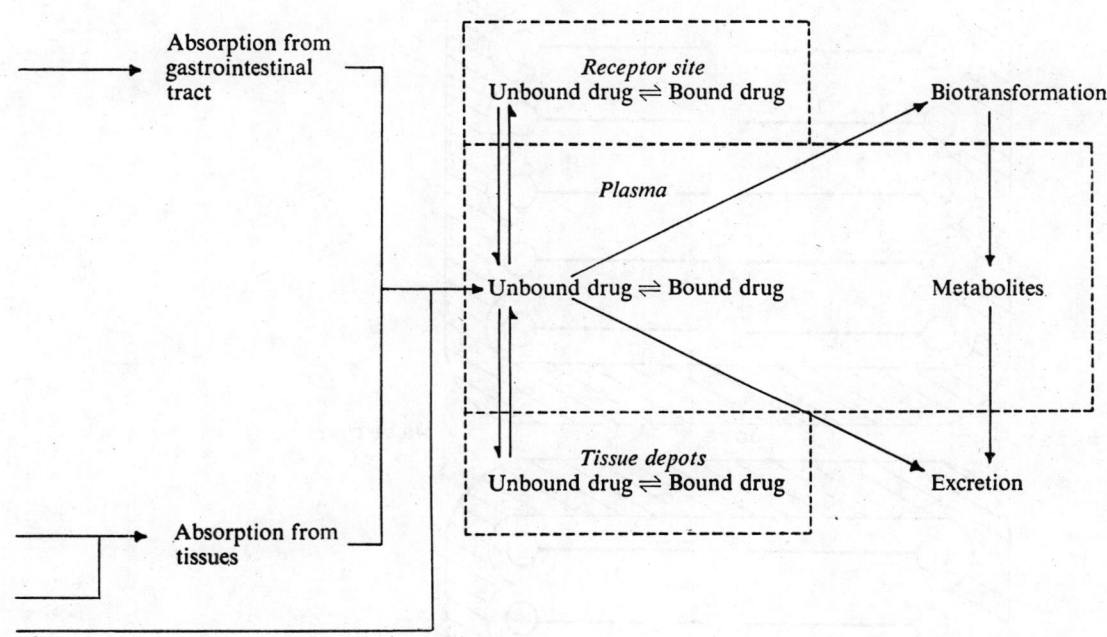

the concentration of a systemically active drug at its receptor site

facing outwards, as shown in Fig. 6.6. These molecules include lecithin, sphingomyelin, cephalin, and cholesterol. The bimolecular layer is stabilised by a layer of unfolded protein molecules, which cover each side. This type of structure therefore constitutes a lipid barrier which separates the aqueous intra- and extra-cellular liquids. The thickness of the membrane is about 75×10^{-7} mm, and the structure is perforated by water-filled pores, which usually have an effective radius of the order of 4×10^{-7} mm. However, in certain specialised membranes this pore size may be about 10 times larger (e.g. in glomeruli of the kidney).

Mechanisms of Drug Transport Across Cell Membranes

1. PASSIVE DIFFUSION THROUGH LIPID BARRIERS

This is a common mechanism that is involved in the transport of drugs *in vivo*. Much of the work in this field has been reviewed by Brodie (1964).

The process of passive diffusion through a lipid barrier initially involves partition of a drug between the aqueous phase on one side of the membrane and the lipid phase that constitutes the membrane. This stage is followed by diffusion across the membrane and a second partition between the lipid phase and the aqueous liquid on the other side of the membrane. The overall rate of transport will therefore be affected by factors that influence these consecutive processes, which are illustrated in Fig. 6.7, where the k values refer to the rate constants of the individual processes. In any reaction that involves consecutive stages, the overall rate of transfer is determined by the rate of transfer in the slowest stage. However, the relative rates of the three stages shown in Fig. 6.7 will depend on the nature of the drug molecules; for example, a molecule that is more soluble in water than in the lipid phase will be taken into the latter phase at a slow rate only but will be released rapidly at the other side after it has diffused across the membrane, hence process (1) in Fig. 6.7 will be the rate-determining

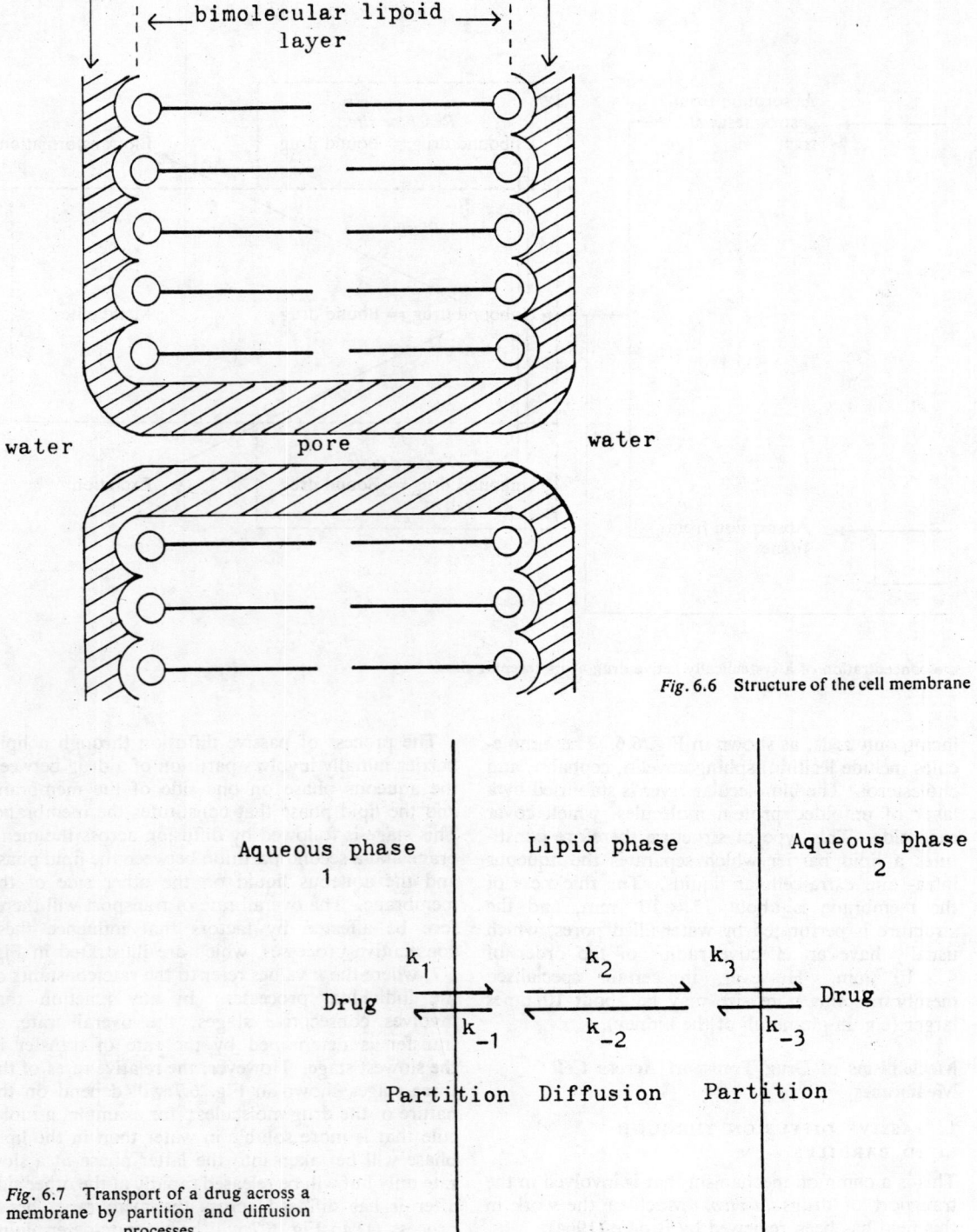

Fig. 6.6   Structure of the cell membrane

Fig. 6.7   Transport of a drug across a membrane by partition and diffusion processes

stage. Conversely, a substance that is more soluble in the lipid phase than in water will enter the lipid stage rapidly but will be released with difficulty at the other side, hence process (3) will now be the rate-determining stage. In compounds with intermediate partition coefficients, the diffusion process (2) may become the limiting stage, when the rate of transfer will be indicated by Fick's law (Eqn 5.5). However, the thinness of the membrane is low enough for this diffusion process to be relatively rapid, when the partition processes may often be the rate-determining stages, as mentioned above. It should be pointed out that the diffusion stage is almost always the rate-determining process in many *in vitro* models that have been used to represent drug transport by this mechanism because the thickness of the organic solvent layer that is used in place of a lipid membrane creates a long diffusion pathway.

It has been assumed in the previous discussion that the drug exists in aqueous solution as a single species with a definite partition coefficient for distribution between water and the lipid phase of the membrane. However, most drugs are weak electrolytes and exist in aqueous solution as a mixture of ionised and unionised forms. The latter are much more soluble in the lipid phase than the water soluble ions so that body membranes tend to be preferentially permeable to unionised forms of drug molecules. In other words, the rate constant k_1 in Fig. 6.7 is extremely low for ions but is much more appreciable for the corresponding unionised molecules.

pK_a Values

The fraction of drug that is ionised in solution is given by the dissociation constant of the drug. Such dissociation constants are conveniently expressed in terms of pK_a values for both acidic and basic drugs.

The equilibrium between unionised molecules of an acidic drug (HA) and the ions produced by dissociation may be represented by Eqn (6.36)

$$HA \rightleftharpoons H^+ + A^- \qquad (6.36)$$

The dissociation constant K_a of this drug is therefore defined by Eqn (6.37), where the square brackets represent concentration terms of the species enclosed within them.

$$K_a = \frac{[H^+][A^-]}{[HA]} \qquad (6.37)$$

Taking logarithms of both sides of Eqn (6.37) yields

$$\log K_a = \log [H^+] + \log [A^-] - \log [HA]$$

and the signs in this equation may be reversed to give

Eqn (6.38)

$$-\log K_a = -\log [H^+] - \log [A^-] + \log [HA] \qquad (6.38)$$

The symbol pK_a is used to represent the negative logarithm of the acid dissociation constant K_a in the same way that pH is used to represent the negative logarithm of the hydrogen ion concentration $[H^+]$, and Eqn (6.38) may therefore be rewritten as Eqn (6.39)

$$pK_a = pH + \log [HA] - \log [A^-] \qquad (6.39)$$

or

$$pK_a = pH + \log \frac{[HA]}{[A^-]} \qquad (6.40)$$

Thus, a general equation, Eqn (6.41), that is applicable to any acidic drug with one ionisable group may be written, where c_u and c_i represent the concentrations of the unionised and ionised species, respectively. This equation is known as the Henderson-Hasselbalch equation.

$$pK_a = pH + \log \frac{c_u}{c_i} \qquad (6.41)$$

The protonation of a basic drug (B) may be represented by the equilibrium shown in Eqn (6.42)

$$B + H^+ \rightleftharpoons BH^+$$

The acid dissociation constant, K_a, of the protonated base is therefore expressed by Eqn (6.43).

$$K_a = \frac{[H^+][B]}{[BH^+]} \qquad (6.43)$$

Taking negative logarithms yields Eqn (6.44)

$$-\log K_a = -\log [H^+] - \log [B] + \log [BH^+] \qquad (6.44)$$

or

$$pK_a = pH + \log \frac{[BH^+]}{[B]}$$

The Henderson-Hasselbalch equation for any weak base with one ionisable group may therefore be written as shown by Eqn (6.45)

$$pK_a = pH + \log \frac{c_i}{c_u} \qquad (6.45)$$

where c_i and c_u refer to the concentrations of the protonated and unionised species, respectively.

The Influence of pK_a *Values on the Transport of Drugs Across Biological Membranes.* Because the ionised forms of acidic and basic drugs have low lipid:water partition coefficients compared to the coefficients for the corresponding unionised molecules, lipid membranes are preferentially permeable to the latter species. Thus, an increase in the fraction of a drug that is unionised will increase the rate of transport of the drug across a lipid membrane. However, the Henderson-Hasselbalch equation indicates that the ratio of unionised:ionised forms ($c_u:c_i$) of a given drug will depend on the pH of the medium and the pK_a value of the drug For example,

(i) the pK_a value of aspirin, which is a weak acid, is about 3·5, and if the pH of the gastric contents is 2·0 then from Eqn (6.41)

$$\log \frac{c_u}{c_i} = pK_a - pH = 3·5 - 2·0 = 1·5$$

so that the ratio of the concentration of unionised acetylsalicyclic acid to acetylsalicylate anion is given by

$$c_u:c_i = \text{antilog } 1·5 = 31·62:1$$

(ii) the pH of plasma is 7·4 so that the ratio of unionised:ionised aspirin in this medium is given by

$$\log \frac{c_u}{c_i} = pK_a - pH = 3·5 - 7·4 = -3·9$$

and

$$c_u:c_i = \text{antilog } -3·9 = \text{antilog } \bar{4}·1$$
$$= 1·259 \times 10^{-4}:1$$

(iii) the pK_a of the weakly acidic drug sulphapyridine is about 8·0 and if the pH of the intestinal contents is 5·0 then the ratio of unionised:ionised drug is given by

$$\log \frac{c_u}{c_i} = pK_a - pH = 8·0 - 5·0 = 3·0$$

and

$$c_u:c_i = \text{antilog } 3·0 = 10^3:1$$

(iv) the pK_a of the basic drug amidopyrine is 5·0, and in the stomach the ratio of ionised:unionised drug is shown from Eqn (6.45) to be given by

$$\log \frac{c_i}{c_u} = pK_a - pH = 5·0 - 2·0 = 3·0$$

and

$$c_i:c_u = \text{antilog } 3·0 = 10^3:1$$

while in the intestine the ratio is given by

$$\log \frac{c_i}{c_u} = 5·0 - 5·0 = 0$$

and

$$c_i:c_u = \text{antilog } 0 = 1:1$$

Equilibrium Concentration Ratios. When an unionised drug attains an equilibrium distribution

across a membrane its concentration is the same on both sides of the membrane. However, if the pHs of the aqueous phases on either side of the membrane are different (e.g. pH_1 and pH_2) then the total concentrations of a partly ionised drug in these aqueous phases will also differ. The ratio, R, of these concentrations (i.e. $R = c_1/c_2$, where c_1 and c_2 are the total concentrations of the drug in the two aqueous phases, respectively) may be calculated from Eqn (6.46), for an acidic drug, and from Eqn (6.47) for a basic drug.

For an acidic drug $R = \dfrac{c_1}{c_2} = \dfrac{1 + 10^{(pH_1 - pK_a)}}{1 + 10^{(pH_2 - pK_a)}}$

$$(6.46)$$

For a basic drug $R = \dfrac{c_1}{c_2} = \dfrac{1 + 10^{(pK_a - pH_1)}}{1 + 10^{(pK_a - pH_2)}}$

$$(6.47)$$

Equations (6.46) and (6.47) can also be used to calculate an unknown pH if all the other factors are known, or an unknown pK_a if all the other factors are known.

Table 6.2
Equilibrium Concentration Ratios of Various Drugs between Gastric or Intestinal Contents (pH 2 or 5, respectively) and Plasma (pH 7)

Type of drug	$c_{gastric}:c_{plasma}$	$c_{intestinal}:c_{plasma}$
Strongly acidic ($pK_a = 3$)	$1 + 10^{-1}:1 + 10^4$	$1 + 10^2:1 + 10^4$
Weakly acidic ($pK_a = 8$)	$1 + 10^{-6}:1 + 10^{-1}$	$1 + 10^{-3}:1 + 10^{-1}$
Strongly basic ($pK_a = 8$)	$1 + 10^6:1 + 10$	$1 + 10^3:1 + 10$
Weakly basic ($pK_a = 5$)	$1 + 10^3:1 + 10^{-2}$	$1 + 1:1 + 10^{-2}$

Table 6.2 shows the equilibrium concentration ratios of acidic and basic compounds with a range of pK_a values between gastric or intestinal contents and plasma. (The pHs of these fluids have been taken as a whole number for the convenience of calculation.) From this table it can be seen that for an acidic drug the $c_{gastric}:c_{plasma}$ ratio is lower than the $c_{intestinal}:c_{plasma}$ ratio; i.e. a greater proportion of the drug is absorbed into the plasma

from the stomach than from the intestine. The reverse is true for basic drugs. It should be pointed out that the figures given in Table 6.2 are theoretical ones based on the assumption that an equilibrium is established. However, such an equilibrium is rarely obtained *in vivo* because the concentrations of drug on either side of the membrane will be affected by other factors; e.g. flow of blood, dilution of gastric contents.

2. DIFFUSION THROUGH PORES IN LIPID BARRIER

The pores in cell membranes are filled with water, and substances may therefore be transported through the pores by diffusion in aqueous solution. The rate of such transport may be affected by the movement of water under the influence of osmosis. In addition, the movement of ions through these pores will be affected by the presence of static charges on the walls of the pores; e.g. small anions may pass through positively charged pores whereas cations may be hindered by electrostatic repulsion (p. 73). The size of pores in membranes is the main factor that affects transport of substances by this mechanism; i.e. a filtration process is involved. The pore size in cell membranes is usually about 4×10^{-7} mm, and since the radius of most drug molecules is greater than this the entry of drugs into individual cells by this mechanism is of little importance. However, certain body membranes consist of sheets of epithelial cells, and the pores between these cells may be as large as 4×10^{-6} mm; e.g. in the glomeruli of the kidney and in the epithelium of capillaries. The importance of the filtration mechanism of drug transport is therefore greater in such membranes. ·

3. SPECIAL TRANSPORT SYSTEMS

Some naturally occurring substances are too large to pass through the pores in cell membranes and too lipid insoluble to be transported by diffusion through the lipid barrier; (e.g. large ions and large monosaccharides). It is therefore supposed that the ready movement of such substances across cell membranes is brought about by special mechanisms which involve compounds that act as carriers for the transported substances. It is suggested that an ion or molecule forms a complex with the carrier at one surface of the membrane, and the complex moves across the membrane. After liberation of the substrate (i.e. the transported substance) at the other side, the cycle is completed by the return of the uncomplexed carrier to its initial position.

If the substrate is moved across a membrane in the opposite direction to a concentration gradient, then energy must be expended in the transference, which is then referred to as an active transport process. This type of transport is inhibited by compounds that interfere with the cellular reactions that provide the required energy for the process.

The rates of transference in all special systems that involve carrier molecules will depend on the available number of these molecules, and a maximum rate will be obtained when all the carrier molecules are being used. It is therefore possible to saturate this type of transport mechanism with an excess of substrate molecules. Furthermore, although carrier molecules usually show some degree of specificity for a particular substrate, other compounds that possess a similar structure to the normal substrate may compete for the available carrier molecules and, therefore, prevent the transport of the normal substrate.

4. PINOCYTOSIS

It is considered that small particles such as microorganisms may be engulfed by macrophages that have migrated through the epithelial lining of the gastro-intestinal tract. The engulfed particles are transported across this membrane, when the macrophages migrate back again into the lymphoidal tissue. This process appears to be more significant at sites in the body where lymphoidal tissue and mucosal epithelium are close together; e.g. the tonsil and pharynx.

The first three transport mechanisms that have been discussed above are involved to some extent in the passage of drugs across all biological membranes. Their relative importance depends on the structure of the particular membrane. In certain cases it is usual to refer to specialised membranes or barriers in the body (e.g. the blood-brain barrier). Such barriers consist of membranes with structures that differ from that of the simple cell membrane or contain specific carriers for the transport of particular compounds.

The Binding of Drugs *in vivo*

In Fig. 6.5 it is shown that a drug is bound in a reversible manner in various parts of the body. The nature of the binding material may vary but, in general, the bound drug is unable to pass through cell membranes because of the size and nature of the complex in which it is involved.

PROTEIN BINDING

The majority of drugs show some form of reversible binding with proteins. Several sites on the protein molecules may be involved and the stability of the drug-protein complex will determine its influence on the activity of the drug.

The formation of a complex, DP, by interaction of a drug, D, with a protein, P, may be represented by Eqn (6.48) where k_1 and k_2 are the rate constants for the forward and reverse reactions.

$$D + P \underset{k_2}{\overset{k_1}{\rightleftharpoons}} DP \qquad (6.48)$$

The amount of drug held in the complex form DP will depend on the concentrations of the drug and protein ([D] and [P], respectively), on the number of binding sites per protein molecule, n, and the affinity of the drug for the binding sites. This latter affinity may be represented by the association constant K for the reaction expressed in Eqn (6.48); (i.e. $K = k_1/k_2$). Goldstein (1949) has shown that if equilibrium is established then the fraction of total drug that is bound to a protein is given by Eqn (6.49)

$$\frac{[\text{Bound drug}]}{[\text{Total drug}]} = \frac{1}{1 + \dfrac{1}{Kn[P]} + \dfrac{[D]}{n[P]}} \qquad (6.49)$$

It can be seen from this equation that the fraction of bound drug increases as K, n and P increase and decreases as D increases.

Albumin is the commonest protein involved in the binding of drugs in plasma, although the α-globulins sometimes show a specificity for particular drugs. However, the binding capacity of the latter is relatively low compared with that of albumin.

The binding of drugs to proteins gives rise to various effects, some examples of which are given below.

1. Protein bound drugs are unable to penetrate membranes and therefore cannot reach the sites where excretion or biotransformation to other compounds occurs. Since the binding to proteins is a reversible interaction, the bound drug acts as a reservoir which releases unbound drug to replace that lost from the system by excretion or biotransformation. This effect is important in maintaining the concentration of unbound drug at a given level and, therefore, in prolonging the duration of action of the drug. For example, the different degrees of protein binding that occur with sulphonamides enable these drugs to be divided into long and short acting types; e.g. strongly bound drugs, such as sulphamethoxydiazine, exhibit a prolonged activity compared with those, such as sulphathiazole, which are only weakly bound to proteins. This effect is also responsible for the more prolonged action of

hydroxocobalamin compared with that of cyanocobalamin.

2. Protein binding may influence the solubility of drugs in the plasma; e.g. the solubility of dicoumarol in plasma is much greater than it is in physiological saline solutions (Gourley, 1967).

3. The response to a drug is caused by the build-up of a particular concentration of the drug at its site of action. Its total concentration in the plasma (i.e. bound + unbound drug) is, however, often used as an estimate of the amount of drug required to produce a particular response because it is much easier to determine this concentration. This procedure is often inaccurate since the different degrees of binding to proteins in the plasma and tissue proteins at the site of action may lead to an unequal distribution of the drug between the plasma and the particular tissue; for example, the strong binding of chlorpromazine to the lipoproteins in brain tissue produces a total concentration of this drug in the brain that is approximately fifty times greater than its total concentration in the plasma (Gourley, 1967).

4. Different substances may compete for the same binding sites on proteins. Such competition may lead to a variety of effects. For example, (a) the displacement of antibiotics from protein binding may be advantageous since a higher concentration of free drug is available to exert the required activity; (b) the displacement of protein bound anticoagulants may produce a high concentration of free drug and may therefore lead to excessive bleeding; (c) the acidic binding sites on albumin in premature babies are usually saturated with bilirubin, because the concentration of albumin is relatively low. The increase in free bilirubin that results when the bound form is displaced by acidic drugs such as salicylates and sulphonamides may cause brain damage (Gourley, 1967).

5. The response produced by a drug is caused by interaction between the drug and a receptor site. This interaction is similar to protein binding except that the latter type of binding involves relatively non-specific interactions while the drug-receptor interaction is very specific. However, substances with a similar structure to naturally occurring compounds may compete for a particular receptor site and so prevent a normal response; e.g. atropine inhibits the effect of acetylcholine by competing for the receptor sites on the cholinergic nerve endings.

BINDING TO OTHER TISSUE CONSTITUENTS

Interaction between the constituents of other tissues and drugs may lead to effects similar to those caused by binding to proteins. For example, very lipid soluble drugs (e.g. thiopentone) may accumulate in the body fat and tetracyclines may accumulate in hard tissues such as teeth, although the nature of the latter interaction is unknown.

Blood Concentrations

The concentration of a drug in the plasma is often related to the level of activity of the drug. It can be seen from Fig. 6.5 that the blood concentration will be affected mainly by the rate at which drug is absorbed into the plasma and by the rate at which the drug is eliminated by excretion or biotransformation. In addition, the distribution of drug between the plasma and other tissues will affect the blood concentration. Measurement of the concentration of a drug in the blood at various times after administration of a single dose produces results that can usually be represented by a curve similar to that shown in Fig. 6.8.

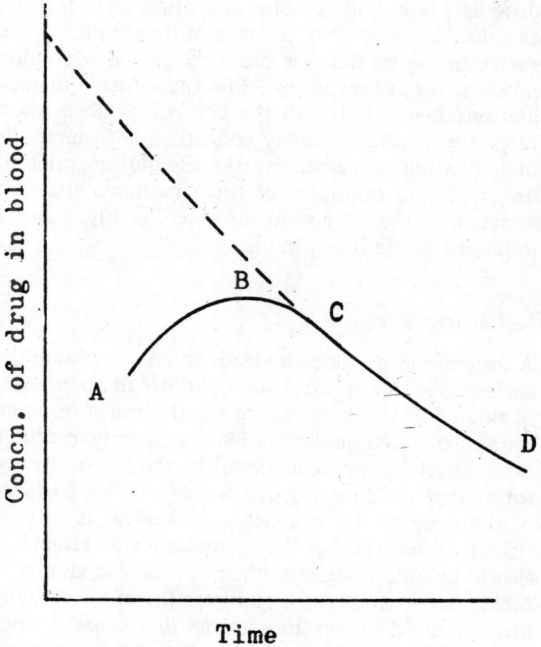

Fig. 6.8 The change in blood concentration of a systemically-active drug after administration of a single dose

The individual points on such a curve represent the difference between the amount of drug that has entered the plasma and the amount that has been eliminated in a given time. The shape of the curve indicates the rate of change in blood concentration (dc/dt), which can be expressed in terms of Eqn

(6.50), where dA/dt and dE/dt are the rates of entry into and elimination from the plasma respectively.

$$\frac{dc}{dt} = \frac{dA}{dt} - \frac{dE}{dt} \qquad (6.50)$$

The initial part, AB, of the curve in Fig. 6.8 indicates that the rate of absorption exceeds the rate of elimination, and this part of the curve is dependent on the nature of the dosage form and the route of administration. Obviously, in intravenous injections this part is absent and the maximum blood concentration is obtained immediately. The effects of other routes of administration and dosage forms that were included in Fig. 6.5 will be discussed later.

The latter part, BD, of the curve indicates that absorption is ceasing and the rate of elimination is now greater, and the smooth section of this part, i.e. CD, may be extrapolated backwards to indicate the apparent concentrations at shorter times, as shown by the dotted line. The elimination curve DC and its extrapolation can often be expressed by the first order kinetics, the linear form of which is given by Eqn (6.51)

$$\log C = \log C_0 - \frac{kt}{2\cdot303} \qquad (6.51)$$

where C is the concentration of drug in the blood, at time t, C_0 is the hypothetical concentration of drug when $t = 0$, and k is the rate constant for elimination of drug from the blood. Thus, a plot of $\log C$ versus t yields a straight line with a slope of $-k/2\cdot303$, and an intercept equal to $\log C_0$ if the disappearance of drug follows first order kinetics.

BIOLOGICAL HALF-LIFE

The rate of disappearance of a drug from body fluids such as blood is often expressed conveniently in terms of its biological half-life, $t_{\frac{1}{2}}$, which is the time taken for its concentration in the fluid to fall to half its initial value, assuming that the disappearance follows first order kinetics. This value is related to the rate constant k in Eqn (6.51), as shown by Eqn. (6.52)

$$t_{\frac{1}{2}} = \frac{0\cdot693}{k} \qquad (6.52)$$

The half-life can also be determined from inspection of graphs (*see* above).

EFFECT OF DOSAGE FORM AND ROUTE OF ADMINISTRATION ON THE BLOOD CONCENTRATIONS OF DRUGS

The rapidity with which maximum blood concentration of a drug is attained is affected markedly by the route of administration. In addition, the proportion of the actual dose administered that is absorbed into the plasma is also affected. In general, in drugs administered as solutions, these differences are dependent on the number and the nature of the membranes across which the drug must be transported before it reaches the plasma. Thus, a drug that is administered intravenously is not subject to any initial transport processes so that the maximum blood concentration is obtained immediately and the complete dose enters the plasma. This route of administration therefore offers the greatest degree of control of blood concentrations.

Absorption of drugs into the plasma after their administration as intramuscular or subcutaneous injections involves transport across membrane barriers. Such absorption is usually more rapid in intramuscular injections than with subcutaneous ones because the skeletal muscles have a better blood supply than subcutaneous tissue. In general both routes provide rapid absorption and involve little loss of drug, so that doses required to achieve a certain blood concentration are less than those in orally administered solutions. It should be borne in mind that the nature of specific drugs may alter these general observations. For example, the binding of phenylbutazone to tissue proteins after intramuscular injection reduces its absorption into the plasma to a considerably slower rate than that obtained after oral administration (Gourley, 1967).

The absorption of dissolved drugs from the stomach and intestine is dependent on the rates at which they are transported across the membrane lining the gastro-intestinal tract. The particular influence of pH on this transport process has already been discussed. The rate of absorption is also affected by the contents of the stomach and intestine and by the rate at which the stomach empties and fills. Rapid emptying will decrease absorption of a drug that is absorbed mainly from the stomach and enhance absorption of a drug that is absorbed readily from the intestine. Since the above effects vary tremendously between individuals, and even in the same individual under different conditions, the control of blood concentrations of orally administered drugs is difficult. Similar effects also apply to the absorption of drugs administered rectally as suppositories or retention enemas, poor control of blood concentrations again resulting.

The above discussion indicates that parenteral administration, particularly intravenous injection, provides the most rapid attainment of maximum blood concentration and allows the most satisfactory control over this concentration. However, the advantages and disadvantages of particular routes of administration must also be taken into account, as indicated by the examples in the following list.

(a) Injections are much less acceptable than oral preparations for self-administration by the patient because of: (i) the inconvenience in administration, (ii) the possibility of sensitisation, (iii) the possibility of discomfort, and (iv) the need for sterility of syringes etc.

(b) Inactivation of drugs by digestive enzymes or by the acid pH in the stomach may preclude oral administration. Parenteral or rectal administration may be used to overcome these effects.

(c) Difficulties in swallowing may prevent the use of oral administration.

When drugs are administered in dosage forms other than solutions the rate of release of drug from a dosage form as a solute in aqueous solution may be more important than its rate of transport across membranes in determining the rate of appearance in the plasma. In oral dosage forms in which the drug is present as a solid (e.g. powders, tablets, capsules, suspensions), the rate of dissolution in the gastro-intestinal fluids is often the rate determining process for absorption. Pharmaceutical manipulations associated with the control of absorption rates are therefore usually concerned with methods of increasing or decreasing the dissolution rates of drugs. Some examples of these methods that are relevant to the dosage forms given in Fig. 6.5 are indicated in the following list.

1. *Particle Size*

A decrease in particle size leads to an increase in the surface area of a powder and therefore to an increase in rate of dissolution. More rapid absorption from the stomach of a slowly soluble or relatively insoluble drug can therefore be achieved by the use of dosage forms that produce suspensions of smaller particles of the drug in the stomach. This effect is of particular importance in the formulation of tablets of slowly soluble materials since the surface area of a tablet is small. Such tablets therefore usually incorporate disintegrating agents that cause disruption of tablets into small particles when in contact with water. The drug is released by dissolution more rapidly from such particles than from the entire tablet. The rate of disintegration may also affect the rate of absorption of drugs administered in tablet form, and the BP includes a test that is designed to limit the time taken for disintegration of official tablets.

The absence of a disintegrating agent in a tablet that consists mainly of a slowly soluble substance produces the converse effect; i.e. a reduced rate of dissolution of the tablet. This effect is made use of in the formulation of tablets that provide a slow release of drug. Such slowly released doses are usually administered together with an initial dose of drug contained in part of the tablet that disintegrates and therefore is made available for rapid absorption. The slow release from the non-disintegrating part of the tablet maintains the concentration of drug in the plasma by allowing sufficient absorption to replace drug lost by excretion or biotransformation.

The increased absorption rate that results from the use of a smaller particle size may increase the efficiency of absorption; i.e. increase the proportion of drug that is absorbed from the administered dose. This effect is demonstrated by the observations of Atkinson *et al.* (1962) which showed that a reduction in the particle size of griseofulvin from 10 to 2·7 μm enabled the required effect of this antibiotic to be obtained with half the original dose.

The increased rate of solubility of chloramphenicol from solid solutions of this drug in urea is attributed to the fact that rapid dissolution of urea from these solid solutions leaves the chloramphenicol in a very finely dispersed form that is more rapidly soluble than normal particles of this drug (p. 30).

The more efficient absorption of salts of poorly soluble, weakly acidic drugs compared with the absorption of the corresponding free acids is attributed to the fact that although the free acids are liberated from their more soluble salts by the action of hydrochloric acid in the stomach, precipitation of the free acids, if it occurs, gives rise to very fine particles only. The latter redissolve rapidly when the concentration of the free acid in solution is decreased by absorption (Gorringe and Sproston, 1964).

2. Changes in Chemical Structure

Desirable changes in dissolution rates can often be achieved by the use of simple derivatives, different polymorphic forms or different hydrated forms of a drug. The effect of using the more soluble salts of sparingly soluble weak acids has already been discussed above. In addition, the use of chloramphenicol palmitate and other fatty acid esters of chloramphenicol instead of the free drug provides an example of the effect of change in solubility obtained from the use of a simple derivate of a drug. Chloramphenicol is extremely bitter and is therefore unsuitable for paediatric suspensions. The fatty acid esters of this drug are so insoluble that they do not stimulate the taste receptors on the tongue and are therefore satisfactory for paediatric use. The free drug is absorbed after liberation from the ester by hydrolysis in the stomach.

The effect of polymorphism is illustrated by the solubilities of the three polymorphic forms of riboflavine, which are 60 mg, 80 mg, and 1200 mg/litre, respectively. The effect of hydration of compounds (i.e. presence of water of crystallisation) usually causes a decrease in the rate of dissolution compared with that of the anhydrous forms; e.g. the anhydrous forms of caffeine and theophylline are more rapidly soluble than their hydrated forms.

3. Properties of Dosage Form

The importance of control of tablet disintegration rates in relation to methods of accelerating or retarding the rates of dissolution of ingredients has already been discussed. Retardation of dissolution rates is also achieved in certain dosage forms intended to provide a prolonged release of drug by the use of physical barriers that usually impede the diffusion of solvent into the dosage form and the outward diffusion of drug in solution. These barriers often consist of water insoluble fats, waxes or plastics and they may be used as a coating around the drugs or as matrices in which the drug is embedded. The rate of penetration of water and aqueous solutions through such barriers depends on the thickness of the diffusion pathway, the nature of the barrier materials (i.e. the more hydrophobic the material the slower the penetration of water), and on the porosity of the barrier. A similar effect is also achieved by the use of ion exchange resins from which bound drug is released when ion exchange occurs in the gastro-intestinal contents. The rate of exchange and the outward diffusion of drug is again dependent on the porosity of the ion exchange beads.

In certain cases the barrier may be insoluble in the gastric fluid but soluble in the intestinal juice. Such barriers, which may consist of shellac or cellulose acetate phthalate, are referred to as enteric coatings and may be used for orally administered drugs that are irritant to the gastric mucosa or that are destroyed by acid pH or gastric constituents.

Drugs administered in the form of suppositories are released into the rectum when the base melts at body temperature (e.g. theobroma oil, Witepsol bases) or when the base dissolves in the aqueous rectal liquid (e.g. polyethylene glycols). The small amount of water usually available in the rectum tends to retard the release of medicaments contained in the latter type of base. The release rates of the former type may be affected by the inclusion of surface active agents in the base. It is suggested that such agents alter the distribution of drugs between the molten fatty bases and aqueous body fluids and may cause emulsification at the interface between these two phases. The latter effect leads to an increase in the interfacial area across which partition can occur and, therefore, increases the rate of release of drug.

BIBLIOGRAPHY

BINNS, T. B. (Ed.) (1964) *Absorption and Distribution of Drugs*. Livingstone, London.

GARRETT, E. R. (1967) *Advances in Pharmaceutical Sciences. Vol. 2*. (H. S. Bean, A. H. Beckett, and J. E. Carless, Eds). Academic Press, London.

HOOVER, J. E. (Ed.) *Remington's Pharmaceutical Sciences* (1970) 14th ed. Mack Publishing Co., Pennsylvania.

KUNIN, R. (1958) *Ion Exchange Resins*. 2nd ed. Wiley and Sons, London.

LUNDBERG, W. O. (Ed.) (1961) *Autoxidation and Antioxidants. Vol. 1*. Interscience, New York.

MARTIN, A. N., SWARBRICK, J. and CAMMARATA, A. (1969) *Physical Pharmacy*. 2nd ed. Henry Kimpton, London.

SAUNDERS, L. (1966) *Principles of Physical Chemistry for Biology and Pharmacy*. University Press, Oxford.

SCOTT, G. (1965) *Atmospheric Oxidation and Antioxidants*. Elsevier, Amsterdam.

TROTMAN-DICKENSON, A. F. and PARFITT, G. D. (1966) *Chemical Kinetics and Surface and Colloid Chemistry*. Pergamon, London.

WILLIAMS, V. R. and WILLIAMS, H. B. (1967) *Basic Physical Chemistry for the Life Sciences*. Freeman and Co., London.

REFERENCES

ATKINSON, R. M., BEDFORD, C., CHILD, K. J., and TOMICH, E. G. (1962) *Antibiotics Chemother.*, **12**, 232–238.

BRODIE, B. B. (1964) *Absorption and Distribution of Drugs*. (T. B. Binns, Ed.). Livingstone, London, 16–48.

GARRETT, E. R. (1967) *Advances in Pharmaceutical Sciences. Vol. 2*. (H. S. Bean, A. H. Beckett, and J. E. Carless, Eds). Academic Press, London, 2–94.

GOLDSTEIN, A. (1949) The interactions of drugs and plasma proteins. *Pharmac. Rev.*, **1**, 102–165.

GORRINGE, J. A. L. and SPROSTON, E. M. (1964) *Absorption and Distribution of Drugs*. (T. B. Binns, Ed.). Livingstone, London. 128–139.

GOURLEY, D. R. H. (1967) *Modern Trends in Pharmacology and Therapeutics. Vol. 1*. (W. F. M. Fulton, Ed.). Butterworths, London, Chapter 1.

GUNN, C. and CARTER, S. J. (1965) *Dispensing for Pharmaceutical Students*. Pitman Medical, London.

HIGUCHI, T. and LACHMAN, L. (1955) Inhibition of hydrolysis of esters in solution by formation of complexes. I. Stabilization of benzocaine with caffeine. *J. Amer. pharm. Ass.*, (*Sci. Ed.*), **44**, 521–526.

JOHNSON, C. A. (1967) *Advances in Pharmaceutical Sciences. Vol. 2*. (H. S. Bean, A. H. Beckett, and J. E. Carless, Eds). Academic Press, London, 224–310.

JONES, W. and GRIMSHAW, J. J. (1963) Accelerated stability testing of pharmaceutical products. Papers 1 and 2. *Pharm. J.*, **191**, 459–465.

MACEK, T. J. (1970) *Remington's Pharmaceutical Sciences*. 14th ed., Mack Publishing Co., Pennsylvania. Chapter 79.

MARTIN, A. N., SWARBRICK, J. and CAMMARATA, A. (1969) *Physical Pharmacy*. 2nd ed. Henry Kimpton, London. Chapter 14.

NACHOD, F. C. and SCHUBERT, J. (1956) *Ion Exchange Technology*. Academic Press, New York.

SAUNDERS, L. (1966) *Principles of Physical Chemistry for Biology and Pharmacy*. University Press, Oxford, Chapter 8.

TOOTILL, J. P. R. (1961) A slope-ratio design for accelerated storage tests. *J. Pharm. Pharmac.*, **13**, 75T–86T.

7

Rheology

RHEOLOGY is the science concerned with the deformation of matter under the influence of stresses, which may be applied perpendicularly to the surface of a body (a tensile stress), tangentially to the surface (a shearing stress), or at any other angle to the surface. The deformations that result from the application of a stress may be divided into two types:

1. spontaneously reversible deformations or elastic deformations, and
2. permanent or irreversible deformations that are referred to as flow and are exhibited by viscous bodies.

The work used in producing an elastic deformation is recoverable when the body returns to its original shape after removal of the applied stress. However, in irreversible deformations the work used in maintaining deformation is dissipated as heat and is not recoverable mechanically when the stress is removed.

The majority of pharmaceutical systems where rheological properties are important range from simple liquids to semi-solids such as ointments, gels, creams, and pastes. Most attention has been paid to the flow properties of these systems, i.e. to their viscous behaviour. The importance of contributions from elastic effects to the rheological properties of semi-solid systems has gained more attention in recent years. However, this chapter is restricted to a consideration of the flow properties of pure liquids and disperse systems containing a liquid continuous phase since the complex nature of the rheological properties of semi-solids is outside the scope of the present discussion; information on these systems may be obtained from the booklist at the end of this chapter and from the review given by Barry and Warburton (1968).

Viscosity

Application of a shearing force to a fluid (i.e. a liquid or a gas) usually causes it to flow because fluid cannot support a strain for very long periods of time. When the force is removed, the fluid does not return to its original state; i.e. irreversible deformation has occurred. Such a deformation may be considered to involve a shearing action between infinitely thin layers (laminae) within the fluid. The deformation that results is expressed in terms of the rate of shear, which is the change in velocity of flow with a distance measured at right angles to the direction of flow. The shear stress that causes a particular rate of shear is obtained by dividing the shearing force by the area of the surface to which the shearing force is tangentially applied. The ratio of the applied shear stress to the rate of shear is known as the coefficient of viscosity. The effect of rate of shear on this ratio varies for different systems which has led to these systems being classified into the following types.

1. Newtonian Fluids

Flow of this type of fluid can be illustrated by Fig. 7.1, which represents two parallel planes each of area A separated by a fluid of depth x. The upper plane is caused to move with a velocity u relative to the lower plane by the application of a shearing force F. This movement causes the fluid in the laminae separating the two planes to be displaced relative to adjacent layers as shown in Fig. 7.1. The rate of movement of the laminae varies from a maximum value in the layer adjacent to the upper plane to a value that is close to zero in the layer adjacent to the lower plane. The mean rate of shear is given by the overall difference in fluid velocity, u, divided by the distance between the two planes, x; (i.e. the mean shear rate $= u/x$). In more general terms, for any point in a layer that is separated by a distance dx from the upper plane the rate of shear is given by du/dx. The shear stress, S, is given by F/A (i.e. the applied force per unit area) and the flow of Newtonian fluids may be expressed quantitatively by the Newton equation, Eqn (7.1)

$$S = \eta \frac{du}{dx} \qquad (7.1)$$

where η is a constant that is known as the coefficient of viscosity or simply the viscosity of the fluid.

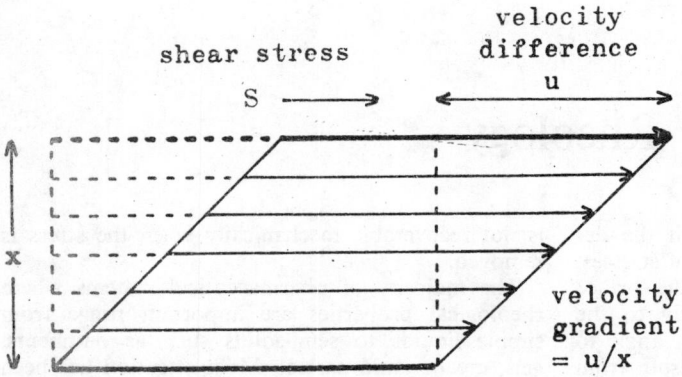

Fig. 7.1 Movement of planar laminae in simple shear

The dimensions of shear stress are force per unit area, and shear rate is measured in terms of reciprocal time: (shear rate = velocity/distance = distance × time^{-1}/distance = time^{-1}). Thus, the dimensions of η are given by Eqn (7.2)

$$\eta = \frac{S}{du/dx} = \frac{F/A}{du/dx} = \frac{\text{force}}{\text{area} \times \text{time}^{-1}} \quad (7.2)$$

However, since

$$\text{force} = \frac{\text{mass} \times \text{length}}{\text{time}^2}$$

and

$$\text{area} = \text{length}^2$$

the dimensions of η that are indicated by Eqn (7.2) reduce to mass/length × time (i.e. $ML^{-1}T^{-1}$).

The basic SI unit is therefore the kg m^{-1} s^{-1}. However, in the cgs system it was usual to express viscosities in units of dyne sec cm^{-2} in accordance with Eqn (7.2) and such units were termed poises in honour of Poiseuille, who was an early worker in this field. A similar derived SI unit is therefore used, the N s m^{-2}. It can be shown that 1 P (poise) = 0·1 N s m^{-2}, and 1 centipoise, cP, which is a convenient unit for use with fluids of low viscosity, is equal to 1×10^{-3} N s m^{-2}.

The rheological properties of liquids are usually expressed in the form of flow diagrams, which consist of graphs showing the variation of shear rate with shear stress. Equation (7.1) indicates that for a Newtonian fluid such a graph should be linear, as shown by line (a) in Fig. 7.2, the slope of which is equal to the reciprocal of viscosity, η, of the fluid, a value referred to as the fluidity, ϕ, i.e.

$$\phi = \frac{1}{\eta} \quad (7.3)$$

The linear nature of the flow diagram for a Newtonian fluid shows that η is, in fact, a true constant unaffected by the value of the rate of shear. Thus, a

single determination of η from the shear stress at any given shear rate is sufficient to characterise the flow properties of a Newtonian fluid. Liquids that show this type of behaviour include water, simple organic liquids, true solutions, and dilute suspensions and emulsions.

2. Non-Newtonian Fluids

Many liquids encountered in pharmaceutical practice (e.g. concentrated suspensions and emulsions) do not follow Eqn (7.1) because the value of η varies with the rate of shear. It is therefore usual to consider the apparent viscosities of these systems at particular rates of shear, where the apparent viscosity, η_{app}, is the ratio of shear stress to shear rate

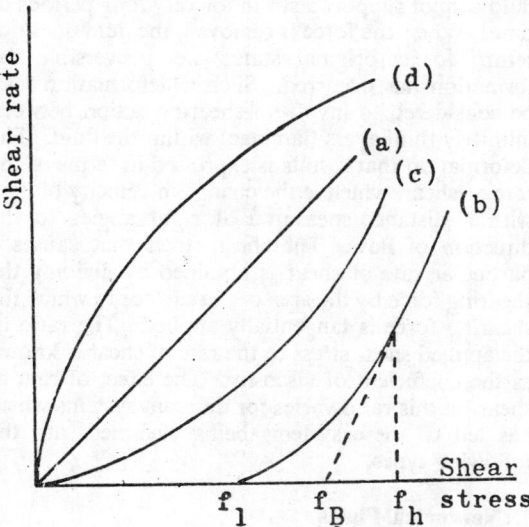

Fig. 7.2 Flow curves for Newtonian and Non-Newtonian systems

(a) Newtonian   (b) Plastic
(c) Pseudoplastic   (d) Dilatant

at a given point on the flow diagram. In addition, the influence of shear on the apparent viscosity may be time-dependent and this effect provides a further variation in the flow properties of some non-Newtonian fluids. The results of such time-dependent effects will be discussed later.

The lines (b), (c), and (d) in Fig. 7.2 represent the flow behaviours of the three common types of non-Newtonian fluid, in which time-dependent effects are absent. These types are referred to as plastic, pseudoplastic, and dilatant flow, respectively. The changing slopes of these three lines indicate that the apparent viscosity varies with rate of shear. A single determination of η_{app} from the shear stress at any given shear rate would therefore be of little use, and the whole flow diagram must be determined in order to characterise these non-Newtonian systems.

(a) PLASTIC FLOW

This is represented by curve (b) in Fig. 7.2 in which it can be seen that the line does not pass through the origin of the graph but arises at some point on the shear stress axis. This indicates that a certain shearing stress must be exerted before flow begins. This stress is termed the yield value, the system behaving like a solid when small stresses that are lower than this value are applied to it; i.e. the system exhibits elastic deformations that are reversible when these small stresses are removed.

Materials that show plastic behaviour are often termed Bingham bodies in honour of Bingham, who carried out many of the early studies on these materials. The quantitative behaviour of these systems is usually expressed in terms of the Bingham equation, Eqn (7.4), where f_B is the Bingham yield value, η_{pl} or U is the plastic viscosity, the other terms being defined as before.

$$U \text{ or } \eta_{pl} = \frac{S - f_B}{du/dx} \qquad (7.4)$$

This equation implies that the flow diagram is a straight line that arises on the shear stress axis at the yield value. In practice, however, flow usually occurs at a lower shear stress, the flow curve gradually approaching the theoretical line shown in Fig. 7.2. It is often more satisfactory to use the lower yield value, f_l, in practical applications of plastic materials since this indicates when actual flow begins. In addition, a higher yield value, f_h, is sometimes used. This corresponds to the shear stress beyond which the flow curve becomes linear. The three yield values are indicated in Fig. 7.2.

(b) PSEUDOPLASTIC FLOW

This type of behaviour is represented by line (c) in Fig. 7.2. It can be seen that the curve arises at the

origin of the graph, i.e. no yield value exists, and flow begins immediately on application of a shearing stress. The slope of the curve gradually increases until it reaches a maximum value. Since the apparent viscosity at any shear rate is given by the reciprocal of the slope it can be seen that the apparent viscosity decreases as the shear rate increases, until a constant value is reached.

Pseudoplastic flow cannot as yet be satisfactorily expressed quantitatively by equations based on fundamental principles. An empirical equation, Eqn (7.5), is often used and this shows reasonable agreement with experimental results except for those obtained over extended ranges of shearing stresses.

$$S^n = k \frac{du}{dx} \qquad (7.5)$$

In this equation k and n are constants for a particular system. If $n = 1$ the equation is similar to the Newtonian equation, Eqn (7.1), but the greater the value of n the more pseudoplastic the behaviour. The values of these constants can be obtained by plotting $\log du/dx$ versus $\log S$. If Eqn (7.5) is applicable, then a straight line is obtained with a slope of n and an intercept on the $\log du/dx$ axis that is equal to $\log k$.

The decrease in apparent viscosity with increasing rates of shear in plastic and pseudoplastic systems results from the breakdown, under the influence of shear, of structures (e.g. aggregates of dispersed particles) in the system. Greater breakdown occurs at higher shear rates, although beyond certain high shear rates no further structural breakdown can occur and the apparent viscosity then becomes constant. When the shear stress is reduced or removed, reformation of the structures in these systems occurs immediately and the flow curve obtained from measurements at decreasing shear rates is superimposable on that obtained from measurements taken at increasing shear rates. The occurrence of a yield value in plastic systems indicates that stronger forces than those in pseudoplastic systems must first be overcome before flow can occur.

To distinguish between plastic and pseudoplastic behaviour it is necessary to obtain measurements at low shear rates. Extrapolation of linear portions of flow curves obtained at high rates of shear should not be carried out to provide possible yield values since the system may, in fact, be a pseudoplastic one. Thus, differentiation between these two types of behaviour often depends upon the sensitivity of the method of measurement at low shear rates.

(c) DILATANT FLOW

This type of behaviour is represented by curve (d) in Fig. 7.2. It can be seen that the slope of this curve gradually decreases to a constant value, which indicates that the apparent viscosity must increase with increase in shear rate up to a maximum value.

A power equation similar to that used for pseudoplastic flow (Eqn 7.5) may be used to describe the behaviour of dilatant materials but in this case the constant n is less than one.

Dilatancy is usually exhibited by concentrated dispersions of deflocculated particles (*see* Chapter 5). It is suggested that in these systems the particles are arranged in a state of close packing and the small amount of liquid present is sufficient to fill the narrow spaces between adjacent particles. These thin liquid films allow the system to flow like a liquid when the rate of shear is low. However, at higher shear rates the particles will become displaced from their close-packed arrangement, which results in the formation of larger void spaces in the system. The liquid continuous medium is now insufficient to fill all the spaces between particles, hence the movement of the latter relative to each other involves a greater amount of friction and the apparent viscosity therefore increases. This effect may be troublesome in high-speed milling processes since the viscosity of dilatant suspensions may increase so much at the high rates of shear involved in the operation of these mills that overloading of the motors may occur.

Time-dependent Effects

In certain cases the breakdown by shearing forces of structures in disperse systems is markedly time-dependent; i.e. the amount of breakdown increases with time so that the apparent viscosity gradually decreases even when the shear rate is maintained constant. The effect may be reversible or irreversible after removal of the shearing stress. If it is reversible, i.e. if the structure reforms on removal of the stress, the reformation process is usually time-dependent also, so that a time lag occurs before the original viscosity is achieved.

The redetermination of a flow curve after an initial determination may be used to indicate the difference in flow properties of a system before and after structural breakdown by shearing forces has occurred; i.e. the two curves are not superimposable and a hysteresis loop is obtained in the flow diagram (*see* Fig. 7.3). The area of such a loop may be used as an indication of the relative amount of structural breakdown that has occurred in the system.

The previous paragraphs have considered only time-dependent effects that result in a decrease in apparent viscosity with increase in shear rate. The reverse process may also occur. The various types of time-dependent effect are as follows.

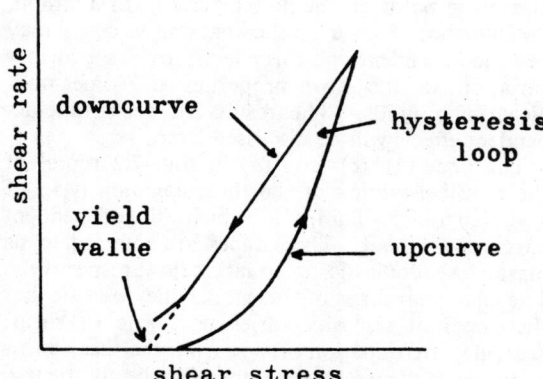

Fig. 7.3   Flow curve for a system that exhibits thixotropy superimposed upon plastic behaviour

(a) THIXOTROPY

This term means 'to change by touch'. It is usually defined as a reversible isothermal transition from a gel to a sol (i.e. a colloidal dispersion). However, it is applied to any reversible time-dependent decrease in apparent viscosity that results from the application of shearing forces. The decrease in viscosity arises from a breakdown of structures (e.g. a gel network) within a system when it is sheared. After the shearing forces are removed a time lag occurs before structural re-formation is complete. Bentonite gel is a good example of a system that exhibits thixotropy, and Fig. 7.3 illustrates the flow diagram of the system. It is believed that the breakdown of the random network (*see* Chapter 5) formed by the hydrated bentonite particles on application of a shearing force is caused by the elongated particles aligning with their long axes parallel to the direction of flow of the continuous aqueous phase. This orderly arrangement causes the interparticle links to be broken; the network therefore disintegrates and the apparent viscosity decreases. On removal of the shearing forces the arrangement of dispersed particles gradually becomes less orderly under the influence of Brownian motion, and the gel network re-forms after a time lag.

A similar effect, referred to as irreversible thixotropy, is sometimes encountered. Application of shearing forces causes breakdown of structures within the system but these structures do not reform on removal of the shear stress, or the time lag is so long that from a practical point of view the effect is irreversible.

(b) RHEOPEXY

The time lag that occurs before a reversible thixotropic system returns to its original state after removal of the shearing stress may often be reduced by applying a gentle rolling or rocking motion. It is suggested this motion provides a mild turbulence that aids the return of dispersed particles to a random orientation when network re-formation can occur.

(c) NEGATIVE THIXOTROPY

The distinction between this effect and rheopexy is confused (Bauer and Collins, 1967). Both effects lead to a time-dependent increase in apparent viscosity on application of a shearing stress. Samyn and Wan (1967) suggest that the negative thixotropy they observed in their studies on clay suspensions was caused by breakdown of relatively large compact floccules, the breakdown leading to an increase in the interparticle contact in the system, which therefore exhibited an increase in apparent viscosity. These workers also observed an effect, analogous to the phenomenon of rheopexy in reversible thixotropic systems, which caused the clay suspensions to become more mobile under the influence of a mild turbulence; they suggested that it be called negative rheopexy.

The frequent occurrence of time-dependent effects in the rheological behaviour of disperse systems, and the long lag times that are often required before an effect is reversed after removal of shearing forces indicate that a knowledge of the histories of these systems is important in any rheological study. Standardised pre-treatments and handling techniques should therefore be employed whenever possible in such studies.

THE DETERMINATION OF FLOW PROPERTIES

Many types of viscometer have been devised for measuring flow properties. Some of these are capable of providing data for calculating viscosities in terms of fundamental units. However, the design of many instruments prevents their use in this manner since they are capable of providing data only in terms of empirical units that cannot be transformed into fundamental ones. These empirical instruments therefore provide relative measurements only; they are often used in quality control processes.

A review of the many types of viscometer that are available commercially is beyond the scope of this chapter, which is therefore limited to a consideration of the general principles of the more common types of instrument and to the methods mentioned in the BP (1968). The most frequently used viscometers involve the measurement of: (a) the rate of flow of liquids through capillary tubes, or (b) the rate of shear or shearing stresses in liquids moving between concentric cylinders or between cones and plates in rotational viscometers. These methods are therefore considered initially in the following sections.

1. Capillary Viscometers

These are the most commonly used instruments for Newtonian liquids. They measure the rate of flow of liquids through capillary tubes under the influence of gravity or an externally applied pressure. Applied pressure increases the range of usefulness of these instruments which can be used for investigating non-Newtonian behaviour.

(a) THE OSTWALD U-TUBE VISCOMETER (Fig. 7.4)

This is the most common type of instrument, in which flow through a capillary occurs under the influence of gravity. It is specified by the British Standards Institution and is described in the BP (1968). Various sizes are designated in the BP for use in determining the viscosity of Liquid Paraffin, Dextran Injection, and Iron Sorbitol Injection.

Liquid is introduced into the viscometer through the arm V until the level reaches the mark G. A fine pipette is used in this operation to avoid wetting the sides of the tube above G. The viscometer is fixed vertically in a thermostatted bath and allowed to attain the required temperature. The sample volume is adjusted and the liquid is sucked or blown into arm W until the meniscus is just above mark E. The suction or pressure is released and the time taken for the bottom of the meniscus to fall from E to F is noted.

(b) THE UBBELOHDE SUSPENDED LEVEL VISCOMETER (Fig. 7.5)

This is one of the many modifications of the U-tube viscometer. It is described in the BP (1968) where it is specified for use in the determination of the viscosity of a standard aqueous solution of Methylcellulose 450. A volume of liquid sufficient to fill bulb C during use is introduced through tube V. This volume must not be too large, otherwise the lower end of the ventilating tube Z will be blocked. The viscometer is fixed vertically in a thermostatted bath and allowed to reach temperature equilibrium. The ventilating tube Z is then closed and liquid is drawn into C by applying suction at W until the meniscus is just above the mark E. The liquid is held at this level by closing W, and Z is opened so that liquid drains away from below the capillary. W is finally opened, and the time taken for the meniscus to fall from E to F is observed. If the end

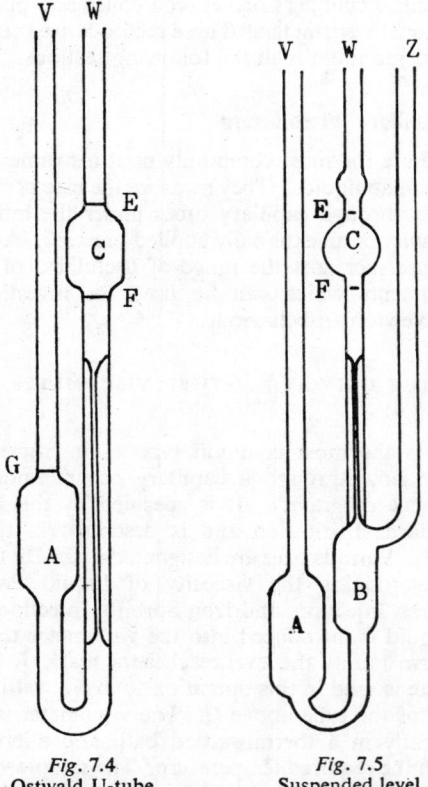

Fig. 7.4
Ostwald U-tube
viscometer

Fig. 7.5
Suspended level
viscometer

of tube Z becomes blocked by the liquid at any time while the liquid is flowing through the capillary the determination must be repeated.

The suspended level viscometer avoids the difficulties associated with readjustment of the volume of liquid in the viscometer when measurements are taken at a series of temperatures, since the lower liquid level is fixed automatically at the bottom of the capillary.

CALCULATION OF RESULTS

The rate of flow of liquids through tubes is given by Poiseuille's equation, Eqn (7.6), where V is the volume of liquid flowing in time t, p is the pressure difference across the ends of the tube, r and l are the radius and length of the tube, respectively, and η is the coefficient of viscosity of the liquid.

$$\frac{V}{t} = \frac{\pi p r^4}{8 \eta l} \qquad (7.6)$$

This equation applies to conditions of streamline flow only; i.e. when Reynolds' number is less than

1000 (*see* p. 146), and the dimensions of a chosen viscometer should therefore ensure that this type of flow does occur in the liquid under test. In a particular viscometer the values of r and l are constant, and Eqn (7.6) may therefore be written as—

$$\frac{V}{t} \propto \frac{p}{\eta} \qquad (7.7)$$

The pressure p will depend on the hydrostatic head of liquid, which depends, in turn, on the difference in heights of the liquid in the two arms of the U-tube viscometer. However, this difference will decrease as the liquid flows from the reservoir through the capillary. If h is the average difference in heights of a liquid with a density ρ, then the average hydrostatic pressure p is given by Eqn (7.8), where g is the gravitational constant.

$$p = h\rho g \qquad (7.8)$$

Substitution for p in Eqn (7.7) yields—

$$\frac{V}{t} \propto \frac{h\rho g}{\eta} \qquad (7.9)$$

However, V and h will be constant for a given viscometer,

$$\therefore \frac{1}{t} \propto \frac{\rho}{\eta} \qquad (7.10)$$

The ratio of viscosity, η, to density, ρ, of a liquid is termed the kinematic viscosity (v); i.e.

$$v = \frac{\eta}{\rho} \qquad (7.11)$$

and it is usually expressed in terms of units known as stokes (St). The SI units are, in fact, $m^2\,s^{-1}$ and $1\,St = 1 \times 10^{-4}\,m^2\,s^{-1}$. Substitution of kinematic viscosity into Eqn (7.10) shows that

$$\frac{1}{t} \propto \frac{1}{v} \qquad (7.12)$$

or

$$v = ct \qquad (7.13)$$

where c is a constant that depends on the dimensions of the viscometer. The value of c can be determined from observations on the rate of flow of a liquid with a known kinematic viscosity. Oils with standard viscosities are available commercially for direct calibration of viscometers. Alternatively, a step-up procedure may be employed in calibrating a series of viscometers of increasing size. This involves using water as a primary standard for calibrating a viscometer with the slowest efflux time. The kinematic viscosity of a more viscous liquid is determined using the same viscometer, the liquid then being used to calibrate the next largest viscometer. The procedure is repeated until all the viscometers in the series are calibrated. However, the method is satisfactory only if the correction terms (see later) are negligible.

EXPERIMENTAL PRECAUTIONS AND CORRECTIONS

A suitable viscometer must be chosen to ensure that: (a) streamline flow occurs in the capillary, and (b) unnecessarily long flow times are avoided. The viscometer must be well-cleaned before use, and air bubbles must be excluded from the liquid inside it. Adequate temperature control should be provided and care should be taken to ensure that the viscometer is fixed vertically.

For accurate determinations corrections should be made to allow for effects that arise from: (i) the changes in velocity that occur when liquid enters a capillary from a reservoir and flows from the capillary into a lower reservoir; (ii) the use of part of the applied pressure to impart kinetic energy to the liquid; and (iii) surface tension, which tends to raise or lower the meniscus of a liquid in a tube and therefore affects the hydrostatic pressure. Details of methods of allowing for these corrections are given in the references cited in the Bibliography at the end of this chapter.

2. Rotational Viscometers

The basic design of this type of viscometer involves the relative rotation of two components, separated by the material under test, about the same axis of symmetry. Many designs are available but the most common geometries are those that involve concentric cylinders or a cone and plate.

(a) CONCENTRIC CYLINDER VISCOMETERS

A simple example of this type of viscometer is shown in Fig. 7.6. The outer cylinder A, which acts as a container for the liquid, can be rotated at different speeds, and the inner cylinder B is suspended freely by a torsion wire. Rotation of A produces movement of the liquid in the gap separating the cylinders, and a torque is transmitted to the inner cylinder. The resultant stress exerted on this latter cylinder is

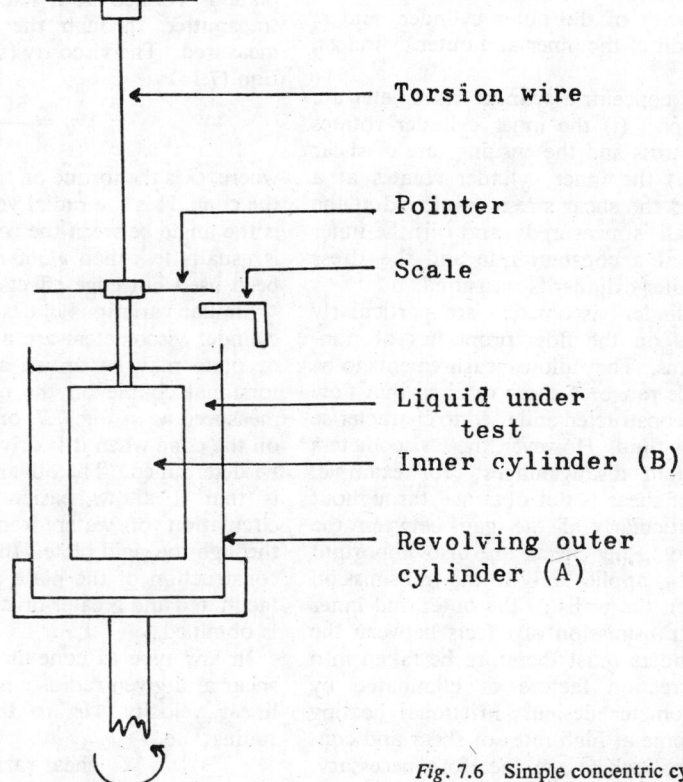

Torsion wire

Pointer

Scale

Liquid under test

Inner cylinder (B)

Revolving outer cylinder (A)

Fig. 7.6 Simple concentric cylinder **viscometer**

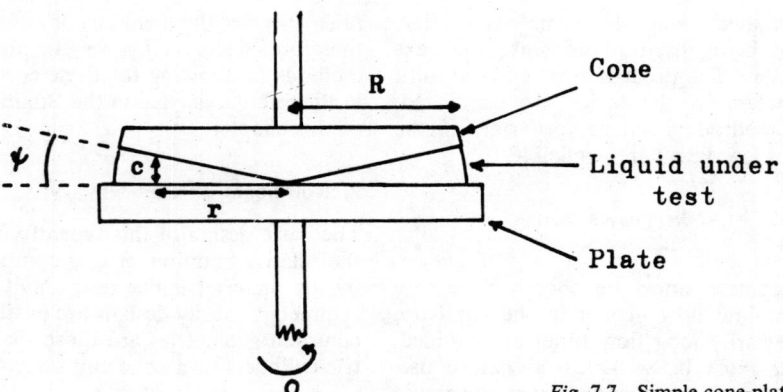

Fig. 7.7 Simple cone-plate viscometer

indicated by the angular deflection, θ, of a pointer which moves past a scale. Provided a steady laminar flow occurs in the liquid then the viscosity may be calculated from Eqn (7.14),

$$c\theta = \frac{4\pi h\omega\eta}{\dfrac{1}{r_1{}^2} - \dfrac{1}{r_2{}^2}} \qquad (7.14)$$

where c is the torsional constant of the wire, h is the height of inner cylinder covered by the liquid, ω is the angular velocity of the outer cylinder, and r_1 and r_2 are the radii of the inner and outer cylinders, respectively.

Other types of concentric cylinder viscometer are available in which: (i) the inner cylinder rotates under constant stress and the ensuing rate of shear is measured; (ii) the inner cylinder rotates at a constant rate and the shear stress developed at the inner cylinder wall is measured; and (iii) the inner cylinder rotates at a constant rate and the stress exerted on the outer cylinder is measured.

Concentric cylinder viscometers are particularly useful in studies on the flow properties of non-Newtonian systems. They allow measurements to be made over a wide range of shear rates so that flow diagrams can be constructed and used to characterise the behaviour of a fluid. However, these viscometers suffer from certain disadvantages; for example, a uniform rate of shear is not obtained throughout the sample, particularly if the gap between the cylinders is large. End effects are also important because Eqn (7.14) applies only to the transmission of torque between the walls of the outer and inner cylinders. The transmission of effects between the ends of the cylinders must therefore be taken into account by correction factors or eliminated by satisfactory viscometer design. Frictional heating may be troublesome at high rates of shear and constant temperature jackets are therefore necessary.

In addition, filling and cleaning are often difficult if the gap width is narrow, and large quantities of liquid may be needed if the gap is wide or if the cylinders are of large dimensions.

(b) CONE-PLATE VISCOMETERS

One type of cone-plate viscometer, illustrated in Fig. 7.7, consists of a slightly conical disc, the apex of which just touches a flat plate. In this type the plate is rotated at a fixed speed and the torque transmitted through the sample to the cone is measured. The viscosity (η) may be calculated from Eqn (7.15)

$$\eta = \frac{3G/2\pi R^3}{\Omega/\psi} \qquad (7.15)$$

where, G is the torque on the cone, R is the radius of the cone, Ω is the radial velocity of the plate, and ψ is the angle between the cone and plate. This angle is usually less than $\pi/360$ rad. Greater angles have been used but edge effects then become important.

Similar variations in design to those of concentric cylinder viscometers are available. Thus, the cone or plate may be driven at a fixed speed and the torsional couple on the other component may be measured as in Fig. 7.7, or the torque that develops on the cone when it is driven at constant speed may be determined. The advantage of this latter design is that it allows easier temperature control by circulation of water from a thermostatted bath through the rigid plate. In addition, the mechanical construction of the plate adjustment mechanism is facilitated and greater precision of gap width control is obtained.

In any type of cone-plate viscometer the rate of shear at a given radius r is equal to the ratio of the linear velocity, Ωr, to the gap width, c, at that radius; i.e.

$$\text{shear rate} = \Omega r/c \qquad (7.16)$$

Since both these quantities are proportional to the radius r it follows that the shear rate is constant throughout the entire sample under test. This is an advantage compared with concentric cylinder viscometers. In addition, only a small amount of liquid is required in cone-plate viscometers, and cleaning is easy.

3. Other Viscometers Specified in the BP

(a) FALLING SPHERE VISCOMETER

This viscometer is based on Stokes' law, which states that a body falling through a viscous medium experiences a resistance or viscous drag that tends to oppose the motion of the body. Thus, when a body falls through a liquid under the influence of gravity, an initial period, during which acceleration of the falling motion occurs, is followed by motion at a uniform terminal velocity when the gravitational force is balanced by the viscous drag. Equation (7.17), in which g represents the acceleration due to gravity, may be applied when this terminal velocity, u, is attained by a sphere of diameter d and density ρ_s falling through a liquid of viscosity η and density ρ_1.

$$3\pi\eta du = \frac{\pi}{6} d^3 g(\rho_s - \rho_1) \qquad (7.17)$$

The left-hand side of this equation represents the viscous drag experienced by the sphere, and the right-hand side represents the force responsible for the downward motion of the sphere under the influence of gravity. Rearrangement of Eqn (7.17) shows that the viscosity may be calculated if the velocity u is measured and r, ρ_s, and ρ_1 are known; i.e.

$$\eta = \frac{d^2 g(\rho_s - \rho_1)}{18u} \qquad (7.18)$$

In addition, since $v = \eta/\rho_1$ then Eqn (7.19) allows the kinematic viscosity (v) of the liquid to be calculated.

$$v = \frac{d^2 g(\rho_s - \rho_1)}{18u\rho_1} \qquad (7.19)$$

In the derivation of these equations it is assumed that the sphere is falling through a medium of infinite dimensions. However, in practice the liquid is contained in a cylinder or fall tube of a finite size. A correction factor, known as the Faxen term, F, must therefore be introduced into these equations to allow for the effect of the walls of the fall tube on the motion of the sphere; e.g.

$$v = \frac{d^2 g(\rho_s - \rho_1)F}{18u\rho_1} \qquad (7.20)$$

The correction factor F may be calculated from Eqn (7.21), where D is the diameter of the fall tube.

$$F = 1 - 2 \cdot 104 d/D + 2 \cdot 09 d^3/D^3 \qquad (7.21)$$

The measurement of u may be carried out in the apparatus illustrated in Fig. 7.8. The liquid is placed in the fall tube, which is clamped vertically

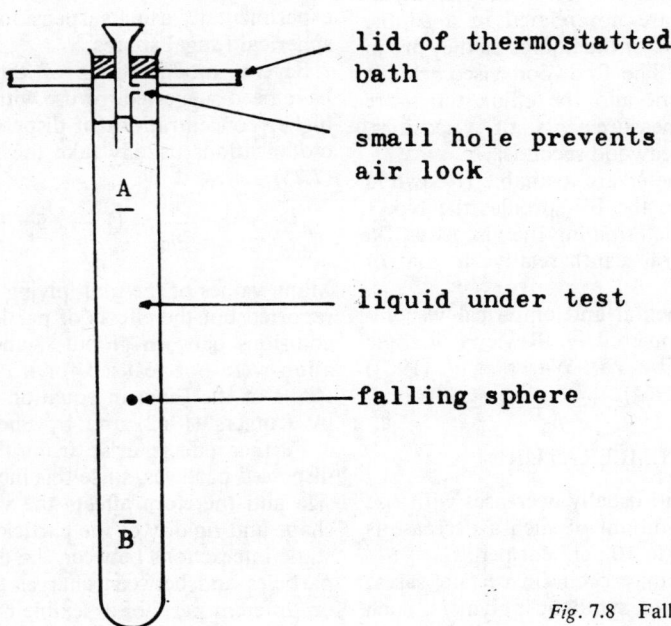

lid of thermostatted bath

small hole prevents air lock

liquid under test

falling sphere

Fig. 7.8 Falling sphere viscometer

inside a constant temperature bath. Sufficient time is allowed for temperature equilibrium to be attained and for air bubbles to be removed from the liquid. A steel sphere is cleaned and allowed to reach the temperature of the test before being introduced into the fall tube through a narrow guide tube. The motion of the sphere is followed by a suitable telescope and the time taken for it to pass between the marks A and B is noted.

If the same sphere and fall tube are used, Eqn (7.20) reduces to

$$\nu = Kt(\rho_s/\rho_l - 1) \tag{7.22}$$

where K is a constant that may be determined from observations using a liquid of known kinematic viscosity.

The falling sphere viscometer is described in the BP (1968), which specifies its use in the determination of the viscosity of a solution of Pyroxylin in acetone.

This type of viscometer is usually employed for Newtonian fluids, and a similar viscometer, known as the rolling sphere viscometer, involves the determination of the velocity of a rolling motion of a sphere down an inclined tube filled with liquid.

(b) REDWOOD VISCOMETER

This involves determining the time taken for a given volume of liquid to flow through a narrow orifice. The geometry of this orifice precludes the application of Poiseuille's equation, Eqn (7.6), to this viscometer and the efflux times are not related in a simple manner to the viscosities of the liquids as they are in capillary viscometers. The Redwood viscometer is an empirical instrument and the efflux times are therefore arbitrary measurements of viscosities, usually expressed as Redwood seconds.

Two sizes of viscometer are available (Redwood No. 1 and No. 2), and the BP specifies the No. 1 instrument for use in determining the viscosity of a standard solution of tragacanth relative to that of water.

Many other fundamental and empirical viscometers are available commercially. Reviews of these instruments are given by Van Wazer et al. (1963) and by Martin et al. (1964).

THE EFFECT OF TEMPERATURE

The viscosity of a liquid usually decreases with rise in temperature. The amount of such a decrease is often of the order of 1 to 10 per cent per °C.

The opposite effect may occur in certain cases; e.g. aqueous solutions of synthetic polymers, such as methylcellulose, which exhibit gel formation when the temperature is increased.

The commonly observed decrease in viscosity with rise in temperature may often be expressed by Eqn (7.23), where A and B are constants for a given liquid, R is the gas constant and T is the thermodynamic temperature.

$$\eta = Ae^{B/RT} \tag{7.23}$$

THE FLOW PROPERTIES OF DISPERSE SYSTEMS

The presence of dispersed particles in a liquid continuous medium causes the streamlines of liquid around the particles to be distorted which, in turn, causes a further dissipation of energy. The viscosity of the system is therefore increased. The Einstein equation (7.24) provides a quantitative expression of this effect.

$$\frac{\eta}{\eta_0} = (1 + 2\cdot5\phi) \tag{7.24}$$

In this equation, η and η_0 are the viscosities of the disperse system and the pure continuous medium, respectively, and ϕ is the volume fraction of the disperse phase; i.e. the volume of the disperse phase divided by the total volume of the system.

The assumptions made in the derivation of Eqn (7.24) restrict its application to dilute disperse systems. In fact, its use is theoretically limited to systems containing disperse particles which consist of rigid spheres. The equation has been verified experimentally using suspensions of glass beads and spherical fungal spores.

Several modifications of the Einstein equation have been suggested for use with systems containing higher concentrations of dispersed particles. These modifications usually take the form shown in Eqn (7.25)

$$\frac{\eta}{\eta_0} = (1 + 2\cdot5\phi + x\phi^2) \tag{7.25}$$

Many values of the multiplying factor, x, have been reported but the effects of particle size distribution, collisions between globules, and degree of flocculation were not realised for a long time. Modified forms of the Einstein equation have been reviewed by Rutgers (1962) and by Sherman (1964, 1968).

Further effects arise from the solvation of the dispersed particles, since this increases their effective size and therefore affects the value of ϕ, from the shape and rigidity of the particles, and from electrostatic interactions between the double layers around particles and between charges that may be present on different parts of a flexible macromolecule.

1. Colloidal Dispersions

The following viscosity coefficients, often referred to in the literature, may be defined with respect to the Einstein equation.

(a) Relative Viscosity (or viscosity ratio)

This is given the symbol η_{rel} and is defined as the ratio of the viscosity, η, of a dispersion to that of its liquid continuous medium, η_0; i.e.

$$\eta_{rel} = \frac{\eta}{\eta_0} = 1 + 2 \cdot 5\phi \qquad (7.26)$$

(b) Specific Viscosity (or viscosity ratio increment)

This is given the symbol η_{sp} and is defined as the relative increase in viscosity caused by the presence of the dispersed phase; i.e.

$$\eta_{sp} = \frac{\eta - \eta_0}{\eta_0} = \frac{\eta}{\eta_0} - 1 \qquad (7.27)$$

$\therefore$ from Eqn (7.26)

$$\eta_{sp} = 2 \cdot 5\phi \qquad (7.28)$$

In addition, since the volume fraction is directly related to the concentration of the disperse phase, then Eqn (7.28) may be written in the form

$$\eta_{sp} = kc \qquad (7.29)$$

where k is a constant and c is the concentration, usually expressed in terms of grammes of disperse phase in 100 cm^3 of total dispersion.

It should be remembered that the above equations apply to dilute systems only. For more concentrated dispersions the last equation is usually written as a power series, Eqn (7.30), where α and β are constants that must be calculated from experimental observations.

$$\eta_{sp} = \alpha c + \beta c^2 + \cdots \qquad (7.30)$$

(c) Reduced Viscosity (or Staudinger's viscosity number)

This is the ratio of specific viscosity to concentration obtained by dividing the previous equation through by c; i.e.

$$\frac{\eta_{sp}}{c} = \alpha + \beta c + \cdots \qquad (7.31)$$

(d) Intrinsic Viscosity (or the Kraemer viscosity number)

This is given the symbol $[\eta]$. It is the intercept obtained by extrapolation of a graph of reduced viscosity versus concentration, as shown in Fig. 7.9.

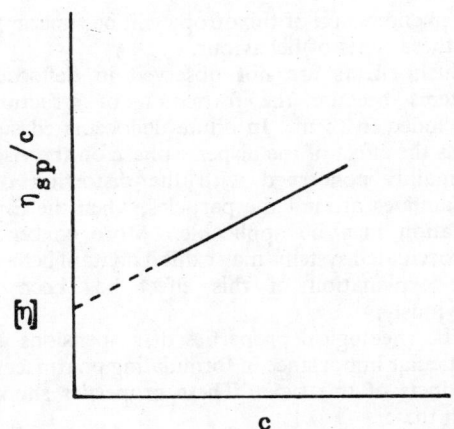

Fig. 7.9 Plot of reduced viscosity versus concentration showing determination of intrinsic viscosity

This coefficient is useful in calculating the average molecular weight, $\bar{M}$, of polymers, to which it is related by Eqn (7.32), where K and a are constants that must be obtained from separate experiments at fixed temperature with a given polymer-solvent system.

$$[\eta] = K\bar{M}^a \qquad (7.32)$$

The determination of intrinsic viscosity is used as a test in the BP for the standardisation of Dextran Injection, which is a plasma substitute, since the average molecular weight of this material will influence its retention in the capillaries.

Suspensions

The rheological properties of suspensions are markedly affected by the degree of flocculation that occurs in a given system. The presence of floccules tends to reduce the amount of free continuous medium, since much of it is entrapped within the floccules. The apparent viscosity of a flocculated suspension is therefore usually higher than that of a similar suspension in which the particles are deflocculated. In addition, marked flocculation produces a considerable amount of structure within a system. If the forces responsible for the formation of such structures are able to withstand weak stresses then the system will possess a yield value, below which it will exhibit the characteristics of solids. When the applied stress is sufficient to overcome the forces responsible for floccule formation a progressively greater amount of structural breakdown will occur as the shear stress is increased. Thus, flocculated suspensions will tend to exhibit plastic or pseudoplastic behaviour. If the breakdown and reformation of floccules is time-dependent, the phenomenon of thixotropy will be superimposed on these types of behaviour.

Such effects are not observed in deflocculated systems because the formation of structures is precluded in them. In dilute deflocculated suspensions the effect of the disperse phase on the viscosity is mainly concerned with the distortion of the streamlines around the particles, when the Einstein equation may be applicable. More concentrated deflocculated systems may exhibit dilatant behaviour. The explanation of this effect has been given previously.

The rheological properties of suspensions are of particular importance in formulating pharmaceutical products of this type. These properties should be such that:

(i) the product is easily administered (e.g. easily poured from a bottle or injected through a syringe needle),
(ii) sedimentation is either prevented, or if it does occur, redispersion is easy, and
(iii) the product has an elegant appearance.

Several methods may be employed to obtain these desired properties.

(a) Deflocculated Particles in Newtonian Vehicles

Sedimentation in these systems will produce a compact sediment or cake that is difficult to redisperse. The rate of sedimentation can be decreased by using a liquid continuous medium that possesses a high Newtonian viscosity. Such a system may introduce problems associated with pourability, and if any sedimentation does occur, redispersion is likely to be even more difficult.

(b) Deflocculated Particles in Non-Newtonian Vehicles

A non-Newtonian dispersion medium that exhibits plastic or pseudoplastic behaviour will retard the sedimentation of small particles since its apparent viscosity will be high at the small stresses associated with sedimentation. In addition, pourability and redispersion are facilitated by the decrease in apparent viscosity that occurs at the higher shear rates involved in these processes.

The commonly used suspending agents such as acacia, tragacanth, methylcellulose, and sodium carboxymethylcellulose impart such properties to aqueous solutions. Suspending agents such as bentonite and similar clays also impart thixotropic properties to aqueous dispersions. The deflocculated particles of a medicament become trapped in the gel network that forms in such dispersions during resting periods, and their sedimentation is retarded. Breakdown of the gel network by shaking reduces the apparent viscosity for a time sufficient to allow easy administration. Subsequent sedimentation is retarded by reformation of the gel network after a time lag.

(c) Flocculated Particles in Newtonian Vehicles

Flocculation of suspended particles will produce large volume sediments with a porous nature that are easy to redisperse. Separation of the product into two layers, i.e. sediment and supernatant liquid, is likely to occur, however, and produces an inelegant appearance. This can sometimes be prevented if flocculation is sufficient to produce a sedimentation volume that occupies the whole system. Careful control of flocculation is necessary to ensure that the product is easy to administer. Such control is usually achieved by using satisfactory concentrations of electrolytes, surface active agents or polymers. Variations in these concentrations will lead to effects that range from complete flocculation to deflocculation. In addition, the observed effect of a given concentration of one of these additives on a particular dispersion will depend on the characteristics of the disperse particles (e.g. specific surface area, presence of trace amounts of impurities). Since these factors are likely to vary between rather wide limits for commercially available materials, the use of controlled flocculation as the sole means of obtaining the desired properties in a pharmaceutical suspension is less satisfactory than using a structured vehicle, for large-scale production.

(d) Flocculated Particles in Non-Newtonian Vehicles

This type of system allows the advantages of the previous two methods to be utilised. In addition, variations in the properties of the material to be suspended are less likely to influence the performance of a product made on a large scale, and less difference will be observed between batches of product made from the same flow sheet.

Further details of these methods are given by Martin and Swarbrick (1966), and the theory of coarse particle suspension formulation has been reviewed by Hiestand (1964).

Emulsions

The flow properties of emulsions have a marked influence on their usefulness as dosage forms for medicinal compounds. Except for very dilute systems, emulsions are non-Newtonian, and in pharmaceutical emulsions the most commonly observed behaviour involves a decrease in apparent viscosity with increase in rate of shear. This may range from pseudoplastic behaviour in emulsions with a moderate concentration of disperse phase to plastic behaviour with considerable yield values in concentrated emulsions and creams. In addition, pharmaceutical emulsions often exhibit some degree of thixotropy. These properties are particularly satisfactory from a user's point of view since they allow easy application of a topical preparation or easy administration of a product intended for oral use. Furthermore, the physical stability of emulsions against the effects of creaming is aided by the high apparent viscosities of these systems at low rates of shear.

Many factors contribute to the rheological properties of emulsions. These have been listed and discussed by Sherman (1964, 1968) and include the effect of the viscosities and chemical natures of the continuous and disperse phases, the volume concentration of the disperse phase and its globule size distribution, and the chemical structures and concentrations of the emulsifying agent and additional stabilising agents. Talman, Davies, and Rowan (1967, 1968) have suggested that the observed rheological properties of emulsions containing a long-chain alcohol as one of the components of a complex interfacial film could be accounted for by the migration of this oil-soluble component into the aqueous phase, where it produces a viscous gel.

BIBLIOGRAPHY

DINSDALE, A. and MOORE, F. (1962) *Viscosity and its Measurement*. The Institute of Physics and the Physical Society, London.

MARTIN, A. N., BANKER, G. S., and CHUN, A. H. C. (1964) *Advances in Pharmaceutical Sciences. Vol. 1.* (H. S. Bean, A. H. Beckett, and J. E. Carless, Eds). Academic Press, London. Chapter 1.

VAN WAZER, J. R., LYONS, J. W., KIM, K. Y., and COLWELL, R. E. (1963) *Viscosity and Flow Measurement*. Interscience, New York.

REFERENCES

BARRY, B. W. and WARBURTON, B. (1968) Some rheological aspects of cosmetics. *J. Soc. cosmet. Chem.*, **19**, 725–744.

BAUER, W. H. and COLLINS, E. A. (1967) *Rheology; Theory and Applications. Vol. IV.* (F. R. Eirich, Ed.). Academic Press, London. Chapter 8.

HIESTAND, E. N. (1964) Theory of coarse suspension formulation. *J. pharm. Sci.*, **53**, 1–18.

MARTIN, A. N., BANKER, G. S., and CHUN, A. H. C. (1964) *Advances in Pharmaceutical Sciences. Vol. 1.* (H. S. Bean, A. H. Beckett, and J. E. Carless, Eds). Academic Press, London. Chapter 1.

MARTIN, A. N. and SWARBRICK, J. (1966) *American Pharmacy*. 6th ed. (J. B. Sprowls and H. M. Beal, Eds). Lippincott, Philadelphia. Chapter 8.

RUTGERS, I. R. (1962) Relative viscosity and concentration. *Rheol. Acta*, **2**, 305–348.

SAMYN, J. C. and WAN, Y. J. (1967) Negative thixotropy in flocculated clay suspensions. *J. pharm. Sci.*, **56**, 188–191.

SHERMAN, P. (1964) The flow properties of emulsions. *J. Pharm. Pharmac.*, **16**, 1–25.

SHERMAN, P. (1968) *Emulsion Science*. (P. Sherman, Ed.). Academic Press, London. Chapter 4.

TALMAN, F. A. J., DAVIES, P. J., and ROWAN, E. M. (1967) The rheology of some oil-in-water emulsions stabilized by complex condensed films. *J. Pharm. Pharmac.*, **19**, 417–425.

TALMAN, F. A. J., DAVIES, P. J., and ROWAN, E. M. (1968) The effect of the concentration of the water-soluble component on the rheology of some emulsions containing long-chain alcohols. *J. Pharm. Pharmac.*, **20**, 513–520.

VAN WAZER, J. R., LYONS, J. W., KIM, K. Y., and COLWELL, R. E. (1963) *Viscosity and Flow Measurement*. Interscience, New York.

PART TWO

Pharmaceutical Technology

8

Formulation and Development

THE materials handled by the present-day pharmacist differ greatly from those used by his predecessors of some twenty years ago. The 'ethical' products of modern pharmacy are produced by a manufacturer on the large scale, and the 'galenical' products still in use by a pharmacist will be made only rarely in the dispensary, the majority being prepared in bulk by the pharmaceutical industry.

The purpose of this section on Pharmaceutical Technology is to outline the procedures involved in developing a new pharmaceutical product, and to discuss the principles of, and the methods employed in the manufacturing processes used by the pharmaceutical industry.

OBJECTIVES OF DEVELOPMENT

The announcement of a new pharmaceutical product is not an infrequent event, indeed inspection of almost any number of a periodical such as the *Pharmaceutical Journal* will reveal advertisements of this type. The appearance of such an article is not the result of a chance decision by a manufacturer, but is the end-product of a long and complex sequence of events, embracing all branches of the pharmaceutical sciences.

The objective of the development process is to translate an idea for a new preparation into a successful product for routine manufacture and commercial marketing. This demands the evolution of a satisfactory formula for the product to enhance the specific therapeutic action of the medicament and, in conjunction with correct packaging, to ensure stability for several years, despite transport and storage under tropical conditions in some cases. Most large pharmaceutical companies maintain organisations in which a systematic search is carried out for new medical products.

Pharmaceutical chemists seek new materials, or modify the structure of existing substances of known action, bearing in mind recent knowledge of the relationship between molecular structure and therapeutic activity. These substances are then screened for pharmacological activity. Occasionally, one will be found that shows possibilities for medicinal use, but for each one that appears to be pharmacologically attractive, many must be rejected because of inactivity or excessive toxicity.

Any material that justifies further investigation is returned to the chemists to obtain additional information about its chemical properties, for isolation of purified forms, or for confirmation of the synthesis, so ensuring that manufacture of the proposed medicament is a practical and economic possibility.

If this proceeds satisfactorily, there follows the pharmaceutical stage, involving the formulation of a stable preparation, the evolution of a suitable packaging method, and investigation of the pharmaceutical problems involved in developing the process from the laboratory bench to the manufacturing scale.

Finally, the pharmaceutical engineer designs and constructs the plant for the manufacture of the product or, in co-operation with the pharmaceutist, adapts the process to existing equipment in the factory.

This outline of the procedure emphasises the important fact that the development of a new product depends on the integration of all branches of pharmacy and not on one specialist section alone. Discussion of the chemical and pharmacological aspects of development is outside the scope of this book, which will be confined to the work of the pharmaceutist and to the manufacturing operations.

STAGES OF DEVELOPMENT

In practice, the development of the new product occurs gradually in all directions but, for convenience, it can be divided into a number of stages, bearing in mind that the starting point may be a completely new idea, when the operator may be left to determine the form of the preparation, or, may be, a request, when the formulation may be required to meet certain specifications.

Search of the Literature

Before any work begins, as much information as possible is obtained through reference books, abstracts, or journals. In addition, it is appropriate at this time to make some investigation of the markets, since an indication of consumer demand may influence the type of product.

Theoretical Formulation

In the light of the information obtained, a preliminary theoretical formulation is devised. Consideration is given to suitable presentation of the medicament, in a form appropriate to the intended method of administration; the aims of formulation should also include stability, acceptable elegance of presentation, and economy of materials and processing.

Practical Formulation

Devising the theoretical formula will show up gaps in the known facts; these are ascertained and the components and proportions of the formula are confirmed by laboratory experiment.

Packaging

Concurrently with the theoretical formulation, attention is given to the packaging method proposed and this, again, is confirmed by laboratory experiment alongside the practical formulation work. The importance of packaging is so great that it is considered separately in Chapter 9.

Small-scale Production

Once a satisfactory formula has been obtained, the next stage is small-scale manufacture to produce batches, probably of several kilogrammes compared with the 50 or 100 gramme quantities used in early tests. Use is made of small-scale plant, rather than hand methods, which acts as a preliminary guide to large-scale procedures. The product is used for further trials.

Clinical or 'Field' Trials

Samples from small-scale production are used in practice, and clinical reports obtained. This information, coming from actual experience, may result in amendment of the original formulation.

Storage Tests

The performance of clinical trials may take some time, which is used for storage tests. Samples are stored in the laboratory under controlled conditions of temperature and humidity, utilising various packaging methods. Again, amendment of formulation, or of packaging may prove to be necessary.

Process Development

At this stage, a successful small-scale formula has been evolved and tested, but this is rarely suitable for scale-up to large production by simple multiplication of the quantities. Many problems will be found in handling the larger amounts, selection of equipment, control of processing times and speeds, and so on. Some problems can be anticipated from experience or from the small-scale production, but others become apparent only when the process is subjected to works trial on production equipment. In some cases it may be necessary to carry out trials on a *pilot plant*, that is, on a scale intermediate between laboratory and production. This has the advantage that production conditions can be simulated, but using smaller quantities of materials and avoiding the need for taking large-scale plant off production.

Manufacturing Directions

Much of the plant work is carried out by unskilled or semi-skilled labour under qualified supervision. It is necessary, therefore, to draw up a complete product specification with accurate manufacturing directions, and to devise suitable process testing, in co-operation with the analytical laboratories.

9

Packaging

REFERENCE has already been made to the importance of packaging (p. 132), and this cannot be over-emphasised. Clearly there is little point in taking great care during the manufacturing process to obtain a product of suitable purity and potency if unsatisfactory packaging permits deterioration to set in before it is used by the patient.

Packaging has other functions also, which can be defined as the art and science of, and the operations involved in, preparing articles for transport, storage, display, and use. Although similar principles apply to packaging extemporaneously dispensed articles, this chapter is directed towards packaging products that have been manufactured on a large-scale, and distributed to the public by retail sale or on prescription, or used in medical practice.

The variety of such products is so great that a detailed treatment of every type of package is impossible in the compass of this book; packaging, therefore, is considered in general terms, with a few illustrative examples, and these principles can then be applied by the reader to packages encountered in practice.

After reviewing the general properties any package must possess, and the range of pharmaceutical products, we shall consider the influence of the product on packaging and the hazards encountered by the package, which permits definition of the particular qualities a pharmaceutical package should possess, with notes also on the packaging media that can be used, and a summary of the types of package used for particular groups of products. Methods of testing packaging materials and packages will be reviewed briefly.

In all aspects of pharmaceutical packaging it must be borne in mind that it is necessary to combine commercial sales appeal with appropriate professional restraint.

LIFE HISTORY OF A PACKAGE

The package passes through a number of stages, beginning with the container manufacturer, thence to the product manufacturer, wholesaler, retailer and, finally, the consumer. During this time, the package will undergo:

Transport, including manual (and possibly mechanical) handling, by road, rail, sea, or air.

Storage, either short term or long term; in some cases there may be intermittent use with intervals of storage between.

Display, during transit, in storage, as a part of retail display, and in the home.

Use of the product, demanding ease of opening and discharge of the contents, with means of re-closing in some instances.

Qualities of the Package

Consideration of the life history and the functions of the package shows that five basic qualities are required.

Protection

Any package should afford protection to the contents and, pharmaceutically, this is of great importance; indeed in certain circumstances the life of the patient may depend upon it. Sometimes the form of the protection may be specified; for example, in legislation relating to poisons or to therapeutic substances or in the *British Pharmacopoeia* or *British Pharmaceutical Codex*.

Some aspects of protection are superficial, such as the wrapping of an outer carton in cellulose film to avoid dust or 'scuffing', but the protection given to the product by the primary package is very important and is considered on p. 136.

Identification

The package must also give clear identification of the product at all stages and, again, the life of the patient may depend upon rapid and correct identification in emergencies. Certain products have labelling specifications in the *British Pharmacopoeia*, the *British Pharmaceutical Codex*, the *British National Formulary*, and the *British Veterinary Codex*. Others are controlled by legislation affecting materials such as poisons, dangerous drugs, therapeutic substances, food and drugs, and methylated spirits.

Often, the package is required to identify the manufacturer to the user by a characteristic house style.

Presentation

Good presentation enhances the product and attracts the consumer during storage or display. In addition, the public can judge the product only by the appearance of the package, so that a dignified and professional presentation will give confidence to the user.

Convenience

The form of the package should be such that it offers convenience at all stages of its life history and the design of the package should be convenient for manufacture, for transport and storage and for use by the consumer. These aspects are considered further on p. 138.

Economical

The economics of packaging are of considerable practical importance; the package cost should be minimal, provided the previous qualities are not prejudiced. In particular, care should be taken to ensure that protection is not sacrificed simply to reduce package costs.

Range of Pharmaceutical Products

The emphasis on the qualities referred to in the previous section varies with different products. Four main groupings can be used:

Drugs

Packages for drugs are essentially utilitarian, with the emphasis on protection, and the scale may vary considerably; for example—

Bulk transport between manufacturers or between manufacturer and wholesaler, using tanker wagons, barrels, wood boxes, sacks, drums or carboys.

Transport to the retailer in smaller bulk; for example, 2·5 or 5 litre bottles, metal boxes or drums and fibre-board cartons.

Sale to the public in small bottles, cartons or boxes.

'Ethical' Products

'Ethical' products are difficult to define precisely, but include products of high quality from reputable manufacturers, often intended for supply to and use by the medical profession or for supply on prescription, rather than sale to the public. Packaging is usually of a high standard and may be expensive, but aims at having a clean and dignified professional appearance.

Proprietary Products

Such products are sold under the trade name of a particular manufacturer and not as official products, although often very similar, if not identical. The purpose is usually direct sale to the public and, while some have similar packaging to ethicals, others have a more commercial character.

Toilet and Cosmetic Products

From the technical point of view, these products are very similar to pharmaceuticals, both categories including creams, emulsions, powders, aqueous and spiritous solutions, for example. Hence, packaging methods are based on similar principles, but the emphasis is on elegant presentation, and package cost is often of little importance.

Choosing the Form of Package

The choice of the package is governed to some extent by the facilities available (pressurised dispensers require special filling equipment, for example) and by the ultimate use of the product (thus, the product may be used by skilled personnel in a hospital or may need to be suitable for use in the home by a patient).

The most important aspects, however, arise from the nature and properties of the product; for example—

The physical form of the product; solid, semisolid, liquid or gas.

The route of administration; oral, parenteral or external.

The stability of the materials; moisture, oxygen, carbon dioxide, light, trace metals, temperature or pressure or fluctuations of these may have a deleterious effect on the product.

The product may react with the package (such as the release of alkali from glass or the corrosion of metals) and, in turn, the product is affected.

Expensive products usually justify expensive packaging, but sometimes an item may have a low cost but be of considerable therapeutic value, hence deterioration could represent a danger to the patient's life.

Hazards Encountered by the Package

Analysis of the many stages in the life-history of a package shows that hazards can be divided into two main groups—mechanical and environmental. The only exception is theft, which can be a serious risk with drugs and may demand special protection in certain cases.

MECHANICAL HAZARDS

Shock

Damage due to shock is usually caused by rough handling or dropping during transport, although it can result also from carelessness in use. Cushioning can be provided and a warning label may be useful.

Compression

Fragile items may be broken, or collapsible articles crushed by compression, the usual procedure then being to protect with a rigid outer package.

Puncture

Soft articles, such as collapsible tubes, may be damaged by the sharp edges of other articles; protection can, again, be given by cushioning or a rigid outer.

Vibration

Considerable vibration may occur during transport, especially with exported items. Damage may be external, such as the 'scuffing' of labels, but some products may be affected, as by the cracking of emulsions, abrasion of tablets, or segregation of mixed powders.

ENVIRONMENTAL HAZARDS

Environmental conditions encountered by the package are likely to vary considerably, especially in articles for export to the tropics. In general, it is extremes of conditions that give rise to problems, and this is especially true of fluctuating conditions.

Temperature

Extreme conditions may cause deterioration, low temperatures leading to aqueous solutions freezing and, hence, to fracture of containers. High temperatures increase diffusion coefficients, accelerating the entry of water vapour into hygroscopic products and the loss of volatile components. In addition, high temperatures increase reaction rates, so that breakdowns such as hydrolysis or oxidation are encouraged.

Pressure

Decrease in pressure, as in mountainous regions or during flight in non-pressurised transport aircraft, may cause thin containers to burst or strip packs to inflate.

Moisture

Although liquid moisture may cause obvious damage, water vapour may penetrate into a package, leading to hydrolysis, without visual changes. It is essential to check the water vapour permeability of materials to be used for packaging moisture-sensitive products; for example, plastics show considerable variation in this property.

Gases

Gases from the atmosphere may diffuse into the package, leading to deterioration. Thus, oxygen will encourage oxidation, while carbon dioxide will precipitate barbiturates from solutions of their sodium salts.

Light

A number of deteriorations are due to photochemical reactions particularly affected by the ultra-violet band of the spectrum. Protection may be given by using ultra-violet absorbing materials for the package. Alternatively, an opaque outer package may be used, with a warning that the inner package should be protected from light; this has the advantage that the latter may be transparent, permitting the contents to be inspected.

Infestation

Packaging materials, particularly those of a cellulosic nature, are liable to attack by various living organisms, from rodents to bacteria. Moulds, in particular, may grow on paper or board in the presence of moisture.

Contamination

The outside of containers is likely to become dirty during transport or storage; although unlikely to affect the contents, it detracts from the appearance, and can easily be prevented by outer wrappers. Plastics are particularly subject to this, due to electrostatic charges that attract dust.

Of greater importance is that the product may become contaminated by the odour of packaging materials, printing inks, or of foreign materials, which may permeate through the package. Again, plastics may show unexpected permeabilities in this respect.

PROTECTION BY THE PACKAGE

The many hazards encountered by a package discussed in the previous section show that protection is the most important package property. Protection may take many forms according to the hazard, but may be divided into two main groups, relating to the materials from which the package is made and the method of closure of the package.

Package Material Properties

To afford the necessary protection, the materials from which the container is to be made must show certain basic properties, which can be divided into four groups—

MECHANICAL PROPERTIES

The materials must give the container sufficient mechanical strength to withstand handling empty, when filling, and when closing (all these are often performed mechanically); processing (labelling, sterilisation, etc.), transport, storage and supply to, and use by, the consumer.

Typical of the care in design needed in this respect are glass containers. The natural form of a blown glass vessel is pear-shaped, which gives a uniform layer of glass. Moulding to other shapes affects the glass distribution, sharp angles giving weak points where the glass is thin and easily damaged. Thus, a glass container will have greatest strength if all corners are rounded.

PHYSICAL PROPERTIES

The material should be impervious to any possible contaminants; for example, solids, liquids, gases, vapours, or micro-organisms.

The container must be able to withstand heat if the processing includes sterilisation.

The surface must be capable of clear labelling, often difficult, for example, with plastics.

The package must have a suitable life; thus, rubber may present problems if it 'perishes'.

The material must protect from light, if necessary; that is, it must be ultra-violet absorbent.

The container must not abstract substances from the product; e.g. absorption of water from creams into cardboard boxes.

CHEMICAL PROPERTIES

The container and the closure should not react together, either alone or in the presence of the product. This can occur with certain combinations of dissimilar metals.

The product should not react with the container or closure, as might happen if alkaline substances are packed in aluminium containers.

Substances must not be abstracted from the product, such as the loss of bactericides from injection solutions to rubber.

The container or closure must not yield substances to the product; for example, alkali from glass or plasticiser from plastics.

BIOLOGICAL PROPERTIES

The material of the container must be able to withstand attack by insects if this hazard is likely to be encountered.

The package should not support mould growth.

In both cases, the risk is greatest with cellulosic substances and, if the use of such materials is unavoidable, the attack may be minimised by impregnation.

Closures

Suitable closing of the container is necessary to—

Prevent loss of material by spilling or volatilisation.

Avoid contamination of the product by the entry of dirt, micro-organisms or insects.

Prevent deterioration due to the effect of the environment; for example, the entry of moisture, oxygen, or carbon dioxide.

Minimise the effect of changes of the surroundings, such as changes of relative humidity, temperature, or pressure.

Closure methods may be *once-only* or *renewable*.

ONCE-ONLY CLOSURES

In these, the container is used on one occasion only, the package then being closed by folding, as with paper and plastic bags or with cartons. More commonly, closing is effected by fusion of the package material, such as the fusion of the glass to seal an ampoule or of plastic to close a polyethylene bag.

RENEWABLE CLOSURES

Renewable closures apply principally to bottles, jars, tubes, and similar containers, and may be:

Plug Type

The plug closure is a push fit into the neck of the container. The cork or the glass stopper were common examples of this type, but both these have been replaced almost entirely by stoppers of plastic, such as polyethylene. The advantages of this change include the fact that the stopper is impervious, unbreakable, and flexible to ensure a good fit.

Cap Type

In this form, the closure is an external cap over the neck. It is used in two forms:

Push-fit Caps. These may have a simple slide fit, as applied to metal boxes or plastic 'pots'; a better seal is obtained in tablet vials, where the neck and the plastic cap are shaped in such a way that the latter must be stretched over the neck and is a snap-on fit.

Screw Closures. The screw closure is probably the most widely used renewable closure and consists of three components: the cap, the wad, and the liner (Fig. 9.1).

It is important that the cap should be screwed on to the correct extent, so that the wad is distorted to provide a suitable seal. If the closure is used with bottles, care must be taken to ensure that no mould marks remain on the neck.

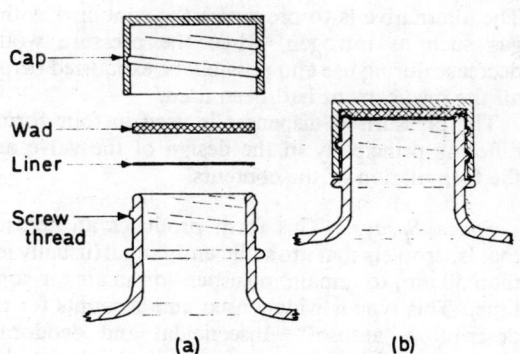

Fig. 9.1 Components of the screw closure
(a) separate (b) in position

The *cap* may be of metal (usually tin-plate or aluminium) and may be *pre-formed* when the container is closed by screwing the cap on the neck. Alternatively, the cap may be *rolled-on*, when a blank cap is dropped over the neck and is formed to the threads on the neck. This procedure has the disadvantage that mechanical methods are essential to form the cap, but the advantages are that the pressure of application (and hence the seal) is uniform, there is no risk of tearing the liner as the cap is tightened, and the cap can include a tamper-proof

seal that must be broken before the cap can be removed.

Caps may also be of plastic materials, which may be of the thermosetting type (such as phenol-formaldehyde or urea-formaldehyde) or thermoplastic (for example, polyethylene or polypropylene). Caps from thermosetting plastics have the advantage of rigidity, the possibility of incorporating colours, and certain varieties have suitable heat resistance to withstand sterilisation. Thermoplastic caps have the advantage of flexibility, but may not always produce a good seal.

Compared with metal caps, plastic caps are capable of resisting corrosion and so do not contaminate the product. A particular feature is that the plastic cap can be moulded to fit special shapes; for example, nozzle tubes.

The *wad* should be resilient to provide a satisfactory seal, and inert to avoid contaminating the product. Ideally, the material should also be impervious, to prevent absorption of product. Rubber or silicone rubber can be used, but, in practice, wads are commonly of cork composition or cardboard.

The *liner* must be inert, and materials that are used include metal foils, plastic films, rubber or silicone rubber or paper, preferably impregnated with a suitable resin, wax, or plastic. If the wad is of a material such as rubber or silicone rubber it is, of course, unnecessary to use a separate liner.

The screw closure in this form has certain disadvantages, namely that material may be lost behind the liner, leading to contamination and possibly mould growth; the liner may be torn; the wad may distort permanently so that it does not re-seal effectively; the seal is dependent on the cap being correctly tightened.

To overcome these difficulties, many different designs of cap are used, a typical variant of which has the form shown in Fig. 9.2. This is made in a plastic material such as polypropylene, the tapered projecting ring giving resilience, distorting into the shape of the neck as the cap is tightened.

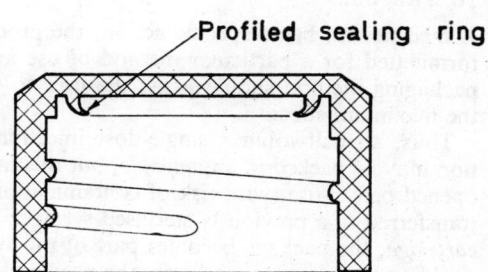

Fig. 9.2 Screw closure: polypropylene

CONVENIENCE OF THE PACKAGE

The package should be convenient to handle and use at all stages of its life history, including:

TO THE PACKAGE MANUFACTURER

The container should be manufactured by a process that is as simple and cheap as possible. Thus, an extruded aluminium container is to be preferred to a tin-plate can with soldered joints.

TO THE PRODUCT MANUFACTURER

The handling, filling, closing, sealing, labelling, and storage should be possible in a convenient manner, with most of the procedures mechanised.

This can be illustrated by the *antibiotic vial* (Fig. 9.3), where the squat form permits the use of a shallow layer of material during freeze drying (*see* p. 279). The vial can then be closed by dropping in the rubber stopper, adding the aluminium sealing ring and pressing the edge of the latter under the lip on the neck of the vial. All these closing procedures can be carried out mechanically.

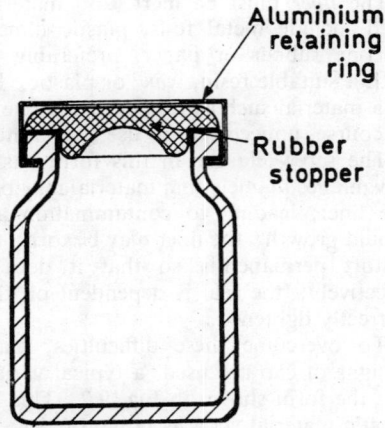

Aluminium retaining ring

Rubber stopper

Fig. 9.3 Antibiotic vial

TO THE USER

A medicament has a specific action, the product is formulated for a particular method of use and the packaging method should assist the user to obtain the maximum effect.

Thus, a small-volume, single-dose injection solution may be packed in an *ampoule*, but this must be opened before use (with risk of contamination) and transferred to a previously sterilised syringe. In the *cartridge*, the package becomes part of the syringe, avoiding transference, and only the needle needs to be sterilised. The *disposable syringe* is even more convenient, since a needle is incorporated in the pack and administration is direct from the package (for further details *see* Gunn and Carter, 1965).

Similarly, nasal sprays can be packed in polyethylene 'squeeze' bottles; use is again direct from the container and replaces the separate bottle and cumbersome glass spray and rubber bulb.

Probably the best example of convenience combined with protection is the *pressurised dispenser* (commonly, but incorrectly known as an 'aerosol'). A section of a typical form is shown in Fig. 9.4, from which it will be seen that it consists of a container capable of withstanding considerable pressure, a dip-tube leading down to the bottom of the vessel, and a spring-loaded valve, whereby the contents can be released, usually in the form of a spray, by pressing the top of the valve.

The medicament is enclosed in the container, together with the *propellant*, which is a suitable liquid with a low boiling point, so that a considerable vapour pressure will be exerted at ordinary temperatures. Examples of substances used for this purpose are some of the chloro-fluoro-methanes and ethanes, which have vapour pressures of the order of 5 to 6 bars at 20°C. The objective of using a propellant of this type is that the pressure remains constant, while any liquid remains in the container, since it is due to the vapour pressure exerted by the liquid. The alternative is to pressurise the container with a gas such as nitrogen, when the pressure would decrease during use and possibly be exhausted before all the medicament had been used.

The pressurised dispenser is used in four forms, differing principally in the design of the valve and the formulation of the contents.

Space Sprays. This form produces an aerosol, that is, droplets that are sufficiently small (usually less than 50 μm) to remain in suspension in air for some time. This type is widely used and accounts for the description 'aerosol'. Insecticidal and deodorant sprays are of indirect pharmaceutical interest, but inhalation sprays are specific medical examples of this variety. A metering valve may be fitted to deliver a measured amount and to assist in obtaining correct dosage.

Surface Sprays. As the name implies, these produce larger droplets (100 to 200 μm) that will wet the surface on which they fall. Everyday examples in this category are paint sprays and hair lacquers, while spray-on burn and wound dressings typify pharmaceutical uses.

Powder 'Sprays'. These sprays are modified forms that allow the method to be used with fine

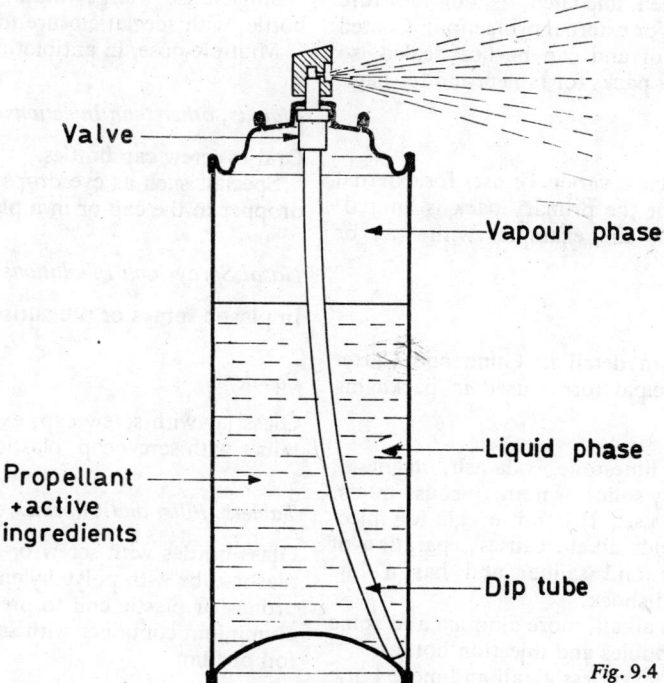

Valve

Vapour phase

Propellant +active ingredients

Liquid phase

Dip tube

Fig. 9.4   Pressurised dispenser

powders; examples include spray-on dusting powders such as antibiotics and hydrocortisone.

Foam Dispensers. These are used for products such as shaving creams and sunburn preparations.

As well as offering convenience, pressurised dispensers have the advantages that contamination by micro-organisms is prevented and that contact with atmospheric oxygen and moisture is avoided.

Packaging Media

Apart from economic aspects, selection of materials for the manufacture of packages is governed by the chemical and physical properties of the material and the product.

All the media used for packaging also have applications for the construction of pharmaceutical plant and are considered in this connection in Chapter 25. This section adds notes on the special packaging aspects of the materials.

Metals

Metal containers are used mainly for dry products, due to the effect of trace metal contamination introduced by corrosion, especially of iron. Aluminium containers are commonest, including extruded

tubes for tablets and collapsible tubes for creams and ointments. Tin is also used for collapsible tubes.

Metal foils, especially aluminium, are used for sachets and unit packs of tablets, etc. These consist of sealing the individual tablets between two sheets of foil, previously coated with a suitable plastic. Thus, each tablet is enclosed in a separate compartment which is opened only when required for administration.

Plastics

Coming into increasing use are—

Phenol-, urea-, and melamine-formaldehyde resins as screw closures.

Polystyrene tubes for tablets, etc.

Polyethylene is widely used for flexible containers, closures, bags, etc. The type is important, depending on the crystallinity of the polymer; low density forms soften at 100 to 110°C, but high density can be sterilised by moist heat.

Polypropylene is similar to polyethylene, but has greater transparency and better heat resistance. It is also more resistant to attack by solvents, but more expensive than polyethylene.

Cellulose acetate is used as films for unit packs of tablets in the same way as foils, but it has lower strength and moisture resistance. Thicker sections are used for moulded packs for suppositories.

Cellulose film, when uncoated, is non-moisture proof and is suitable for external protection. Coated film is moisture proof and can be heat-sealed, so that it is used for unit packs for tablets and for bags.

Paper and Board

Papers and *boards* have a variety of uses for external packages, but use for the primary pack is limited; usually impregnated, for example, with wax or plastic.

Glass

Glass is dealt with in detail in Gunn and Carter (1965) but the principal forms used in packaging are—

Soda glass (silica, limestone, soda ash, magnesia, alumina) used for dry solids or non-aqueous liquids, for oral or external use. It is unsuitable for injections, because it yields alkali, causes separation of flakes with citrates and saline, and has a low resistance to thermal shock.

Neutral glass (less alkali, more alumina and some boric oxide) for ampoules and injection bottles.

Borosilicate glass (even less alkali and more boric oxide) is excellent, but usually too expensive for packaging.

Treated glass, where surface alkali is neutralised during annealing with an acidic substance such as sulphur dioxide. It is satisfactory for many purposes and cheaper than borosilicate. The *British Pharmacopoeia* has a test to limit alkalinity of glass. The surface of glass may also be treated with silicones to aid drainage and reduce foaming.

Glass may have additives to absorb light, particularly ultra-violet.

Rubber

Rubber is needed in a specialised form for closures for injection containers.

Packaging Examples

To illustrate the range of pharmaceutical packaging, the following summary indicates the general groups of products, with typical methods of packaging.

It will be noted that glass is very widely used, since it possesses important properties of protection, convenience, and presentation.

Injections

Single-dose, small-volume, in ampoules, cartridges or disposable syringes.

Single-dose, large-volume, in screw-cap glass bottle, with special closure to fit administration set.

Multiple-dose, in antibiotic type vial.

Liquids, other than Injections

Oral in screw cap bottles.

Special, such as eye drops in glass bottles with a dropper in the cap or in a plastic container.

Nasal Sprays and Inhalations

In plastic sprays or pressurised dispensers.

Powders

Glass jar with screw cap, extruded aluminium container with screw cap, plastic bag in carton.

Tablets, Pills, and Capsules

Glass bottles with screw or snap-on caps; glass or plastic tube with polyethylene closure, possibly with prongs or plastic coil to prevent rattling; extruded aluminium container with screw cap; unit packs in foil or film.

Suppositories

Partitioned, slip-on lid or slide box; moulded cellulose acetate packs.

Ointments, Creams, and Pastes

Screw-cap glass jars; slip-lid plastic pots; collapsible tubes.

Surgical Dressings

Sealed paper wraps; metal tins or spools.

Surgical Ligatures and Sutures

Glass tubes; plastic sachets

Package Testing

Page 132 refers to the testing of packages during development of new products, and testing forms a part of the quality control procedure of routine production.

Of the package properties discussed in this chapter, only protection demands scientific evaluation, the remainder being tested by more empirical methods. Conditions in the laboratory can never reproduce precisely those encountered in practice, indeed the laboratory conditions are often deliberately exaggerated in order to accelerate the results of the test; interpreted with care, however, laboratory tests can yield useful information.

Testing procedures may be divided into two groups according to whether the test is applied to the packaging material in isolation or to the entire package.

TESTING MATERIALS

Tests applied to packaging materials may be—

Chemical

The pH value of materials, chloride and sulphate in paper or board, alkalinity of glass, compatibility tests with chemicals or medicaments are typical of the chemical tests.

Mechanical

Standard tests are available for properties such as the bursting strength and the tensile strength of papers, films, and foils, and for the effect of creasing, folding, and so on.

Environmental

Materials may be tested by standard methods for absorption of water, permeability to water vapour, gases, oils, odours, etc., and for characteristics such as light transmission.

TESTING PACKAGES

The test procedures for packages fall into similar groups to those applied to the packaging materials; the chemical tests are virtually identical and will not be considered further.

Mechanical

Mechanical tests apply principally to outer packaging for protection from journey hazards and consist of the use of a standardised test procedure to compare the effect of different protective materials to prevent damage to the contents.

Typical are tests for drop, impact, compression, and vibration.

Study of an actual journey can provide useful information with regard to handling hazards, but complete observation is very difficult, if not impossible. PIRA (the Research Association for the Paper and Board, Printing and Packaging Industries) has devised a drop recorder which produces a record of the number and intensity of the impacts received by the package during the journey, enabling the degree of protection to be assessed.

Environmental

Packages are subjected to conditions that reproduce the environment, and some evaluation is made at suitable intervals.

Such procedures may be applied to testing closures for water vapour transmission, for example. Desiccant is placed in the container, the absorption of water measured by weighing at intervals, and a 'closure efficiency' calculated by comparison with a standard.

Packages may also be tested for the effect of the product on the container, such as the corrosion of metal pressurised dispenser containers by medicaments, propellants, or other additives. Similarly, products may be examined for any effects due to the packaging materials, such as metallic contamination or the leaching of plasticiser.

Often, it is useful to be able to accelerate the effect of the environment, and elevated temperatures are used in particular. This aspect is discussed in detail in relation to the stability of medicaments in Chapter 6.

BIBLIOGRAPHY

BULL, A. W. (1955) Plastics in containers and equipment. *J. Pharm. Pharmac.*, **7**, 806–815.

CHILD, C. L. (1955) Nature and properties of plastics. *J. Pharm. Pharmac.*, **7**, 793–805.

DIMBLEBY, V. (1953) Glass for pharmaceutical purposes. *J. Pharm. Pharmac.*, **5**, 969–989.

EVANS, D. M. (1961) The micro-organisms and insects affecting packaging materials. *Pharm. J.*, **187**, 241–243.

FOWLER, H. W. (1959) Modern packaging. *Pharm. J.*, **183**, 357–359.

GUNN, C. and CARTER, S. J. (1965) *Dispensing for Pharmaceutical Students.* 11th ed. Pitman Medical, London.

PAINE, F. A. (Ed.) (1962) *Fundamentals of Packaging.* London, Blackie.

SHOTTON, E. (1955) Packaging in relation to stability. *Pharm. J.*, **174**, 389–391.

STEPHENSON, D. (1953) Some experiences with containers and closures in the pharmaceutical industry. *J. Pharm. Pharmac.*, **5**, 999–1007.

10

Introduction to Industrial Processing

CHAPTER 8 has indicated that the emphasis in making pharmaceutical preparations has moved from the individual dispenser to the large-scale manufacturer; the reasons for the change will be considered in this chapter.

Anyone who has visited a large pharmaceutical factory will know that it can seem to be both complex and confusing, but the full manufacturing process can be broken down to a number of stages, each of which can be individually examined and the underlying principles studied.

Reasons for Increasing Large-scale Manufacture

Economic Reasons

As the scale of manufacturing batches increases so, proportionally, does the cost of production decrease. Fewer manual methods are employed, and efficiency increases with the use of mechanical equipment for handling and processing materials.

Accuracy

The larger the quantities of materials involved so, proportionally, is the accuracy of measurements increased. Furthermore, larger organisations can support analytical laboratories for control during manufacture and for testing the final product.

Greater Scope

The increasing complexity of modern therapy has made it virtually impossible to prepare many medicaments on a small scale; for example, antibiotic production is feasible only on a large scale. Furthermore, large organisations can maintain staff and facilities for research work and the development of new products.

Changed Character of Medicaments

The product of research by a pharmaceutical manufacturer is marketed in a 'proprietary' form in order to recover the expenditure involved in its discovery and development. These proprietaries are then prescribed by medical practitioners instead of traditional prescriptions which have to be prepared extemporaneously. This has led to an extensive change in the prescribing habit of medical practitioners and, in turn, to a complete change in pharmaceutical practice.

Nationally Standardised Formulae

The formulae of pharmaceutical preparations began in the writings of individuals in Egyptian, Greek, and Roman times and progressed to recognised standards, first for cities, then nationally, and now internationally.

It is, therefore, now general practice for standard preparations to be made in bulk by pharmaceutical manufacturers to recognised formulae—the *British Pharmacopoeia*, *British Pharmaceutical Codex*, and *British National Formulary* in the United Kingdom—and distributed to pharmacists throughout the country.

Breakdown of Processes

The first impression of a pharmaceutical factory, like many other industries, is of great complexity with a maze of pipes, many complicated and noisy machines, and no apparent order.

In fact, this is a false impression, the appearance of confusion being due to the physical arrangement of the plant to fit it into a compact working area, and to ancillary equipment with many pipes carrying 'services' such as water, steam or compressed air.

If each item of plant is represented symbolically in a diagram, the layout spread to a two-dimensional form, and details of services omitted, then quite a complicated process can be reduced to a simple *flow sheet*.

Flow sheets for the manufacture of a number of pharmaceutical products are shown in Figs. 10.1 to 10.4, from which it will be seen that the processes can be simplified to diagrams representing the

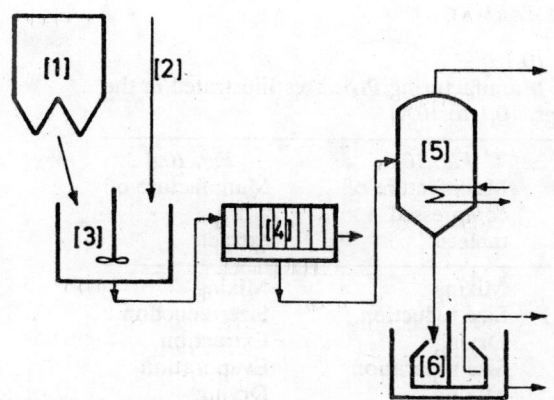

Fig. 10.1 Flow sheet: purification of a substance by crystallisation

(1) storage hopper   (2) solvent feed
(3) mixing vessel   (4) filter press
(5) evaporator   (6) centrifuge

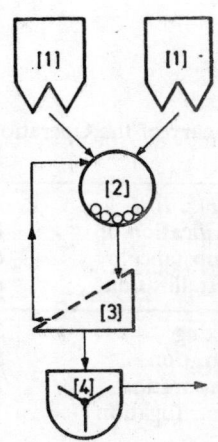

Fig. 10.2 Flow sheet: manufacture of a mixed powder

(1) storage hoppers   (2) ball mill
(3) sifter   (4) powder mixer

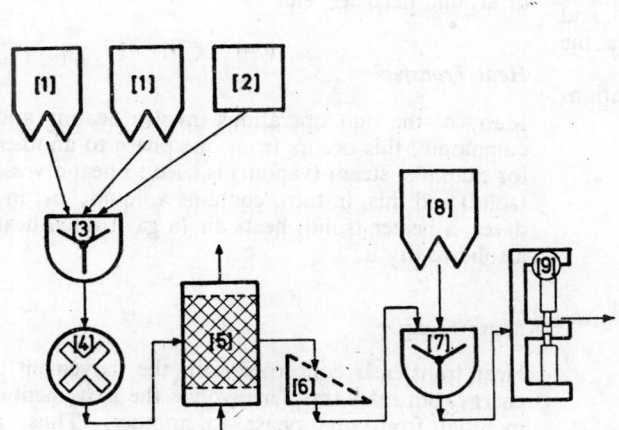

Fig. 10.3 Flow sheet: manufacture of compressed tablets

(1) storage hoppers
(2) granulating liquid storage tank
(3) mixer
(4) granulator
(5) fluidised bed dryer
(6) sifter
(7) mixer
(8) storage hopper
(9) tablet machine

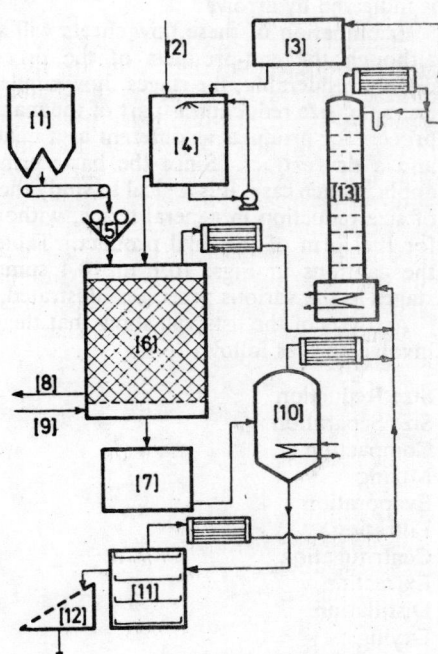

Fig. 10.4 Flow sheet: manufacture of a dry extract

(1) drug storage hopper   (2) water supply
(3) ethanol storage tank   (4) circulating mixer
(5) crushing mill   (6) extraction vessel
(7) extractive storage tank   (8) exhausted drug discharge
(9) steam supply   (10) evaporator
(11) vacuum oven   (12) sifter
(13) fractionating column

Table 10.1

Summary of the Operations Involved in the Manufacturing Processes Illustrated in the Flow Sheets (Figs. 10.1 to 10.4)

Fig. 10.1 Purification of a substance by crystallisation.	Fig.10.2 Manufacture of a mixed powder.	Fig. 10.3 Manufacture of compressed tablets.	Fig. 10.4 Manufacture of a dry extract.
Mixing Filtration Evaporation Centrifugation	Size reduction Size separation Mixing	Mixing Size reduction Drying Size separation Mixing Compaction	Mixing Size reduction Extraction Evaporation Drying Size separation Distillation.

treatment of material in a number of stages in particular pieces of equipment. Material entering or leaving the process, or moving from stage to stage, is indicated by arrows.

Examination of these flow sheets will show that, although the end-products of the processes may differ considerably, the stages show similarities; for example, size reduction is part of the manufacturing process for products as different as a mixed powder and a dry extract. Since the basic principles will apply in each case, it is logical to study the operation of size reduction in general terms, without concern for the form of the final product. Table 10.1 and the captions in Figs. 10.1 to 10.4 summarise the stages in the various processes illustrated.

Analysis of the lists will show that the operations involved are as follows:

Size Reduction
Size Separation
Compaction
Mixing
Evaporation
Filtration
Centrifugation
Extraction
Distillation
Drying

Hence, complete processes will not receive attention at this stage, but the emphasis will be placed on the individual operations that make up the whole. Since these are only a part of something larger, the title *Unit Operations* is used.

Basis of Unit Operations

Although it is convenient to break down the processes for the manufacture of pharmaceutical products into unit operations, these are not fundamental. All unit operations involve and are controlled, to a greater or lesser extent, by one or more of the following—

Fluid Flow

Bearing in mind that the term 'fluid' is being used generally to describe liquid, vapour or gas, certain aspects of all the unit operations employ the movement of a fluid through pipes or channels or between or around particles, etc.

Heat Transfer

Many of the unit operations involve heating and, commonly, this occurs from one phase to another; for example, steam (vapour) is used to heat a vessel (solid) and this, in turn, contains a liquid; or, in a dryer, a heater (solid) heats air (a gas) which heats a solid to dry it.

Mass Transfer

Heat transfer is concerned with the movement of energy, but mass transfer involves the movement of material from one phase to another. Thus, in drying a wet solid, the liquid is converted to vapour and carried away in that form. Similarly, when a drug is extracted with a solvent, soluble material passes from the solid phase into solution and is taken away in the liquid phase.

It will be noted that the transfer of both heat and mass occurs, generally, from one phase to another. Since, of the three phases—solid, liquid, and vapour—two are fluid, the characters and behaviour of fluid materials is basic to all the unit operations.

BIBLIOGRAPHY

BOURTON, K. (1967) *Chemical and Process Engineering, Unit Operations: a Bibliographical Guide.* London, Macdonald.

COULSON, J. M. and RICHARDSON, J. F. (1964) *Chemical Engineering, Vol. I, Fluid Flow, Heat Transfer and Mass Transfer*, 2nd ed. Oxford, Pergamon.

COULSON, J. M. and RICHARDSON, J. F. (1968) *Chemical Engineering, Vol. II, Unit Operations*, 2nd ed. Oxford, Pergamon.

CREMER, H. W., DAVIES, T. and WATKINS, S. B. (1956–1965) *Chemical Engineering Practice*, 12 vols. London, Butterworth.

FOUST, A. S., WENZEL, A. L., CLUMP, C. W., MAUS, L., and ANDERSON, L. B. (1960) *Principles of Unit Operations.* New York, Wiley.

PERRY, R. H., CHILTON, C. H., and KIRKPATRICK, S. D. (Eds.) (1963) *Chemical Engineers' Handbook.* 4th ed. New York, McGraw-Hill.

MEAD, W. J. (1964) *The Encyclopedia of Chemical Process Equipment.* New York, Reinhold.

11

Fluid Flow

THIS chapter is concerned with the characteristics of fluids that affect their flow properties, with particular reference to flow through pipes and channels, as will occur in process plant.

Descriptions of some experimental work refer to water, but the considerations apply equally to any fluid, remembering that the term can be applied to any substance that does not offer permanent resistance to distortion. Thus, liquids, gases and vapours will be included.

Mechanism of Fluid Flow

When a fluid flows through a pipe or channel, the character of the flow can vary according to the conditions.

The forms of flow can best be visualised by reference to a classical experiment on the flow of water through a circular tube, first carried out by Osborne Reynolds in 1883.

In Reynolds' Experiment a long, glass tube was connected to a reservoir providing a constant head of water, with a control at the outlet so that the rate of flow could be varied. In the inlet of the tube a jet was inserted which allowed a coloured liquid to be injected into the centre of the tube. The arrangement is illustrated diagrammatically in Fig. 11.1.

Reynolds studied the effect of varying the conditions on the character of flow and on the appearance of the thread of coloured liquid. This can be illustrated, for example, by varying the *velocity* of the water through the tube.

When the velocity is *low*, the thread of coloured liquid remains undisturbed in the centre of the water stream and moves steadily along the tube, without mixing. The situation can be visualised if the water is thought of as moving in a series of concentric layers, like the draw-tubes of a telescope or the extending leg of a camera tripod. This condition is known as *streamline*, *viscous*, or *laminar flow*.

At *moderate* velocities, a point is reached (the *critical velocity*) at which the thread begins to waver, although no mixing occurs. This is the phase of *transitional flow*.

As the velocity is increased to *high* values eddies begin to occur in the flow, so that the coloured liquid mixes with the bulk of the water immediately after leaving the jet. Since this is a state of complete turbulence, the condition is known as *turbulent flow*.

An analogy may assist in giving a clearer mental picture of these various states of flow. Imagine that the situation is magnified millions of times, so that the 'smooth' surface of the tube can be represented as a cobbled street and the molecules become rubber balls. Large numbers of these rubber balls are moving along the street and, when the movement is slow, they will roll along with little disturbance of their relative positions and the 'flow' is streamlined. When the movement is rapid, however, the balls bounce off the cobbles and off each other and their relative positions change continually, giving turbulent flow.

As a result of his experiments, Reynolds found that flow conditions were affected by four factors:

Diameter of pipe
Velocity of fluid
Density of fluid
Viscosity of fluid

It was discovered, furthermore, that these were connected together in a particular way and could be grouped into a particular expression, known now as *Reynolds Number:*

$$\text{Re} = \frac{\rho u d}{\mu} \qquad (11.1)$$

where Re = Reynolds Number, ρ = density of fluid, u = velocity of fluid, d = diameter of pipe, μ = viscosity of fluid.

It is important to remember that this is a number and has no dimensions, provided consistent units of mass, length, and time are used. Thus;

$\rho = \text{kg/m}^3$
$u = \text{m/s}$
$d = \text{m}$
$\mu = \text{kg/m s}$

146

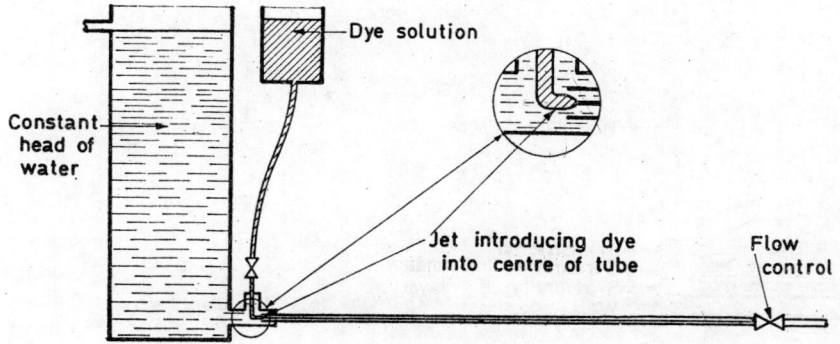

Constant
head of
water

Dye solution

Jet introducing dye
into centre of tube

Flow
control

Fig. 11.1
Reynolds' apparatus

Hence:

$$\text{Re} = \frac{\text{kg}}{\text{m}^3} \times \frac{\text{m}}{\text{s}} \times \text{m} \times \frac{\text{m s}}{\text{kg}}$$

It can be seen that all the units cancel out; i.e. Re is dimensionless.

Significance of Reynolds Number

Later, it will be shown that it can be very important in practice to know whether flow is streamline or turbulent, and the special significance of Reynolds Number is that it can be used to predict the character of flow in a particular set of circumstances.

In general, if the Reynolds Number is less than 2000 the flow will be streamline and if the number exceeds approximately 4000 the flow will be turbulent. Between these two values, the type of flow will depend on the form of the flow channel. If there is no disturbance of any sort the flow pattern may be unbroken and streamline flow may persist at Reynolds Numbers well in excess of 2000. On the other hand, if the pipe surface is rough or if there are bends or other pipe fittings, flow may be turbulent at Reynolds Numbers less than 4000, possibly lower even than 2000.

The important difference to remember between the two types of flow is that, in streamline flow there is no velocity component at right angles to the direction of flow. Hence, there is no movement of the fluid between the centre and the walls, which accounts for the thread of coloured liquid remaining in the centre of the tube in the Reynolds Experiment. When the flow is turbulent, however, there is a great deal of movement across the direction of flow, eddies are set up, and mixing occurs.

Distribution of Velocities Across the Tube

When a fluid flows along a tube, not all parts are moving at the same velocity, so that, for example,

a portion near the walls will not travel at the same velocity as fluid near the centre.

This can be demonstrated in a simple manner with Reynolds' apparatus by allowing a mass of the coloured solution to collect near the entrance and then to move slowly through the tube. The fluid in the centre travels at the highest velocity and that at the walls at the lowest, so that the coloured liquid acquires an elongated streamline form.

More elaborate apparatus with methods of measuring fluid velocities at various points over a cross-section would show a parabolic *velocity profile* in streamline flow, as illustrated in Fig. 11.2.

The reason for this will be apparent if the fluid is again visualised as a series of concentric tubes, remembering the analogy of the draw-tubes of a telescope or the extending leg of a camera tripod. The outer 'layer' is held back by drag against the wall, while frictional forces exist between the various layers (the viscosity of the fluid). Thus, the fluid in the centre can move at the highest velocity, with the frictional forces causing a continual decrease in velocity towards the walls. If measurements are

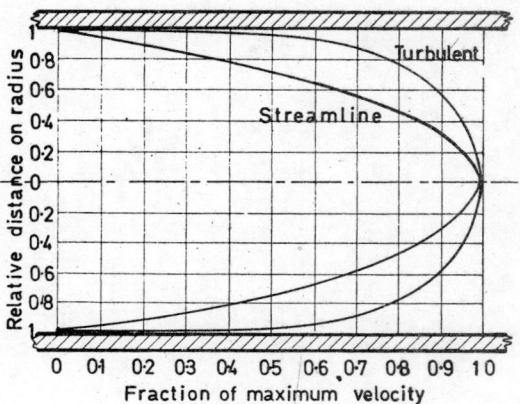

Fig. 11.2 Velocity distributions across a pipe

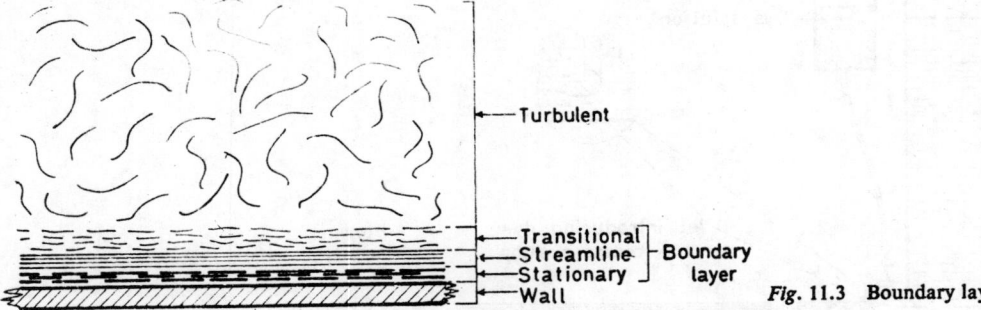

Fig. 11.3   Boundary layers

made of velocities across the tube, it is found that the average velocity is 0·5 of the maximum.

In turbulent flow, however, there is movement at right angles to the direction of flow. Thus, the fluid 'keeps together' over the cross-section, so that a rounded velocity profile is found (*see* Fig. 11.2) and the average velocity is 0·8 of the maximum.

Boundary Layers

Examination of the velocity profiles illustrated in the previous section will show that the velocity reaches very low values near the walls, in fact there will be a layer that is stationary.

Consider, then, a fluid in turbulent flow. These conditions will apply through the bulk of the fluid, but approaching the wall the velocity will decrease until, ultimately, it becomes zero at the wall itself. Reynolds Number is proportional to the velocity so that there will be a similar decrease in the value of the local Reynolds Number. This means that there will be a change from turbulence, through a transitional region to a sluggish streamline region and,

finally, to a stationary film on the wall. This is represented diagrammatically in Fig. 11.3, where, for clarity, the layers are given sharply defined boundaries; in practice, however, there will be a gradual transition from one region to another. These are referred to collectively as the *boundary layer*.

It is essential that there should be a clear mental picture of the boundary layer, which exists at any interface involving a fluid and is of very great practical importance, as will be shown in succeeding chapters.

It must be emphasised, too, that boundary layers can never be eliminated. Increasing the velocity of the fluid over the surface will *reduce* the thickness of the layer, but it will never be *removed* entirely.

BIBLIOGRAPHY

LEWITT, E. H. (Ed.) (1958) *Hydraulics and Fluid Mechanics*, 10th ed. London, Pitman.

BENNETT, C. O. and MYERS, J. E. (1962) *Momentum, Heat and Mass Transfer*. New York, McGraw-Hill.

12

Heat Transfer

MANY pharmaceutical processes involve heating of materials and this chapter will consider the methods by which heat can be transferred, with special reference to the heating of liquids.

Of the various heating media, steam is the most important, and the properties and use of steam will receive attention.

Methods of Heat Transfer

Heat transfer can take place by three methods—

Conduction

In conduction, the energy transfer occurs by transmission of momentum of individual molecules. No mixing action is involved, so that conduction is limited to solids and to fluids that are 'bound' in some way that prevents free movement.

Convection

In convection the heat flow results from mixing or turbulence, which can occur in fluids only.

Radiation

Heat transmission by radiation occurs by energy transfer through space by electromagnetic radiation. Thus, a hot body acts as an emitter, the energy being transmitted through the intervening space to a receiving body where it is absorbed and is manifested as heat.

Heat Transfer by Conduction

When heat is flowing under steady-state conditions, the quantity of heat transferred is given by:

$$Q = \frac{kA(t_1 - t_2)\theta}{L} \qquad (12.1)$$

or

$$q = \frac{kA(t_1 - t_2)}{L} \qquad (12.2)$$

where Q = quantity of heat, A = area, $(t_1 - t_2)$ = temperature difference, θ = time, L = thickness, q = quantity of heat transferred in unit time, k = constant for the material.

The constant, k, which is characteristic for any material, is known as the *coefficient of thermal conductivity* and can be defined by putting all other factors in Eqn (12.1) equal to one. Thus, the coefficient of thermal conductivity is the heat passing in unit time from one face of a cube of unit side to the opposite face, the temperature difference being kept at one unit. Since any units can be used, these must be given when values are quoted. Thermal conductivities vary considerably, ranging from metals that have high values, through non-metallic solids and liquids to gases that have the lowest values.

Typical thermal conductivities for a range of materials are given in Table 12.1. Equation (12.1) or (12.2) enables the heat flow to be calculated for a particular set of circumstances.

Table 12.1

Material	Thermal conductivity W/mK
Copper	379
Aluminium	242
Steel	43
Stainless steel	17
Borosilicate glass	1
Water	0·6
Boiler scale	0·09 to 2·3
Diatomite	0·07
Glass wool	0·06
Air	0·03

Example

Calculate the amount of heat that will flow through a sheet of steel 10 mm in thickness, 0·6 m wide and

1 m long, in 30 minutes with a temperature of 70°C on one side and 30°C on the other.

$$Q = \frac{kA(t_1 - t_2)\theta}{L}$$

$$k = 43 \text{ W/mK}$$

$$A = 0.6 \times 1 = 0.6 \text{ m}^2$$

$$(t_1 - t_2) = 70 - 30 = 40 \text{ K}$$

$$\theta = 30 \text{ min} = 1800 \text{ sec}$$

$$L = 10 \text{ mm} = 0.01 \text{ m}$$

$$Q = \frac{43 \times 0.6 \times 40 \times 1800}{0.01}$$

$$= 185.76 \text{ MJ}$$

However, a difficulty arises in a compound layer of several materials of different thermal conductivities, since the overall conductivity cannot be obtained simply by adding together the individual conductivities. The problem can be overcome by re-arranging Eqn (12.2) into the following form:

$$q = (t_1 - t_2)\Big/\frac{L}{kA} \qquad (12.3)$$

This is the specific case for heat transfer by conduction of the general expression representing any rate process:

$$\text{rate} = \frac{\text{driving force}}{\text{resistance}} \qquad (12.4)$$

Thus, the temperature difference is the driving force for heat transfer, and it will be realised that the resistance to conduction will increase for greater thicknesses and will decrease as the coefficient of thermal conductivity increases and as the area becomes larger.

Recalling the theory of electricity, conductivities cannot be added together to obtain the total conductivity of a circuit, but the overall resistance of a number of resistances in series is obtained by taking their sum. Furthermore, the resistance and the conductivity bear a simple relationship to each other, being inversely proportional. Applying the electrical analogy to heat transfer means that the overall resistance to heat transfer of a number, n, of layers can be obtained by adding the reciprocals of their thermal conductivities, that is—

$$\text{resistance} = \frac{1}{k_1} + \frac{1}{k_2} + \cdots \frac{1}{k_n} \qquad (12.5)$$

This assumes that the layers are each of unit thickness, which is very unlikely, so that allowance must be made for this.

$$\text{Resistance} = \frac{L_1}{k_1} + \frac{L_2}{k_2} + \cdots \frac{L_n}{k_n} \qquad (12.6)$$

Generally, the area for conduction will be the same for each layer, but if it is not, an additional area term can be included.

To calculate heat transfer we need to know the overall thermal conductivity, which can be obtained by reversing the process, that is by taking the reciprocal of the overall resistance. Usually, this is

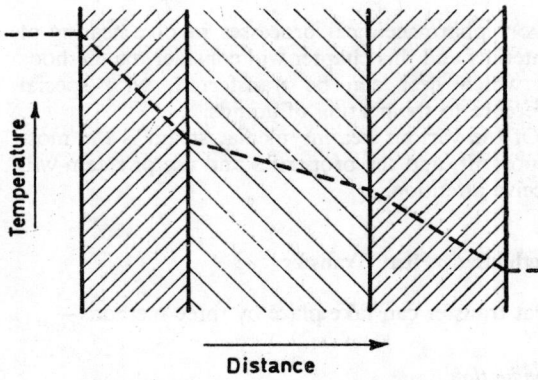

Fig. 12.1   Temperature gradients through solids

known as the *overall coefficient of heat transfer* and is represented by U.

$$U = 1\Big/\frac{L_1}{k_1} + \frac{L_2}{k_2} + \cdots \frac{L_n}{k_n} \qquad (12.7)$$

To calculate heat transfer, U is used instead of k/L in (12.2), so that:

$$q = UA(t_1 - t_2) \qquad (12.8)$$

The situation in a compound layer may be represented in a convenient graphical form using temperature and thickness of layer as ordinates, so that the relative slopes of the various sections of the temperature gradient will be dependent upon the thermal conductivity of the material of each layer, as shown in Fig. 12.1.

Heating of Fluids

When a liquid is to be heated, the process is commonly carried out in a steam-heated vessel, similar to the jacketed pan described in Chapter 14. At first sight it might appear that there would be a simple temperature gradient through the wall between the steam and the liquid. Referring back to p. 148, however, it will be recalled that whenever a fluid contacts a surface there will be a boundary layer and, being stationary, heat must be *conducted* through this layer to the bulk of the liquid. Also, it is likely that some scale will have been deposited on

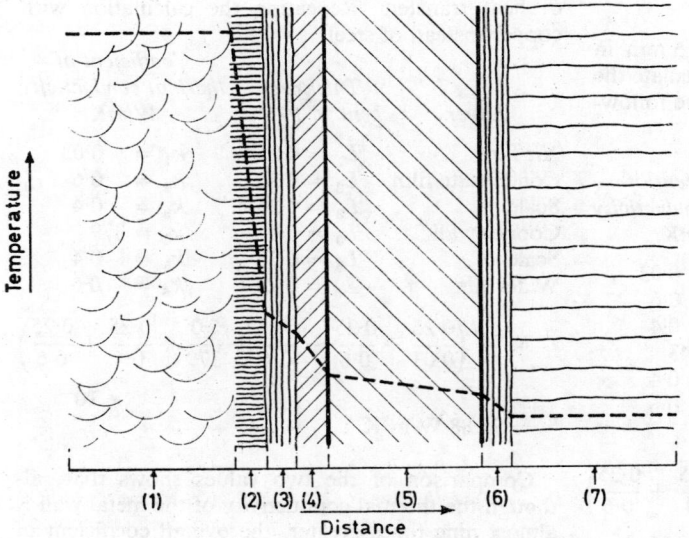

Fig. 12.2 Temperature gradients through heating surface and fluids, idealised

(1) steam   (2) air film
(3) condensate film   (4) scale
(5) metal wall   (6) liquid film
(7) liquid

the surface of the metal wall, and heat must be conducted through this.

When steam gives up its latent heat, water will condense on the surface of the vessel. Again, the heat must be conducted through this water film.

Furthermore, as explained on p. 160, air exists in the jacket before heating begins, and some may remain with the steam. The air will not remain as a clearly defined film, but there will be a greater number of air molecules adjacent to the surface. For the sake of simplicity, therefore, it will be assumed

that the air is present as a stagnant film through which heat must be conducted.

The situation is rather more complicated than a first impression of Fig. 12.2 suggests, the diagrammatic form of Fig. 12.3 being nearer to the truth.

The temperature gradients of Fig. 12.3 suggest that the various layers are likely to exert a considerable effect on heat transfer, the extent of which can best be seen from a numerical example. The values assigned to the thicknesses of the various layers are hypothetical, but are of the correct order.

Fig. 12.3 Temperature gradients through heating surface and fluids, actual

(1) steam   (2) air film
(3) condensate film   (4) scale
(5) metal wall   (6) liquid film
(7) liquid

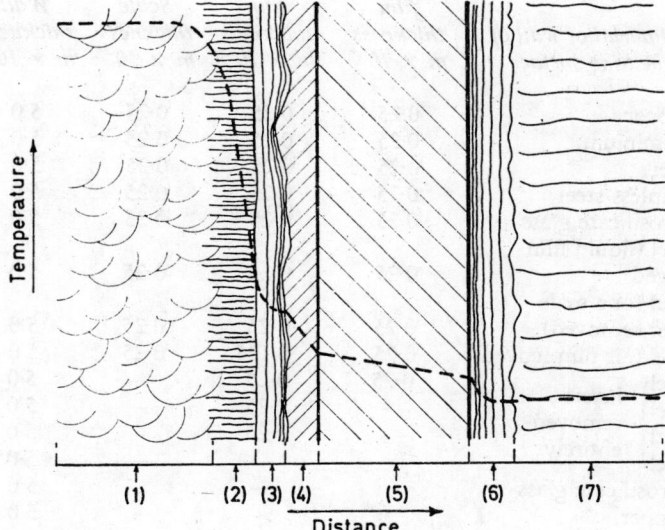

Example

A steam-jacketed pan with a steel wall, 5 mm in thickness, is being used to heat water. Calculate the overall coefficient of heat transfer, using the following data:

Layer	Thickness $m \times 10^{-3}$	Coefficient of thermal conductivity W/mK
Air film	$L_1 = 0 \cdot 25$	$k_1 = 0 \cdot 03$
Condensate film	$L_2 = 0 \cdot 25$	$k_2 = 0 \cdot 6$
Scale	$L_3 = 0 \cdot 25$	$k_3 = 0 \cdot 4$
Steel wall	$L_4 = 5 \cdot 0$	$k_4 = 43$
Scale	$L_5 = 0 \cdot 25$	$k_5 = 0 \cdot 4$
Water film	$L_6 = 0 \cdot 25$	$k_6 = 0 \cdot 6$

Substituting in Eqn (12.7):

$$U = 1 \left/ \left(\frac{0 \cdot 25}{0 \cdot 03} + \frac{0 \cdot 25}{0 \cdot 6} + \frac{0 \cdot 25}{0 \cdot 4} + \frac{5 \cdot 0}{43} + \frac{0 \cdot 25}{0 \cdot 4} + \frac{0 \cdot 25}{0 \cdot 6} \right) \right. \times 10^{-3}$$

$$= 94 \cdot 94 \ W/m^2K$$

Clearly, a value of about 95 W/m^2K for a wall 5 mm in thickness is very low when it is considered that steel has a thermal conductivity that can conduct 4300 W/mK for a wall 10 mm in thickness.

Other metals are better conductors of heat, for example copper, which has a thermal conductivity of 379 W/mK, and substitution of a copper wall should increase the value of the overall coefficient of heat transfer. Repeating the calculation with copper instead of steel:

Layer	Thickness $m \times 10^{-3}$	Coefficient of thermal conductivity W/mK
Air film	$L_1 = 0 \cdot 25$	$k_1 = 0 \cdot 03$
Condensate film	$L_2 = 0 \cdot 25$	$k_2 = 0 \cdot 6$
Scale	$L_3 = 0 \cdot 25$	$k_3 = 0 \cdot 4$
Copper wall	$L_4 = 5 \cdot 0$	$k_4 = 379$
Scale	$L_5 = 0 \cdot 25$	$k_5 = 0 \cdot 4$
Water film	$L_6 = 0 \cdot 25$	$k_6 = 0 \cdot 6$

$$U = 1 \left/ \left(\frac{0 \cdot 25}{0 \cdot 03} + \frac{0 \cdot 25}{0 \cdot 6} + \frac{0 \cdot 25}{0 \cdot 4} + \frac{5 \cdot 0}{379} + \frac{0 \cdot 25}{0 \cdot 4} + \frac{0 \cdot 25}{0 \cdot 6} \right) \right. \times 10^{-3}$$

$$= 95 \cdot 88 \ W/m^2K$$

Comparison of the two values shows that, although the thermal conductivity of the metal wall is almost nine times greater, the overall coefficient of heat transfer has changed from 94·94 to 95·88, a negligible increase. Obviously, factors other than the metal wall are involved, and the answer lies in the other layers on the wall. Table 12.2 shows the effect of using various materials for the wall and of reducing or removing the various layers.

Examination of the values of the overall coefficient of heat transfer listed in Table 12.2 emphasises the influence of the surface layers and films on heat transmission. Note especially the considerable

Table 12.2

Material of wall of heating surface	Condensate film thickness $m \times 10^{-3}$	Air film thickness $m \times 10^{-3}$	Scale thickness $m \times 10^{-3}$	Wall thickness $m \times 10^{-3}$	Scale thickness $m \times 10^{-3}$	Liquid film thickness $m \times 10^{-3}$	U (W/m^2K)
Copper	0·25	0·25	0·25	5·0	0·25	0·25	95·88
Aluminium	0·25	0·25	0·25	5·0	0·25	0·25	95·80
Steel	0·25	0·25	0·25	5·0	0·25	0·25	94·94
Stainless steel	0·25	0·25	0·25	5·0	0·25	0·25	93·36
Borosilicate glass	0·25	0·25	0·25	5·0	0·25	0·25	64·87
Steel (liquid film halved)	0·25	0·25	0·25	5·0	0·25	0·125	96·85
Steel (one scale layer removed)	0·25	0·25	0·25	5·0	—	0·25	100·93
Steel (air film halved)	0·25	0·125	0·25	5·0	0·25	0·25	157·08
Steel ⎫ layers	0·25	0·25	—	5·0	—	0·25	107·72
Steel ⎬ removed	—	0·25	—	5·0	—	0·25	112·79
Steel ⎪ entirely	—	0·25	—	5·0	—	—	118·34
Steel ⎭	—	—	—	5·0	—	—	8 620·69
Borosilicate glass	—	—	—	5·0	—	—	200·00
Copper	—	—	—	5·0	—	—	76 923·00

change in the value of U when the air film is halved, and the dramatic increase when it is eliminated entirely.

The material of the wall has a negligible effect, unless it is of very low thermal conductivity (borosilicate glass, for example) or unless the various films and layers can be removed completely, which is impossible in practice.

This will be understood if the thermal conductivity of air is compared with metals, when it will be found that the resistance to heat transfer of an air film 0·25 mm in thickness is the same as 360 mm of steel, 2 m of aluminium, and more than 3 m of copper.

Film Coefficients

The calculation of overall coefficients of heat transfer in the previous section used the resistance of each layer, expressed as L/k, but in practice this is impossible. While the thermal conductivity of the material may be known, clearly the thickness of a liquid or air film cannot be defined. Hence, these two are combined in the *film coefficient* which replaces the expression k/L in Eqns such as (12.1) or (12.2). The film coefficient represents, therefore, the thermal conductivity of a particular film of a fluid, whereas the usual coefficient of thermal conductivity refers to unit thickness of the material.

Film coefficients may be determined practically or may be calculated theoretically and used in the conduction equations; for example, Eqn (12.2) for a single layer is:

$$q = hA(t_1 - t_2) \qquad (12.9)$$

where h = film coefficient.

For a solid wall with two fluid layers, the overall coefficient of heat transfer would be given by:

$$U = 1 \left/ \frac{1}{h_1} + \frac{L}{k} + \frac{1}{h_2} \right. \qquad (12.10)$$

Design of Heating Equipment

Consideration of the factors affecting heat transfer shows that a number of precautions must be observed in designing equipment for operations involving heating, especially when steam is the source of heat.

AREA

Heating should take place over as large a surface area as possible.

TEMPERATURE GRADIENT

A suitable temperature gradient should be employed and theory suggests that this should be as great as possible, but this is not so in practice. First, many pharmaceutical substances are thermolabile and would be damaged or destroyed by contact with a surface at high temperature. This is discussed further in connection with evaporation in Chapter 14. Secondly, liquids boiling on a hot surface form irregular streams of vapour bubbles and, because each stream originates from a point on the surface, this is called *nucleate boiling*. Above a certain critical surface temperature, however, evolution of vapour is so rapid that it cannot escape and the surface acquires a blanket of vapour, which forms an additional resistance to heat transfer. This condition is known as *film boiling*.

MATERIALS OF CONSTRUCTION

The plant should be made from materials of suitable thermal conductivity.

GENERAL DESIGN

The design of the plant should be such that resistances due to surface layers are minimised.

Air Removal

Elimination, as far as possible, of air in steam is of extreme importance and is discussed in more detail later in this chapter, on p. 160.

Cleanliness

The surfaces of the vessel should be kept clean and free from deposits of solids or scale.

Condensate Removal

The system should be arranged to permit correct drainage and removal of the condensate formed as the steam gives up its heat. Methods of ensuring this are considered later (*see* p. 158).

Liquid Circulation

Liquid movement should be arranged to ensure turbulent flow by avoiding awkward shapes where stagnation might occur, and using forced circulation if natural circulation due to density or viscosity changes is inadequate. The importance of this will be apparent if it is realised that, if the velocity of the fluid is V, then, when flow is streamline, heat transfer is proportional to $V^{0.33}$ while for turbulent flow the heat transferred is proportional to $V^{0.8}$

Convection

Heat transfer by convection will not be considered in detail partly because of the complexity of the subject, but the principal reason is that convection is rarely the controlling factor in equipment operation. Heat transfer to a fluid begins by conduction through the boundary layers, as discussed in preceding sections. In the bulk of the fluid, the rise in temperature causes change in density and viscosity, setting up convection currents the form of which will depend upon the surroundings; for example, whether the liquid is passing through a pipe or over banks of tubes. If natural convection is inadequate, forced circulation may be induced by the use of a pump or stirrer.

It must be emphasised that transfer of heat through the boundary layers to the fluid is related to the vigour of the movement of the fluid, as this influences boundary layer thickness (*see* p. 148).

Radiant Heat Transmission

A hot body emits energy in the form of electromagnetic waves, this radiation proceeding in all directions with virtually no loss to the intervening atmosphere. If it falls on another body, some of the radiation may be transmitted, some reflected and part absorbed, the relative proportions depending on the properties of the body.

A black body is the perfect emitter and absorber, but all bodies radiate to some extent, the amount and the quality of the emission being dependent upon the Absolute temperature. This can be summarised in three expressions:

TOTAL ENERGY

The total energy emitted, E, is given by:

$$E \propto T^4 \qquad (12.11)$$

where T = Absolute temperature.

This emission is distributed in a spectrum between the wavelengths 1 to 100 μm, which is above the visible red, hence the commonly used term 'infrared'. In practice, the useful wavelengths lie between 1 and 10 μm.

PEAK WAVELENGTH

The emission of energy is not distributed uniformly over this band of the spectrum, there being a peak wavelength, Z, at which the intensity of radiation is greatest:

$$Z \propto 1/T \qquad (12.12)$$

INTENSITY

Once more, the Absolute temperature controls the intensity of the radiation, I, at the peak wavelength

and is given by:

$$I \propto T^5 \qquad (12.13)$$

Thus, as the temperature of the emitter is raised, the total radiated energy is increased, the peak wavelength becomes shorter, and the radiation at the peak wavelength is of greater intensity. This is illustrated graphically in Fig. 12.4.

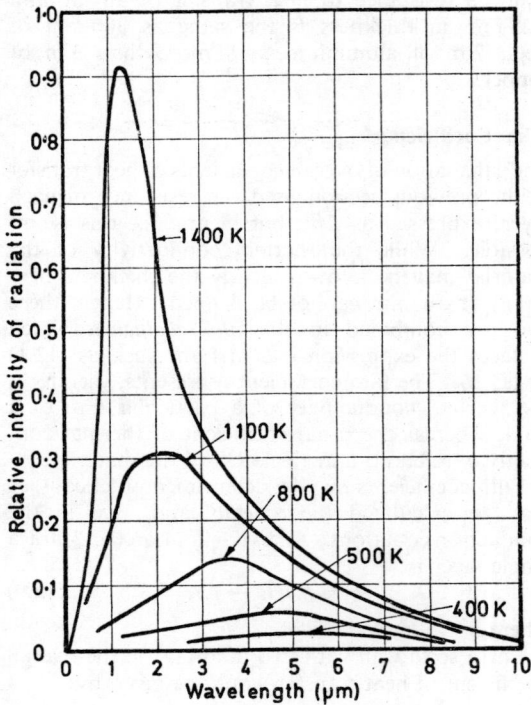

Fig. 12.4   Radiant energy distributions

USE OF RADIANT HEAT TRANSMISSION

The character of radiant energy means that, when used in practice for heat transfer, the heating effect depends upon the temperature of the emitter and the absorption into the material to be heated.

Forms of emitter include infra-red lamps in which the filament operates at approximately 1000°C giving a peak wavelength of about 1 μm, and ceramic rods or panels heated by gas or electricity. The latter work at lower temperatures, usually from 800°C down to 500°C, with peak wavelengths between 2 and 4 μm. This means that the latter may be preferable when pharmaceutical materials that are thermolabile and likely to be affected by the greater intensity of emission of the infra-red lamp are involved.

A special feature of this form of heat transmission is that the radiant energy penetrates a short distance (1 to 2 mm) into materials so that the heating effect occurs below the surface. This property can be of considerable importance where the material is being heated in thin layers or films; for example, in a film of a solution being dried by radiant heat, where the energy will pass through the film and be absorbed into the supporting medium. Hence, the film is heated from below outwards, thus possibly avoiding the surface skin which can retard the drying process when convection methods are used.

Absorption of the energy into a substance will depend on the properties of the material, but, in general, more energy will be absorbed into dark-coloured, opaque, rough-surfaced media, and least into light-coloured, transparent, smooth-surfaced substances.

Combination of Heat Transfer Methods

It is stated commonly that heating occurs by a particular method of heat transfer; for example, an oven with forced circulation of the hot air by a fan transfers heat by convection. While this is the principal method of heat transfer, it must not be forgotten that an object in an oven receives heat also by conduction from the shelf on which it stands and by radiation from the hot walls of the oven.

Steam as a Heating Medium

Of the various means of heating pharmaceutical materials to effect operations such as evaporation or drying, steam is used most commonly. In addition, steam has important uses in pharmacy for sterilisation.

Among the reasons for the widespread use of steam, are:

steam has a very high heat content;

the heat is given up at constant temperature;

the raw material—water—is cheap and plentiful.

Steam is clean, odourless and tasteless, so that the results of accidental contamination of a product are not likely to be serious. Alternative heating media, such as oils, could be very dangerous if any entered a product.

Steam can be used at high pressure to generate electric power, and the low-pressure exhaust steam used for process heating.

Steam is easy to generate, distribute, and control.

From the kinetic theory of heat, it will be recalled that a vapour contains heat in two 'forms'—*sensible heat* and *latent heat*. Sensible heat is heat that can be detected by the senses, that is, a temperature change is caused when sensible heat is taken up or given out. 'Latent' means concealed or invisible, so that latent heat is not detected as a temperature change. Thus, latent heat is taken up or given out at constant temperature as a change of phase occurs between solid or liquid or vapour. The sensible and latent heat contents are very important properties of steam.

Properties of Steam

The properties can be visualised if one kilogramme of water is imagined in a cylinder enclosed by a frictionless piston at a constant pressure P bars and at a temperature of $0°C$.

If heat is added until a change of state occurs, that is, the water starts to boil, it will take place at a temperature t_s and the amount of heat required is $h = t_s - 0$ kilojoules. The heat, h, is the sensible heat of the water.

If more heat is added, a fraction of the water, q, will be vaporised. If the latent heat of vaporisation is L kJ/kg, then the amount of heat added is qL kJ and the total heat content of the wet steam (that is the steam-water mixture) is $h + qL$ kJ. q is known as the *dryness fraction* of the wet steam and can be expressed as a percentage or as a decimal part of one. Thus, steam may be spoken of as 85 per cent dry or 0·85 dry.

As further heat is added, a point will be reached when $q = 1$, that is, all the water has been evaporated and the steam is dry. The total heat now added is $h + L = H_s$ kJ, but it must be remembered that the temperature will still be t_s.

Clearly, the kilogramme of water occupies a small volume, but the steam will occupy a considerably greater volume. One kilogramme of dry steam at a temperature t_s will occupy a volume V_s cubic metres. V_s is known as the *specific volume* and can be defined as the volume occupied by one kilogramme of dry steam.

When steam is in this condition, all the water is vaporised, so that the steam is dry, and is exerting its full saturated vapour pressure, hence the description *dry saturated steam*.

Any additional heat added cannot be used as latent heat of vaporisation, and therefore must enter as sensible heat, which causes the temperature of the vapour to rise, when the steam is said to be *superheated*. Thus, the temperature reaches a value t_{sup}, the volume increases (approximately in accordance with the Gas Laws), and the total heat content is $H_s + H_{sup}$.

These data are published in the form of 'Steam Tables', which tabulate the following information:

P = pressure

t_s = saturation temperature at pressure P

h = sensible heat

L = latent heat of vaporisation

H_s = total heat of dry saturated steam

V_s = specific volume

H_{sup} = superheat for specified number of degrees of superheat

It should be noted that 0°C is used as the datum temperature.

Examples from Steam Tables

From the list in the previous section it will be seen that Steam Tables enable us to calculate the sensible heat in water at any temperature, the total heat of wet and dry saturated steam (if the dryness fraction is known), and of superheated steam.

A few examples of the heat contents of steam under various conditions will illustrate the information that can be derived from Steam Tables and, also, certain important properties of steam.

Example 1

Determine the temperature, t_s, and the total heat, H_s, of dry saturated steam at 2 bars.

$$t_s = 120.2°C$$
$$\text{Sensible heat } (h) = 505 \text{ kJ/kg}$$
$$\text{Latent heat } (L) = 2\,202 \text{ kJ/kg}$$
$$\text{Total heat } (H_s) = \overline{2\,707} \text{ kJ/kg}$$

Example 2

Determine t_s and H_s for any saturated steam at 15 bars.

$$t_s = 198.3°C$$
$$h = 845 \text{ kJ/kg}$$
$$L = 1\,947 \text{ kJ/kg}$$
$$H_s = \overline{2\,792} \text{ kJ/kg}$$

Example 3

Determine t_s and H_s for saturated steam at 15 bars, dryness fraction, $q = 0.95$.

$$t_s = 198.3°C$$
$$h = 845 \text{ kJ/kg}$$
$$qL = 0.95 \times 1\,947 = 1\,850 \text{ kJ/kg}$$
$$H_s = \overline{2\,695} \text{ kJ/kg}$$

Example 4

Determine the total heat, H, for superheated steam at 2 bars with 80°C superheat.

From superheated steam tables:

$$t_s = 120.2°C \text{ at 2 bars}$$
$$t_{sup} = 120.2 + 80 = 200.2°C$$
$$H = 2830 \text{ kJ/kg}$$

DISCUSSION OF EXAMPLES

From Example 1 it will be seen that approximately one-fifth of the heat content of steam at 2 bars is sensible heat, while about four-fifths is latent heat. It must be remembered that, if it is to be used for process heating, the steam (at its saturation temperature) will be brought into contact with the surface to be heated. Heat will be transmitted to the cold surface and, as the steam was at its saturation temperature, the heat given up will be the latent heat, that is, part of the steam will condense. This will continue, either until all the steam has been condensed or the surface has been brought up to the steam temperature. In practice, the transferred heat is used for a process such as evaporation and the steam is replaced continually, so that the process can go on indefinitely. Two conclusions must be emphasised: first, that this process will occur at the saturation temperature of the steam, dependent upon the pressure, i.e. 100°C at 1 bar, 115°C at 1·7 bars, 121°C at 2 bars and so on; secondly, that the latent heat is the *useful* heat of the steam. Only when all the steam has been condensed will the temperature begin to fall and sensible heat be liberated.

Comparison of Examples 1 and 2 shows that the saturation temperature of steam at 15 bars is about 200°C against 120°C at 2 bars, which means that the sensible heat is 340 kJ/kg higher in the first case. Total heat, however, is only 85 kJ/kg higher, due to a decrease in the latent heat from 2202 kJ/kg at 2 bars to 1947 kJ/kg at 15 bars. This may appear surprising, since school work in physics often leaves the impression that the latent heat of steam is constant at 2258 kJ/kg (540 cal/g). In fact, this is the value for atmospheric pressure and it is a variable dependent upon pressure.

The reason for this variability will be understood easily if the situation is considered in terms of the kinetic theory of heat. In a liquid, the molecules vibrate and are able to make some movement relative to each other, but they do not have complete freedom, due to intermolecular attractive forces. These forces may cause molecules to aggregate into groups, especially near the surface, leading to a 'skin' effect (surface tension). When the liquid vaporises, sufficient energy has been imparted to the molecules (as latent heat) to allow them to overcome these attractive forces. Thus, the molecules can expand to fill the available volume, moving freely with random movements in all directions. Since the specific volume of the steam decreases as the pressure increases, it follows that the molecules will need less energy to expand to fill the available volume at high pressure compared with that necessary at lower pressures; in other words, the higher the pressure, the smaller the specific volume and the lower the latent heat of steam. To give some idea of the difference, the specific volume of steam at 2 bars, from Steam Tables, is 0·8856 m³/kg, while at 15 bars it is 0·1317 m³/kg. The ultimate case will occur, of course, at the critical pressure (221·2 bars) when one kilogramme of steam occupies the same volume as one kilogramme of water and the latent heat of vaporisation is zero.

The conclusion to be reached from these observations is that, since the latent heat is the useful heat, steam should be used at the lowest pressure that will give a suitable temperature gradient.

Turning to Example 3, it will be seen that steam at 15 bars, which is 0·95 dry, contains *less heat* than dry saturated steam at 2 bars, and that the useful latent heat is considerably less, although, the 15 bars steam will still be at the higher temperature, of course. Since heat is lost from steam pipes, it will be realised that a great deal more than 5 per cent of the steam can be condensed, constituting a costly loss of heat. Thus, it is important that precautions should be taken to keep the steam as dry as possible, by minimising heat losses.

Example 4 should be compared with Examples 1 and 2, when it will be seen that steam at 2 bars with 80°C superheat contains only about 123 kJ/kg more than dry saturated steam at that pressure, although the temperature is considerably higher. The temperature will, in fact, be about the same as that of dry saturated steam at 15 bars, but the important difference to realise is that dry saturated steam at 15 bars will liberate its latent heat at 200°C, but the superheated steam of the example will liberate only 123 kJ of sensible heat in cooling from 200°C down to 120°C, when the latent heat will become available.

These conclusions lead us to three important rules for using steam for process heating:

Steam Pressure

Steam should be used at the lowest pressure that will give a suitable temperature gradient.

Steam Dryness

Great care should be taken to keep steam dry by minimising heat losses.

Steam Saturation

Saturated steam and not superheated steam should be used in equipment.

Practical Aspects of the Use of Steam

In practice, it is usual for steam to be generated centrally in the factory and distributed to the various items of process plant.

GENERATION OF STEAM

The method of generating the steam in a central boiler house at high pressure has a number of advantages. The high pressure steam can be used to drive a turbine for generating electric power, and the low pressure exhaust steam for process heating.

Central generation is more economical in fuel.

Having high pressure steam available means that higher temperatures are available, if required, for special purposes.

More steam is stored in the boiler if high pressures are used. Although Boyle's law applies only to a perfect gas at constant temperature, it gives an approximate indication of the behaviour of steam, which means that, if the pressure is doubled, the boiler will hold about twice as much steam. This will be found to be true if specific volumes are looked up in Steam Tables, for example, V_s at 2 bars = 0·8856 m³/kg and V_s at 4 bars = 0·4623 m³/kg. Hence, a better reserve of steam is provided to allow for fluctuations in the demand.

Expansion of the high pressure steam to low pressure at the plant will help to dry the steam (*see* p. 158).

The pressure provides the driving force for distribution of the steam.

DISTRIBUTION

From the boiler, the steam will be distributed through piping which should be of adequate size to carry the required quantities of steam and as short as possible to minimise heat losses. To reduce loss of heat further, the pipes should be *lagged*, that is, covered with a layer of porous, poor conducting material, such as kieselguhr, asbestos, or glass wool. The most important property of lagging is that it should be porous, to trap a stagnant layer of air round the pipe, since air is such a very poor conductor of heat. As an alternative, several layers of aluminium foil can be applied and this is very effective for insulation, the surface of the foil preventing radiation losses and the air trapped between the layers minimising convection losses.

Since some heat losses are inevitable, arrangements should be made for the condensate to be drained off at low points.

PRESSURE REDUCTION

In general, process plant uses steam at a pressure of 1·7 to 2 bars, so that a reduction from the boiler pressure is necessary. This is carried out by a reducing valve, the principles of which are shown in Fig. 12.5.

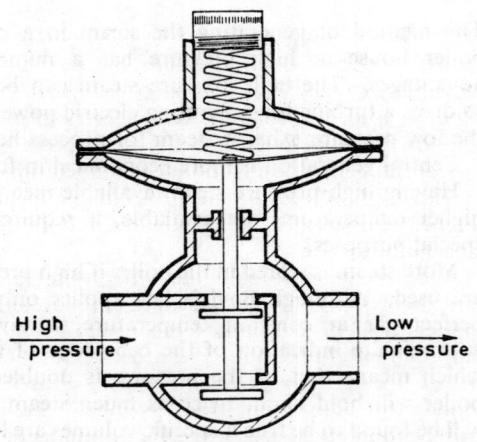

High pressure → ← Low pressure

Fig. 12.5 Pressure reducing valve

The pressure of a spring attempts to open the valve against the high pressure steam. The closing of the valve is caused by the low pressure steam, so that, when this reaches a pre-determined value, a balance will be reached in which the low pressure steam acting on the diaphragm closes the valve against the spring pressure.

In practice, an equilibrium is set up in which the valve is open slightly, sufficient steam passing through from the high pressure to maintain the desired level on the low-pressure side.

Expansion at the plant has the advantage also that some drying of the steam can take place due to the higher value of the latent heat of vaporisation at 'lower pressures. This process is known as 'throttling or 'wire-drawing' and the effect can be seen by a numerical example, using Steam Tables.

Consider steam at 2·7 bars and dryness fraction 0·99, being expanded to 1·7 bars.

At 2·7 bars:

$$h = \quad 546 \text{ kJ/kg}$$
$$L = 2\,174 \times 0.99 = 2\,153 \text{ kJ/kg}$$
$$H = 2\,699 \text{ kJ/kg}$$

At 1·7 bars:

$$h = \quad 483 \text{ kJ/kg}$$
$$L = 2\,216 \text{ kJ/kg}$$
$$H = 2\,699 \text{ kJ/kg}$$

This means that the water in the steam will be vaporised and will become dry saturated steam at 1·7 bars.

There is a risk, however, that the steam may become superheated if expanded to a pressure that is too low; for example, suppose the steam at 2·7 bars and 0·99 dry is expanded to 1 bar. From Steam Tables, H for dry saturated steam at 1 bar is 2675 kJ/kg and from tables for superheated steam, 2699 kJ/kg at 1 bar gives 12°C superheat.

In general, though, steam that has been transmitted any distance through pipes is likely to have a dryness fraction lower than 0·99 and expansion will be insufficient to dry it completely. Mechanical methods are used, therefore, in which the steam is caused to change direction suddenly, the greater momentum of the liquid droplets causing separation. Centrifugal methods or baffles may be used.

USE OF STEAM IN THE PLANT

The use of the steam at the plant may be *direct* or *indirect*. In the first case, the *live* steam is blown directly into the material. It has the advantage of greater efficiency of heat transfer with no boundary layer resistance to overcome, but the disadvantage that the condensate enters the material. It is a useful method of heating liquids if this dilution is not important, but the special applications are in steam distillation and for sterilisation (*see* Gunn and Carter, 1965).

When the steam is used indirectly there is a barrier between the steam and the material to be heated. This may be effected by means of a jacket round the piece of plant or by having a steam coil or tubes throug! the vessel. The use of a steam jacket is convenient but has the limitation that, as the vessel increases in size, the heating area decreases relative to the volume. This will be understood easily if the simple case is taken of a spherical vessel, when the volume is proportional to the cube of the diameter, whereas the surface area is proportional only to the square of the diameter. A steam coil or tubes permits the use of larger areas and may increase the heat transfer coefficient by promoting turbulence but may make cleaning of a vessel difficult.

CONDENSATE REMOVAL

Indirect methods of using steam in jackets or tubes must use closed systems to maintain the steam pressure and prevent loss of steam. This means, therefore, that the condensate that forms as the steam gives up its latent heat will accumulate and waterlog the system, unless some arrangements are made for condensate removal. Thus, the system must include a *steam trap*, which is a device to distinguish between water and steam, allowing the former to be discharged and the latter retained.

The steam traps in common use can be divided into two main classes: *mechanical* and *thermostatic*. The former depend on the physical difference between steam and water, that is between vapour and liquid, while the thermostatic variety rely on the fact that condensate can lose sensible heat and so will be at a lower temperature than the steam.

Mechanical traps have the advantage of possessing greater strength and the ability to operate under a greater variety of conditions than thermostatic traps; for example, if the temperature difference between the steam and the condensate is small, or if the pressure or the amount of condensate changes.

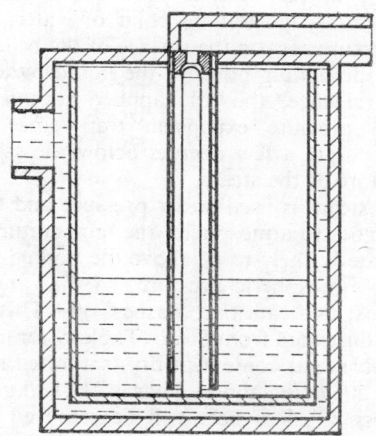

Fig. 12.7   Bucket type steam trap

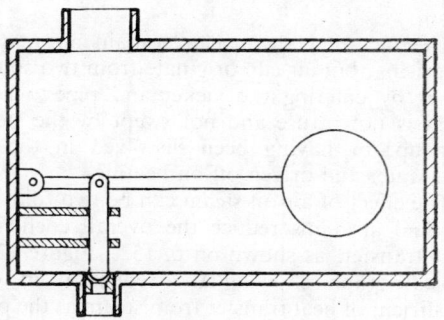

Fig. 12.6   Float type steam trap

On the other hand, thermostatic traps differ from mechanical traps by opening when the plant is not in use, allowing condensate to drain away and air to be swept out of the system when starting up. Thermostatic traps also vent air when operating, because of the reduction of temperature of steam when contaminated with air (*see* p. 160), whereas mechanical traps are unable to distinguish between air and steam.

Typical examples of these traps are shown in Figs. 12.6 to 12.8. The *float trap* in Fig. 12.6 is a mechanical trap in which the outlet is opened by the float as the condensate level rises. As the condensate is discharged, the float falls and the outlet closes. In the *bucket trap* (Fig. 12.7) the outlet is closed when the bucket floats in the condensate. As more condensate drains down into the trap, some overflows into the bucket until the latter sinks and opens the outlet. The condensate is blown out by the

pressure of the steam until the bucket recovers its buoyancy and floats up to close the outlet once more.

Thermostatic traps can take the form of a simple thermostatic device which can be set to open at a particular temperature appropriate to the steam pressure, but this has the disadvantage that a slight variation in the steam pressure (and hence the temperature) may cause the trap to stay either open or closed until the setting has been altered to meet the new conditions.

This difficulty is overcome in the *balanced pressure expansion trap*, illustrated in Fig. 12.8. A capsule in the form of a bellows contains a liquid having a boiling point a few degrees below the boiling point of water. Thus, when surrounded by steam, the liquid in the capsule boils, causing the bellows to expand and close the outlet. Condensate cools the capsule, the liquid then ceases to boil, and the bellows contract, opening the outlet and discharging the condensate. When all the condensate is removed, steam causes the trap to close again. A particular

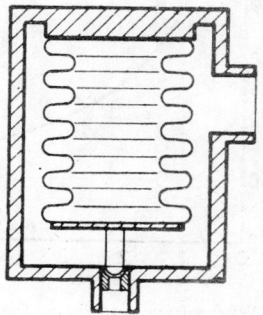

Fig. 12.8   Balanced pressure steam trap

advantage of this trap is that increase of steam pressure raises the boiling point of water, but the same pressure acts on the surface of the bellows and elevates the boiling point of the liquid by a similar amount. Hence, the title applied to this type— balanced pressure expansion trap—since it will always operate a few degrees below the saturation temperature of the steam.

When steam is used under pressure and the condensate goes to atmosphere, the temperature of the condensate is likely to be above the boiling point of water at atmospheric pressure, so that any excess heat is lost as steam that 'flashes' off. This, again, may be illustrated from Steam Tables; for example, the sensible heat content of dry, saturated steam at 2 bars is 505 kJ/kg and at 1 bar is 417 kJ/kg, so that the excess 88 kJ of heat will be removed as *flash steam*. This heat can be recovered if the condensate is discharged into a suitable vessel; in fact, if this vessel is operated at a pressure below atmospheric a further advantage can be gained. Thus, using a pressure of 0·15 bar the sensible heat content is 226 kJ/kg. Under these conditions, therefore, 279 kJ can be recovered from each kilogramme of condensate.

Use can still be made of the condensate, since it has a purity equivalent to distilled water. Hence, it is returned to the boiler as feed water, thereby reducing costs and helping to minimise the amount of scale formed.

AIR IN STEAM

Reference has been made in the previous section to air venting, a subject that is of great importance

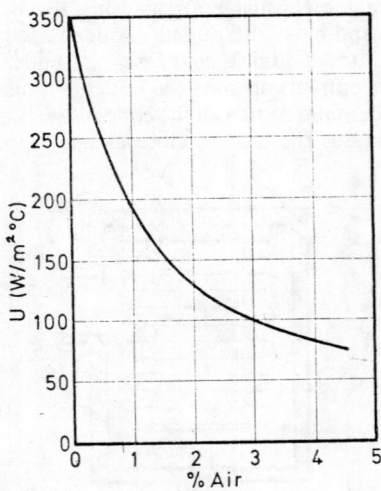

Fig. 12.9   Effect of air in steam on the coefficient of heat transfer

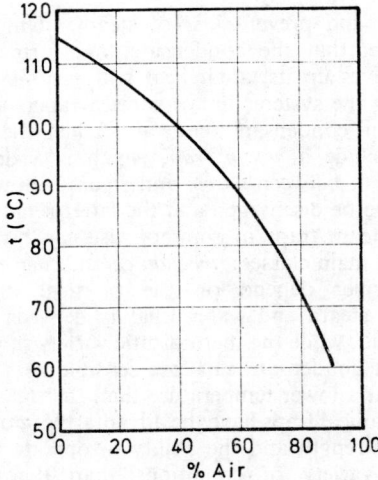

Fig. 12.10   Effect of air on steam temperatures

since the presence of even small proportions of air can have considerable effects on the properties of steam.

The fact that steam can contain air may seem surprising, but air can originate from two sources— either by entering the jacket and pipes when the plant is not in use and not swept by the steam at start-up, or having been dissolved in the boiler feed water and driven off on heating.

The effect of air on steam can be two-fold. First, residual air films reduce the overall coefficient of heat transfer, as shown on p. 152. Figure 12.9 is a typical graph showing the reduction in overall coefficient of heat transfer from steam as the proportion of air increases, from which it will be seen that as little as 4 per cent of air reduces the overall coefficient of heat transfer to about one quarter of the value for air-free steam. The second effect is that the pressure due to a mixture of air and steam will consist of a partial pressure of air and a partial pressure of steam. From Dalton's law of 'partial pressures', the pressure due to the steam will be the pressure it would exert if it occupied the whole volume. This means that the temperature of a mixture of air and steam will be lower than the temperature of saturated steam at the same pressure. The temperature will depend on the proportion of air and this relationship at 1·7 bars is shown in the graph in Fig. 12.10. From this it will be seen, for example, that the temperature of steam containing 40 per cent of air at 1·7 bars is the same as the temperature of dry saturated steam at 1 bar, that is, 100°C.

Clearly, this will be of importance in heating processes where the temperature gradient will be

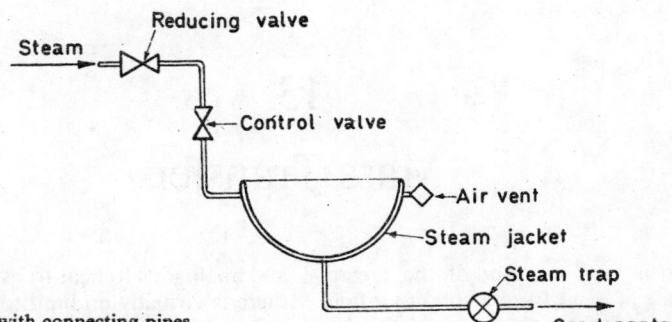

Fig. 12.11 Steam pan with connecting pipes

lower than expected. It is of greatest significance, however, in sterilisation processes where the lower temperature may make sterilisation ineffective. This is discussed fully by Gunn and Carter (1965).

Air may be removed by use of the thermostatic type of trap which will operate when the proportion of air lowers the steam temperature sufficiently. In addition, air vents can be used that are similar in principle to balanced pressure expansion traps.

The position of air vents is important and it has been suggested that they should be located at the lowest point, as air/steam mixtures are denser than steam. In practice, this is not always true and, in general, the air vents should be at a point or points furthest from the steam inlet, so that as much air as possible is swept out as the steam enters when the plant is started up and before the vent closes.

Special cases, such as autoclaves, may require several vents to deal with 'dead spots', an aspect considered in detail by Gunn and Carter (1965).

CONCLUSION

To summarise the considerations of the practical use of steam, Fig. 12.11 shows diagrammatically the connections to a vessel such as a jacketed pan.

In practice, the size of the plant and its economics will govern whether the steam trap will discharge to atmosphere or whether the flash steam is recovered.

BIBLIOGRAPHY

GUNN, C. and CARTER, S. J. (1965) *Dispensing for Pharmaceutical Students.* 11th ed. London, Pitman Medical.

HSU, S. T. (1963) *Engineering Heat Transfer*, Princeton, N.J., Van Nostrand.

LYLE, O. (1947) *The Efficient Use of Steam.* London, H.M. Stationery Office.

MAYHEW, Y. R. and ROGERS, G. F. C. (1967) *Thermodynamic and Transport Properties of Fluids, SI Units.* 2nd ed., Oxford, Blackwell.

13

Mass Transfer

THIS chapter gives a brief account of the factors affecting the transfer of mass from a solid to a fluid and from a fluid to a fluid, with emphasis on the effect of the boundary layer and the influence of mass transfer phenomena on the unit operations.

Solid/Fluid Mass Transfer

Consider a crystal of a soluble material immersed in a solvent in which it is dissolving. A situation will exist, shown diagrammatically in Fig. 13.1, where the crystal is surrounded by a stationary boundary layer of the solute, with the bulk of the fluid able to move. Such movement could be natural convection, arising from temperature or density changes, or forced convection resulting from agitation.

Hence, transport of the molecules of the dissolving solid will take place in two stages. First, the molecules move through the boundary layer by *molecular diffusion*, with no mechanical mixing or movement, a process that is analogous to heat transfer by conduction. Once material has passed through the boundary layer, mass transfer takes place by bulk movement of the solution, known as *eddy diffusion*,

and analogous to heat transfer by convection. Since there is virtually no limit to the vigour of the movement of the bulk of the fluid, the controlling factor in the rate of solution of the crystal will be the molecular diffusion through the boundary layer. It will be appreciated that this continues the analogy with heat transfer where the limitation was the rate at which heat could be conducted through the boundary layer. Eddy diffusion will not be considered further since, in general, molecular diffusion is the controlling process. As would be expected, mass transfer by the latter process can be represented in a similar manner to conduction heat transfer, as shown in Fig. 13.2, but with a concentration gradient instead of a temperature gradient.

It will be recalled that the term fluid includes gases and vapours as well as liquids, and the preceding discussion can refer equally to mass transfer from a solid to a gas. As an example, if a solid is drying in air, the vapour molecules must diffuse through the air boundary layer to the atmosphere. The driving force in this case will be the partial vapour pressure gradient through the air boundary layer.

Mass transfer by molecular diffusion can be represented by an equation, similar to conduction

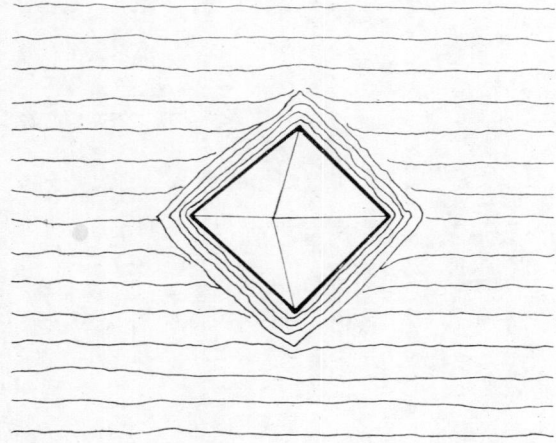

Fig. 13.1 Crystal immersed in solvent

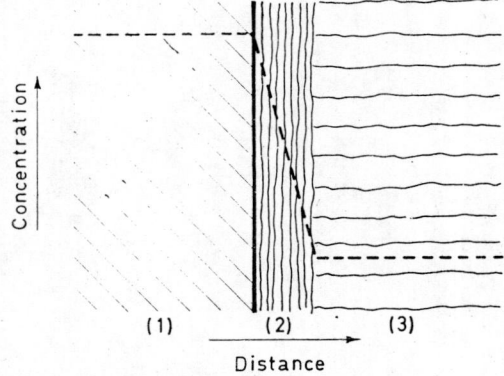

Fig. 13.2 Concentration gradients in solid/fluid system
(1) solid (2) fluid film (3) fluid .

heat transfer, in which:

$$W = \frac{DA(C_1 - C_2)\theta}{L} \qquad (13.1)$$

or

$$w = \frac{DA(C_1 - C_2)}{L} \qquad (13.2)$$

where W = weight of solute diffusing; w = weight of solute diffusing in unit time; D = diffusion coefficient; A = area; θ = time; C_1 = concentration of solute at interface; C_2 = concentration of solute in bulk; L = film thickness.

A similar equation can be written for a vapour:

$$w = \frac{DA(P_1 - P_2)}{L} \qquad (13.3)$$

where P_1 = partial pressure of vapour at interface; P_2 = partial pressure of vapour in the atmosphere.

As in heat transfer, films of unknown thickness can be dealt with as film coefficients, and for multiple layers an overall coefficient of mass transfer can be derived.

Fluid/Fluid Mass Transfer

An equivalent situation occurs when mass transfer takes place between two immiscible fluids, which may be two liquids or a liquid and a gas (or vapour).

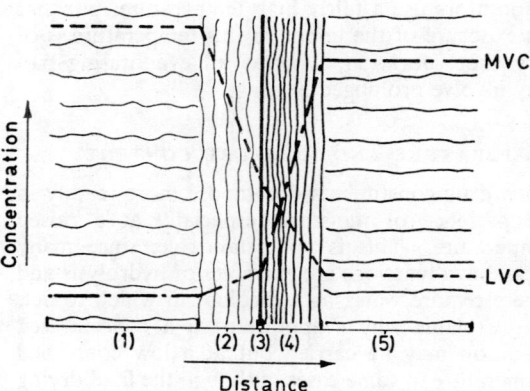

Fig. 13.3   Concentration gradients in fluid/fluid system

(1) vapour (2) vapour film (3) interface (4) liquid film (5) liquid

MVC = more volatile component
LVC = less volatile component

In this case there will be boundary layers of both fluids on each side of the interface, as shown in Fig. 13.3, where the slope of the concentration gradients depends on the diffusion coefficients in the two materials.

Influence on Unit Operations

Mass transfer theory outlined briefly above can be applied to any operation in which material changes phase, whether it is solid/liquid, solid/vapour (or gas), liquid/liquid, or liquid/vapour (or gas).

The effect can be seen in simple operations, such as the making of a solution of a solid in liquid, where the rate of solution can be increased by:

Agitation, which reduces the thickness of the boundary layers and disperses any local concentrations of solution, so increasing the concentration gradient.

Elevated temperatures (which will increase the solubility of most materials) but which increase the diffusion coefficient and decrease the viscosity of the liquid, so reducing boundary layer thickness.

Size reduction of the solid, which increases the area over which diffusion can occur.

Similar principles will apply when solvent extraction of a drug takes place, and a parallel situation exists with solid and vapour when drying a solid in a stream of air.

Probably the most complex case arises when a liquid of two components is required to reach equilibrium with a vapour consisting of the same two components in different proportions. This may occur in distillation and can involve counter-current diffusion, that is both components may diffuse in opposite directions to each other. Distillation additionally includes simultaneous heat and mass transfer, which complicates the situation further. (*See* Fig. 13.3 and Chapter 23.)

Design of mass transfer equipment must take account, therefore, of similar considerations to heat transfer, that is, turbulent flow conditions, maximum concentration or partial pressure gradients and the largest possible surface area.

BIBLIOGRAPHY

BIRD, R. B., STEWART, W. E., and LIGHTFOOT, E. N. (1960) *Transport Phenomena.* New York, Wiley.
TREYBAL, R. E. (1968) *Mass Transfer Operations.* New York, McGraw-Hill.

14

Evaporation

Definition

IT is desirable to begin consideration of any unit operation with a definition in order to establish a basis for understanding the principles and practice of the operation.

Theoretically, evaporation means simply vaporisation from the surface of a liquid. Thus, no boiling occurs and the rate of vaporisation depends on the diffusion of vapour through the boundary layers above the liquid. The principles of mass transfer, as discussed in Chapter 13, will apply, with the partial pressure as the driving force.

In practice, however, this would be too slow, so that the liquid is boiled, causing vapour to be liberated in the form of bubbles from the bulk of the liquid. Thus, a practical definition of evaporation is: the removal of liquid from a solution by boiling the liquor in a suitable vessel and withdrawing the vapour, leaving a concentrated liquid residue.

This means that heat will be necessary to provide the latent heat of vaporisation and, in general, the rate of evaporation is controlled by the rate of heat transfer. Evaporators are designed, therefore, to give maximum heat transfer to the liquid, as discussed on p. 153, with the largest possible area, a suitable temperature gradient and boundary layers reduced by all possible means.

It must be remembered, however, that there may be a limit to heat transfer in practice and, apart from the economic reasons which are outside the scope of this book, there are a number of pharmaceutical and technical factors arising from the properties of the materials being handled. These may demand special consideration in the design or selection of evaporators.

Factors Affecting Evaporation

TEMPERATURE

Apart from the significance of temperature as a factor that affects the rate of evaporation, its effect on drug constituents is of great importance. Reference has been made already to the thermolability of many medicinal principles, and, during the evaporation, temperatures that will cause the least possible decomposition must be used. Many glycosides and alkaloids are decomposed at temperatures below 100°C and some others, for example hormones, enzymes and antibiotics, are even more heat sensitive. Extremely heat-sensitive substances may require special treatment if decomposition is to be avoided during concentration. Malt Extract, for example, is prepared by evaporation under reduced pressure to avoid loss of enzymes, and for some antibiotics the only possible method is freeze drying.

TEMPERATURE AND TIME OF EVAPORATION

Exposure to a relatively high temperature for a short period of time may be less destructive of active principles than a lower temperature with exposure for a longer period. It will be shown later that film evaporators use a fairly high temperature, but that the exposure of the liquor to this temperature is of very short duration, whereas an evaporating pan may involve prolonged heating.

TEMPERATURE AND MOISTURE CONTENT

Some drug constituents decompose more readily in the presence of moisture, especially at a raised temperature. This is understandable, since many breakdown reactions are examples of hydrolysis and others require water as a medium in which to act. This explains why evaporation to a concentrated condition may be carried out at a low controlled temperature in some cases, although the final drying can be performed at higher temperatures when little moisture remains. Belladonna Dry Extract is an example of this type.

TYPE OF PRODUCT REQUIRED

The type of product required will often decide which method and apparatus should be employed for evaporation. Evaporating pans or stills will produce liquid or dry products, but film evaporators will yield only liquid products. Hence, if a dry product is required a choice must be made between a method that will form a suitable product directly (even if the method has certain technical disadvantages) and one in which a preliminary concentration is carried out, with the process completed by another method.

EFFECT OF CONCENTRATION

As the liquor becomes concentrated, the increasing proportion of solids results in elevation of the boiling point of the solution. This leads to a greater risk of damage to thermolabile constituents and to reduction of the temperature gradient, which is the driving force for heat transfer. In general, concentrated solutions will have increased viscosity, causing thicker boundary layers, and many will deposit solids that may build up on the heating surface and reduce heat transfer. Both these problems may be minimised by ensuring turbulent flow conditions.

EVAPORATORS

The equipment used in evaporation may be classified conveniently according to the form of the movement, as this is very important in heat transfer, and can be divided into three main groups:

natural circulation evaporators;
forced circulation evaporators;
film evaporators.

There are many commercial varieties of evaporators and typical examples will be discussed in the following sections. While types other than those described here may be seen in operation in pharmaceutical plants, if their construction and principles are examined it will be found that they may be fitted into one or other of these groups.

Although various methods of heating can be used, steam is the commonest in pharmaceutical practice and all the evaporators illustrated here are steam-heated.

Natural Circulation Evaporators

Evaporators in this category are those in which the movement of the liquid results from convection currents set up by the heating process.

EVAPORATING PANS

The simplest form of natural circulation evaporator is the *evaporating pan*. As shown in Fig. 14.1, the apparatus consists of a hemispherical, or shallower, pan, constructed from a suitable material such as copper or stainless steel and surrounded by a steam jacket. The hemispherical shape gives the best surface/volume ratio for heating, and the largest area for disengagement of vapour. The pan may have a mounting permitting it to be tilted to remove the product, but the shallow form makes this arrangement somewhat unstable, and an outlet at the bottom, as shown in the illustration, is commoner.

Advantages

(a) It is simple and cheap to construct.
(b) It is easy to use, clean and maintain.

Disadvantages

(a) Having only natural circulation, the overall coefficient of heat transfer will be poor and solids are likely to deposit on the surface, leading to decomposition of the product and a further deterioration in heat transfer. Also, many products give rise to foaming when boiled under conditions of natural convection.

(b) All the liquor is heated all the time, which may be unsatisfactory with thermolabile materials.

(c) The heating surface is limited and decreases proportionally as the size of the pan increases (*see* p. 153). Furthermore, the heating area will decrease as concentration of the product occurs.

(d) The pan is open, so that vapour passes to the atmosphere, which can lead to saturation of the

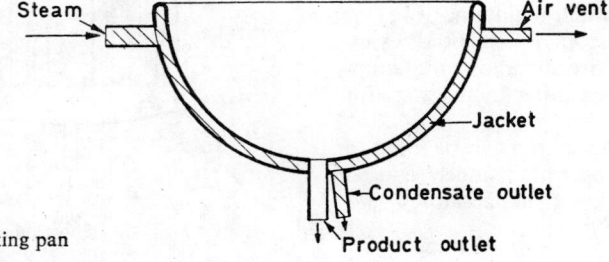

Fig. 14.1 Evaporating pan

atmosphere, slowing evaporation as well as causing discomfort. Furthermore, it limits the evaporating pan to use with aqueous liquids only. The open design means also that reduced pressure cannot be used, so that the temperature of boiling cannot be lowered.

The evaporating pan can, therefore, be used only for the concentration of aqueous and thermostable liquors, for example, extracts of liquorice. Since many pharmaceutical materials are thermolabile or dissolved in organic solvents, such as ethanol, the evaporating pan is limited in its applications.

EVAPORATING STILLS

This type of evaporator is known commonly as a still, since it is essentially a vessel similar to the evaporating pan, with a cover that connects it to a condenser, so that the liquid is distilled off.

Typical construction is shown in Fig. 14.2, although any type of condenser referred to on pages

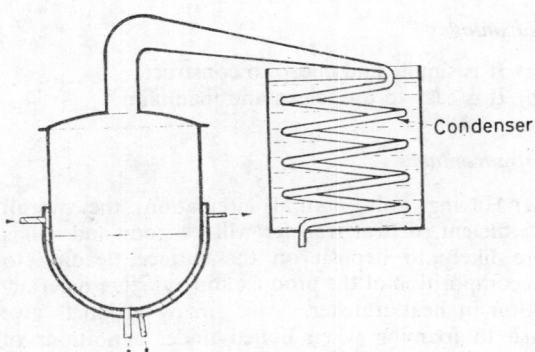

Fig. 14.2   Evaporating still

172 and 173 may be used. Often, a quick-release system of clamps which allows the cover to be removed easily for access to the interior of the vessel for cleaning or removal of product may be used.

Advantages

(a) Like the evaporating pan, it is quite simple to construct and easy to clean and maintain.

(b) The vapour is condensed, which speeds evaporation, reduces inconvenience and allows the equipment to be used for solvents other than water, for example, ethanol.

(c) A receiver and vacuum pump can be fitted to the condenser, permitting operation under reduced pressure and, hence, at lower temperatures (*see* p. 172).

Disadvantages

(a) natural convection only;
(b) all the liquor is heated all the time;
(c) the heating surface is limited.

As the advantages show, the still can be used for evaporating liquors in general, with aqueous or other solvents. Thermolabile materials can be evaporated under reduced pressure, while the easy removability of the still head makes it convenient for evaporating extracts to dryness.

The method is used widely in the pharmaceutical industry where it may be necessary to deal with small batches of a variety of materials. The technical disadvantages are outweighed by the ease with which the plant can be opened and cleaned for transference to another job.

SHORT TUBE EVAPORATOR

As the size of evaporators increases, heating by means of an external steam jacket becomes inadequate. The *short tube evaporator,* as the name implies, uses steam-heated tubes instead of surrounding the vessel by a steam jacket.

General construction and operation are illustrated in Fig. 14.3, where it is seen that the lower portion of the evaporator consists of a *nest* of tubes, with the liquor inside and the steam outside. These tubes are from 1 to 2 m in length and from 40 to 80 mm in

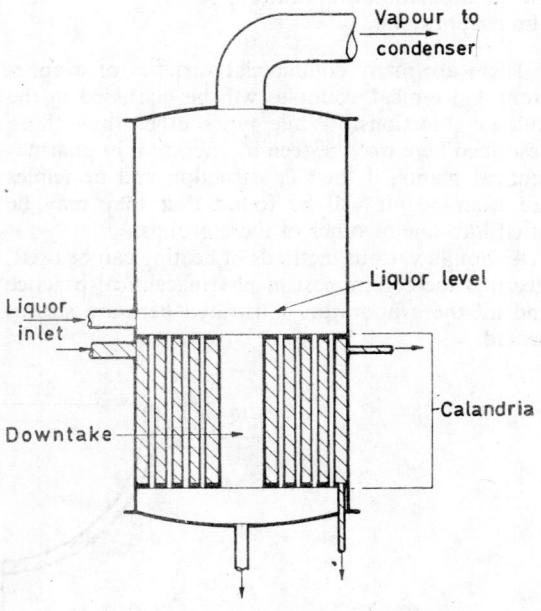

Fig. 14.3   Short tube evaporator

diameter, with the tubes up to 1000 in number in a vessel up to 2·5 m or more in diameter. This part of the evaporator is known as the *calandria*.

The liquor is maintained at a level slightly above the top of the tubes, the space above this being left for the disengagement of vapour from the boiling liquor.

In operation, the liquor in the tubes is heated by the steam and begins to boil, when the mixture of liquid and vapour will shoot up the tube in a similar manner to that of a liquid that is allowed to boil too vigorously in a test-tube.

This sets up a circulation, with boiling liquor rising up the smaller tubes of the calandria and returning down the larger central *downtake*.

Advantages

(*a*) Use of a tubular calandria increases the heating area, possibly by a factor of 10 or 15 compared with that of an external jacket.

(*b*) The vigorous circulation reduces boundary layers and keeps solids in suspension, so increasing the rate of heat transfer. As a result, overall coefficients of heat transfer are from 3 to 5 times greater than those found in evaporating pans.

(*c*) Like the still, a condenser and receiver can be attached, giving the advantages referred to under the evaporating still.

Disadvantages

(*a*) Since the evaporator is filled to a point above the level of the calandria, a considerable amount of the liquor is heated for a long time. The effect of this continual heating can be reduced to some extent by removing strong liquor slowly from the outlet at the bottom of the vessel.

(*b*) The plant is much more complicated, making it expensive to construct and increasing the difficulty of cleaning and maintenance compared with the simple still.

(*c*) The head of liquor increases pressure at the bottom of the vessel and, in large evaporators where the liquor depth may be of the order of 2 m, this may give rise to a pressure of about 0·25 bar, leading to elevation of the boiling point by 5 or 6°C. This reduces the effective temperature gradient and may affect heat-sensitive materials.

Clearly, this type of equipment will be most useful for products manufactured on a large scale, where the process can be operated continuously on one type of material. The complexity of the plant makes it much less suitable for changing from one product to another. The method can be used, for example, for extracts manufactured in large quanti-

ties, such as cascara, or for more general products, such as sugar, salt or caustic soda. It must be emphasised that the short-tube evaporator does not differ *fundamentally* from the evaporating still, since it is merely a larger vessel with a calandria instead of a jacket, to give improved heat transfer rates.

Forced Circulation Evaporators

In general, forced circulation evaporators are natural circulation evaporators with some added form of mechanical agitation; indeed, in its simplest form, an evaporating pan in which the contents are agitated by a stirring rod or pole could be described as a forced circulation evaporator.

Alternatively, a mechanically operated propeller or paddle agitator can be introduced into an evaporating pan or still, or into the downtake of a short-tube evaporator. Special forms of forced circulation evaporator can be used, a typical example being shown in Fig. 14.4.

As indicated, the liquor is circulated by means of the pump and as it is under pressure in the tubes, the boiling point is elevated and no boiling takes place. As the liquor leaves the tubes and enters the body of the evaporator there is a drop in pressure and vapour flashes off from the superheated liquor.

Compared with natural-circulation types, evaporators with forced circulation have the advantage that the rapid liquid movement improves heat transfer, especially with viscous liquids or materials that deposit solids or foam readily.

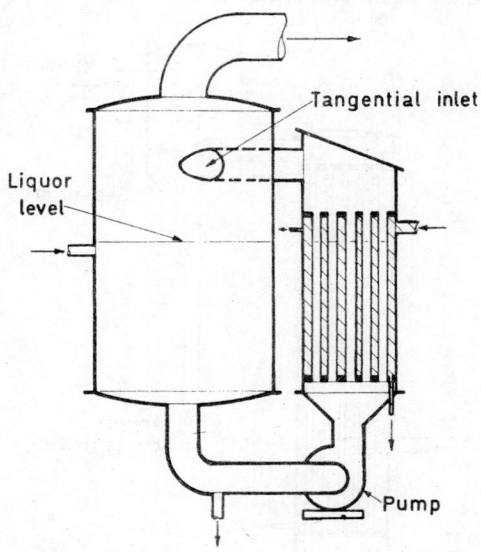

Fig. 14.4   Forced circulation evaporator

The equipment is particularly suitable for operation under reduced pressure, as the forced circulation overcomes the effect of the greater viscosity of liquids when evaporated under reduced pressure, as discussed on p. 172. This fact, together with the rapid evaporation rate, makes the method suitable for thermolabile materials; for example, it is used in practice for the concentration of insulin and liver extracts.

Film Evaporators

All the evaporators discussed above are operated by boiling the liquor in a vessel, the vapour escaping as bubbles from the bulk of the liquor. Film evaporators, as the name implies, spread the material as a film over the heated surface, and it is important to realise that this basic difference between the two groups greatly influences the rate of heat transfer (and so of evaporation) and the suitability of the method for particular purposes.

As with conventional evaporators, the film may be formed naturally or by mechanical means.

LONG-TUBE EVAPORATORS

In this type of evaporator, the heating unit consists of steam-jacketed tubes, having a length to diameter ratio of about 140 to 1, so that a large evaporator may have tubes 50 mm in diameter and about 7 m in length.

In the commonest form, illustrated in Fig. 14.5, the liquor to be evaporated is introduced into the

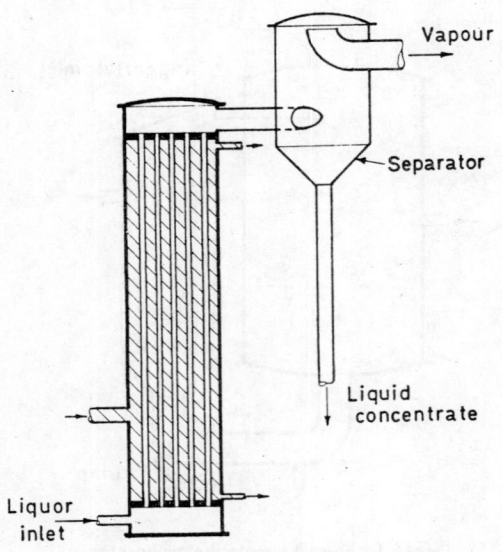

Fig. 14.5 Climbing film evaporator

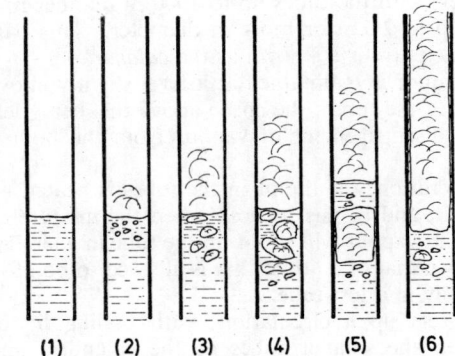

Fig. 14.6 Principles of climbing film evaporator

bottom of the tube, a film of liquid forms on the walls and rises up the tubes, hence the title *climbing film evaporator*. At the upper end, the mixture of vapour and concentrated liquor enters a separator, the vapour passing on to a condenser, and the concentrate to a receiver.

The fact that the film of liquid 'climbs' up the tube through a distance of 5 or 6 metres without mechanical assistance may seem improbable, but the explanation is as follows. The various stages from start-up are illustrated in Fig. 14.6, which represents a part of the tube about one fifth of the way from the bottom.

Cold or pre-heated liquor is introduced into the tube (1). Heat is transferred to the liquor from the walls, and boiling begins (2), increasing in vigour (3) and (4). Eventually, sufficient vapour has been formed for the smaller bubbles to unite to a large bubble, filling the width of the tube and trapping a 'slug' of liquid above the bubble (5). As more vapour is formed, the slug of liquid is blown up the tube, the tube is filled with vapour, while the liquid is spread as a film over the walls (6). This film of liquid continues to vaporise rapidly, the vapour escaping up the tube and, because of friction between the vapour and liquid, the film also is dragged up the tube. Some idea of the rate of vaporisation can be gained from the fact that the liquid film travels up the tube at velocities of the order of 6 or 7 metres/second.

It must be emphasised that this is the sole reason for the liquor travelling up the tube, and that reduced pressure, for example, does not affect this mechanism, although it is sometimes stated incorrectly that the vacuum 'draws' the liquid up the tube. While it is true that such evaporators are used commonly under reduced pressure, the climbing film evaporator will function equally well at atmospheric pressure.

Clearly, the mechanism of this process differs greatly from the evaporators discussed earlier, leading to a number of special advantages:

(a) The very high film velocity reduces boundary layers to a minimum giving improved heat transfer.

(b) The use of long narrow tubes provides large areas for heat transfer.

(c) Because of the increased efficiency of heat transfer, a small temperature difference is sufficient, with less risk of damage to thermolabile materials.

(d) The time of the contact between the liquor and the heating surface is very short. Even allowing for the pre-heating period, the total time a given portion of the liquor is in the evaporator is of the order of 20 seconds, of which about one second only is occupied in climbing the tube in the boiling film. The advantage of this method for heat-sensitive materials will be realised when this time is compared with the hours of continuous boiling the liquor may receive in other evaporators.

(e) Despite the short heating time, the evaporation rate is very high, since the film formation gives an extremely large surface area in relation to the volume of the liquid.

(f) The mixture of liquid and vapour enters the separator (usually of the cyclone type, see p. 198) at high velocity, which improves the separation efficiency and makes the method especially suitable for materials that foam.

(g) Although the tubes are very long, they are not submerged, as in the short-tube evaporator, so that there is no elevation of boiling point due to hydrostatic head.

The equipment has the disadvantage that it is expensive to manufacture and is difficult to clean and maintain. From the operational point of view the feed rate is critical. If too high, the liquor may be concentrated insufficiently, whereas if the feed rate is too low, the film cannot be maintained and dry patches may form on the tube wall.

Because of the rapid evaporation, minimum temperature gradient and short heating time, this method approaches most nearly the perfect method for pharmaceutical products. Even thermolabile materials can be processed in film evaporators and they have been used successfully for the concentration of solutions such as insulin, liver extracts, and vitamins.

An alternative form of the long-tube evaporator is the *falling film evaporator*, which resembles the climbing form but is inverted as shown in Fig. 14.7, so that the feed liquor enters over a weir at the top of the tubes and the concentrate and vapour leave from the bottom. The special advantage of this arrangement is that the movement of the liquid

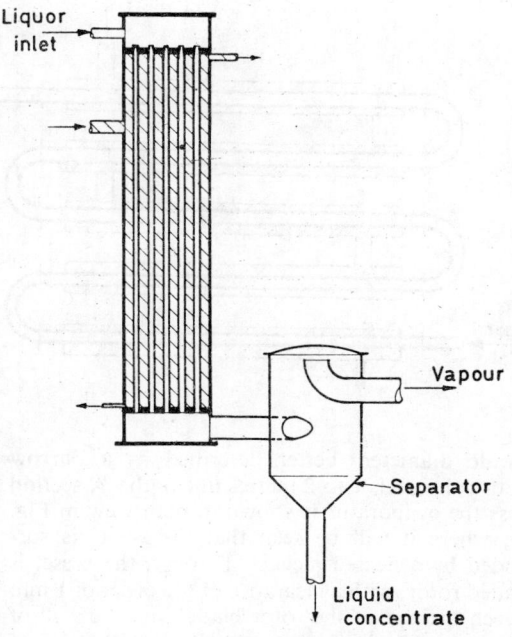

Fig. 14.7 Falling film evaporator

film is assisted by gravity, enabling more viscous liquids to be handled.

In some cases, climbing and falling film units are combined, so that the weak liquor is concentrated partially in the climbing film unit and the evaporation completed as the liquor returns down the falling film unit. The method is used where a high percentage evaporation is required and where the concentrated liquor is viscous. It can be useful also where the plant is located on one floor, since the product is returned to the same level as the starting point.

Where space is important and a small, versatile film evaporator is required to serve a similar purpose to a steam pan, the horizontal film evaporator can be useful. The arrangement is illustrated in Fig. 14.8 where it will be seen that it is, in effect, a climbing film evaporator that has been 'folded up' and occupies, therefore, a very small space, needing little head-room. Since most forms have only one tube, and the U-bends can be removed easily, it can be used safely with small batches of different materials.

WIPED FILM EVAPORATORS

A form of film evaporator coming into increasing use is the *wiped film evaporator* or *rotary film evaporator*, which consists of a single, short tube

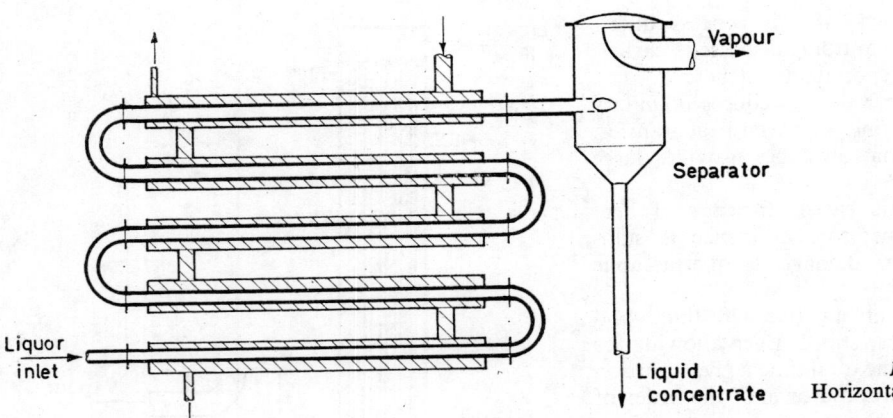

Fig. 14.8
Horizontal film evaporator

of wide diameter, better described as a narrow cylindrical vessel, 1 to 2 metres in length. A section across the evaporator is shown in plan view in Fig. 14.9, where it will be seen that the vessel is surrounded by a heated jacket. Through the vessel is a bladed rotor, with a clearance of the order of 1 mm between the tips of the rotor blades and the wall of the vessel. The liquor is introduced at the top of the vessel and is spread as a film over the heated wall by the action of the rotor. Evaporation occurs as the liquor passes down the wall, vapour is taken off to a condenser and the concentrated liquor withdrawn at the bottom of the vessel.

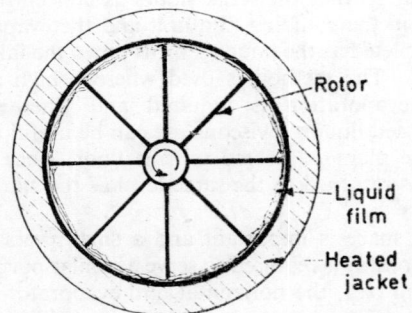

Fig. 14.9   Section through wiped film evaporator

The evaporator is, therefore, a form of single tube, falling film evaporator in which the film is formed and agitated mechanically. Because of this, good heat transfer is obtained, the method being especially useful with liquids that are too viscous to be processed in units in which the film is formed naturally.

Improvement of Efficiency of Evaporation

In theory, each part by weight of water vaporised in an evaporator will require an equal weight of

steam. In practice, more is required because of variations in specific heat and to allow for heat losses.

Modifications of the normal method will allow efficiency to be improved.

MULTIPLE EFFECT EVAPORATION

The *single effect* evaporators described previously use steam to supply heat to the liquor and provide latent heat of vaporisation. This vapour is then taken off to a condenser, where the latent heat is given up to the cooling water, which commonly then goes to waste. Recalling that the latent heat of vapour is considerable (*see* p. 156) it will be realised that a great deal of heat goes, quite literally, 'down the drain'.

In the simplest case of multiple effect evaporation, two evaporators are connected together, with piping arranged so that the calandria of the first effect is heated by steam; the vapour from the first effect is used to heat the calandria of the second effect. In other words, the calandria of the second effect is used as a condenser for the first effect, so that the latent heat of vaporisation is used to evaporate a further quantity of the liquor instead of going to waste. The vapour from the second effect is then taken to a condenser in the ordinary way. The arrangement is shown diagrammatically in Fig. 14.10.

Theoretically, any number of evaporators could be connected in this way with increasing economy, but in practice the number of effects is limited for two reasons:

1. It is necessary to have the evaporators operating at decreasing temperatures in order to provide the temperature gradients necessary for heat transfer in each effect. Thus, the first effect might operate at atmospheric pressure, so that water will boil at

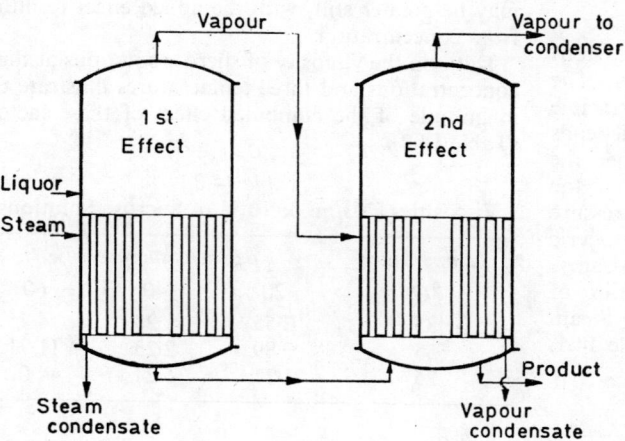

Fig. 14.10   Multiple effect evaporation

100°C. If the calandria is heated by steam at 2 bars (with a temperature of approximately 120°C) the temperature gradient will be about 20°C. The vapour from the first effect is taken to the calandria of the second effect, still at 100°C. Hence, this unit must operate at a pressure below atmospheric in order to lower the boiling point of the liquid. A pressure of 0·5 bar will lower the boiling point of water to about 80°C, again providing a temperature gradient of about 20°C.

Clearly, the result is a limitation on the number of effects that can be arranged so that each has a suitable temperature gradient.

2. The number of effects will be controlled also by the economics of the process and the relative cost of the additional effects compared with the saving of steam. In general, if fuel is expensive or the product is cheap the maximum economy is necessary and more effects will be used. If fuel is cheap, however, or the product expensive, fewer effects can be justified.

As a result of these factors, two or three effects are used commonly, quadruple effect occasionally, but rarely is this number exceeded.

VAPOUR RECOMPRESSION

When vapour recompression is used on an evaporator, some of the vapour from the process is returned to the calandria to provide heat to vaporise more of the liquor. Since the pressure will need to be increased to provide the necessary temperature gradient, the vapour is compressed by means of a pump or by the injection of a certain amount of high pressure steam. The latter method is commonest and is shown diagrammatically in Fig. 14.11. The use of a compressor is most advantageous in situations where power is cheaper than heat; for example, if hydro-electric power is available.

The use of vapour recompression allows an economy in heat to be made, and in the example illustrated in Fig. 14.11 unit mass of steam will evaporate about 1·75 times its weight of water. Compared with multiple effect, it has two advantages:

1. Evaporation can be carried out at low temperatures, whereas the earlier effects of multiple effect systems may have to operate at temperatures too high for thermolabile materials.

2. Only one evaporator unit is needed, which reduces the capital cost of the equipment.

It should be borne in mind that both multiple effect evaporation and vapour recompression can be applied to any type of enclosed evaporator. The illustrations show short-tube evaporators, but both modifications are used to great advantage with long-tube evaporators.

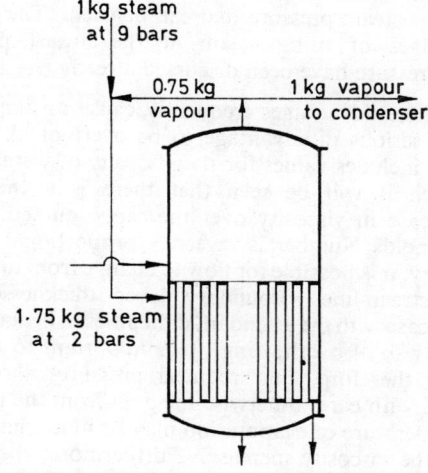

Fig. 14.11   Vapour re-compression evaporator

Evaporation under Reduced Pressure

Reference has been made on a number of occasions to the use of reduced pressure in evaporation. The application of this method is based on the principle that the vapour pressure exerted by a liquid depends on the temperature, and the liquid boils when the vapour pressure is equal to the pressure of the surrounding atmosphere. If, therefore, the pressure in an evaporator is reduced below atmospheric pressure, an aqueous liquid will boil at a temperature less than 100°C. The extent of the reduction of boiling point of water can be obtained from Steam Tables, and some values are quoted in Table 14.1.

Table 14.1

Pressure (bars)	Boiling point of water (°C)	Viscosity of water ($N s/m^2 \times 10^{-3}$)
1	100	0·28
0·7	90	0·31
0·47	80	0·35
0·31	70	0·40
0·12	50	0·54
0·10	45	0·59
0·07	40	0·65
0·03	25	0·89

Consideration of the data in Table 14.1 shows that the use of reduced pressure has three advantages:

1. Evaporation occurs at a lower temperature, with less risk of damage to heat-sensitive materials.
2. A lower operating temperature gives higher temperature gradients, without the need for excessive steam pressures.
3. The lower the operating temperature, the lower the steam pressure that can be used. The advantages of using steam at the lowest possible pressure have been discussed already (*see* p. 157).

These advantages frequently cause an important and serious disadvantage to be overlooked. Table 14.1 includes values for the viscosity of water, from which it will be seen that there is a three-fold increase in viscosity over the range quoted. Since Reynolds Number is inversely proportional to viscosity, it is possible for flow to change from turbulent to streamline. Boundary layer thicknesses will increase with the attendant difficulties in heat transfer and risk of overheating. It is important to remember, therefore, that reduced pressures should be used with care, otherwise the gain from the lowered temperature of evaporation may be more than offset by the viscosity increase. Furthermore, the values for water are quoted and the increases for solutions

may be greater still, with the added effect resulting from concentration.

Data on the viscosity of sucrose solutions at three concentrations and three temperatures illustrate the magnitude of the combined effect of these factors (Table 14.2).

Table 14.2
Viscosities ($N s/m^2 \times 10^{-3}$) of Sucrose Solutions

Temperature °C	per cent sucrose w/w		
	20	40	60
85	0·55	1·23	4·75
55	0·89	2·23	11·71
25	1·71	5·21	44·02

These figures emphasise the danger of overheating in thick boundary layers resulting from the effect of concentration on viscosity, especially at lower temperatures. The value of the long-tube evaporator will be appreciated in this situation, since rapid film movement helps to overcome the effect. The wiped film evaporator can help to reduce the controlling influence of viscosity to an even greater extent.

Vapour Condensation

All evaporators, except open evaporating pans, use condensers for removing vapour. No discussion of theory is necessary since, in principle, a condenser is identical to an evaporator with the objective reversed, that is, an evaporator uses a vapour (steam) to heat a liquid, and a condenser uses a liquid to cool a vapour.

Condensers used in practice can be divided into two main groups:

INDIRECT OR SURFACE CONDENSERS

In this type there is no direct contact between coolant and vapour, that is, the latter is condensed on to a cooled surface.

On the large scale, multi-tubular condensers are commonest and Fig. 14.12 shows the general arrangement, vapour usually being inside the tubes and cooling water outside, although these can be reversed. The special point to note is that these condensers operate by *counter-current flow*, that is, the vapour and the water move in opposite directions; the condensed liquid, as it leaves the condenser, is cooled by the entering cold water, while the water leaves immediately after meeting the entering vapour. Thus, the water carries away as much heat as possible.

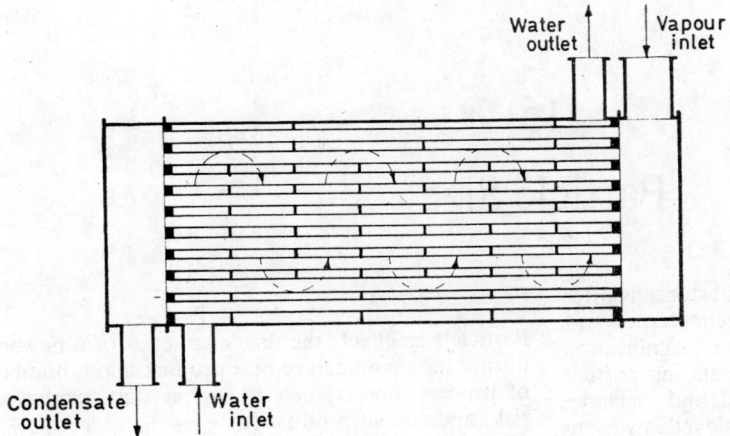

Fig. 14.12 Tubular condenser

DIRECT, CONTACT OR JET CONDENSERS

As the names imply, the vapour and cooling water are brought into direct contact, a procedure comparable with the use of live steam for heating. Since condensed vapour and water are mixed, it is applicable only to condensers for evaporators handling aqueous liquids.

The exact form of the equipment can vary considerably, but in the example shown in Fig. 14.13 the vapour enters a vessel where it is brought into contact with jets of water (hence the alternative titles of *contact* or *jet condensers*).

Condensation of the vapour lowers the pressure and so assists the reduced pressure operation of the evaporator, but vacuum pumps can be connected to the top of the vessel, as indicated.

To prevent water being drawn into the vacuum pump, the condensate/cooling water mixture escapes through the *barometric leg*. This is simply a piece of pipe of greater length than the water barometer, that is, about 10 or 11 metres, dipping into a reservoir. The vacuum pump is, therefore, unable to lift the water to the height of the condensing vessel. This length of pipe may seem inconvenient but it is very cheap and can often be located alongside the evaporator without difficulty, especially in long-tube evaporators.

In general, surface condensers are used for organic solvents in all cases and in smaller installations for dealing with aqueous liquids also. Jet condensers are used with large evaporators to condense water vapour only.

BIBLIOGRAPHY

REAVELL, B. N. and GOODWIN, G. A. (1958) Evaporation of Heat-Sensitive Materials. *Chem. and Ind.*, 1450–1458.

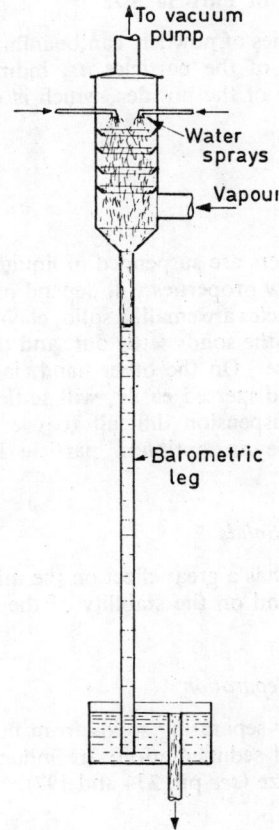

Fig. 14.13 Jet condenser

15
Particle Size

The size of the particles of a solid substance is often of considerable importance. This chapter reviews the factors that make particle size of significance, discusses the problems involved in stating particle size and the methods that can be used, and concludes by stating some of the principles employed in various methods of particle size analysis.

Significance of Particle Size

The properties of powders can be influenced directly by the size of the particles or, indirectly, by the surface area of the powder, which is dependent on the size.

SIZE

Suspensions

When powders are suspended in liquids, the behaviour and flow properties will depend on the particle size. If particles are small, a solid, clay-like sediment will form as the solids settle out, and this is difficult to re-disperse. On the other hand, large particles, although re-dispersed easily, will settle rapidly and make the suspension difficult to use. There will, therefore, be an optimum particle size for any suspension.

Mixtures of Solids

Particle size has a great effect on the mixing of solid substances and on the stability of the mixture (*see* p. 203).

Solid/Fluid Separation

Processes for separating solids from fluids, such as filtration and sedimentation, are influenced greatly by particle size (*see* pp. 234 and 197).

Granule Size in Tablets

Successful tablet manufacture requires careful control of the size of granules from which the tablets are compressed.

Process Factors

Particle size affects the flow characters of a powder during the manufacture of a product and a number of process aspects such as loss as dust, explosion risk, and cost of production.

SURFACE AREA

As particle size decreases, the surface area of the particles increases. This will be understood easily by reference to Fig. 15.1, where one cube-shaped particle is represented; when the particle is cut in two, the original surfaces remain but two new surfaces are formed. Similarly, a further cut adds two more surfaces, and so on. The same principle will apply when irregular particles are size reduced. Thus, particle size influences material properties which depend upon surface area.

Mass Transfer Processes

It has been shown (*see* p. 163) that the equation expressing mass transfer includes a term for surface area. This means that operations such as solution, extraction, and drying will be influenced indirectly by particle size.

Adsorption

From the discussion of adsorption in Chapter 4, it will be seen that it is a surface phenomenon. This means that the adsorptive capacity of a material will increase as particle size decreases.

Absorption of Drugs

A good deal of work has been done in recent years on the absorption of drugs, parenterally, orally, and externally. It will be seen in Chapter 6, where aspects of drug action are discussed, that particle size is of considerable significance.

Definition of Particle Size

It is important to consider the meaning and the significance of the term 'particle size'. In practice,

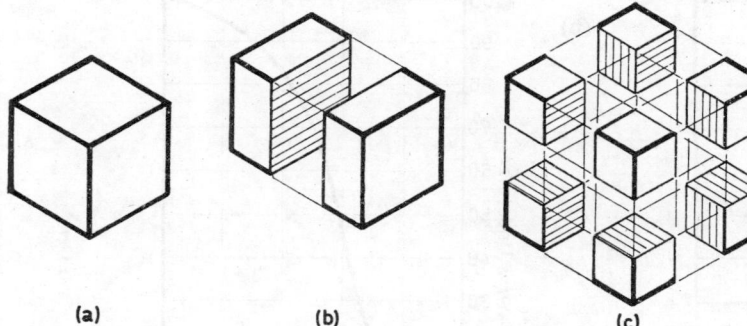

(a)   **(b)**   **(c)**

Fig. 15.1 Surface area of cut cube

Relative surface areas: (*a*) 6A, (*b*) 8A, (*c*) 12A

a large consignment of a powder may be supplied, with the statement that it has a mean particle size of 20 μm. While this indicates one fact clearly—that the material consists of a fine powder and not large pieces—it must be remembered that the statement attempts to characterise a very large number of *irregular, three-dimensional* objects in terms of *one linear* dimension. By analogy, one might state that the average size of a building in the United Kingdom is *x* metres, but the information this provides is very limited. Clearly, the statement of a powder as one linear dimension can be strictly true only if the particles are spherical and are all of the same diameter, which is extremely unlikely in practice.

Referring again to the analogy, the dimension of the buildings could be based on a character of special significance for a particular situation, for example, the concern may be with low-flying aircraft, when height is the important consideration; if working space is needed, then the dimension could be derived from floor area or, if storage space is of interest, it could be based on the volume of the building.

Similarly, particle dimensions can be derived from various characters; for example, a diameter may be expressed in terms of weights, volumes, surface areas, projected areas or sedimentation velocities of particles. This means, therefore, that the 'particle size' quoted is the diameter of a sphere equivalent to the particle in weight, volume, surface area, projected area or sedimentation velocity.

The method of stating the diameter will depend on two factors:

1. The form of the data from the test procedure used; for example, sieving gives weights, permeability methods depend on surface areas, and sedimentation velocities are given by sedimentation methods.

2. The purpose for which the powder is to be used; if it is to be used for adsorption the surface mean diameter is most useful, while if it is to be used in a suspension the Stokes diameter (derived from sedimentation velocity) is more satisfactory.

In addition to the various particle characters on which the particle size can be based, a number of different statistical means can be used to weight the data for particular purposes. A detailed discussion of these is outside the scope of this book, but, as well as the usual arithmetic mean, geometric or harmonic means can be used or the median diameter (the diameter for which 50 per cent of the particles are less than the stated size: *see* Fig. 15.2(*a*)) or the mode diameter (the size occurring with the greatest frequency: *see* Fig. 15.2(*c*)). Further information is obtainable in specialist texts on this subject, but the conclusion to be borne in mind is that the same powder tested by different methods or the result stated by different statistical methods can yield values over a considerable range.

Particle Size Distribution

In many circumstances a knowledge of the distribution of sizes is more important than the mean. The reason for this will be apparent if it is recalled that the volume of a sphere is proportional to the cube of the diameter. Hence, one particle 100 μm in diameter will have the same volume as 1000 particles 10 μm in diameter, and 1 000 000 particles of 1 μm diameter.

Some means is needed, therefore, of expressing the range of the particle size in the group and the distribution of the sizes within the range. This may be done in various ways by statistical methods, such as standard deviations, but the reader is referred again to books on statistics.

The simplest method is graphical and Fig. 15.2 illustrates several forms in which data from a particle size analysis can be presented. The test will yield a series of fractions of various size ranges which can be plotted as cumulative curves. They may be

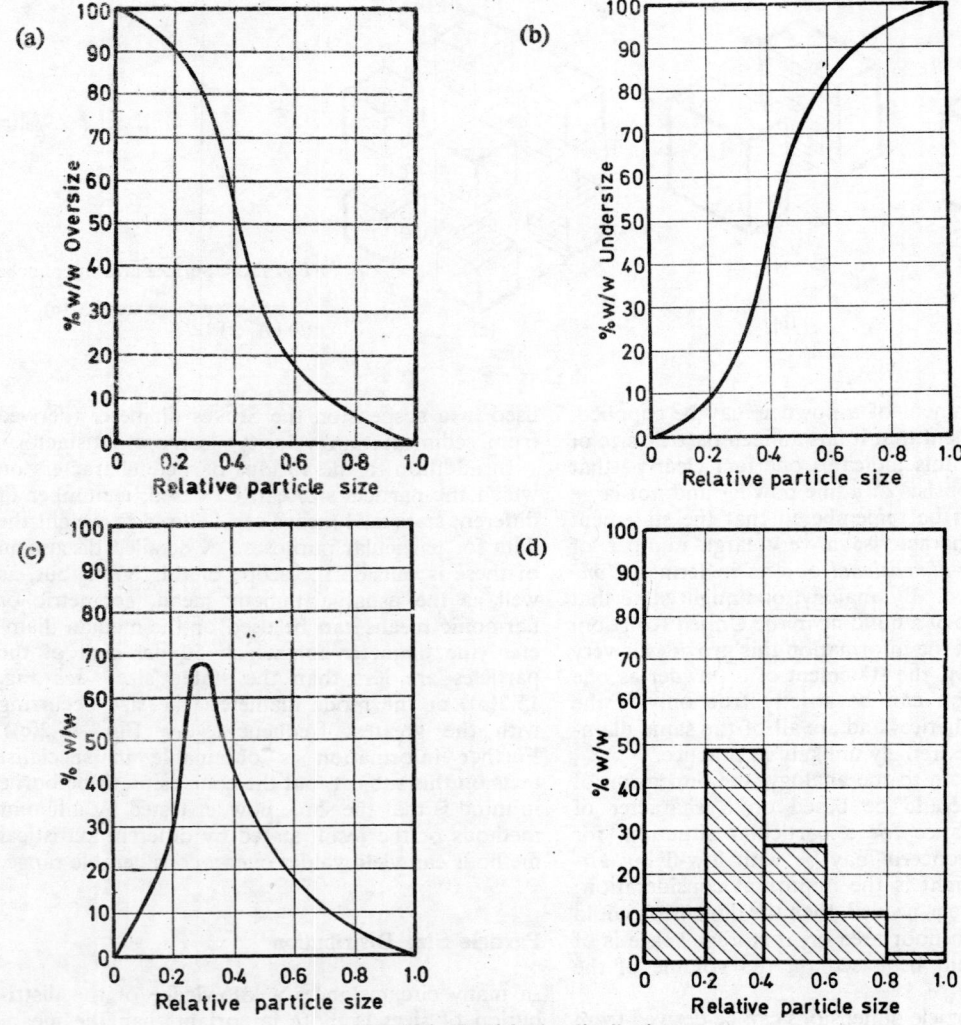

Fig. 15.2   Particle size distribution curves

(*a*) oversize, (*b*) undersize, (*c*) distribution, (*d*) histogram

oversize, as in Fig. 15.2(*a*), to represent all particles larger than the specified size, or *undersize* as in Fig. 15.2(*b*), which is the converse.

Alternatively, the graph can show the frequency with which each size occurs, that is, the data are plotted as a distribution curve of the type illustrated in Fig. 15.2(*c*). If the test yields insufficient fractions to plot a smooth curve with confidence, a histogram may be used, as in Fig. 15.2(*d*), which indicates the limitations of the data, for example, to show that a certain percentage of the powder lies between two sizes, but that the size distribution between these limits is unknown.

Particle Size Analysis

The methods used for analysing particle size are numerous and various in principle. This great variety arises from endeavours to find solutions to the problem, discussed previously, of expressing the 'size' of an irregular, three-dimensional particle in terms of one linear dimension.

Although there is no upper limit to the size of particles, the discussion will be confined to 'powders' as defined in B.S.2955, that is, with a particle size of less than 1000 micrometres.

It is essential that the test should be carried out

on a sample representative of the whole. Generally, it is not sufficient to remove a small amount from the top of a container, since segregation may have occurred during transport. Preliminary mixing of the contents can be of assistance, but special sampling techniques are available. Furthermore, it must be remembered that one container may not be typical of an entire batch. In some cases, a manufacturing batch may fill many containers and segregation may occur during filling. Again, statistical methods can be used but are outside the scope of this book. This chapter refers only to the general principles underlying the various processes. Where official methods and standards apply to powders, these are discussed in the chapter on Size Separation.

Sieving

In the sieving process the powder is passed over a perforated screen, so that particles sufficiently small will pass through, while those that are oversize will be retained on the sieve.

Sieving is, therefore, a simple 'go/no go' test which divides the powder into two fractions above and below a specified size. To obtain a distribution of particle size it is necessary to carry out a series of tests with sieves of different sizes, although these can be performed simultaneously by using a nest of sieves; that is, a number of sieves that fit into each other in a tier. The coarsest sieve is placed on top so that the powder is passed successively over finer sieves and a series of fractions obtained.

Sieves may consist of a mesh made from wire, or other material such as nylon, or a plate perforated with holes. Test sieves used for particle size analysis are normally of the wire mesh type.

Sieving is the normal method for larger particle sizes, but is limited by the smallest size of sieves that can be produced. In practice, this is the size referred to as 300 mesh (the standard for sieves is based on the number of meshes in a length of 25·4 mm) which means that the mesh opening is of the order of 50 micrometres.

It is difficult to obtain accurate results from a sieve analysis for a number of reasons:

1. Particles can be attracted electrostatically to form aggregates that will not pass through the mesh, although the individual particles would do so.

2. Humidity can affect particles of hygroscopic materials and lead to aggregation.

3. Particle shape has a very great influence, since only a sphere requires no special orientation to pass through the mesh. Clearly, then, the further a particle departs from the spherical shape the greater the difficulty it will have in passing through the aperture. Typical extreme cases will be plate-like particles where the breadth of the plate is similar to the diagonal of the mesh, or long fibrous particles where the cross-section is similar to the area of the mesh. In both cases the particles must be tilted into an upright position to pass the mesh.

From this it will be concluded that a sieve will classify a particle as less than the dimension of the mesh, provided that the particle is less than the mesh size in *one plane* and that the sifting process is carried on for sufficient time for the particle to become suitably orientated to the mesh opening.

4. The sieving process is affected considerably by the particle size distribution, since particles that are well below the mesh size will pass through easily, while those that are greatly oversize will not block the meshes. Experiment has shown that particles that are more than 0·75 of the mesh opening tend to obstruct the mesh while becoming aligned in order to pass through. Similarly, particles up to 1·5 times the mesh size attempt to pass the mesh, but are unable to do so and block the aperture.

5. Linked with the previous factors is the shape of the aperture. Generally, wire mesh sieves have square apertures, but rectangular shapes can be used. Perforated sieves commonly have circular openings, but, again, squares or rectangles are used occasionally or even special forms such as herring-bone slots.

6. It is necessary to cause some disturbance of the bed of particles to allow sieving to occur and this affects the way in which material passes through the meshes. Shaking or vibration are typical examples, but the methods are referred to in more detail on page 196.

7. Standardisation of technique is essential if sieving is used as a method of particle size analysis, especially with regard to the end point, since it is virtually impossible to sieve to completion. This is especially true if the particles are irregular in shape or in a close size range. Various end points can be used; for example, to use a standard time or to continue the process until the weight of powder passing through the sieve in unit time is less than a certain proportion of the original sample or of the oversize powder left on the sieve.

In any case, it should be borne in mind that prolonged sieving is likely to lead to the formation of some fine particles by attrition of the coarser particles between each other and against the sieve.

Results of sieve analyses are best presented in the form of a cumulative oversize curve or as a histogram, since the size ranges are usually too wide to plot a size distribution curve. A convenient method is to use *semi-log* graph paper, whereby the particle size is on the logarithmic scale and the proportion of material passing through is plotted on the arithmetic scale. A typical design is shown in Fig. 15.3, which illustrates a form of graph paper that can be obtained, with the appropriate ranges, sieve sizes and particle sizes printed in.

Fluid Classification Methods

A number of size analysis methods for powders in the sub-sieve range depend on the movement of the particles in a fluid.

The behaviour of a sphere in a fluid can be expressed by Stokes's law (p. 75).

It is essential to realise that this law applies to a single spherical particle falling under streamline flow conditions in a stagnant fluid and, in practice, a powder suspended in a fluid will consist of a large number of irregular particles of variable size. Furthermore, effects can arise from eddy currents in the fluid, rotation of the particle, Brownian movement or from electrical charges leading to aggregation of particles. Nevertheless, Stokes's law is adequate to give an estimate of the particle size.

In any one set of circumstances, the density of the solid and the density and viscosity of the fluid will be constant, so that the important conclusion from Stokes's law is that the terminal velocity of any particle is proportional to the *square* of the diameter of the particle.

If the flow conditions are turbulent, however, Newton's law applies; this is similar to Stokes's law except that the viscosity of the fluid no longer has influence. The important difference is that the rate of fall is proportional to the *square root* of the particle diameter.

Although all methods depend on Stokes's law for the interpretation of the results, there are many ways of determining the settling velocity. All use a sampling technique, whereby the concentration of particles at a particular level can be observed. This is compared with the starting concentration and the settling velocity determined.

Methods that can be used may be *cumulative*; that is, measure the total amount of material that has settled out since the beginning of the test, or *incremental*, when the amount of material that has sedimented in a particular time increment can be determined.

CUMULATIVE METHOD

A suitable method of the cumulative type is the sedimentation balance in which the bottom of the settling column consists of a balance pan. Hence the weight of the material that settles out can be determined.

INCREMENTAL METHODS

The methods in this category are numerous and varied, including:

Pipette Sampling

A sample of the suspension is removed from a known depth below the surface by means of a pipette, and the solids determined, usually gravimetrically.

Hydrometer Methods

As the solid settles out, the density of the suspension decreases. This can be observed by means of a special hydrometer or by the use of *divers*. These are small floats of suitable density which sink as the density of the suspension changes.

Pressure Methods

A sensitive manometer is attached to the side of the settling column at a known distance below the surface. As the solids settle past that point, the density of the column changes and shows as a decrease in the manometer reading.

Turbidimetric Methods

If a beam of light is passed through the suspension, some of the light will be scattered by reflection from the surface of the particles.

The amount of light transmitted through the suspension can be measured by means of a photoelectric cell and a galvanometer. Hence, the change in galvanometer reading is indicative of the light absorbed and this, in turn, is related to the surface area of the particles. As the settling time and distance are known, the particle size can be determined. The method has the special advantage that the suspension is not disturbed in any way, as it is, for example, in pipette sampling or hydrometer methods.

Centrifugal Methods

When particles are very small, normal sedimentation methods are very slow and factors such as Brownian movement interfere with the results. This can be overcome by applying the same basic principles, but utilising centrifugal force instead of gravitational force, when settling velocities can be increased greatly. Thus, a particle of quartz, 0·5 micrometres in diameter, will take approximately 250 kiloseconds to fall through a distance of 50 millimetres in water, under the influence of gravity. The same particle, under centrifugal force at a

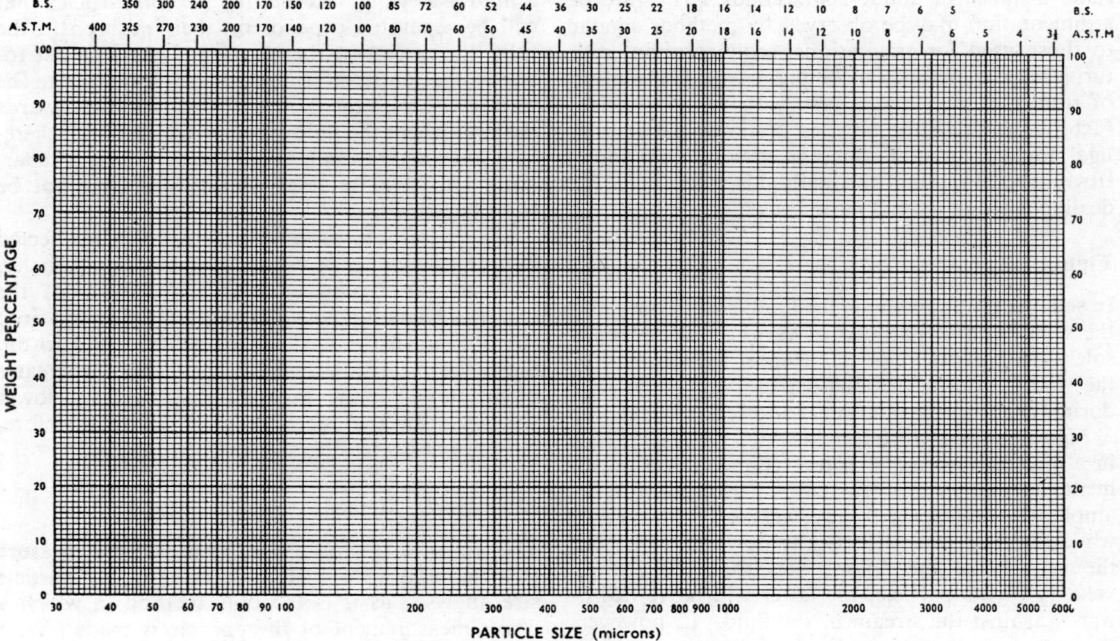

Fig. 15.3   Sieve analysis

(Courtesy Endecotts (Test Sieves) Ltd.)

rotational frequency of 70 s^{-1} will move through the same distance in about 200 seconds. The rate of sedimentation may be observed by methods similar to those used for gravitational sedimentation, with turbidimetric methods to be preferred. Calculation of results is by Stokes's law, with an appropriate factor to indicate the number of times the centrifugal force is greater than the gravitational force. It will be realized that the method is most useful for dealing with very small particles.

Elutriation

In sedimentation methods the fluid is stationary and the separation of particles of various sizes depends solely on particle velocity. Hence, the division of the particles into fractions depends upon the *time* during which sedimentation is allowed to occur.

Elutriation is a procedure in which the fluid moves in a direction opposite to the sedimentation movement, so that in the gravitational process, for example, the particles will move vertically downwards while the fluid travels vertically upwards. If, then, the velocity of the fluid is less than the settling velocity of the particle, the latter will move downwards against the stream of the fluid. If, however, the reverse applies, the settling velocity of the particle will be insufficient to overcome the velocity of the fluid, and the particle will be carried upwards.

In this case, the separation depends on the *velocity* of the fluid and is independent of time.

Elutriation and sedimentation are compared in Fig. 15.4 where the arrows are vectors, that is, they show the direction and the magnitude of the movement.

This figure suggests that if particles are suspended in a fluid moving up a column there will be a clear cut into two fractions of particle size. In practice this is not so since, as is shown in Chapter 11, there is a distribution of velocities across the tube in which a fluid is flowing. Hence, the size of particles that will be separated depends on their position in the tube, the largest in the centre and the smallest towards the outside. In practice, particles can be seen to rise with the fluid and then to move towards the wall where the fluid velocity is lower and, therefore, they start to fall. Thus, there will be a separation into two fractions, but the cut will not be sharply defined.

Separation into several fractions may be effected by using a number of vessels of increasing diameter, with the suspension entering the bottom of the narrowest column, overflowing from the top into the bottom of the next widest column, and so on. Since the mass flow remains the same, the greater diameter will cause the fluid to flow at a lower velocity. As the tubes become wider, therefore, particles of decreasing size will be separated.

Microscopic Methods

The use of a microscope to examine and measure particles is a very effective procedure for particle size analysis, as it is the only method in which a direct measurement of the particle is made. With optical microscopes there is a theoretical limit of resolution, making the smallest measurable particle size about 0·2 micrometres, but in practice the limit of measurement is nearer 1 micrometre. Greatest accuracy of measurement can be obtained with an *image-shearing eyepiece*, that is, a special eyepiece by means of which a second image, which can be moved until its left-hand edge just touches the right-hand edge of the first image, can be obtained. The extent of the movement can be read from a setting head on the eyepiece.

Smaller particles can be measured by use of the electron microscope, when the lower limit is of the order of 0·01 micrometres.

Despite the advantage of direct measurement, microscopic methods have a number of disadvantages:

Shape

Again, it is necessary to decide on one linear dimension to represent the particle and, usually, it is preferable to estimate the diameter of a circle of the same area as the projected area of the particle.

Particle Position

A particle will assume the position of maximum stability on the microscope slide. This means that particles that are laminar or plate-like in shape will

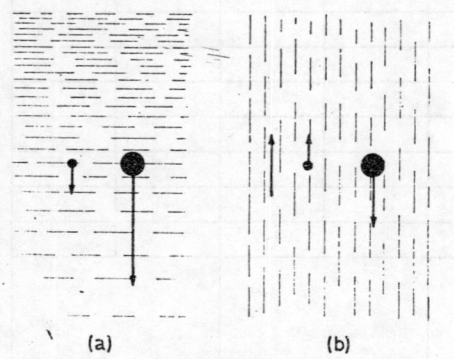

(a)   (b)

Fig. 15.4 Comparison of
(a) sedimentation, and (b) elutriation

appear to be considerably larger than they would be if tested by other methods.

Aggregation

If particles aggregate on the slide, anomalous results will be obtained, the effect being greater than it is with other methods.

Speed of Method

The method is very slow, since large numbers of particles must be measured and many fields examined in order to obtain reliable results.

Sampling

A further effect of measuring a relatively small number of particles is that special sampling techniques must be used and, like the counting and measuring procedures, must be rigidly standardised to ensure that the few particles measured are typical of the bulk.

It will be realised, therefore, that the microscopic method demands considerable skill and care. Automatic scanning procedures which increase the speed and reliability are available.

Surface Methods

Under certain circumstances a powder will adsorb a mono-molecular layer of a liquid or a gas. This can be measured to give a value for the surface area of the powder and this, in turn, will give a mean particle size. The methods are considered in Chapter 4, but will not be pursued further in this context as they are capable of giving mean values only.

Permeability Methods

If a fluid is caused to flow through a packed bed of particulate solids, the rate of flow will be described by Darcy's law as discussed in Chapter 20. Among the factors that control the rate of flow is the permeability of the bed, which depends on the particle size. Measurement of the flow rate of the fluid enables a mean particle size to be calculated but, as the method does not yield information on the size distribution, it will not be considered further.

Conductivity Methods

One of the more recent particle size analysis procedures to be developed is the *Coulter Counter* in which the particles are suspended in an electrically conductive fluid. The suspension flows through a suitable aperture with an immersed electrode on either side and the particle concentration is arranged so that only one particle travels through the aperture at a time (Fig. 15.5).

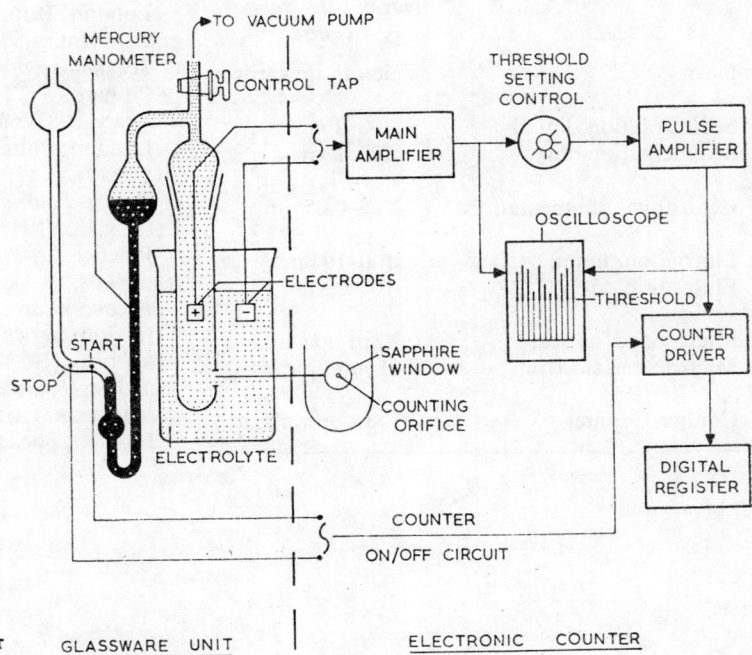

Fig. 15.5 Diagram of Coulter Counter

As the particle passes through the aperture, some electrolyte is displaced and changes the resistance between the electrodes which causes a pulse in the voltage. The magnitude of the pulse will be proportional to the volume of the particle. This is a unique feature of the Coulter Counter, since it is the only method that measures a property having a direct relationship to the *volume* of the particle. The changes in voltage are amplified and impulses above a predetermined threshold value are counted, so that the recorder provides a count of the number of particles over a certain size. The process is repeated with different threshold values, the Coulter Counter carrying out counts of particles which are oversize to a series of pre-determined values.

The method possesses a number of special advantages:

(*a*) The results are expressed in terms of particle volume from which it is a simple matter to calculate the diameter of the sphere of equivalent volume.

(*b*) The instrument can operate with particles between 0·5 and 1000 micrometres.

(*c*) Operation is very rapid, a single count usually taking less than 30 seconds and a ten-point size distribution determination occupying only about 600 seconds.

Table 15.1
Summary of Particle Size Analysis Methods

Method	Normal size range (μm)
Sieving	50 μm upwards
Sedimentation, liquid	200–2 μm
Sedimentation, air	100–1 μm
Centrifugal sedimentation	5–0·05 μm
Elutriation, liquid	100–10 μm
Elutriation, air	100–2 μm
Microscope, optical	0·2 μm upwards
Microscope, electron	0·01 μm upwards
Coulter Counter	0·5 μm upwards

(*d*) Since a large number of particles are counted, the results are more reliable than the data obtained from many other methods.

(*e*) The operational simplicity of the method reduces operator variables, enabling reproducible results to be obtained.

The principal disadvantage is that the material must be suspended in an electrolytic liquid, but non-aqueous electrolytes are available for water-soluble materials. Also, care must be taken to avoid dispersion or flocculation effects on the particles. Nevertheless, it is probably the best method for pharmaceutical powders.

BIBLIOGRAPHY

BRITISH STANDARD 410 (1962) with amendments. *Test Sieves*. London, British Standards Institution.

BRITISH STANDARD 1796 (1952) *Methods for the Use of British Standard Fine-Mesh Test Sieves*. London, British Standards Institution.

BRITISH STANDARD 2955 (1958) with amendment. *Glossary of Terms Relating to Powders*. London, British Standards Institution.

BRITISH STANDARD 3406 *Methods for the Determination of Particle Size of Powders*. *Part I (1961) Sub-division of Gross Sample down to 0·2 ml. Part II (1963) Liquid Sedimentation Methods. Part III (1963) Air Elutriation Methods. Part IV (1963) Optical Microscope Methods*. London, British Standards Institution.

DALLA VALLE, J. M. (1948) *Micro-meritics; the Technology of Fine Particles*, 2nd ed. New York, Pitman.

HERDAN, G. (1960) *Small Particle Statistics*. 2nd ed. London, Butterworth.

HEYWOOD, H. (1963) The Evaluation of Powders. *J. Pharm. Pharmac.*, **15**, 56T–74T.

LEES, K. A. (1963) Fine Particles in Pharmaceutical Practice. *J. Pharm. Pharmac.*, **15**, 43T–55T.

RICHARDS, J. C. (Ed.) (1966) *The Storage and Recovery of Particulate Solids*. London, The Institution of Chemical Engineers.

ROSE, H. E. (1953) *The Measurement of Particle Size in Very Fine Powders*. London, Constable.

SCI MONOGRAPH NO. 14 (1961) *Powders in Industry*. London, Society of Chemical Industry.

16

Size Reduction

THE term *size reduction* is largely self explanatory, but a suitable description of this unit operation is the reduction of materials to smaller pieces, to coarse particles, or to powder. The reason for including in the definition three terms suggesting different degrees of size reduction will be apparent when the various methods of attaining these objects are considered.

An alternative name for the operation is *comminution*, derived from the Latin *minuere*, meaning less, but size reduction is to be preferred as a more straightforward title.

The chapter considers the objectives of size reduction, the factors that affect the process, the mechanism of size reduction, typical examples of equipment used in pharmaceutical practice, and a discussion of the factors governing the selection of a method for a particular material and purpose.

Objectives of Size Reduction

The significance of particle size has been discussed in Chapter 15, hence it will be clear that the function of size reduction may simply be to produce smaller particles (for example, in the preparation of suspensions or to facilitate the mixing of powders) or to increase surface area (for example, to increase adsorptive properties or mass transfer coefficients).

Size reduction may, however, have special functions, as in drugs that are crushed to expose cells prior to extraction. Another example is where it is desired to reduce the bulk of a material, since shipping charges may be based on volume. 'Even-ised' cascara is an example where the volume occupied is less than the hollow quills of the whole drug.

Factors Affecting Size Reduction

The operation of size reduction is well standardised in many industries; for example, flour, cement, and coal. The pharmaceutical industry, however, uses a great variety of materials, including chemical substances, animal tissues, and vegetable drugs. The last-named may be hard (such as seeds), fibrous (barks or roots) or spongy (peels, for example); hence, the methods of size reduction are numerous, and selection of the appropriate method involves consideration of the material properties that may influence the process.

The properties that can affect size reduction include:

HARDNESS

It is important to understand that *hardness* is a *surface* property of the material, although it is frequently confused with a property that could be better described as strength. Thus, it is possible for a material to be very hard, but if it is brittle also, then size reduction may present no special problems.

In connection with size reduction, an arbitrary scale of hardness has been devised. Known as *Moh's Scale*, a series of mineral substances has been given hardness numbers between 1 and 10, ranging from graphite to diamond. Up to 3 are known as *soft* and can be marked with the finger nail. Above 7 are *hard* and cannot be marked with a good pen-knife blade, while those between are described as *intermediate*.

In general, the harder the material the more difficult it is to reduce in size, although this is linked with the next property.

TOUGHNESS

A property that can best be described as *toughness* is often more important than hardness, so that a soft but tough material may present more problems in size reduction than a hard but brittle substance; compare, for example the ease with which a stick of blackboard chalk can be broken and the difficulty of attempting to break a rubber.

Toughness is encountered in many pharmaceutical materials, particularly in fibrous drugs, and is often related to moisture content. In this connection, compare the toughness of a 'green' twig with the brittleness of a dry one.

For special cases, toughness can be reduced by treating the material with a liquefied gas such as liquid nitrogen. By this means, substances can be cooled to temperatures lower than -100 to $-150°C$, when even rubber becomes brittle and will break like glass. The method has additional advantages, in that there is a reduction in the decomposition of thermolabile materials, in the loss of volatile materials, in the oxidation of constituents, and in the risk of explosion. In practice, the procedure is little used, partially due to the cost, but also due to engineering problems; for example, the metals of the machinery also become brittle at such low temperatures, and normal lubricants solidify.

ABRASIVENESS

In general, *abrasiveness* is a property of hard materials, particularly those of mineral origin, and may limit the type of machinery that can be used. It has been reported that during the grinding of some very abrasive substances the final powder has become contaminated with more than 0.1 per cent of metal worn from the grinding mill.

STICKINESS

Although an unscientific term, *stickiness* is self-explanatory. It is a property that may cause considerable difficulty in size reduction, for material may adhere to the grinding surfaces, or the meshes of screens may become choked. Pharmaceutical substances that are gummy or resinous may be troublesome, particularly if the methods used for size reduction generate heat. Complete dryness may help, and the addition of inert substances may sometimes be of assistance. Manufacturers tend to be reticent about any inert substances they may employ, but the addition of kaolin to sulphur and to DDT has been quoted, and the results were stated to be advantageous.

The reverse of this property, which can be described as *slipperiness*, for want of a better term, can also give rise to size reduction difficulties, since the material acts as a lubricant and lowers the efficiency of the grinding surfaces.

SOFTENING TEMPERATURE

Many of the size reduction processes result in the generation of heat, which may cause some substances to soften, and the temperature at which this occurs can be important. Waxy substances, such as stearic acid, or drugs containing oils or fats are examples that may be affected. With some methods it may be possible to cool the mill, either by a water jacket or by passing a stream of air through the equipment. Another alternative is to use liquid nitrogen, as discussed above.

MATERIAL STRUCTURE

Some substances are homogeneous in character, but the majority show some special structure; for example, mineral substances may have lines of weakness along which the material splits to form flake-like particles, while vegetable drugs have a cellular structure often leading to long fibrous particles.

MOISTURE CONTENT

Moisture content has an important influence on a number of the properties that affect size reduction; for example, hardness, toughness or stickiness. In general, materials should be dry or wet and not merely damp. Usually, less than 5 per cent of moisture is suitable if the substance is to be ground dry, or more than 50 per cent if it is being subjected to wet grinding (*see* p. 190).

PHYSIOLOGICAL EFFECT

Some substances are very potent (e.g. podophyllum resin or hormone drugs) and small amounts of dust may have an effect on the operators. In such cases, enclosed mills must be used to avoid dust; special air extraction systems are desirable, and wet grinding also, if possible, as it eliminates the problem entirely.

PURITY REQUIRED

Certain types of size reduction apparatus cause the grinding surfaces to wear, and such methods must be avoided if a high degree of purity of product is needed. Similarly, some machines will be unsuitable if cleaning between batches of different materials is difficult.

RATIO OF FEED SIZE TO PRODUCT SIZE

Generally speaking, machines that produce a fine product require a fairly small feed size. Thus, it may be necessary to carry out the size reduction process in several stages with different equipment; for example, preliminary crushing, followed by coarse grinding and then fine grinding.

BULK DENSITY

The capacities of most batch mills depend on volume, whereas processes usually demand solid materials by weight. Hence, all other factors being equal, the output of the machine is related to the bulk density of the substance.

Energy Requirements of the Size Reduction Process

Only a very small amount of the energy put into a machine actually effects size reduction. This has been estimated at 2 per cent at the most, the remainder being lost in many ways, including deformation of particles without fracture, deformation of particles to produce fracture, distortion of the machine, friction between particles, friction in the machine, heat, vibration, and noise.

A number of theories have been advanced to predict the energy requirements of a size reduction process, but none gives accurate results. Best known are Rittinger's law which states that the energy used is proportional to the new surface area produced, and Kick's law which proposes that the energy used is proportional to the ratio of the initial and the final particle diameters. Later theories combine both these laws and incorporate a *work index* to take account of the variation in the properties of the material to be size reduced and the size reduction method.

Mechanisms of Size Reduction

There are four main methods of effecting size reduction, involving different mechanisms:

Cutting. As the name implies, the material is cut by means of a sharp blade or blades.

Compression. In this method, the material is crushed by application of pressure.

Impact. Impact occurs when the material is more or less stationary and is hit by an object moving at high speed or when the moving particle strikes a stationary surface. In either case, the material shatters to smaller pieces. Usually both will take place, since the substance is hit by a moving hammer and the particles formed are then thrown against the casing of the machine.

Attrition. In attrition, the material is subjected to pressure as in compression, but the surfaces are moving relative to each other, resulting in shear forces which break the particles.

The four mechanisms are shown diagrammatically in Fig. 16.1 and examples are given of everyday items that illustrate the use of such forces.

METHODS OF SIZE REDUCTION

Cutting and compression have limited uses in pharmaceutical practice, but will be illustrated by one example of each Impact and attrition are used much more widely, both separately and in combination, and there is a great variety in each type. The term *mill* is used normally for machines for size reduction. It should be appreciated that many forms, other than those described, are in use but these will be found to fit into one or other of the classifications.

Cutting

On the small scale, size reduction by cutting can be effected by a knife or by a *root cutter* which is a simple form of guillotine.

On a large scale a *cutter mill* is used.

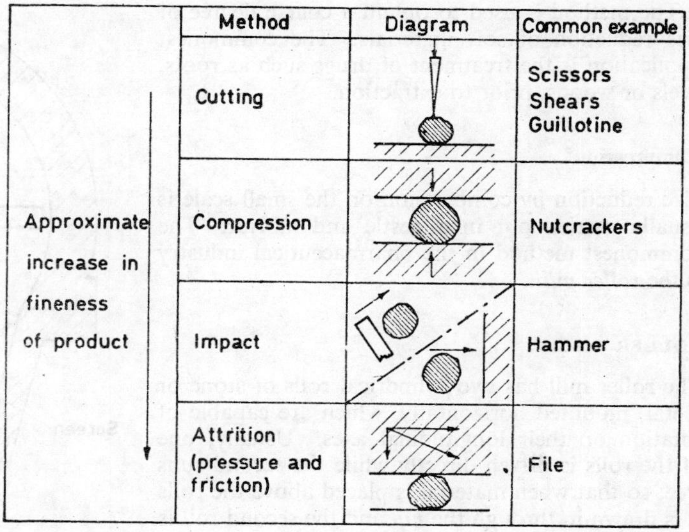

	Method	Diagram	Common example
Approximate increase in fineness of product	Cutting		Scissors Shears Guillotine
	Compression		Nutcrackers
	Impact		Hammer
	Attrition (pressure and friction)		File

Fig. 16.1 Mechanisms of size reduction

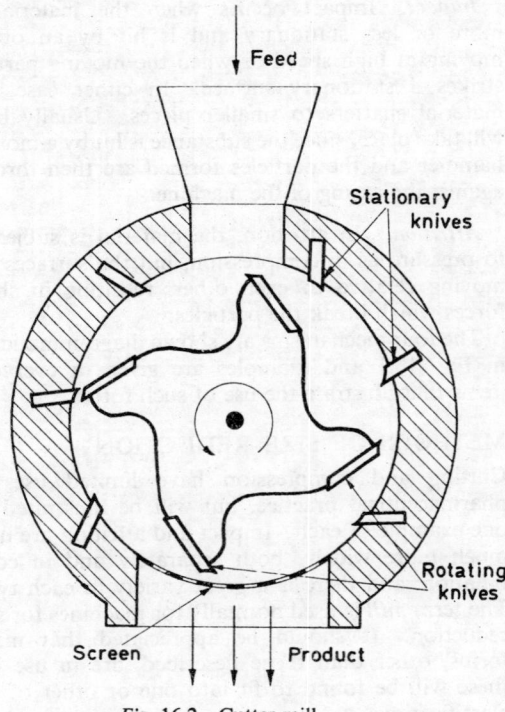

Fig. 16.2   Cutter mill

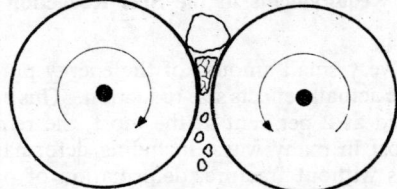

Fig. 16.3   Roller mill

CUTTER MILL

As illustrated in Fig. 16.2, knives are attached to a rotor and act against stationary knives in the casing. The lower part consists of a screen, so that material is retained in the mill until a sufficient degree of size reduction has been effected.

The method is used to obtain a coarse degree of size reduction of soft materials. The commonest application is the treatment of drugs such as roots, peels or woods, prior to extraction.

Compression

Size reduction by compression on the small scale is usually carried out in a pestle and mortar. The commonest method in the pharmaceutical industry is the *roller mill*.

ROLLER MILL

The roller mill has two cylindrical rolls of stone or metal, mounted horizontally, which are capable of rotation on their longitudinal axes. Usually, one of the rolls is driven directly while the second runs free, so that when material is placed above the rolls it is drawn in through the *nip* and the second roll is

rotated by friction. The rolls may be from a few centimetres up to a metre or more in diameter and the gap between the rolls can be adjusted to control the degree of size reduction. The principle of operation is shown diagrammatically in Fig. 16.3.

The roller mill is used for crushing, such as cracking seeds prior to extraction of fixed oils, or bruising soft tissues (often after cutting) to aid solvent penetration in extraction.

This form of the roller mill should not be confused with the type used for milling ointments (*see* p. 187) where both rolls are driven, but at different speeds, so that size reduction is by attrition.

Impact

There is no 'hand' method of effecting size reduction by impact, apart from the shattering of brittle substances with a hammer or with a pestle and mortar. Laboratory equipment takes the form of miniature versions of industrial-scale machines.

HAMMER MILL

As shown in Fig. 16.4, the *hammer mill* consists of a stout metal casing, enclosing a central shaft to

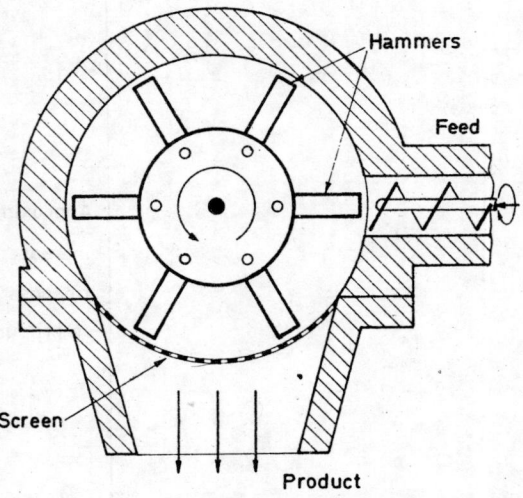

Fig. 16.4   Hammer mill

which four or more *hammers* are attached. These are mounted with swivel joints, so that the hammers swing out to a radial position when the shaft is rotated. The lower part of the casing consists of a screen through which material can escape, when sufficiently size reduced, and be collected in a suitable receiver. The screen can be changed according to the particle size required, although the latter is not related directly to the mesh size since particles are carried round by the hammers and approach the meshes tangentially. In general, therefore, particles are smaller than the mesh sizes would indicate, the difference being greater with circular meshes, and for this reason squares, rectangular slots or herring-bone slots are often used.

According to the purpose of the operation, the hammers may be square-faced, tapered to a cutting edge, or have a stepped form.

An alternative form with rigid beaters is known usually as a *disintegrator*, but this type of machine is more likely to be damaged by any hard material in the feed.

The interior of the casing may be undulating in shape, instead of a smooth circular form, with the object of increasing efficiency by ensuring repeated impacts as the particle is thrown back and forth between the hammers and the casing.

The rotor operates at fairly high frequency, usually up to about 80 s^{-1}, although the actual speed will depend on the diameter, which may be from 0·1 to 1 metre.

Advantages

(*a*) It is rapid in action, and is capable of grinding many different types of materials.

(*b*) The product can be controlled by variation of rotor speed, hammer type, and size and shape of mesh.

(*c*) Operation is continuous.

(*d*) No surfaces move against each other, so that there is little contamination of the product with metal abraded from the mill.

Disadvantages

(*a*) The high speed of operation causes generation of heat that may affect thermolabile materials or drugs containing gum, fat or resin. The mill may be water-cooled, if necessary, to reduce this heat damage.

(*b*) The rate of feed must be controlled carefully, otherwise the mill may be choked, resulting in decreased efficiency or even damage.

(*c*) Because of the high speed of operation, the hammer mill is susceptible to damage by foreign objects such as stones or metal in the feed. Magnets may be used to remove iron, but the feed must be checked visually for any other contamination. The disintegrator is even more likely to be damaged, since its rigid beaters, unlike the swing hammers of the hammer mill, cannot absorb the shock of hitting a hard object.

The hammer mill is capable of producing intermediate grades of powder from almost any substance, apart from sticky materials that choke the screen. Applications include the powdering of barks, leaves, roots, crystals, and filter cakes. With cutting edges to the hammers, the method has proved to be especially useful for granulation, the damp masses being cut to granules by the hammers when they are found to produce greater uniformity than is obtained by sieve granulation.

Attrition

Size reduction by attrition can be effected in the laboratory by using pestle and mortar or, if a small-scale mechanical method is required, the *roller mill* can be used.

ROLLER MILL

The roller mill uses the principles of attrition for the size reduction of solids in suspensions, pastes, or ointments.

Two or three rolls, usually in metal but possibly in porcelain, are mounted horizontally with a very small, but adjustable, gap between. The rolls rotate at different speeds, so that the material is sheared as it passes through the gap and is transferred from the slower to the faster roll, from which it is removed by means of a scraper. The method is very effective for size reducing and dispersing solids in semi-solid media.

Combined Impact and Attrition

The mechanisms of impact and attrition can be combined in two forms of mill. In the *ball mill* the particles receive impacts from balls or pebbles and are subjected to attrition as the balls slide over each other. In *fluid energy mills* the impacts and attrition occur between rapidly moving particles.

BALL MILL

The ball mill consists of a hollow cylinder mounted in such a way that it can be rotated on its horizontal longitudinal axis, as shown in Fig. 16.5. Some models are very large, with cylinders 3 m in

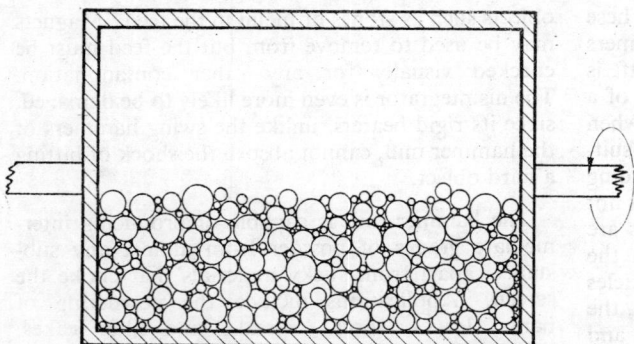

Fig. 16.5 Ball mill

diameter, but about 1 m is more common in pharmaceutical practice. The cylinder contains balls that occupy 30 to 50 per cent of the mill volume, the ball size being dependent on the size of the feed and the diameter of the mill. Usually a mill 1 m in diameter will use balls of approximately 75 mm, larger versions using balls of 150 mm diameter. In practice, the balls are worn away, so that a range of sizes exists from about 20 mm upwards. This gives a better product, in fact, since the larger balls crush the feed and the smaller ones form the fine product.

The cylinder may be of metal, porcelain or of rubber, to reduce abrasion. The balls may be of metal, porcelain or, occasionally, pebbles are used, when the mill may be described as a *pebble mill*. The amount of the material in the mill is of considerable importance, too much exerting a cushioning effect and too little leading to loss of efficiency and to abrasion.

The factor of greatest importance in the operation of the ball mill is the speed of rotation, illustrated in Fig. 16.6. At low speeds, the mass of balls will slide or roll over each other and only a negligible amount of size reduction will occur. At high speeds, the balls will be thrown out to the wall by centrifugal force and no grinding will occur. At about two-thirds of the speed at which centrifuging just occurs, it is found that movement takes place as shown in Fig. 16.6(c), that is, the balls are carried almost to the top of the mill and then fall in a cascade across the diameter of the mill. By this means, the maximum size reduction is effected by impact of the particles between the balls and by attrition between the balls. The rotational frequency will depend upon the diameter of the mill, but is usually of the order of 0·5 s^{-1}.

Advantages

(*a*) It is capable of grinding a wide variety of materials of differing character and of different degrees of hardness.

(*b*) It can be used in a completely enclosed form, which makes it especially suitable for use with toxic materials.

(*c*) It can produce very fine powders.

(*d*) It can be used for continuous operation, and a classifier can be used in conjunction with the mill, so that particles of suitable size are removed while oversize particles are returned.

(*e*) It is equally suitable for wet or dry grinding processes.

Disadvantages

(*a*) Wear occurs, principally from the balls, but partially from the casing and this may result in the product being contaminated; with abrasive materials this may exceed 0·1 per cent, but even ordinary substances may be contaminated with 0·03 per cent metal after grinding. In some cases, this may not be significant, but in others it may be of great importance.

(*b*) Soft or sticky materials may cause problems by caking on the sides of the mill or by holding the balls in aggregates.

The ball mill is a very noisy machine, particularly if the casing is of metal, but much less so if rubber is used.

Ball mills are applicable to a wide variety of materials, large ones being used for grinding ores prior to manufacture of pharmaceutical chemicals and small versions for the final grinding of drugs or for grinding suspensions.

Variants of the simple ball mill include the *Hardinge Mill* in which the cylinder has a conical end towards a discharge point. In this mill the balls become segregated, the largest collecting in the cylindrical portion, and those of decreasing size towards the apex of the cone. As a result, the coarser grinding is carried out by the large balls, the particle size decreasing as the material works its way towards the smaller balls. The product is finer and more uniform than that produced by a simple cylindrical model.

The *Tube Mill*, as its name implies, has a long narrow cylinder and can grind to a finer product than the conventional ball mill.

The *Rod Mill* has rods, which extend the length of the mill, instead of balls and is useful with sticky materials, since the rods, unlike balls, do not adhere to form aggregates.

A recent variation on the ball mill is to use a vibratory movement instead of rotation, known, therefore, as *vibration milling*. The casing is on a sprung mounting and connected to an off-balance flywheel, which sets up vibration, the mill moves through a circular path, with an amplitude of vibration up to about 20 mm and a rotational frequency of 15 to 50 s^{-1}.

Advantages Compared with Conventional Ball Milling

(*a*) Grinding is faster and it has been claimed that only one tenth of the time or even less is needed.

(*b*) For most materials, a closer size range is produced.

(*c*) The power requirements are lower.

(*d*) Although the rotating ball mill is unlikely to be replaced in large equipment, for example the crushing of ores, vibration milling shows considerable advantages for medium and small-scale applications.

FLUID ENERGY MILL

A typical form of the fluid energy mill is shown in Fig. 16.7. It consists of a loop of pipe, which has a diameter of 20 to 200 mm, depending on the overall height of the loop which may be up to about 2 m. A fluid, usually air, is injected at high pressure through nozzles at the bottom of the loop, giving rise to a high velocity circulation in a very turbulent condition. Solids are introduced into the stream and, as a result of the high degree of turbulence, impacts and attritional forces occur *between the particles*. A classifier is incorporated in the system, so that particles are retained until sufficiently fine.

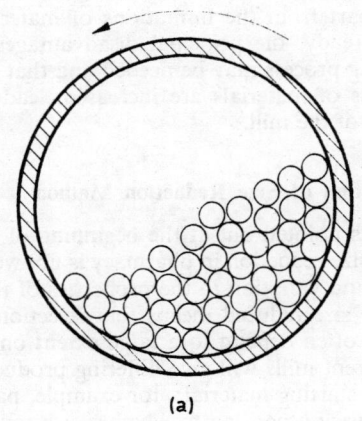

(a)

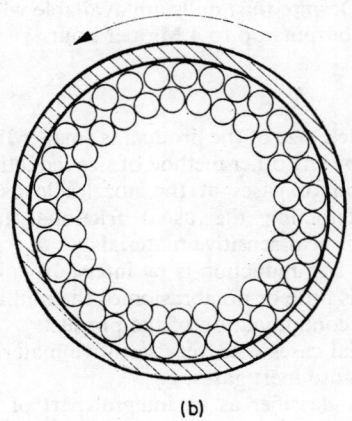

(b)

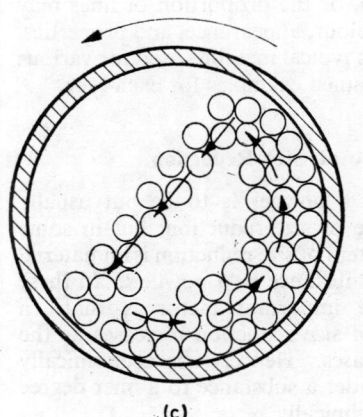

(c)

Fig. 16.6 Ball mill operation
(*a*) low speed with sliding
(*b*) high speed with centrifuging
(*c*) correct speed with cascading

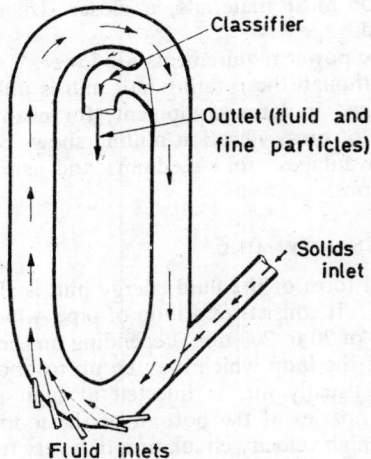

Fig. 16.7 Fluid energy mill

The feed to the mill needs to be pre-treated to reduce the particle size to the order of 100 mesh, enabling the process to yield a product as small as 5 μm or less. Despite this, mills are available which are capable of outputs up to 4 Mg per hour.

Advantages

(*a*) The particle size of the product is smaller than that produced by any other method of size reduction.

(*b*) Expansion of gases at the nozzles leads to cooling, counteracting the usual frictional heat which can affect heat-sensitive materials.

(*c*) Since the size reduction is by inter-particulate attrition there is little or no abrasion of the mill and so virtually no contamination of the product.

(*d*) For special cases with very sensitive materials it is possible to use inert gases.

(*e*) Having a classifier as an integral part of the system permits close control of particle size and of particle size distribution.

The method is used where especially fine powders are required, and antibiotics, sulphonamides and vitamins are typical examples.

WET GRINDING

Reference has been made to wet grinding as an alternative procedure in size reduction. Instead of processing dry materials, the size reduction is carried out on a paste of the substance, hence the title *wet grinding*. An alternative description is *levigation*, derived from the Latin—*levis*, meaning smooth.

Wet grinding is of limited application, since it demands a material that is already of small particle size and is insoluble in the liquid used. It is obvious that it will be most useful where a substance is produced as a suspension, for example after precipitation in a chemical reaction, and needs to be size reduced, or where dry material has to be ground to manufacture a suspended product. In general, therefore, a paste that is being wet ground will consist of at least 50 per cent liquid, often water, but any liquid may be used.

Advantages

(*a*) The powdered substance contains less fines, in fact often 20 or even 30 per cent less.

(*b*) The capacity of the plant is greater.

(*c*) Materials are easier to handle in the form of suspensions and in many cases will flow under gravity or can be pumped.

(*d*) The problem of dust is eliminated.

(*e*) If grinding is to be followed by screening or sieving, the wet process is more efficient.

(*f*) For products in the form of suspensions, the size reduction and mixing operations are combined.

Apart from the limitations of materials referred to already, the principal disadvantages are that a drying process may be needed and that the abrasive effects of materials are increased, leading to more wear of the mill.

Selection of Size Reduction Method

It was pointed out at the beginning of this chapter that size reduction in pharmacy is not well standardised and variation in the properties of the materials to be size reduced means that selection of method must often depend to a large extent on experience. Different mills will give differing products from the same starting material; for example, particle shape may vary according to whether size reduction is by impact or attrition, or the proportion of fines may vary, so altering colour, appearance, and properties.

Table 16.1 shows typical methods used for various size ranges, with named examples for each type.

Selection of Degree of Size Reduction

The use to which a powder is to be put usually controls the degree of size reduction, but in some cases the precise extent of size reduction is immaterial provided that the substance is 'a powder'. In these circumstances, the important factor is that, in general, the cost of size reduction increases as the particle size decreases. Hence, it is economically undesirable to powder a substance to a finer degree than is required technically.

Table 16.1
Use of Size Reduction Methods

Degree of size reduction	Typical methods	Examples
Large pieces	Cutter or compression mills	Rhubarb
Coarse powders	Impact mills	Liquorice, cascara
Fine powders	Combined impact and attrition mills	Rhubarb, belladonna
Very fine powders	Fluid energy mills	Vitamins, antibiotics

By way of illustration, if a substance is to be used directly in the form of a powder, for example, the components of indigestion powders or an external powder (such as a dusting powder) then a fine powder is needed. Incidentally, the fineness of the powder also aids the mixing process (*see* p. 203).

When a drug is suspended in a liquid it should be in the form of a very fine powder, for example Light Kaolin, and this is especially important if the suspension is to be injected, as in the case of procaine penicillin.

When extraction is the objective, a soft drug such as Gentian need only be sliced or crushed, while harder drugs such as Liquorice or Belladonna should be in coarse to moderately coarse powders. Special characters may exert an effect; for example, the constituents of Ipecacuanha are of low solubility so that a fine powder is used to improve the penetration of the solvent into the particles. Cascara is usually extracted with water and swells when moistened, making a coarse powder preferable as finer grades would form an impenetrable mass.

The degree of size reduction may affect properties in special cases, for example, the viscosity of mucilage of tragacanth decreases with finer powders, but the opposite is often true with acacia, where low grade gums may be improved by grinding.

Adsorption is a surface property, so that the adsorptive power of a substance can usually be improved by grinding. On the other hand, if a drug contains volatile oils, the greater surface area and the additional heat generated in grinding to a finer powder is likely to increase the loss of oil considerably.

In conclusion, it should be borne in mind that a number of size reduction procedures, particularly those involving attrition, are of value in the unit operation of mixing (*see* Chapter 18). This is especially true where powders are being mixed or where solid/liquid dispersion has to be effected and aggregates of particles have to be broken down.

BIBLIOGRAPHY

NORTH, R. (1954) Grinding Practice as Related to the Characteristics of the Material to be Pulverised. *Trans. Instn. Chem. Engrs.*, **32**, 54–60.

ROSE, H. E. and SULLIVAN, R. M. E. (1958) *A Treatise on the Internal Mechanics of Ball, Tube and Rod Mills*. London, Constable.

ROSE, H. E. and SULLIVAN, R. M. E. (1961) *Vibration Mills and Vibration Milling*. London, Constable.

17

Size Separation

CHAPTER 15 considered the significance of particle size and the principles involved in separating a powder into fractions of known particle size. Chapter 16 dealt with the methods of reducing particle size and in this chapter the standards that are applied to powders, and the methods by which size separation can be achieved on the industrial scale, will be discussed.

Large pieces of material are usually estimated visually, difficulties arising only in the estimation of powders.

Standards for Powders

Standards for powders for pharmaceutical purposes are laid down principally in the *British Pharmacopoeia* which states that the degree of coarseness or fineness of a powder is differentiated and expressed by the size of the mesh of the sieve through which the powder is able to pass.

The BP specifies five grades of powder and these are shown in Table 17.1 which gives the name by which the grade of powder is known and the number of the sieve through which *all* the particles must pass.

Table 17.1
British Pharmacopoeia Powders

Grade of powder	Sieve through which all particles must pass
Coarse	10
Moderately coarse	22
Moderately fine	44
Fine	85
Very fine	120

A little thought will indicate that this is an inadequate definition for powders, since particles that will pass through a 120 sieve will also pass through a 10 sieve. Hence, the very fine powder meets the same definition as a coarse powder! Clearly a limit must be placed on 'fines' in the coarser grades of powders and it is obvious that this

can be done by specifying two sieves for each powder—a larger size through which all particles must pass and a smaller size through which the particles will not pass. This is not practicable, however, since a size reduction process (especially to produce a coarse grade of material) inevitably produces particles finer than is intended. The 'slack' produced when a large lump of coal is broken into smaller pieces is an everyday example of this.

Because of this, the BP specifies a second, smaller size of sieve for the coarser powders but states that not more than 40 per cent shall pass through. This means that the objective is to obtain a powder with all the particles between specified maximum and minimum sizes but, because of practical size reduction difficulties, at least 60 per cent of the powder between those sizes is acceptable. It must not be forgotten, however, that although it is permitted that 40 per cent of the powder may pass through the finer of the two sieves, the ideal remains that *none* shall pass through.

The relevant grades of powder and sieve numbers are shown in Table 17.2.

Thus, the full definition of Coarse Powder is that it is powder all the particles of which pass through a No. 10 sieve and not more than 40 per cent through a No. 44 sieve. For convenience, this is usually referred to as a 10/44 powder. Other grades are expressed in a similar way.

Table 17.2
British Pharmacopoeia Powders

Grade of powder	Sieve through which all particles must pass	Sieve through which not more than 40 per cent of particles pass
Coarse	10	44
Moderately coarse	22	60
Moderately fine	44	85
Fine	85	Not specified
Very fine	120	Not specified

A better idea of the degree of divergence of these powders can be obtained by comparing the areas of the particles, based on the maximum particle size for each grade, that is, on the upper or coarser limit. Coarse Powder is represented as unity and the other grades are shown in Table 17.3:

Table 17.3
Comparison of Powder Sizes

Coarse powder	1
Moderately coarse powder	1/6
Moderately fine powder	1/24
Fine powder	1/90
Very fine powder	1/200

No limit is placed on 'fines' in the two finer grades of powder, since this would not serve any useful purpose.

It will be appreciated that the pharmacopoeial standards are approximate when the specifications are considered in the light of the discussion in Chapter 15 of the efficiency of the sieving process. Thus, factors such as the method of sieve movement can affect the amount of the powder passing through the sieve, so that it is possible for a powder to pass if tested by one method and to fail by another. The alternative is to impose rigid specifications for the test, but this would be very complicated and the standards are, in fact, adequate for the purposes for which the coarser grades of powder are intended, such as, for extraction (*see* Chapter 22).

The *British Pharmacopoeia* makes two statements with regard to these 'official' grades of powders in practice:

1. It is required that, when a powder is described by a number, *all* particles must pass through the specified sieve.

2. When a vegetable drug is being ground and sifted, *none* must be rejected.

The reason for this will be apparent if the character of a vegetable drug is compared with a chemical substance. The latter is a homogeneous material so that, if a certain quantity of a powder is required, an excess may be ground, a sufficient amount of the desired size range obtained by sieving, and the oversize particles (known as *tailings*) may be discarded.

A vegetable drug, however, consists of a variety of tissues of different degrees of hardness, so that softer tissues will be ground first and tailings obtained by sifting will contain a higher proportion of the harder tissues. In many cases, constituents are not distributed uniformly through vegetable tissues; for example, in digitalis the glycosides are

concentrated in the mid-rib and veins. Hence, if tailings are discarded when grinding and sifting the drug, it is likely that a high proportion of the active constituents will be lost.

The Pharmacopoeia does, however, permit tailings to be withheld from a batch of drug that is being ground provided an approximately equal amount of tailings from a preceding batch is added before grinding. The object of this is to allow a batch mill to be used efficiently since, without this concession, it would be necessary to grind a batch completely, and any tailings, even if the quantity were very small, would have to be ground separately and the mill would be operating at much less than its correct capacity for a considerable amount of the time. The addition of tailings to the mill permits operation at full capacity all the time.

A useful precaution to observe when batch grinding drugs in the preparation of a standard grade of powder is to stop the mill at frequent intervals, sieve the powder, and return the tailings. The significance of this is that it is easy to grind the soft tissues, and excessive amounts of fines may be obtained. In addition, fines will cushion the grinding action and so decrease the size reduction efficiency of the mill.

Since segregation will occur during grinding and sifting, it is important to ensure that the powder is thoroughly mixed at the end of the process.

In addition to the grades of powder specified by the *British Pharmacopoeia*, the *British Pharmaceutical Codex* details a further grade known as *Ultra-fine Powder*. In this case, it is required that the maximum dimension of at least 90 per cent of the particles must be not greater than 5 μm and none must be greater than 50 μm. Determination of particle size for this grade is carried out by a microscopic method.

Sieves

The standardisation of powders by means of sieves demands that specifications must be stated for these also, and sieves for test purposes are the subject of a British Standard.

Most of the sieves used are of the wire mesh type, the number of the sieve indicating the number of meshes included in a length of 25·4 mm (1 inch) in each direction parallel to the wires. It should be noted that it is the number of *meshes* that is specified and not the number of *wires*. Thus, a No. 10 sieve has 10 meshes per inch in each direction, but it will be realised that if there were 10 wires there would be 9 meshes only.

The simple statement of the number of meshes per unit length is not sufficient, however, as the size

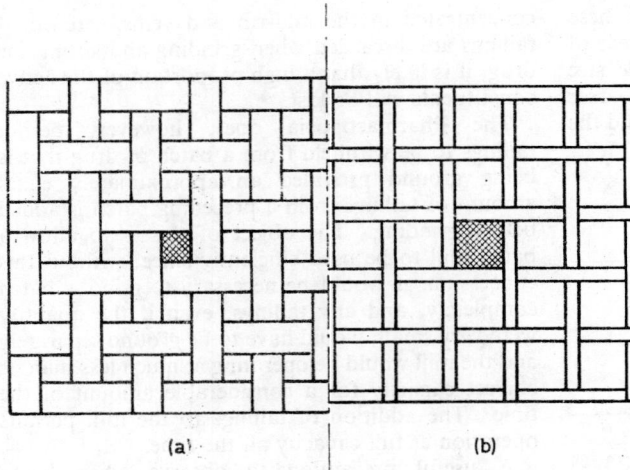

(a)   (b)

Fig. 17.1 Effect of wire diameter on sieve mesh size

of the particle that will pass the sieve will depend on other factors, principally the diameter of the wire, as shown in Fig. 17.1.

The *British Pharmacopoeia* quotes the full details from the British Standard.

STANDARDS FOR SIEVES

It is required that wire-mesh sieves shall be made from wire of uniform, circular cross-section and for each sieve the following particulars are stated:

Number of Sieve

This is the number of meshes in a length of 25·4 mm (1 in.), in each direction, parallel to the wires.

Nominal Size of Aperture

This is the distance between the wires, so that it represents the length of the side of the square aperture. While it is the diameter of the largest sphere that would pass the mesh, it is not necessarily the maximum dimension of the particle, since plate-like particles will pass through diagonally and long fibrous particles require only suitable orientation.

Nominal Diameter of the Wire

This dimension and the number of meshes form the basic standards for the sieve. The wire diameter has been selected to give a suitable aperture size, but also to have sufficient strength to avoid distortion. The wire is stated also in terms of a Standard Wire Gauge, which is a system for representing certain diameters by means of numbers.

Approximate Screening Area. This standard expresses the area of the meshes as a percentage of the total area of the sieve. It is, of course, governed by the size of wire used for any particular sieve number and, as far as possible, is kept within the range 35 to 40 per cent. This gives suitable strength to the sieve, but leaves adequate area of meshes since these are obviously the useful area of the sieve.

Aperture Tolerance Average

Some variation in the aperture size is unavoidable and this variation, expressed as a percentage, is known as the aperture tolerance average. The term tolerance is used in engineering practice to mean the limits within which a particular quantity or dimension can be allowed to vary and still be acceptable for the purpose for which it is required. Finer wires are likely to be subject to a greater proportional variation in diameter than coarse and, also, fine meshes cannot be woven with the same accuracy as coarse meshes. Hence, the aperture tolerance average is smaller for sieves of 5 or 10 mesh than is the case for 300 mesh.

PERFORATED PLATE SIEVES

Sieves may also be made by drilling holes in metal plate, so that this type will have *circular* apertures as against the *square* apertures of the wire mesh sieve. In general, these sieves are used in the larger sizes and can be made with greater accuracy than wire-mesh sieves, as well as being less susceptible to distortion in use. This type is commonly used also as screens in impact mills (*see* p. 186). Usually, the holes are spaced with their centres arranged at the apices of equilateral triangles, so that all the apertures are equidistant, as shown in Fig. 17.2.

Similar standards are laid down with the appropriate equivalent specifications for *plate thickness* and *nominal width of the bridge* (dimension *A* in Fig. 17.2) which control the strength of the sieve in the same way as wire diameter in wire mesh sieves.

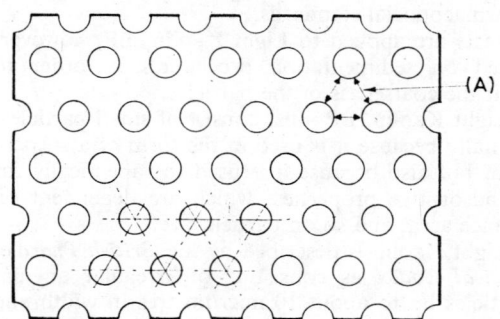

Fig. 17.2   Perforated plate sieve

Materials Used for Sieves

The only official specification for materials for the construction of sieves is that the wire should be of uniform, circular cross-section. In addition, however, the material should have suitable strength to avoid distortion and be resistant to corrosion by any substances that may be sifted.

Although described usually as wire sieves, both metals and non-metals may be used.

METALS

Iron

Iron wire has the advantage of being cheap, but the disadvantage that rusting occurs very readily and iron contamination of products is usually undesirable.

Coated Iron

Iron wire may be coated as a protection from corrosion by galvanising or tinning, but there is a tendency for the diameter to become variable. Some sieves are coated after manufacture, which increases the protection against corrosion and increases the strength also, but is likely to lead to some variation in the mesh size. Like all coatings, it remains effective only if it is not damaged.

Copper

Copper wire is readily available and is used commonly, having the advantage of avoiding the risk of iron contamination, but it is a soft metal and the meshes can be distorted easily.

Copper Alloys

A number of alloys of copper, for example brass and phosphor-bronze, resemble copper in possessing good resistance to corrosion by most materials but their strength is very much greater so that there is less risk of the meshes being distorted in use.

Stainless Steel

Although the most expensive of the metals from which sieves are made, stainless steel is the most satisfactory, having good resistance to corrosion by all materials that are likely to be sieved, as well as adequate strength. Sieves with stainless steel meshes are recommended, therefore, for pharmaceutical purposes.

NON-METALS

Sieves with meshes from non-metals are used when it is important that all risk of metallic contamination be avoided. Non-metals are used also for sieves with fine meshes, since many non-metal fibres are stronger than a metal wire of comparable thickness.

Materials of natural origin, for example hair and silk, were used originally, but synthetic fibres have proved to be more satisfactory. Man-made fibres, such as nylon and terylene, are excellent, having considerable strength and resistance to corrosion. In addition, these materials can be extruded in all diameters, enabling a wide variety of sieves to be made.

Sieving Methods

Sieves should be used and stored with care, since a sieve is of little value if the meshes become damaged or distorted. With the exception of the use of sieves for granulation (*see* Chapter 19), material should never be forced through a sieve. Particles, if small enough, will pass through a sieve easily if it is shaken, tapped, or brushed. There is a procedure laid down in a British Standard relating to the testing of sieves, which attempts to ensure a uniform method of treatment for each test.

MECHANICAL SIEVING METHODS

Mechanical sieving devices are usually based on methods that agitate or brush the sieve or use centrifugal force.

Agitation Methods

Sieves may be agitated in a number of different ways, for example—

Oscillation. The sieve is mounted in a frame that oscillates back and forth. The method is simple, but the material may roll on the surface of the sieve, and fibrous materials in particular tend to 'ball'.

Vibration. In this case, the mesh is vibrated at high speed, often by means of an electrical device using the 50 Hertz alternations of alternating electric current. The rapid vibration is imparted to the particles on the sieve and the particles are less likely to 'blind' the mesh.

Gyration. The gyratory method uses a system in which the sieve is on a rubber mounting and connected to an eccentric flywheel. Thus, the sieve is given a rotary movement of small amplitude, but of considerable intensity, giving a spinning motion to the particles. This increases the chances of a particle becoming suitably orientated to pass through the mesh, so that the output is usually considerably greater than that obtained with oscillating or vibratory sieves.

Agitation methods may be made continuous, by inclination of the sieve and the provision of separate outlets for undersize and oversize particles. This applies irrespective of the method of agitation.

Brushing Methods

A brush can be used to move the particles on the surface of the sieve and to keep the meshes clear.

A single brush across the diameter of an ordinary circular sieve, rotating about the mid-point, is effective, but in large-scale production a horizontal cylindrical sieve is employed, with a spiral brush rotating on the longitudinal axis of the sieve.

Centrifugal Methods

Mechanical sieves of this type normally use a vertical cylindrical sieve with a high-speed rotor inside the cylinder, so that particles are thrown outwards by centrifugal force. The current of air created by the movement assists sieving also, and is especially useful with very fine powders.

WET SIEVING

The methods described above use the powder in the dry state, which may lead to difficulties with some materials. As in size reduction, wet sieving is more efficient than the equivalent dry process, particles being suspended readily and passing easily through the sieve with less blinding of the meshes. The process has obvious limitations, however.

FLUID CLASSIFICATION

The principles of fluid classification discussed in Chapter 15 do not have application in the general pharmacopoeial standards.

Tests are applied to Light Kaolin, BP, however, based on sedimentation procedures in order to limit the coarseness of the particles.

Light Kaolin, BP must consist of small particles, partially because it is used in the form of a suspension, but also because it is used therapeutically for its adsorptive properties, which are dependent on surface area, and so on particle size.

Light Kaolin is described by the *British Pharmaceutical Codex* as consisting of irregular angular particles up to about 10 micrometres in width and innumerable minute fragments 1 to 2 micrometres in width. Other forms of kaolin may contain much larger particles; for example, Heavy Kaolin is stated by the *British Pharmaceutical Codex* to consist of particles of approximately 60 micrometres.

The *British Pharmacopoeia*, therefore, places three limits on the particle size of Light Kaolin: on 'coarse' particles, on particles larger than 10 micrometres, and on particles larger than 3 micrometres. Full details of these tests can be found in the *British Pharmacopoeia*, but an outline here will show how these are related to sedimentation theory.

Light Kaolin

Test for Coarse Particles

A sample is placed in a stoppered cylinder of specified dimensions with a stated volume of 1 per cent sodium pyrophosphate solution, which acts as a peptising agent (*see* p. 57), shaken and allowed to stand for five minutes.

Most of the suspension is then pipetted off from a stated depth (5 cm) below the surface and discarded, so removing all particles that have not settled below the sampling point in five minutes.

The residual suspension is made up to the original volume with water, shaken, stood for 5 minutes, and pipetted off, as before.

The process is repeated until 8 quantities have been removed.

The residue will consist only of particles that have been able to settle below the sampling point on each occasion. These particles are dried and weighed and should not exceed 0·5 per cent of the starting weight of the sample.

Some idea of the minimum size of a 'coarse particle' can be obtained by assuming a theoretical particle that can settle from the surface to the sampling point in the standing time used in the test, that is, 5 cm in 5 min, and substituting this velocity in Stokes' law.

Stokes' law (Eqn. 5.10) can be expressed as:

$$d = \sqrt{\left\{\frac{18\eta u}{(\rho_s - \rho_l)g}\right\}} \qquad (17.1)$$

If it is assumed that:

$u = 5$ cm/5 min
$\quad = 1$ cm/1 min
$\quad = 0·167 \times 10^{-3}$ m/s
$\eta = 0·001$ Ns/m^2
$\rho_s = 20$ kg/m^3
$\rho_l = 10$ kg/m^3
$g = 9·807$ m/s^2

then:

$$d = \sqrt{\left\{\frac{18 \times 0·001 \times 0·167 \times 10^{-3}}{(20 - 10) \times 9·807}\right\}}$$

$$= 17·5 \times 10^{-6} \text{ m}$$

$$= 17·5 \ \mu\text{m}$$

Test for Particles Larger than 10 μm in Diameter

A sample of specified weight is shaken in a stated volume of water and allowed to stand for 20 minutes, a sample being removed by pipette from a specified depth.

The weight per millilitre is determined and must be less than a given limit, since if there are too many particles above a certain size the number settling below the sampling point will be greater, giving a low value for the weight per millilitre.

Test for Particles Larger than 3 μm in Diameter

The test is carried out in the same way as for 10 μm particles but the standing time is 3·5 h. The value of the weight per millilitre specified for this test is, of course, different from that stated for the 3 μm test.

The difference between the times used for sedimentation in these two tests may seem surprising, but the reason will become apparent if a comparison is made, again making use of Stokes' law:

From Stokes' law:

$$\text{Settling velocity} \propto d^2 \qquad (17.2)$$

But velocity = distance/time, so that for the same distance:

$$\frac{1}{t} \propto d^2 \qquad (17.3)$$

so that:

$$t \propto \frac{1}{d^2} \qquad (17.4)$$

For 10 μm particles:

$$d^2 = 100 \quad \therefore \quad \frac{1}{d^2} = 0·01 = t_{10}$$

For 3 μm particles:

$$d^2 = 9 \quad \therefore \quad \frac{1}{d^2} = 0·111 = t_3$$

$$\therefore \quad \frac{t_{10}}{t_3} = \frac{0·01}{0·111} = \frac{1}{11·1}$$

But the times used in practice are:

$$T_{10} = 20 \text{ minutes}$$

and

$$T_3 = 3·5 \text{ hours} = 210 \text{ minutes}.$$

$$\therefore \quad \frac{T_{10}}{T_3} = \frac{20}{210} = \frac{1}{10·5}$$

Hence, the times used in practice show close agreement with times predicted theoretically on the basis of Stokes' law.

Large-scale Fluid Classification Methods

Industrial methods of particle size separation, like the analytical procedures discussed on pp. 178, 180, may be based on sedimentation or on elutriation.

SEDIMENTATION METHODS

Sedimentation Tank

A suspension of the solids in a fluid, usually a liquid, and most commonly water, is placed in a tank and allowed to stand for a suitable time. The upper layer is then removed, giving a single separation, or the suspension may be collected as a number of fractions by arranging for the pump inlet to remain just below the surface. The suspension pumped out will then contain successively coarser particles.

Although a very simple process, it has the disadvantage of being a batch process only and that, also, it does not give a clean split of particle sizes. This occurs because some small particles will be near the bottom of the tank at the beginning of the process and so will be removed with the coarse particles.

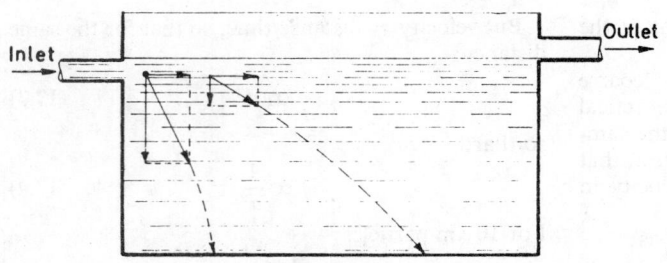

Fig. 17.3 Continuous sedimentation tank

Continuous Sedimentation Tank

A shallow tank is arranged with inlet and outlet pipes as shown in Fig. 17.3. Particles entering the tank will be acted upon by a force that can be divided into two components: a horizontal component due to the flow of the fluid that carries the particle forward, and a vertical component due to gravity, which causes the particle to fall towards the bottom of the tank. The latter will depend on Stokes's law, so that the velocity of fall is proportional to the diameter. Thus, particles will settle to the floor of the tank at a point that depends on particle size, the coarsest particles being nearest to the inlet and the finest nearest to the outlet.

In some tanks, partitions are arranged on the floor, enabling particular size fractions to be collected continuously. In other tanks, the flow is arranged so that only coarse particles will settle out, fine particles being carried through to the overflow and collected elsewhere by sedimentation or filtration.

Although the apparatus is still simple and inexpensive, the method has the merit of being continuous in operation and gives a clean separation of particles into as many size fractions as may be required.

Cyclone Separator

The cyclone separator consists of a cylindrical vessel with a conical base, as shown in Fig. 17.4. The suspension is introduced tangentially at fairly high velocity, so that a rotary movement takes place within the vessel, and the fluid is removed from a central outlet at the top. The rotatory flow within the cyclone causes the particles to be acted on by centrifugal force, solids being thrown out to the walls, thence falling to the conical base and out through the solids discharge.

Cyclones can be used with liquid suspensions of solids, but the most common application is with suspensions of a solid in a gas, usually air.

The separator is still a form of sedimentation, but with centrifugal force used instead of the gravitational force. Hence, depending on the fluid velocity,

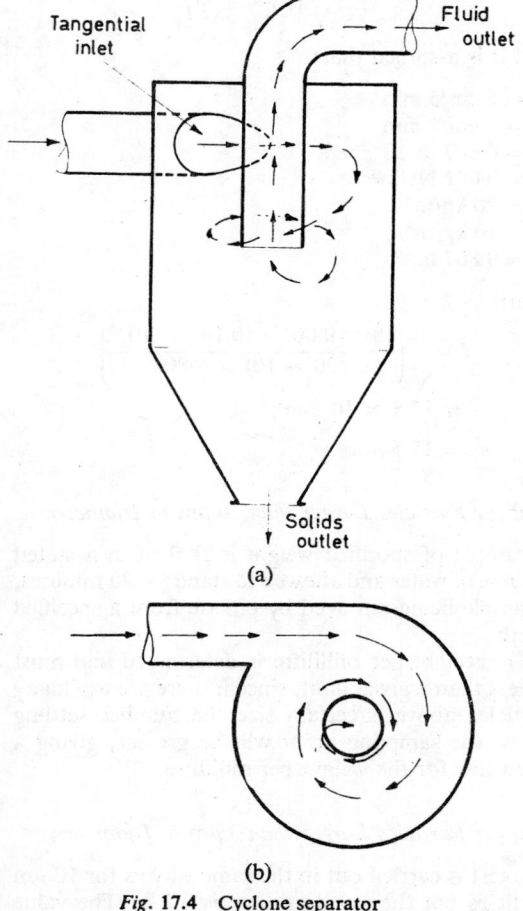

Fig. 17.4 Cyclone separator
(*a*) elevation
(*b*) plan

the cyclone can be used to separate all particles or to remove only coarser particles and allow fine particles to be carried through with the fluid.

Mechanical Air Classifier

Mechanical air separation methods use similar principles to the cyclone separator, but the air movement is obtained by means of a rotating disc and vanes, and separation is improved by the use of stationary vanes. By controlling these vanes and the speed of rotation, it is possible to vary the size at which separation occurs. Often, the method is used in conjunction with mills to separate and return oversize particles for further size reduction.

ELUTRIATION METHODS

As indicated on p. 180, elutriation depends on the movement of a fluid against the direction of sedimentation of the particles. For the gravitational system, therefore, the apparatus consists simply of a vertical column (Fig. 17.5) with an inlet near the

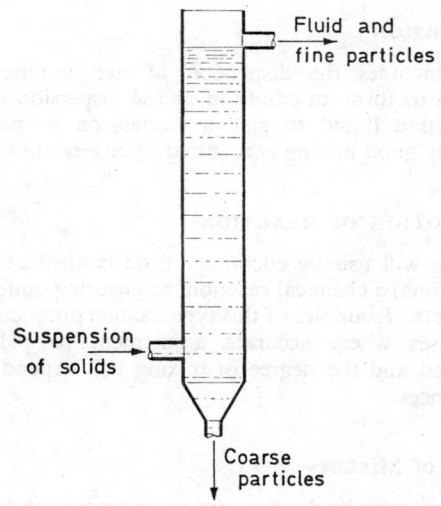

Fig. 17.5 Elutriation

bottom for the suspension, an outlet at the base for coarse particles, and an overflow near the top for fluid and fine particles. One column will give a single separation into two fractions, but it must be remembered that this will not give a clean cut, since there is a velocity gradient across the tube, resulting in the separation of particles of different sizes according to the distance from the wall.

If more than one fraction is required, a number of tubes of increasing area of cross-section can be connected in series. With the same overall flow-rate, the velocity will decrease in succeeding tubes as the area of cross-section increases, giving a number of

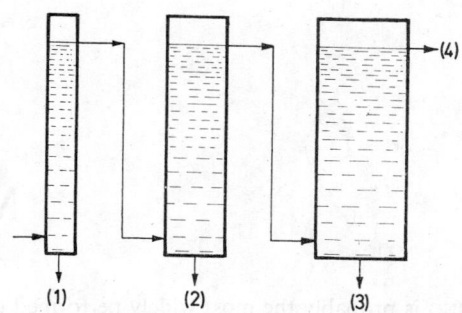

Fig. 17.6 Multi-stage elutriator
(1) to (4) are fractions of decreasing particle size

fractions. The process is shown diagrammatically in Fig. 17.6.

Advantages

(*a*) The process is continuous.
(*b*) As many stages can be used as necessary.
(*c*) The separation is quicker than with sedimentation, so that the apparatus is more compact.

The principal disadvantage is that the suspension has to be dilute, which may sometimes be undesirable.

APPLICATIONS OF SEDIMENTATION AND ELUTRIATION

Both methods are used for similar purposes, usually following a size reduction process, with the object of separating oversize particles, which may be returned for further grinding, used for other purposes, or discarded according to the circumstances.

With liquids, the techniques are applicable to insoluble solids, such as kaolin or chalk, which are often subjected to wet grinding followed by sedimentation or elutriation with water.

With gases, the methods are applicable to finer solids that would separate too slowly in liquids, to water-soluble substances, or where dry processing is required. Thus, a cyclone or mechanical air separator is often incorporated in circuit with a ball mill or hammer mill to separate and return oversize particles.

BIBLIOGRAPHY

POOLE, J. B. and DOYLE, D. (Eds) (1966) *Solid/Liquid Separation: a Review and a Bibliographical Guide.* London, H.M. Stationery Office.

18

Mixing

MIXING is probably the most widely performed unit operation in pharmaceutical manufacturing, in fact, it is difficult to find a product where mixing is not involved in some stage of the process.

The operation has, however, little theoretical basis, largely because of the great variety of materials involved, ranging from mobile liquids to viscous liquids, semi-solids and solids. In addition, it is difficult to know what is meant by the term 'mixed' or what degree of mixing is required in particular circumstances and how it is to be assessed.

This chapter considers the objectives of the mixing operation, types of mixtures, the theory of mixing and the methods by which mixing may be effected.

Definition and Objectives

Mixing may be defined as an operation in which two or more components in a separate or roughly mixed condition are treated so that each particle lies as nearly as possible in contact with a particle of each of the other ingredients.

This degree of mixing is not normally practicable, is frequently unnecessary, and sometimes undesirable. How nearly the mixing should attempt to approach this theoretical ideal will depend on the purpose of the product and the objective of the mixing operation. The objectives of mixing may be broadly classified, as follows.

SIMPLE PHYSICAL MIXTURE

This may be simply the production of a blend of two or more miscible liquids or two or more uniformly divided solids. In pharmaceutical practice, the degree of mixing must commonly be of a high order, as many such mixtures are dilutions of a potent substance, and correct dosage must be ensured.

PHYSICAL CHANGE

Mixing may aim at producing a change that is physical as distinct from chemical, for example the solution of a soluble substance. In such cases, a lower efficiency of mixing will often be acceptable because the mixing merely accelerates a process that could occur by diffusion, without agitation.

DISPERSION

This includes the dispersion of two immiscible liquids to form an emulsion or the dispersion of a solid in a liquid to give a suspension or paste. Usually good mixing is required to ensure stability.

PROMOTION OF REACTION

Mixing will usually encourage (and control at the same time) a chemical reaction, so ensuring uniform products. Examples of this type include products or processes where accurate adjustment to pH is required and the degree of mixing will depend on the process.

Types of Mixtures

Mixtures may be divided into three types that differ fundamentally in their behaviour:

POSITIVE MIXTURES

Positive mixtures are formed from materials such as gases or miscible liquids, where irreversible mixing would take place, by diffusion, without the expenditure of work provided time is unlimited. In general, such materials do not present any problems in mixing.

NEGATIVE MIXTURES

Suspensions of solids in liquids are examples of negative mixtures that require work for their formation, and the components of which will separate unless work is continually expended on them. Negative mixtures are more difficult to form and a higher degree of mixing efficiency is required.

NEUTRAL MIXTURES

Neutral mixtures are static in their behaviour, the components having no tendency to mix spontaneously, nor do they segregate when mixed. Many pharmaceutical products are examples of this type; for example, pastes, ointments and mixed powders.

Within these main groups many variations occur owing to the different physical properties of the components of the mixture. Such factors will include viscosity (which may change during mixing), the relative densities of the components, particle size, ease of wetting of solids, surface tension of liquids, while other factors such as the proportions of the components and the required order of mixing may exert an influence. Some of these factors that have relevance to particular circumstances will be considered later.

For convenience, mixing will be dealt with in three categories: liquids, solids (powders), and semi-solids. In practice, the divisions are not well defined, the materials that have to be mixed in pharmacy lying in a continuous range from mobile liquids to solids, wet and dry.

Liquid Mixing

In general, the mixed condition is not difficult to achieve with two or more mobile liquids or with mobile liquids and solids, although the latter mixture is unlikely to be permanent.

The mixing operation has two requirements:

1. Localised mixing, sufficient to apply shear to the particles of the fluid.

2. A general movement, sufficient to take all parts of the bulk of the material through the shearing zone and to ensure that a uniform final product is obtained.

In some cases, flow alone may be sufficient; for example, if the process aims simply at producing a blend of two liquids that are readily miscible or is assisting the solution of a solid in a liquid. Flow is unlikely to prove adequate, however, to produce an emulsion from two immiscible liquids, shear forces being essential.

Liquid mixing is usually performed with a mixing element, commonly a rotational device, which provides the necessary shear forces, but is of suitable shape to act as an impeller to produce an appropriate flow pattern in the mixing vessel. Typical forms of the impeller will be considered later.

The movement of the liquid at any point in the vessel will have three velocity components and the complete flow pattern will depend upon variations in these three components in different parts of the vessel.

The three velocity components are:

Radial components, acting in a direction vertical to the impeller shaft.

A *longitudinal* component, acting parallel to the impeller shaft.

A *tangential* component, acting in a direction that is a tangent to the circle of rotation round the impeller shaft.

A satisfactory flow pattern will depend on the balance of the components. Assuming that the impeller shaft is vertical, excessive radial movement, especially if solids are present, will take materials to the container wall, whence they fall to the bottom and may rotate as a mass beneath the impeller. If the tangential component is dominant, a vortex forms and may deepen until it reaches the impeller, when aeration occurs. If the longitudinal component is inadequate, liquids and solids may rotate in layers without mixing. This stratification may occur even when rotation is rapid and in the presence of vortexing, when it would appear that mixing is vigorous and satisfactory.

The flow pattern will be influenced by factors such as the form of the impeller and its position; for example, whether it is high or low in the vessel, whether mounted centrally or to one side, or whether the shaft is vertical or inclined. Container shape and the presence of baffles will have an effect also.

Liquid properties will also affect the flow pattern and thereby influence the design and operation of the mixing unit. Thus, it has been found that the optimum speed of rotation of the mixing element and the ratio of the diameter of the container, D, to the diameter of the mixing element, d, are both inversely proportional to the apparent viscosity of the liquid. Hence, a liquid of low viscosity will use an impeller with a D/d value of the order of 20 and rotating at high speed. On the other hand, a liquid of high viscosity, such as a paste, will need a D/d ratio of 1 and low speed of rotation; that is, use blades that move slowly and scrape the side of the vessel.

Powder Mixing

As would be expected from the fact that, in general, powders are neutral mixtures (*see* above), the character of the powder mixing operation is quite different from that of liquids.

The process can be illustrated diagrammatically by representing particles from two powders that are to be mixed as black and white squares. In Fig. 18.1(*a*) 200 particles of each of the two powders are shown in a completely segregated form before mixing begins. From the theoretical definition of mixing

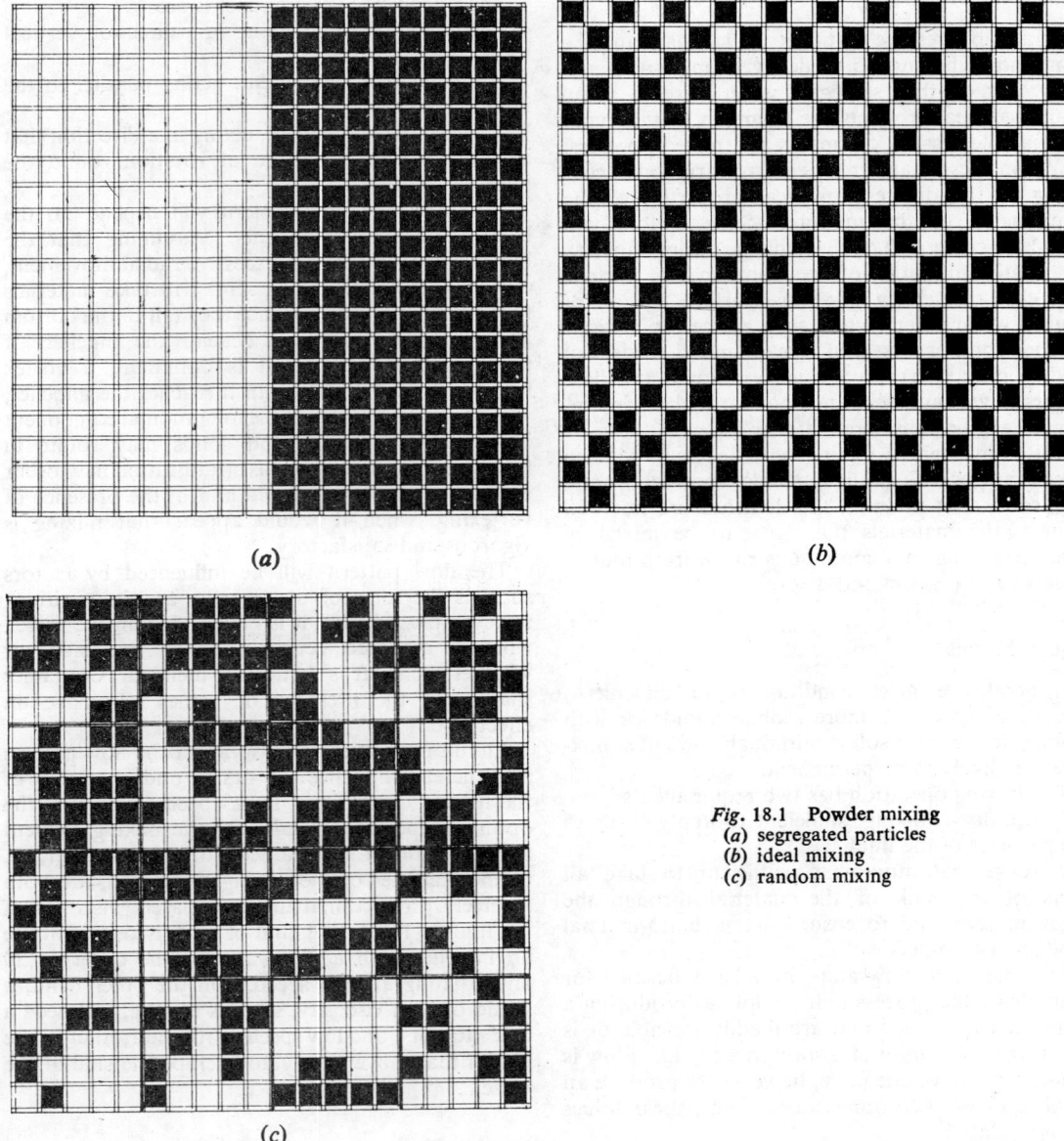

(a)

(b)

(c)

Fig. 18.1   **Powder** mixing
   (*a*) segregated particles
   (*b*) ideal mixing
   (*c*) random mixing

(*see* p. 200) we derive Fig. 18.1(*b*) where each particle lies in an ordered manner adjacent to a particle of the other ingredient.

Powder mixing is a chance process, however, and, while the situation shown in Fig. 18.1(*b*) could arise in this way, the odds against it are so great that for all practical purposes it can be regarded as impossible. This is particularly true when it is remembered that the diagram is two-dimensional only, and a solids mixture will be three-dimensional.

Hence, the practical result of mixing is a random distribution, with the particles arranged as shown in Fig. 18.1(*c*). The artificial randomisation in the diagram is based on random numbers in statistical tables.

It will be seen that there is no longer a condition of full mixing in accordance with the theoretical definition, but, if the overall view is taken, the particles can be described as mixed. Even so, this sample has not been given the correct proportions, there being only 48·5 per cent of black particles instead of the theoretical 50 per cent. From examination of Fig. 18.1(c) and of Table 18.1 it will be seen that 5 only of the smaller squares, each representing 25 particles, approach as nearly as possible to the theoretical 50 per cent (that is, either 12 or 13 black particles in 25). The remainder show considerable variation from the mean of 48·5 per cent, with the standard deviation being 11·85 and the range from 24 to 72 per cent.

These results lead to three conclusions, which are of great importance in the mixing of powders.

Table 18.1
Percentage of Black 'particles' in Various Blocks of Squares in Fig. 18.1(c)

Arrangement of squares:

1 A	1 B	2 A	2 B
	1		2
1 C	1 D	2 C	2 D
3 A	3 B	4 A	4 B
	3		4
3 C	3 D	4 C	4 D

Theoretical percentage = 50

Sample number	Number of squares in sample	Per cent blacks
Overall	400	48·5
1 and 3	200	49·5
2 and 4	200	47·5
1 and 2	200	52·5
2 and 4	200	43·5
1	100	55
2	100	52
3	100	44
4	100	43
1 A	25	52
1 B	25	64
1 C	25	60
1 D	25	44
2 A	25	44
2 B	25	52
2 C	25	72
2 D	25	40
3 A	25	52
3 B	25	60
3 C	25	24
3 D	25	40
4 A	25	48
4 B	25	48
4 C	25	36
4 D	25	40

DEGREE OF MIXING

Commonly, the object of the mixing operation is to produce a bulk of mixture that is subdivided to individual doses, and it is important that *each article* should contain the correct proportions.

Thus, a mixture of 86 per cent of sodium potassium tartrate and 14 per cent of sodium bicarbonate would be subdivided into 17·5 gramme quantities in the manufacture of Double Strength Seidlitz Powders, but the distribution of the two components within the 17·5 gramme quantity is unimportant, provided the correct proportions are present. On the other hand, 17·5 grammes of tablet granules may produce as many as $350 \times 0·05$ gramme tablets of a potent medicament and *each tablet* must contain the correct dose. Thus, the degree of mixing must be suitable to ensure that every unit of dose contains the correct proportions of each component. The size of this unit governs the closeness with which the mixture must be examined; it is known as the *scale of scrutiny* and would be 17·5 grammes in the first case and 0·05 gramme in the second case.

EVALUATION OF MIXTURES

Assessment of the degree of mixing and checking of the final product usually involves sampling and analysis and Fig. 18.1(c) shows the importance of sample size. If it is assumed that 400 squares represents the minimum amount for analysis, but the dose units are represented by 25 squares, then the analysis would show a result of 48·5 per cent, which would probably be acceptable. Individual dose units, however, would range from 24 to 72 per cent, which would be quite unacceptable. Examples can be found in the Pharmacopoeia where the analytical sample consists of a number of tablets, although modern analytical techniques of greater sensitivity can often be applied permitting the use of smaller samples. Ideally, the sample should be the same as the scale of scrutiny, with sufficient replication to ensure representative results. If a large sample is unavoidable, statistical techniques should be applied to the sampling methods and to the interpretation of the results.

PARTICLE SIZE

A third conclusion from Fig. 18.1(c) concerns the effect of particle size on mixing. The discussion has been based on *numbers* of particles, whereas in practice the samples will be based on *weights*. Thus, for a given weight, a reduction in particle size will increase the number of particles and lead to an improvement in the chances of obtaining the correct 50 : 50 proportions.

MECHANISM OF POWDER MIXING

Under the influence of gravity, a static bed of particles will adopt the closest form of packing, illustrated in Fig. 19.19(*b*), which is known as *rhombohedral packing* and has a porosity of the order of 25 per cent. Mixing demands movement of the particles, so that *cubical packing* is brought about, where the porosity is about 50 per cent, as shown in Fig. 19.19(*a*). Hence, dilation of the bed occurs, that is, there is an increase in the total volume occupied by the powder.

The actual mixing will be analogous to the mixing of liquids, discussed on page 201, since localised shear forces will be necessary to bring about the change to open packing and movement of the particles relative to each other, while a general circulation brings the material through the intense mixing zone.

The localised shear forces may be brought about in two ways:

By tilting the material beyond its angle of repose (*see* Chapter 19), so that gravitational forces cause the upper layers to slip, and the moving particles to mix. This gives rise to small-scale movement and, because of the resemblance to molecular diffusion of liquids and gases, it is known as *diffusive mixing*.

By creating shear forces in the material by using an agitator arm or a blast of air. This is referred to as *shear mixing*.

In both cases, a general convective movement must occur, also.

PRACTICAL MIXING

The previous discussion of the theory has been based on the mixing of equal numbers of particles, identical in all respects and distinguished only by colour. In practice, dissimilarities will occur, some of which will favour the mixing operation and some that will oppose it.

Material Density

If the components are of different density, the denser material will sink through the lighter one, the effect of which will depend on the relative positions of the materials in the mixer. If the denser particles form the lower layer in a mixer at the start of a mixing operation, the degree of mixing will increase gradually until an equilibrium is attained, not necessarily complete mixing. If the denser component is above, the degree of mixing increases to a maximum, then dropping to an equilibrium as the denser component falls through the lighter one, so that segregation has started. This factor is of practical significance in charging and operating a mixer.

Particle Size

Variation in particle size can lead to segregation also, since smaller particles can fall through the voids between the larger particles. There will be a critical particle size that can just be retained in the mixed condition, which will depend upon the packing. When the bed of particles is disturbed, dilation occurs and the greater porosity of open packing allows a larger size of particle to slip through the voids, leading to segregation.

Particle Shape

The ideal particle is spherical in shape, and the further particles depart from this theoretical form, the greater the difficulty of mixing. On the other hand, irregular shapes can become interlocked, decreasing the risk of segregation once mixing has been achieved.

Particle Attraction

Some particles exert attractive forces, arising from such causes as adsorbed liquid films or electrostatic charges, such particles tending to aggregate. Since these are surface properties, the effect increases as particle size decreases.

Proportions of Materials

The theory has considered the mixing of equal numbers of black and white particles, which represents the best conditions for mixing. In this case, if two particles change places there is the greatest chance that they will be different, that is, a black will be replaced by a white or vice versa, so that mixing takes place. In practice, however, it is necessary frequently to make mixtures when 1 per cent or less of a substance has to be dispersed in a diluent.

The usual practical method is to mix the component in the lesser amount with an equal quantity of the diluent. Then a further amount of diluent is added, equal to the previous concentrated mixture and so on until all has been added. Thus, although this procedure must have arisen empirically in the first place, it is supported by theory, since each stage is carried out in 50:50 proportions, which ensures that mixing is taking place under the best possible conditions.

Figure 18.2 is a diagram, similar in principle to Fig. 18.1(c) based on random numbers for a 10:90 distribution. The full analysis is not given, but it represents an average that comes out to 11·75 per cent, with limits of 0 per cent and 32 per cent in the smaller samples. This illustrates the danger of proceeding directly to a 10 per cent dilution, and the situation will be worse with the lower proportions encountered in practice.

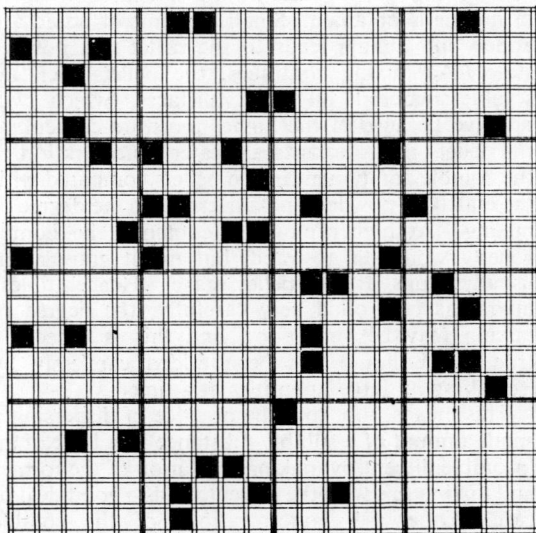

Fig. 18.2   Powder mixing: 10 per cent random mixing

Mixing techniques or apparatus can be tested easily in practice by dispersing a highly coloured material in a white diluent. It is then worth bearing in mind that a dilution of a small amount of a potent white medicament in a white diluent will require similar treatment, although there is no easy method of visual evaluation.

CONDITIONS FOR MIXING

The theory shows four conditions that should be observed in the mixing operation.

Mixer Volume

The mixer must allow sufficient space for dilation of the bed. Overfilling reduces the efficiency and may prevent mixing entirely.

Mixing Mechanism

The mixer must apply suitable shear forces to bring about local mixing and a convective movement to

ensure that the bulk of the material passes through this area.

Mixing Time

Mixing must be carried out for an appropriate time, since the degree of mixing will approach its limiting equilibrium value asymptotically. Hence, there is an optimum time for mixing for any particular situation, bearing in mind that the equilibrium condition may not represent the best mixing if segregation has occurred.

Handling the Mixed Powder

When the mixing operation is completed, the mixer should stop and the powder should be handled in such a way that segregation is minimised. Also, the vibration caused by subsequent manipulation, transport, handling or use is likely to cause segregation. Hence, a bulk powder that has been stored or transported should be re-mixed before removing a part of the contents.

Mixing Semi-solids

The mechanisms involved in mixing semi-solids depend on the character of the material, which may show considerable variation. There is very little difference between liquids at the upper end of the viscosity range and semi-solids capable of flow. Also, when a powder and liquid are mixed, at first they are likely to resemble closely the mixing of powders.

The rheological properties of non-Newtonian materials, discussed elsewhere (*see* Chapter 7), may have an important effect on the mixing operation. Thus, dilatant or plastic materials are usually much more difficult to mix than Newtonian liquids, but thixotropy may make the mixing process easier.

THEORY OF MIXING SEMI-SOLIDS

It has been found that, in mixing an insoluble powder with a liquid, a number of stages can be observed as the liquid content is increased:

Pellet and Powder State

Addition of a small amount of liquid to a bulk of dry powder causes the solid to ball up and form small pellets. The pellets are embedded in a matrix of dry powder, which has a cushioning effect and makes the pellets difficult to break up. From the overall point of view, the solid is free-flowing and the rate of homogenisation is low.

Pellet State

Further addition of liquid results in the conversion of more dry powder to pellets until, eventually, all the material is in this state. The mass has a coarse granular appearance, but the pellets do not cohere and agitation will cause aggregates to break down into smaller granules. The rate of attainment of homogenisation is even lower than in the pellet and powder stage and it is the state aimed at in moistening powders for tablet granulation.

Plastic State

As the liquid content is increased further, the character of the mixture changes markedly: aggregates of the material adhere, the granular appearance is lost, the mixture becomes more or less homogeneous and of a clay-like consistency. Plastic properties are shown, the mixture being difficult to shear, flowing at low stresses but breaking under high stresses. Homogenisation can be achieved much more rapidly than in the previous cases. This is the state obtained when making a pill-mass, for example.

Sticky State

Continual incorporation of liquid causes the mixture to attain the 'sticky' state; the appearance becomes paste-like, the surface is shiny, and the mass adheres to solid surfaces. The mass flows easily, even under low stresses, but homogeneity is attained only slowly. Kaolin Poultice exemplifies the sticky state.

Liquid State

Eventually, the addition of liquid results in a decrease of consistency until a fluid state is reached. In this state, the mixture flows under its own weight and will drain off vertical surfaces. The rate of homogenisation is rapid, and the behaviour of the mixture is described by the theory discussed in connection with liquid mixtures (*see* p. 201).

The mechanisms involved in mixing liquids with powders can give rise to situations potentially dangerous, unless controlled carefully. Consider a potent soluble substance with a small dosage that is to be granulated by the moist granulation process. If an insoluble diluent such as starch is used, the process will begin by mixing the soluble and insoluble powders together until a satisfactory degree of mixing is obtained. Small amounts of liquid are added and mixing leads to the pellet and powder state. As mixing continues, the pellets pick up soluble material on their surfaces, which will dissolve because of the higher moisture content of the pellets. This leads to a greater concentration of the soluble component in the pellets compared with the matrix of powder, and a decrease in the degree of mixing. At higher moisture contents, the homogeneity would be restored, but tablet granulation usually stops at the pellet stage. Hence, unless mixing is controlled very carefully, the degree of mixing may be very poor, and this is especially true if the liquid has been added carelessly by 'splashing in' large quantities at a time.

This means, too, that the practice of dispersing a small amount of a soluble substance in a bulk of an insoluble diluent by making a solution of the former and mixing this with the diluent needs a good deal of care. Otherwise, concentrations of the soluble material are likely to occur in the pellets.

As with the mixing of powders, it is useful to evaluate the mixing procedure that is being used, by testing with a coloured material.

MIXING IN THE PLASTIC STATE

Mixing a plastic material takes place in a manner represented diagrammatically in Fig. 18.3, having four stages that occur repeatedly. Considering a quantity of the materials represented by two black

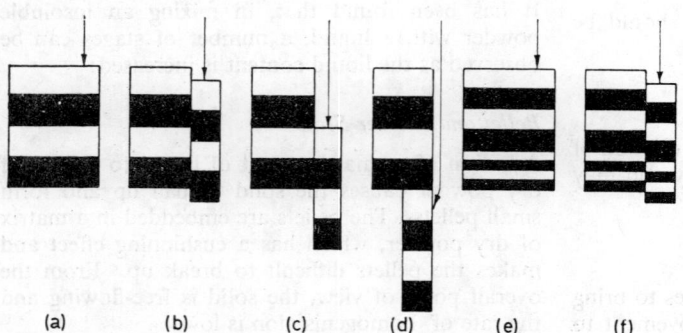

(a)   (b)   (c)   (d)   (e)   (f)   *Fig.* 18.3 Mixing of plastic solids

and two white rectangles, (Fig. 18.3(a)), the application of shear forces will cause movement of a part of the material (b). This is displaced by a shearing action (c), and the continuing forces circulate the material (d). Distortion of the mass (e), followed by further shearing (f), starts the cycle again.

ASSESSMENT OF DEGREE OF MIXING SEMI-SOLIDS

Many semi-solids form neutral mixtures with no tendency to segregation, although sedimentation may occur with suspensions in fluid media and emulsions may separate. The former may be minimised by the use of thixotropic suspending agents (see p. 126) which enable mixing to be effected readily, but the increase in consistency when mixing has ceased helps to reduce sedimentation. The bentonite gel used in Calamine Lotion, BP illustrates the method.

The discussion of scale of scrutiny and the degree of mixing in connection with powders (see p. 203) is applicable equally to semi-solids. The degree of mixing of disperse systems such as emulsions may be evaluated by globule counts or globule size distributions (see p. 81), provided that care is observed in the sampling techniques. Similar methods may be applied to dispersions of particles and a microscopic method is specified in the *British Pharmaceutical Codex*.

Mixing Equipment

The limited theoretical basis to mixing and the great variety of materials and of mixing requirements encountered in practice has given rise to the commercial development of a vast number of mixers. This leads to difficulties in classification of the machinery used for mixing and, for convenience, the mixing equipment will be divided broadly into the same three groups used when the theory of mixing was considered. It must be emphasised that these must not be regarded as clear cut divisions; for example, certain forms of paddle mixers are suitable for use with liquids, solids, and semi-solids.

Because of this variety, the mixers will be discussed in general terms only, without details of construction or dimensions. Mixers observed in practice will be found to have characters that relate them to particular groups.

LIQUID MIXERS

Shaker Mixers

Mixers in this category cause the container material to be agitated, either in an oscillatory or a rotary movement. Oscillatory movement is applicable to small-scale working only, but rotary movement can be applied to large vessels, which are usually cylindrical in shape and rotated in a similar manner to the ball mill (see p. 187). Mixing efficiency is very variable, depending on the degree of turbulence, which is affected by factors such as the properties of the liquid (viscosity, for example) or by constructional characters like the use of baffles within the vessel. For these reasons, mixers of this type find limited use in practice.

Propeller Mixers

Propeller mixers (Fig. 18.4) are probably the most widely used form of mixer for liquids. The propeller usually resembles the ordinary marine propeller in shape, is small in relation to the container (a propeller to container ratio of 20 is satisfactory for mobile liquids), and operates at high speeds, up to 8000 rev/min. The propeller accentuates the longitudinal movement of the liquid and is, therefore, most suitable when the energy imparted by the propeller to the fluid is sufficient to set up a satisfactory flow pattern and when little shear is needed. The propeller mixer is not normally effective with liquids of viscosity greater than about 5 N s/m^2, which is somewhat greater than the viscosity of glycerin or castor oil.

To avoid undesirable vortexing and aeration (air bubbles may be difficult to remove from the product and the air may encourage oxidation in some cases) the propeller should be deep in the liquid, and symmetry should be avoided. This can be done in a number of ways: for example, the propeller shaft may be off-set from the centre or mounted at an angle (a), (b); the shaft may enter the side of the vessel (c); or a vessel of a shape other than cylindrical may be used, although this is liable to give rise to 'deadspots' in corners.

Vortexing may be avoided also by the use of a *push-pull* propeller (d), in which two propellers of opposite pitch are mounted on the same shafts, so that the rotary effects are in opposite directions and cancel each other. The simplest method of preventing the formation of a vortex is to use one or more baffles, which are usually vertical strips attached to the wall of the vessel (e).

The propeller will perform most mixing duties with liquids when used correctly, but the longitudinal movement imparted by a propeller makes it the best unit to use when strong vertical currents are required, as in the suspension of solids in a liquid. It is not normally suitable when considerable shear is needed, as in emulsification.

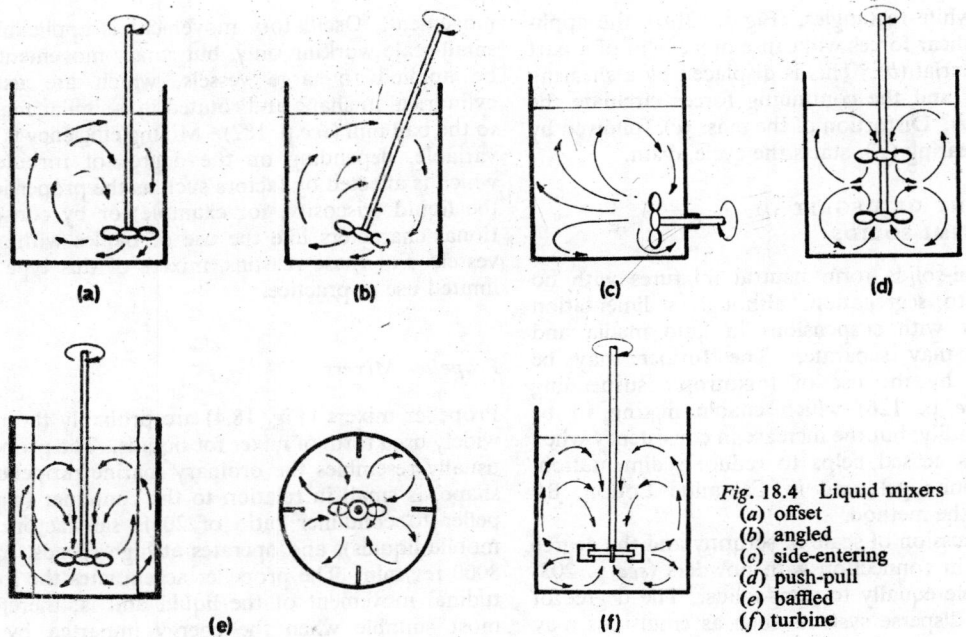

Fig. 18.4 Liquid mixers
(a) offset
(b) angled
(c) side-entering
(d) push-pull
(e) baffled
(f) turbine

Turbine Mixers

The turbine mixer (Fig. 18.4(*f*)) uses a circular disc impeller, to which are attached a number of short, vertical blades, which may be straight or curved. The turbine impeller is usually rotated at a somewhat lower speed than the propeller type and the ratio of the impeller and container diameters is usually lower also.

The blades may have a pitch giving some axial flow, but most turbine impellers have flat blades. In such cases, there is very little axial or tangential flow, the liquid being moved rapidly in a radial direction. Turbine-type impellers give rise to greater shear forces than propellers and these forces can be increased further by fitting a *diffuser ring*. This is a stationary perforated or slotted ring which surrounds the impeller, so that the discharged liquid must pass through the apertures. The diffuser reduces rotational swirling and vortexing, but is most useful in increasing shear forces.

Turbine mixers are satisfactory with mobile liquids, but, because of the greater shearing effect, they can deal with more viscous liquids than the propeller mixer, having a range up to 100 N s/m²— approximately the consistency of liquid glucose.

The absence of marked vertical flow means that the standard turbine mixer is less suitable than the propeller for suspending heavy solids, although special heads can be used. The higher shear forces and the greater viscosity range give it a special

application in the mixing of liquids that may stratify with a propeller and, particularly, in the preparation of emulsions of immiscible liquids.

Paddle Mixers

Paddle mixers use an agitator consisting, usually, of flat blades attached to a vertical shaft and rotating at a low speed of the order of 100 rev/min. For liquids of low viscosity simple flat paddles are used and the emphasis is on radial and tangential movement, with very little longitudinal effect which, however, can be increased by using paddles with a slight pitch.

Paddles for more viscous liquids generally have a number of blades, often shaped to fit closely to the surface of the vessel, avoiding 'dead-spots' and deposited solids.

Low speeds of rotation do not normally demand baffles, but at higher speeds it is necessary to use them to avoid swirling and vortexing. An alternative design for the more viscous range of liquids is the *planetary motion mixer*, which has a smaller paddle that rotates on its own axis, but travels, also, in a circular path round the mixing vessel. Thus, the term 'planetary' is analogous to the movement of a planet round the sun while rotating on its own axis. The agitator is shaped to the side of the vessel, again to eliminate 'dead-spots'. The width of the agitator is not more than half to two-thirds of the diameter of the vessel, which calls for less power than that needed for a full width central agitator, improves the circulation in the vessel, and increases mixing efficiency. A variety of agitator shapes are available according to the character and viscosity of the product.

POWDER MIXERS

Size reduction equipment (*see* Chapter 16) can be used for mixing, the attrition type of mill giving good shearing action near the moving surfaces. In general, these are not good mixers, however, because the batch is small, the material is not dilated, and there is very little convective movement. Impact mills (such as hammer mills) are effective in dealing with aggregates, but the hold-up is too small to permit bulk mixing. Such methods are useful as a preliminary, but must be followed by a general mixing process. These mills will not be considered further.

Agitator Mixers

Agitator mixers for powders can take a similar form to paddle mixers for liquids, but their efficiency is low. Planetary motion mixers are more effective, but special designs are to be preferred.

These are most commonly in the form of a trough in which an arm rotates and transmits shearing action to the particles. General mixing requires an end-to-end movement which can be obtained by fitting helical blades to the agitator, as shown in Fig. 18.5. Generally, shear forces are not high, so that aggregates may remain unbroken and the movement may encourage segregation due to density or size differences.

This type of mixer is most suitable for blending free-flowing materials, with components that are of uniform size and density. Special designs have been developed with modified agitators and vessels to overcome these limitations. One form, for example, uses an agitator resembling plough-shaped shovels which pick up the material and then spill it back, particles intermingling as the material falls. Shear

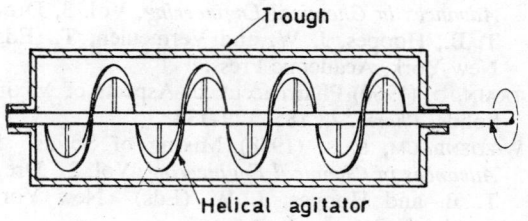

Fig. 18.5   Agitated powder mixer

forces are increased by introducing perforated baffles which act as rubbing or grinding elements and break down aggregates. Any effect due to density or size differences is eliminated by rotating the vessel at a lower speed than the shovels.

As an alternative to mechanical agitators, air movement may be used. The materials are contained in a vertical cylindrical vessel and intermittent blasts of air are admitted at the base of the cylinder, the inlets being arranged at an angle so that a spiral movement is imparted to the powder. The admission of the air must be intermittent and not continuous, otherwise the material would become fluidised and permit the segregation of denser or larger particles. The special feature of this method is the shortness of the mixing time, only a limited number of short blasts being needed. A typical procedure is to use eight air blasts, each of two seconds duration with a one second interval between, giving a total mixing time of twenty-four seconds. Air filters are needed to prevent loss of material, making the apparatus somewhat bulky, but the short mixing time means that the equipment has a high through-put.

Tumbling Mixers

In tumbling mixers, rotation of the vessel imparts movement to the materials by tilting the powder until the angle of the surface exceeds the angle of repose when the surface layers of the particles go into a slide.

Simple forms use a cylindrical vessel rotating on its horizontal axis, but shear forces are low and end-to-end movement is slight. This may be overcome by including *flights* (a form of baffle), or the shape of the vessel may be altered to avoid symmetry. Many different designs are used, such as a cylinder rotating about its mid-point on an axis at right angles to the longitudinal axis, a cube rotating about a diagonal and double-cone, V-shape, Y-shape or diamond shaped vessels, together with baffles where appropriate.

Shapes such as these give effective three-dimensional movement, and shearing takes place as the charge flows. In addition, the particles hit against the wall and are deflected, causing considerable velocity and acceleration gradients. The repeated reversal of the direction of flow makes the tumbling mixer preferable where differences in density or particle size occur.

The speed of rotation is important and it is likely that there is a critical speed, as in the ball mill (*see* p. 188). Thus, too low a speed will cause sliding only, while too high a speed will give rise to centrifuging, with cascading taking place at the correct speed.

The method of charging the load into a tumbling mixer may be important in some cases. In a simple drum mixer, for example, if the material is loaded in two layers, the diffusive movement will affect the upper layer only and no mixing will take place for some time. If the components are loaded side-by-side, mixing starts immediately, the ideal method being to add the ingredients together by running them into the mixer in intermingling streams.

To assist in breaking down aggregates, these mixers may incorporate an agitator within the vessel, rotating in the opposite direction or at a different speed from the shell. In this way, the advantages of the agitator and the tumbling types of mixer can be included in one piece of equipment.

MIXERS FOR SEMI-SOLIDS

Mixers for semi-solids may be divided into three main groups:

Agitator Mixers

These are similar in principle to the agitator mixers used for liquids and for powders, indeed the planetary motion mixer is often used for semi-solids. Mixers designed specifically for semi-solids are usually of heavier construction to handle materials of greater consistency. The agitator arms are designed to give a pulling and kneading action and the shape and movement is such that material is cleared from all sides and corners of the mixing vessel.

One form in common use for handling semi-solids of plastic consistency is known as the *sigma-arm mixer*, since the mixer uses two mixer blades, the shape of which resembles the Greek letter, sigma. The two blades rotate towards each other and operate in a mixing vessel which has a double trough shape, each blade fitting into a trough. The two blades rotate at different speeds, one usually about twice the speed of the other, resulting in a lateral pulling of the material and division into the two troughs, while the blade shape and difference in speed causes end-to-end movement. Being of sturdy construction and high power, this form of mixer can handle even the heaviest plastic materials, and products such as pill masses, tablet granule masses, and ointments are mixed readily (*see* Fig. 19.7).

One of the problems encountered in the mixing of semi-solids is the entrainment of air. The sigma-arm mixer can be enclosed and operated under reduced pressure, which is an excellent method for avoiding entrainment of air and may assist in minimising decomposition of oxidisable materials, but it must be used with caution if the mix contains volatile ingredients.

As with many other mixers, the vessel is jacketed for heating or cooling and, in this case, the blades can be hollow for the same purpose. This can be very useful in practice, since some semi-solids may be reduced in viscosity by heating, while with other materials it may be necessary to dissipate the heat resulting from the energy put into the mixing process.

Shear Mixers

Once again, machines designed for size reduction (*see* p. 187) can be used for mixing (e.g. roller mills) but although shear forces are good, the general mixing efficiency is poor.

Rotary forms may be used and the *colloid mill* has a stator and a rotor with conical working surfaces. The rotor works at speeds of the order of 3000 to 15 000 rev/min and the clearance can be adjusted between 50 and 500 μm. A roughly mixed suspension or dispersion is introduced through a funnel and is thrown out between the working surfaces by centrifugal force.

Ultrasonic Mixers

An effective method for dealing with certain forms of mixing problems is to subject the material to ultrasonic vibration. This has a special application in mixing in the preparation of emulsions and is discussed in that connection (*see* p. 85).

MATERIALS OF CONSTRUCTION

No reference has been made to the materials used for the construction of mixers. In practice, any material of sufficient strength and corrosion resistance may be used, but stainless steel is favoured for most pharmaceutical applications. Monel metal is a suitable alternative if ferrous metals are to be avoided.

BIBLIOGRAPHY

FOWLER, H. W. (1961) Liquid Mixers. *Manf. Chem.*, **32**, 490–494. Powder Mixers. *ibid.*, **33**, 5–11. Mixers for Semi-solids. *ibid.*, **33**, 104–109.

HYMAN, D. (1962) Mixing and Agitation. In *Advances in Chemical Engineering*, Vol. 3, Drew, T. B., Hoopes, J. W. and Vermeulen, T. (Eds). New York, Academic Press.

TRAIN, D. (1960) Pharmaceutical Aspects of Mixing Solids, *Pharm. J.*, **185**, 129–134.

WIEDENBAUM, S. S. (1958) Mixing of Solids. In *Advances in Chemical Engineering*, Vol. 2. Drew, T. B. and Hoopes, J. W. (Eds). New York, Academic Press.

19

Powder Flow and Compaction

BECAUSE of the popularity of compressed tablets and capsules as unit dose forms the flow and compaction of powdered materials are operations of considerable importance in pharmaceutical manufacturing. As it is both convenient and logical to consider tablet manufacture as an operation involving both the flow and compression of powders and granules, this chapter will open with an account of the production of compressed tablets.

Compressed Tablets

These are small compressed masses containing a medicament or medicaments, officially circular in shape. They may be flat or bi-convex. In most instances they contain additional substances necessary for their manufacture, disintegration, or appearance.

The manufacture of compressed tablets for medicinal use dates back to the first half of last century, when, in 1843, a Mr Brockedon took out a patent for 'shaping pills, lozenges, and black lead by pressure dies'. The general manufacture of compressed tablets, however, assumed considerable proportions only at the beginning of this century, when many new machines were devised and a considerable amount of investigation into methods of preparation was carried out.

Today, the use of medicinal tablets is very extensive, as they have largely replaced powders and cachets. In addition, many formulae, formerly dispensed as pills, are now dispensed in tablet form.

The following types of compressed tablets are in use for medicinal purposes—

1. Tablets that disintegrate readily when swallowed; e.g. Aspirin Tablets. In such cases fairly rapid absorption is required.
2. 'Lozenge' tablets. These do not disintegrate readily and are intended for slow solution in the mouth, usually to produce a local action on the throat.
3. Tablets to be dissolved in water for administration, either:
   (a) orally, or
   (b) by external application, or
   (c) by parenteral injection.

The term 'Solution-tablet' or 'Solvella' is used in the *British Pharmaceutical Codex* to designate a tablet that is to be dissolved in water to form a solution for external use.

4. Tablets that are to be chewed. These include Aluminium Hydroxide Tablets, in which mastication ensures thorough breaking up of the mass, and diffusion of the antacid, which acts mainly by adsorption. Also included in this group are Phenolphthalein Tablets, since this substance is absorbed mainly in the mouth.
5. Buccal tablets are placed in the buccal pouch where they dissolve or disintegrate slowly and are absorbed directly without passing into the alimentary canal. Certain steroids are presented in this way; e.g. Ethisterone Tablets.
6. Sublingual tablets to be placed under the tongue. where they dissolve or disintegrate quickly and are absorbed directly without passing into the alimentary tract. Glyceryl Trinitrate Tablets are used in this way. The BP states that 'they dissolve slowly in the mouth'. The USP XVIII gives a disintegration time of 2 minutes.
7. Implants. These may be made by heavy compression but are normally made by fusion. They are inserted subcutaneously by means of a minor surgical operation and are slowly absorbed. They are packed singly in sterile containers. Official examples are Deoxycortone Acetate Implants and Testosterone Implants.

THE COMPRESSION PROCESS

The compression of medicinal materials into tablets is normally carried out by means of a machine that stamps out the tablets in a die between punches. For reasons that will be discussed later it is necessary to prepare the material in the form of small granules.

Before dealing with this and other aspects of tablet manufacture, it is helpful to have a clear idea of the actual compression process. This can perhaps best be obtained by considering the construction and operation of the tablet machines in common use.

Hand Tablet Machines

A typical hand tablet machine is shown in Fig. 19.1. It is operated by turning the driving wheel manually, but a power operated model is available. The machine incorporates a single punch and die assembly shown in section in Fig. 19.2. The compression cycle can be traced easily by reference to Fig. 19.3, the stages of which are as follows.

1. On turning the driving wheel (clearly seen in Fig. 19.1), the upper punch rises and the hopper rotates on its swivel nut until it is over the die.

2. The lower punch then drops to a position set by the capacity regulating screw. This 'depth of fill' governs the tablet weight. Raising the bottom punch decreases the volume of granules required to fill the die and vice versa (Figs. 19.2, 19.3, 19.4A). To set the machine initially, the operator fills a quantity of granules equal to the tablet weight into

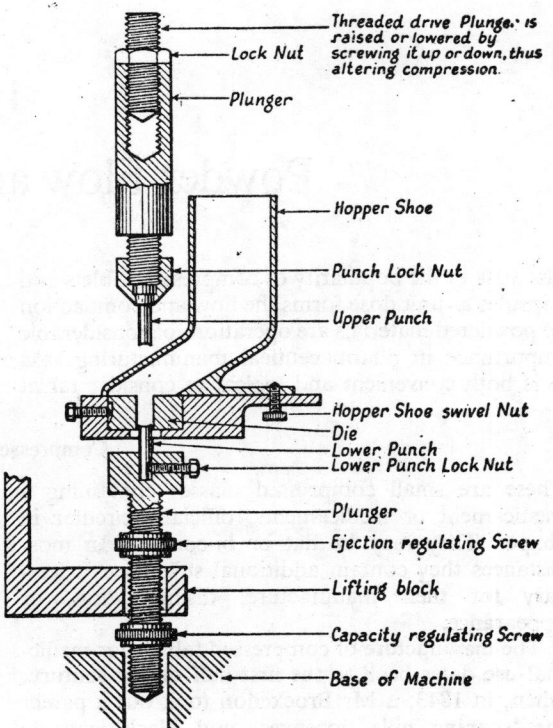

Fig 19.2 Diagram of part of a single-punch hand tablet machine

the die, with the bottom punch in its lowest possible position. On turning the driving wheel slowly the bottom punch moves upwards and pushes the granules flush with the die surface. The capacity regulating screw is then set so that it rests on the base of the machine. In subsequent cycles this setting will then ensure that the bottom punch always drops to its correct level.

3. The hopper shoe moves aside leaving the die filled with granules flush with the die surface. The bottom punch remains stationary while the top punch descends compressing the granules into a tablet (Fig. 19.4B). The degree of compression, and hence the hardness of the tablet, can be varied by screwing down the top punch in its plunger. When well screwed down the top punch will enter the die for a greater distance and compress the granules into a smaller volume. The compression should be adjusted until a tablet of adequate hardness and mechanical strength is produced, but too much compression may cause the machine to stall or the tablet to fail the test for disintegration (p. 221). Note that the degree of compression will not affect the tablet weight since this is fixed solely by the volume of granules contained in the die.

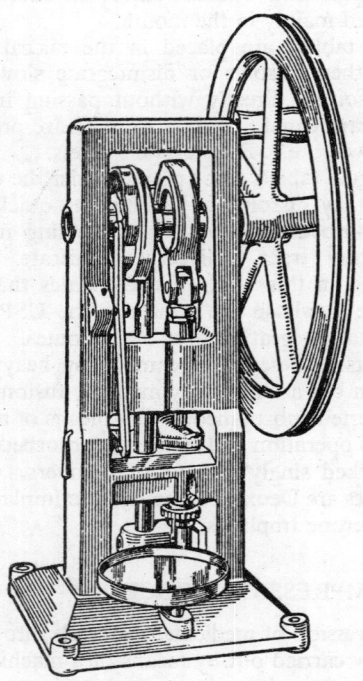

Fig. 19.1 Hand-operated tablet machine
The capacity regulating screw is concealed by the circular tray

(*Courtesy Manesty Machines Ltd*)

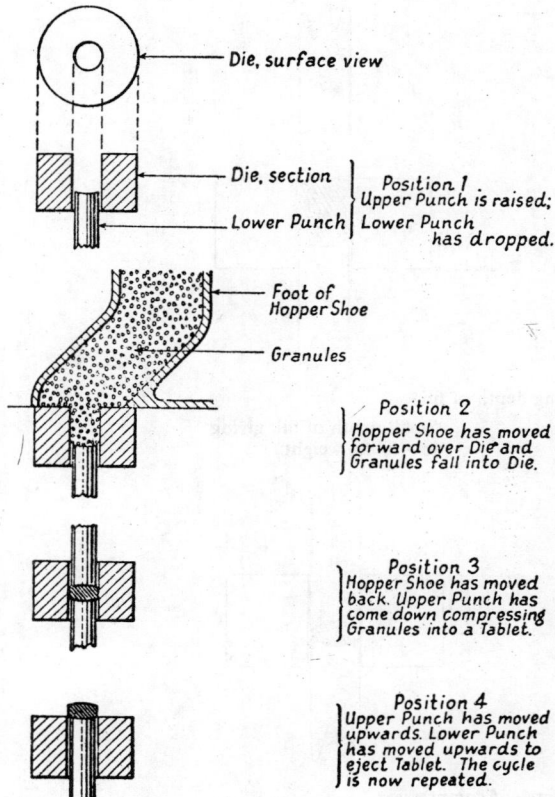

Position 1.
Upper Punch is raised;
Lower Punch has dropped.

Die, surface view

Die, section

Lower Punch

Foot of Hopper Shoe

Granules

Position 2
Hopper Shoe has moved forward over Die and Granules fall into Die.

Position 3
Hopper Shoe has moved back. Upper Punch has come down compressing Granules into a Tablet.

Position 4
Upper Punch has moved upwards. Lower Punch has moved upwards to eject Tablet. The cycle is now repeated.

Fig. 19.3   Movements involved in compression

4. The upper punch rises clear of the die and the lower punch also rises to eject the tablet. The ejection regulating screw is set to ensure that the bottom punch rises flush with the die surface. Thus, it completely ejects the tablet but does not foul the hopper shoe as it rotates over the die to knock the finished tablet aside.

5. The bottom punch falls, the die refills with granules and the whole cycle is repeated.

Some slight adjustment to the compression and tablet weight may be required at intervals when a large batch of tablets is prepared. This variation may be due to a change in packing arrangement leading to a variation in the weight of granules filling the die (p. 226) or to segregation occurring in the hopper (p. 227).

Rotary Type Tablet Machines

The single punch tablet machine, even if power operated, has an output seldom exceeding 100 tablets a minute. Although this may seem large, it is a quite inadequate rate when long runs involving millions of tablets are contemplated. The majority of tablet machines to be found in pharmaceutical factories are therefore of the much faster rotary type which can have outputs of up to 1500 tablets a minute.

A photograph of a typical modern rotary machine is shown in Fig. 19.5. The essential feature is the circular rotating head carrying a number of punch and die assemblies and constructed in three sections:
(*a*) an upper part carrying the upper punches,
(*b*) a central part carrying the dies, and
(*c*) a lower part carrying the lower punches.

All are arranged around the circumference of the rotating head. Portions of the stems of the upper and lower punches can be seen clearly in Fig. 19.5. Note the large hopper which can contain a large quantity of granules and give an extended run before refilling is required. The hopper delivers the granules to the 'feed frame' placed over the central part containing the dies. The object of the feed frame is to confine the granules in position immediately over the die track. As the head revolves, the dies come under the feed frame in succession, and are filled. Compression is effected by the upper and lower punches passing between rollers that gradually compress the granules.

The cycle of events in one revolution of the rotary head is shown diagrammatically in Fig. 19.6, where the circular punch track is shown 'opened out'.

An overload mechanism is incorporated in these machines to 'cushion' excess strain if foreign matter enters the dies or excessive pressure is applied.

The Preparation of Material for Tabletting

It will be evident that successful tabletting depends largely on a uniform flow of material from the hopper to the die. Some factors governing the flow of powders will be considered later but it may be stated now that very few powders will flow sufficiently well to make successful tablets unless special means are employed. For this and other reasons (summarised in Table 19.1) it is normally necessary to convert such powders into spherical granules 1 to 2 mm in diameter. The process is known as granulation, three methods of which are in common use, namely—
(*a*) dry granulation,
(*b*) moist granulation, and
(*c*) granulation by preliminary compression.

DRY GRANULATION

Some substances can be purchased in the form of small crystals, or as larger crystals that can easily be

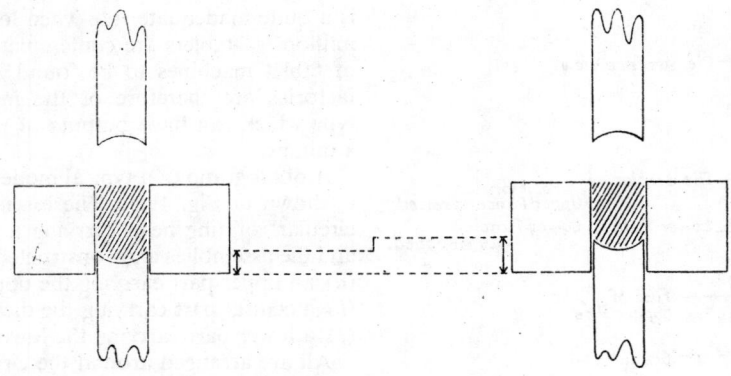

Fig. 19.4A   Illustrating depth of fill

Large depth of fill, giving   Small depth of fill, giving
high tablet weight   low tablet weight

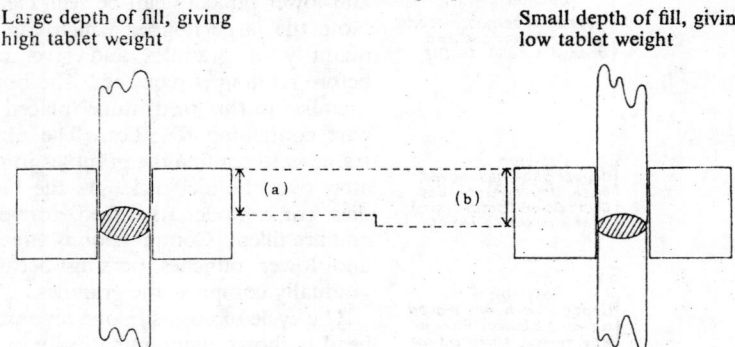

Fig. 19.4B   Illustrating degree of compression

The punch enters die by a distance (a),   Top punch enters die by a distance (b),
giving low tablet compression   giving high tablet compression

reduced to smaller size. The only preparation necessary in such cases is to crush the crystals if too large so that they just pass through a suitable sieve (No. 20 for average size tablets) and to reject any fine powder. The *British Pharmacopoeia* describes this process as dry granulation.

MOIST GRANULATION

This is by far the most common method since it is applicable to most powdered materials. It is effected by using suitable fluid granulating agents of which there are many, including water, mucilages of acacia and tragacanth, and various alcohols.

On a small scale, the powder is moistened with granulating agent to render it coherent but by no means wet. It is then passed through a suitable sieve and the sifted material, which is now in the form of granules, is dried at a temperature not exceeding 60°C.

The drying usually causes 'caking', so the mass is again passed through a sieve to break it up. If the operation is properly performed, a negligible quantity of fine powder should be present. Some of the granules may be quite small, and it is an advantage to have up to 15 per cent of this fine material present since it makes for a more uniform weight of tablet. No. 8 or 10 sieves may be used for granulation of the moistened material while the dry granules may be passed through a No. 20 sieve.

LARGE SCALE MOIST GRANULATION

This operation affords an excellent illustration of several of the unit operations described in previous chapters. It may be subdivided into the following stages.

Mixing and Granulation

Powders are mixed in one or other of the powder mixers described in Chapter 18. A Sigma arm mixer (Fig. 19.7) is a popular choice. These mixers may also be used to moisten the powders. When the mass is of suitable consistency it is transferred to a mechanical granulator which takes the place of

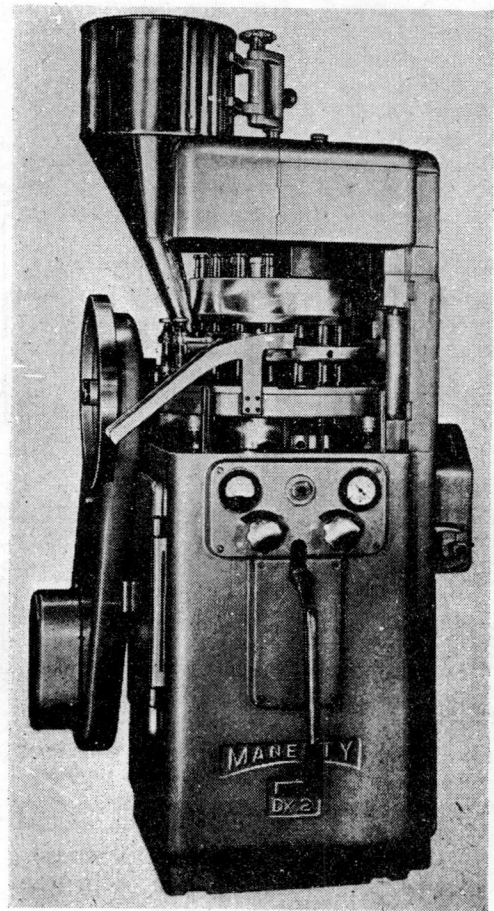

Fig. 19.5   Manesty DX2 rotary tablet machine
(*Courtesy Manesty Machines Ltd*)

advantages of this type over the cabinet dryers formerly used extensively are discussed on p. 276.

There is some attrition of the granules in this type of dryer but as each granule is 'cushioned' from its neighbours by the air flow through the bed, the effect is not too serious. Nevertheless, some fine powder is formed and has caused dust explosions on a number of occasions. It is essential to earth the dryer to prevent build-up of static charge sufficient to produce a spark that could ignite the dust/air mixture.

An interesting extension of the fluidised-bed technique has been reported by Scott *et al.* (1964). They describe a pilot scale installation where the operations of mixing, granulation, and drying are all performed in sequence in the same fluidised bed. Commercial equipment using this principle has recently become available. For an excellent account of the use of fluidised beds in the pharmaceutical industry see Ridgway and Segovia (1966).

Final Additions

Any other substances required may be added at this stage by gently tumbling them with the dry granules in a drum mixer.

GRANULATION BY PRELIMINARY COMPRESSION

'Double compression', 'precompression', and 'slugging' are terms also used to describe this process. It is done by first compressing the dry powder into large tablets or 'slugs', as they are called, by means of a tablet machine adapted for powder feeding. The slugs are then broken up into suitable granules in an oscillating granulator.

It has been said that fine powders do not flow well enough to make tablets, but for this purpose the tablets need not be perfect so long as they are hard. The use of large dies and punches assists in feeding the powder to the die, and to ensure uniform feeding excess powder is fed into the die and the surplus scraped away by means of a mechanical device. Compression is slow to allow entrapped air to escape. By this process two possible causes of decomposition are avoided, namely moisture and heat, and there is little loss of volatile matter if this is present.

It may occur to the student to enquire if the process could not be improved so as to produce an acceptable tablet directly. The F. J. Stokes Corporation has in fact produced a suitable machine. The method involves the force feeding of powder into the dies of a rotary-type tablet machine by means of a special shoe which performs a horizontal orbital

the sieves used in small-scale work. The oscillating granulator (Fig. 19.8) consists of a hopper leading to a chamber containing a powerful oscillating rotor which forces the material through a screen. Screens are of various sizes, No. 8 mesh being commonly used. All parts coming into contact with the materials are of stainless steel. The comminuting machine, Fig. 19.9, works on a different principle. It consists of a chamber through which passes an axle carrying a number of swinging blades, sharp on one edge and flat on the other. The moist mass is cut up into granules by the sharp edge of the blades and falls through a screen at the base of the chamber.

Drying of Wet Granules

The use of a fluidised-bed-type dryer for this purpose is now almost universal (Chapter 24). The

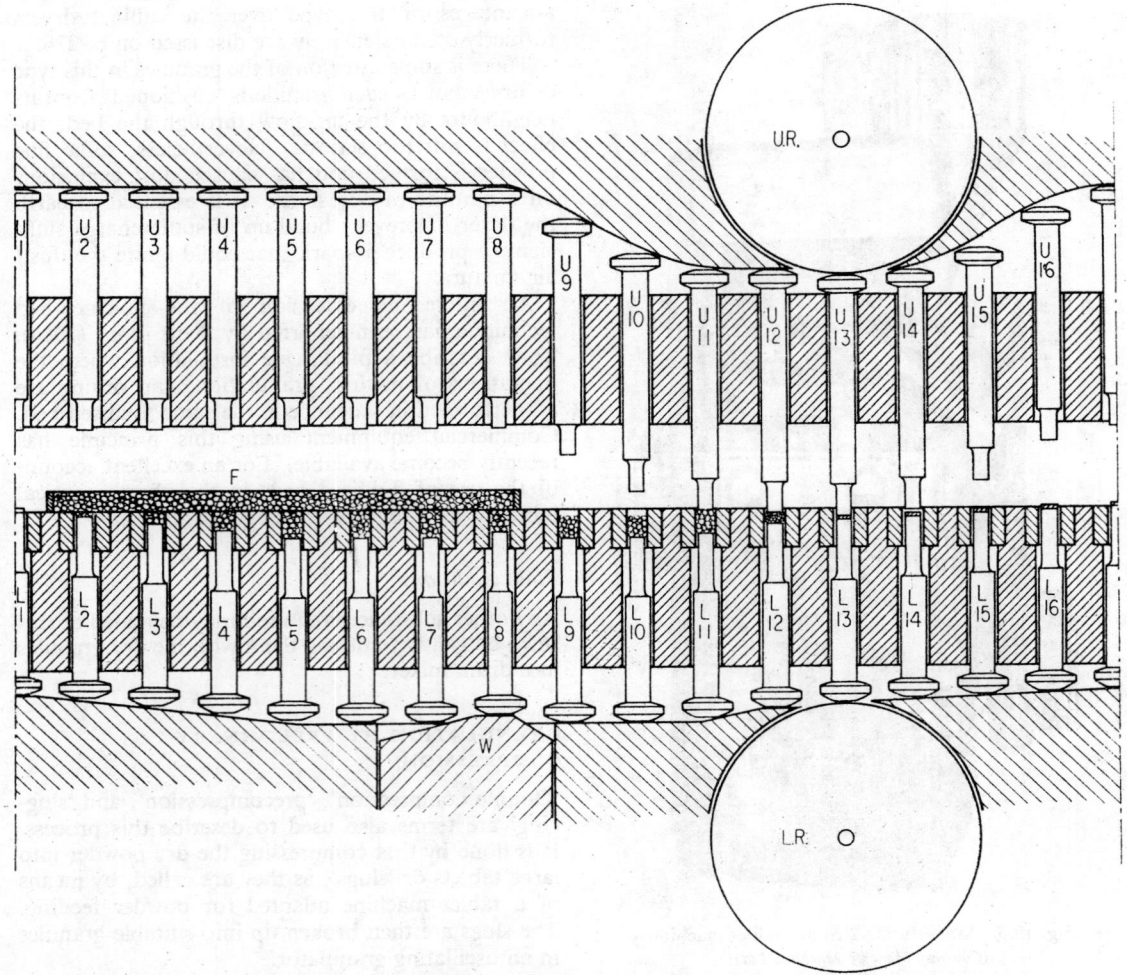

Fig. 19.6   Diagram of punch tracks of rotary tablet machine opened out to show cycle of one revolution

U.R. = upper roller   W = capacity adjuster
L.R. = lower roller   F = feed frame with granules

(1) U1 to U8 — upper punches in raised position
(2) L1 — lower punch at top position; tablet ejected
(3) L2 to L7 — lower punches dropping to lowest position and filling die with granules to an overfill at L7
(4) L8 — lower punch raised to expel excess granules giving correct capacity
(5) U9 to U12 — upper punches lowering to enter die at U12

(6) L9 to L12 — synchronised with U9 to U12 lower punches rising prior to compression
(7) L13 and U13 — upper and lower punches pass between rollers, and granules are compressed to a tablet
(8) U14 to U16 — lower punch rising to completely eject tablet at L16
(9) U1 and L1 — beginning of cycle

movement over the die track. This action develops sufficient pressure to force the powder into the dies and produce the required 'packing density'. The necessity for this is explained further on p. 227.

OTHER INCLUSIONS

In addition to the medicaments and granulating agents, some other inclusions are normally required in a tablet granule formulation.

Disintegrating Agents

Tablets consisting entirely of insoluble substances would, in many cases, fail to disintegrate when swallowed. To ensure the tablet breaking up in the stomach, a disintegrating agent is used. Three types are in use—

1. Substances that swell up on contact with moisture
2. Substances that melt at body temperature.

Table 19.1

Fine powder	*Granules*
1. Fine Powder does not normally flow evenly from the hopper into the die, resulting in uneven tablet weight.	Granules flow and pack down easily (p. 227). This leads to much less variation in tablet weight.
2. A powder containing two or more components may segregate (p. 205). The denser components or those of smaller particle size separate to the bottom of the hopper, the effect often being aggravated by the vibration of the tablet machine.	Granules are of uniform size and composition if properly prepared. Segregation is not serious, although a certain proportion of fine material cannot be avoided. This does not normally exceed 15%.
3. Pressure transmission through a powder mass is very poor due to low packing density (*see* p. 227). Therefore particles do not 'knit' together, unless special methods are employed (p. 215).	Granules pack down rapidly and readily transmit the compression forces. Bond to form a strong tablet.
4. Fine powder tends to blow out of the die at the top and to seep downwards round the stem of the lower punch, causing sticking.	The granules being heavier do not blow out of the die and do not clog the lower punch.

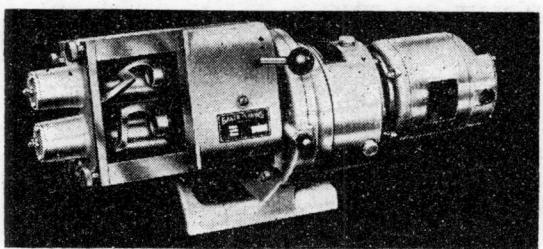

Fig. 19.7 Laboratory mixer
(*Courtesy Baker Perkins Ltd*)

3. Substances that react, with effervescence, on contact with moisture.

Starches are examples of the first type, maize and potato starch being commonly used. Starches are by far the most common type of disintegrant.

Cocoa butter, which melts below body temperature, is an example of the second type. This is used in the form of a solution in ether.

Disintegration may be effected by adding a small quantity of tartaric acid to half the material and a chemical equivalent amount of sodium bicarbonate to the remainder. The two parts are granulated and dried separately, and then mixed before compression. The effervescence occurring on contact with moisture causes disintegration. Wetting agents may also be used to hasten disintegration. Cooper and Brecht (1957) give an account of the use of various surfactants for this purpose.

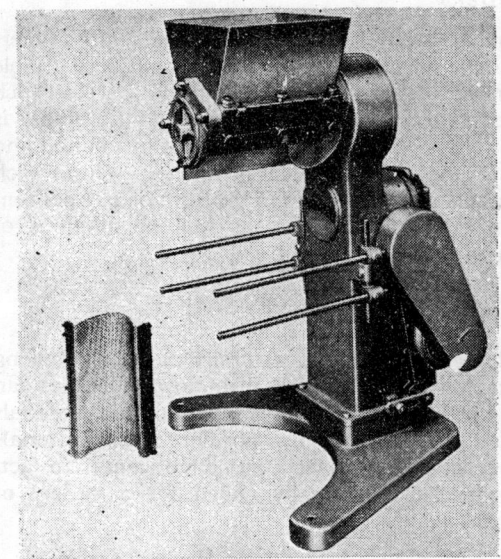

Fig. 19.8 Oscillating granulator
(*Courtesy Manesty Machines Ltd*)

DILUENTS

If the weight of medicament in each tablet is very small, a quantity of inert substance such as lactose is added to increase the bulk. Tablets are required to be of minimal size.

The selection of a suitable diluent is generally left to the pharmacist but the Pharmacopoeia gives

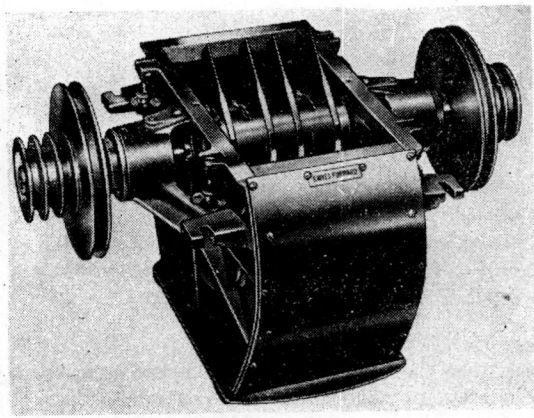

Fig. 19.9 Comminuting machine
(Courtesy Manesty Machines Ltd)

the formula for one diluent, namely, chocolate basis.

BINDERS

Some substances when granulated with water, alcohol, or other simple solvents produce friable granules which easily crumble to powder. In such cases a 'binder' is used. Normally, the binder is included with the granulating agent in solution and this is the most satisfactory method. Gums such as acacia and tragacanth in the form of a 20 per cent solution are often used, as well as solutions of gelatin and sucrose.

LUBRICANTS

Although granules are naturally more free flowing than powdered material, their flow properties can be improved by coating them with certain materials added in the form of fine powder. These materials are often known collectively as lubricants. In fact, a lubricant is normally added for a variety of reasons—

1. To improve the flow properties.
2. To reduce friction between the tablet and the die wall so that the ejection is facilitated.
3. Often to improve the bonding of the granules so as to form a better and stronger tablet.
4. To reduce the tendency for the granules to adhere to the punch surface. If this occurs the tablet may well have a pitted appearance. This fault is known as 'picking'. Strictly the 'lubricant' is functioning as an anti-adherent if it prevents this occurring.

Some authorities prefer to use the term 'glidant' for an inclusion that improves granule flow properties and to reserve the term 'lubricant' for an inclusion that serves the other purposes. There is some justification for this since a substance such as powdered talc is a good glidant but a poor lubricant.

Lubricants are usually added, in a proportion of 1 or 2 per cent, to the dried granules by gently tumbling them together in a drum-type mixer. The aim is to coat the granule surface lightly without causing the granule to disintegrate. Provided the powder is fine enough it is adsorbed on the granules and there is no tendency to segregate.

The most popular lubricants are stearates of divalent metals such as calcium and magnesium. Other long chain fatty acids and their salts are almost as good as the stearates. Other substances in common use include powdered talc (despite its rather low efficiency), liquid paraffin, and boric acid. Boric acid, because it is completely soluble, is a useful lubricant for solution tablets.

In recent years a good deal has been discovered about the mode of action of lubricants and glidants. This work is briefly discussed on page 231.

TABLET COATING

There are two methods in common use—

1. Pan coating
2. Press coating

In addition, fluidised bed techniques have some application, particularly in the process of film coating described below.

PAN COATING

Pan coating of tablets has developed from the much older process of pill coating (Gunn and Carter, 1965). Sutaria (1968) has given a detailed account of sugar coating, which is the traditional process. Practice may vary slightly but usually the coating is carried out in a rotating, tilted, copper pan in which the cascading tablets can be treated with the coating materials (Fig. 19.10). The following stages may be involved.

Sealing

This is sometimes necessary to 'waterproof' the tablets against the aqueous syrups used later. A solution of a resin such as shellac, or a synthetic acrylic in a suitable solvent, is added to the tablet mass in the pan.

Subcoating

Subcoating adds the required coat thickness by building it up with layers of a powder usually based

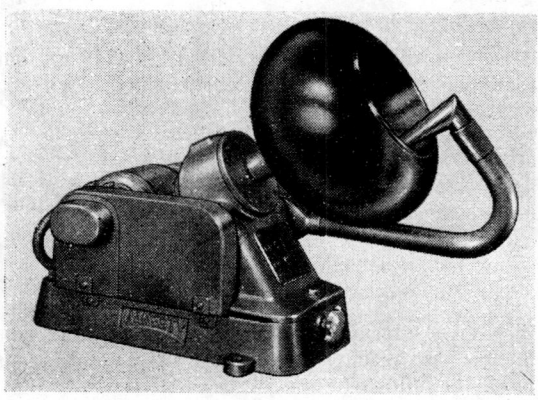

Fig. 19.10 Tablet coating pan
(Courtesy Manesty Machines Ltd)

on talc and starch. Enough syrup is added to render
the tablet mass tacky. The dusting powder adheres
to the moist tablets, and drying is speeded up by
means of a current of warm air blown into the pan.
Alternate quantities of a 'syrup' (such as gelatin
solution) and powder are added until the coating is
built up to the required thickness. Usually the
weight of the tablet has been doubled at this stage.

Smoothing

Towards the end of the process a smooth surface is
ensured by adding thinner syrups without dusting
powder. Colouring may be added to the syrups
both now and during the preceding stage.

Polishing

A special polishing pan lined with wax may be used
to polish the coated tablets but often a dispersion of
polishing wax or resin is simply added to the tablets
in the original pan.

Tablets having a pronounced 'edge' (Fig. 19.11(a)) do
not cascade easily in the pan and the ideal shape is
elliptical (Fig. 19.11(b)). The punch profile required
to form tablets of this shape has a thin edge and
wears very rapidly. In practice, a compromise shape
is used (Fig. 19.11(c)) with a very short edge.

Traditional sugar coating is still very largely an
art. The experienced operator can judge the correct
rate at which to apply syrup and powder, when to
employ warm air and for how long, plus a host of
other details that can be acquired only by experience.
Sutaria (1968) quotes the case of an operator who
produced inferior results when the angle of tilt
of the coating pan was altered slightly. The process
thus requires constant attention for up to three days,
and attempts have been made to automate it.

An installation employing a spraying nozzle to
add the syrup with programmed spraying and drying
times is now available commercially and has been
described recently (Anon., 1967). The saving in
time and labour is very appreciable.

FILM COATING

As an alternative to sugar coating, tablets may be
protected by means of a thin film of a suitable
material laid down by a similar process. Many of
these coatings are based on cellulose such as carboxy-
methyl cellulose or on polymers such as polyvinyl
pyrrolidone. They are added as a solution in a
suitable solvent, which may pose difficulties if it is
toxic or inflammable. However, the process is much
quicker than sugar coating and is gaining in popularity. Enteric coatings, usually based on cellulose
acetate phthalate, may be built up in this way.

Tablets suspended in a fluidised bed were successfully spray-coated by Singiser and Lowenthal (1961)
and commercial equipment based on this method is
available.

PRESS COATING

The principle of this process is that a layer of dry
coating material is pressed on to a pre-formed
tablet. This is done by placing the tablet to be
coated (the core tablet) in the die of a tablet machine,
in which there is a layer of coating material in
granular form, covering the tablet with another
layer of coating granules, and compressing to form
a skin around the tablet.

The idea is not new, a British patent having been
taken out as early as 1896. Whitehouse (1954) gives
an account of some of the earlier processes.

Two types of press coating machines in use in this
country are the Prescoter introduced by Evans
Medical Supplies Ltd, of Speke, Liverpool (Whitehouse, 1954) and the DryCota of Manesty Machines
Ltd, also of Speke, Liverpool (Anon., 1955).

In the Prescoter, core tablets are fed from a
hopper to the dies of a press coating machine in
which there is already a layer of coating granules.

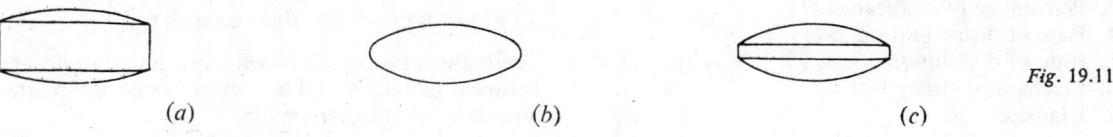

Fig. 19.11

(a)   (b)   (c)

i

A mechanical device centres the tablets, and another layer of coating granules is introduced above them. The punches then compress the coating on to the tablets. It is claimed that an interval between preparing the core tablet and applying the coat is desirable for the following reasons—

A day, or two, is required for the core tablet to attain stable dimensions.

Export tablets may require a sub-coat of varnish before applying the final dry coat.

The core tablet may be analysed and 'passed' before coating, thus avoiding possible waste.

In the DryCota, two rotary tablet machines are used side by side, one to make the core tablets and the other to apply the coating. The coating process follows immediately after the core tablet compression. It is claimed that by this method contamination is avoided, and that soft core tablets can be used. A transfer mechanism, situated between the two machines, carries the core tablets to the coating machine. This mechanism consists of radially disposed fingers each supporting a transfer cup and locating with the dies of each machine. The newly compressed core tablet is picked up by a finger and carried to the coating machine. The transfer unit and rotating turret of the coating machine travel at the same speed, and for a short period each finger is immediately over a die. During this time the finger places the tablet in the centre of the die, which already contains a layer of coating granules. A second layer is now added and the coating is compressed on the tablet.

MULTILAYER TABLETS

This type of tablet, illustrated in Fig. 19.12, has increased in popularity in recent years. Two and

Fig. 19.12   Multilayer tablets

three layer tablets are commonly made. The process in use at Wyeth Laboratories Incorporated is briefly as follows (Anon., 1968).

The tablets are prepared on a rotary-type machine with separate hoppers and feed frames for the different constituents in granular form. The first layer of granules is fed into the dies and undergoes preliminary compaction at a very low compaction pressure. As the turret rotates, granules for the second layer flow on top of the first layer and, again, they are lightly precompressed. The process can be repeated if a third layer is to be added. A final hard compression gives a tablet with a very sharp demarcation line between the layers.

One of the big practical problems of this technique lies in preventing intermingling of the different granules on the die table. Excess granules are scraped off by means of a table scraper and any that escape its action are removed by an air suction device.

Standardisation of Compressed Tablets

Early methods of standardisation were made, or omitted, at the discretion of the maker, and in many cases no serious attempt was made to ensure uniformity. The result was that many tablets on the market were extremely unsatisfactory; the weight, size, shape, and rate of disintegration varying considerably in batches of tablets from different manufacturers. The *British Pharmacopoeia 1932, Addendum VII 1945*, introduced official standards.

The following variables have been investigated by various workers with a view to standardisation—

1. Shape
2. Weight of tablet
3. Percentage of medicament
4. Rate of disintegration
5. Rate of dissolution
6. Mechanical strength
7. Diameter

1. SHAPE

It should be noted that shape is defined in the *Pharmacopoeia* as 'circular with either flat or biconvex faces'.

2. WEIGHT

Small variations in the weights of individual tablets are inevitable and admissible, and, accordingly, accepted limits are officially specified for uncoated tablets.

The *Pharmacopoeia* gives details of the permitted deviation which depends on the size of the tablet and the number taken for the test.

3. PERCENTAGE OF MEDICAMENT

There are various reasons why a variation of dosage between individual tablets must occur no matter how carefully they are made.

1. Even if the mix is perfectly random there is always a variation between samples taken from the bulk of the powder. The tablet granules made from this powder must therefore also vary in a similar manner.
2. Variation in tablet weight as explained above.

In addition, errors due to the limitation of accuracy of the assay process and permitted variation in the purity of the drug must be allowed for. The *Pharmacopoeia* therefore allows some deviation on either side of the stated contents of medicament. Usually the percentage of medicament when determined on a bulk sample of 20 tablets is required to lie between 90 and 110 per cent of the stated value. These limits may be widened if less than 20 tablets are available for assay.

Train (1960) has pointed out that the official requirements allow considerably more than ±10 per cent variation in individual tablets. In a sample of 20, a gross deficiency in some tablets may be compensated by a large excess in others so that the bulk sample may still comply. He quotes digoxin tablets, where a possible ±40 per cent variation in individual tablets may occur.

4. RATE OF DISINTEGRATION

Tablets containing an insoluble or slightly insoluble ingredient may be slow to disintegrate when swallowed, and the inclusion of disintegrants such as starch to hasten the process has been noted previously. It is possible for a badly formulated tablet to pass through the alimentary tract completely whole and thus be useless therapeutically. To guard against this possibility the pharmacopoeial requirements may include a test for the rate of disintegration. For obvious reasons the test is waived for lozenge type, chewing, buccal, and sublingual tablets (p. 211). If the medicament is soluble, disintegration in solution is usually complete and rapid, and this type of tablet is also exempted from the test. There are, however, special cases such as sodium citrate tablets used for citrating milk, where an unusually rapid disintegration rate is required. A disintegration time of three minutes is therefore laid down for this tablet.

Tablets may remain in the stomach for four hours or more, but the *Pharmacopoeia* normally requires them to disintegrate within fifteen minutes, when tested as described below. Some 'difficult' tablets may be allowed a longer time; e.g. phenobarbitone tablets are considered satisfactory if they disintegrate within thirty minutes.

THE OFFICIAL DISINTEGRATION TEST

This test is standardised in the following ways—

(*a*) Water is used at around body temperature. It has been found that there is little or no advantage in using simulated gastric juice.
(*b*) A regular degree of movement is involved.
(*c*) If necessary, a slight pressure is applied to the tablets.
(*d*) Disintegration is judged on final particle size.
(*e*) A time limit is involved.

The essential apparatus is a glass or plastic cylinder closed at its lower end by a No. 10 mesh rustless wire gauze. This tube is suspended in water at 35 to 39°C, the temperature being maintained thermostatically (Fig. 19.13(*a*)). The tube is raised and lowered at a constant rate through a standard distance. Commercial equipment complying with the BP requirements can be purchased.

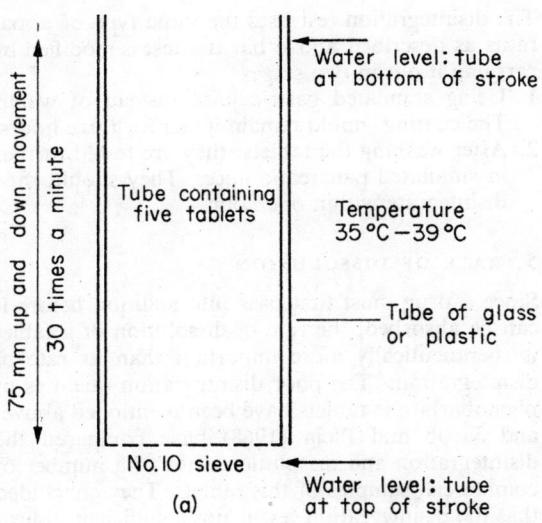

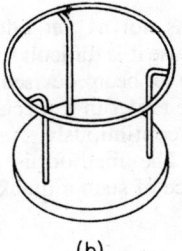

Fig. 19.13

(*a*) Diagram of disintegration tests
(*b*) Guided disc

At the highest point the wire gauze just breaks the surface of the water, thus giving a turbulent effect, and at the lowest point the top of the tube is still above the surface of the water. Five tablets are used for the test, when they should disintegrate and pass through the sieve within the official time.

If the tablets do not disintegrate readily, the test is repeated using a plastic disc which imparts a slight pressure to the tablet. This disc is kept horizontal in the tube by a guide ring supported on three pins (Fig. 19.13(*b*)). The disc assists in breaking up a persistent 'hard core' which is often noted. A possible explanation for this core is given on page 232.

Disintegration Test for Enteric-coated Tablets

These tablets are required to pass through the stomach unchanged and to disintegrate in the intestine. They are usually prepared by coating the tablets with a film of resistant material (p. 219).

The disintegration test uses the same type of apparatus as described above but the test is modified by carrying it out in two stages.
1. Using simulated gastric juice instead of water. The coating should remain intact for three hours.
2. After washing the tablets, they are tested further in simulated pancreatic juice. They should then disintegrate within one hour.

5. RATE OF DISSOLUTION

Since a drug must first pass into solution before it can be absorbed, the rate of dissolution of a tablet is therapeutically more important than its rate of disintegration. The poor disintegration qualities of phenobarbitone tablets have been mentioned above, and Jacob and Plein (1968) have compared the disintegration and dissolution rates of a number of commercial samples of this tablet. They concluded that the disintegration test is not a sufficient indication of quality for this tablet and should be replaced by a dissolution test.

The *Pharmacopoeia* has not as yet adopted this type of test, perhaps because it is difficult to perform. Continuous methods have been devised whereby water is passed round the tablet in a special cell and the solution analysed continuously, usually by spectrographic means. The method is obviously dependent on the existence of such a quick and easy analytical method.

6. MECHANICAL STRENGTH

Although there are no official standards for mechanical strength of tablets, manufacturers normally employ tests to ensure that their tablets will withstand the normal risks of handling and transporting. These are either simple qualitative tests for 'wear and tear' or tests for strength, using mechanical devices of some kind. It has long been the practice to test tablets as they come off the machine by crushing them between the fingers, which can be a good guide to quality if done by an experienced operator, since it is quick and can be used immediately to correct the compression on the tablet machine.

To eliminate the personal factor, a number of methods have been adopted. They fall under three headings—

1. Tests on breaking strength.
2. Abrasion tests.
3. Penetration tests.

Tests on Breaking Strength

A hardness tester in common use designed by the Monsanto Chemical Co. Ltd, is illustrated in Fig. 19.14. In this design the tablet to be tested is placed between the spindle and anvil, and pressure is applied by turning the knurled knob just sufficiently to hold the tablet in position. The reading of the pointer on the scale is then adjusted to read zero. The pressure is then increased as uniformly as possible until the tablet breaks, when the pointer will read the pressure required to break the tablet. The 'hardness factor' is taken as the average of several determinations. The instrument does not entirely eliminate the personal factor since the pressure of setting at zero and the rate of application of pressure can vary.

More sophisticated machines are power-operated and apply the load at constant rate. Brook and Marshall (1968) have reported on four different types of tester, including the Monsanto type.

Abrasion Tests

Rolling or shaking tests of a simple empirical nature have been described by Smith (1949) and Webster and Van Abbé (1955). These consist of mechanical devices which subject the tablets to shaking or

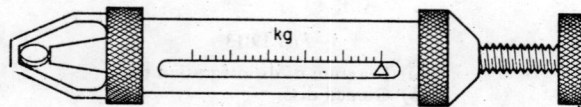

Fig. 19.14 Monsanto hardness tester

tumbling effects. After periods, the abraded material is sifted from the tablets and the percentage estimated. The speed and period of shaking or tumbling must, of course, be standardised.

An interesting point in connection with abrasion tests is the effect of tablet shape. Flat tablets with sharp edges are not so good as flat tablets with chamfered edges, and the most satisfactory shape is bi-convex.

Penetration Tests

These tests have been adapted from those in common use in the engineering industry, and Smith (1949) has described experiments with the Vickers Diamond Hardness Testing Machine. With this machine the impression made with a ball or diamond pointed indenter is measured either in area or in depth according to the type of machine. Hardness is expressed by

$$\frac{\text{applied load (in kg)}}{\text{area of indentation (in mm}^2)} = \text{hardness value}$$

7. DIAMETER

Although the *Pharmacopoeia* does not insist on a standard weight for official tablets, it nevertheless specifies their diameter. The thickness is not directly controlled, but in practice most manufacturers make uncoated tablets of thickness equal to half the diameter since this results in an elegant and pleasing shape. If the diameter and thickness are both defined, the volume and weight of tablet are obviously fixed, and there is now very little variation in the dimensions of official tablets produced by different manufacturers.

The *Pharmacopoeia* permits some slight deviation, usually ±5 per cent from the nominal diameter.

The Flow Properties of Powders and Granules

The preceding account of tablet compression has emphasised the importance of a regular flow of powder or granules from the hopper to the die of the machine. Practically every solid used in pharmacy must be handled as a powder at some stage, and this handling is greatly facilitated if the powder is free flowing. It is essential that preparations such as dusting powders flow easily, and some ways of ensuring this were considered by Gunn and Carter (1965). Enough has now been said to indicate that the factors that promote or hinder the flow of powdered material have appreciable practical importance, but it is only in recent years that they have received the attention they merit.

The study of the flow and deformation of powders is the science of powder rheology and is analogous in some respects to the rheology of liquid systems. However, since a powder mass consists of discreet particles, there is an absence of the continuity found in liquids, and the factors that influence the rheological properties of a powder mass (such as particle size, shape, and distribution) are capable of great variation. At present it is not possible to predict the flow property of powders with any certainty from measurements made on a static mass of powder but some appreciable progress has been made towards this goal.

Cohesion and Other Factors Affecting the Flow of Powders

A few powdered materials will flow easily under gravity. The sand in a domestic egg-timer is an excellent example. However, the majority of powders are not free flowing unless specially treated to make them so, and their poor flow properties may be due to one or more of the following reasons.

1. Surface forces exist between the particles, causing cohesion. Van der Waals, surface tension, and electrostatic forces are the most important. The same forces may cause the particles to adhere to the surface of the container.
2. There may be appreciable interparticulate friction especially if the particle surfaces are rough and pitted.
3. Particles may interlock causing 'bridging' and 'arching'. This is especially likely if they are of irregular shape.

These factors act to confer a certain rigidity on a powder mass that must be broken down before it will flow freely. For many powders the force of gravity is insufficient to do this, such powders being termed cohesive or sticky. Since cohesion is only one of the factors involved, the latter term is preferred. Nevertheless, cohesion predominates if the powder consists of near spherical particles which do not interlock. Fine powders are particularly cohesive.

DEFINITION AND MEASUREMENT OF COHESION

Since it is difficult, though not impossible, to measure the cohesive force existing between individual particles, cohesion is usually defined as the stress

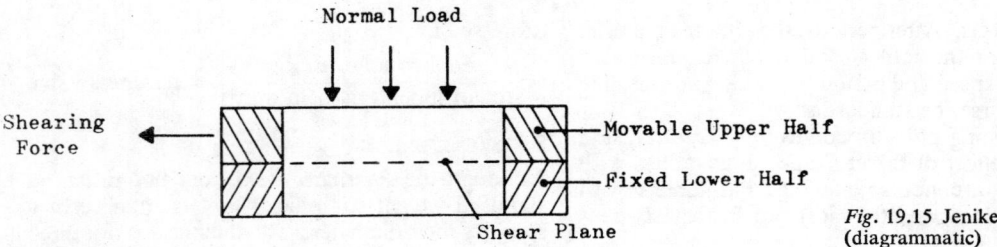

Fig. 19.15 Jenike cell
(diagrammatic)

necessary to shear a bed of the powder under conditions of zero normal load. A brief description of one method of determining this quantity will perhaps help to make this definition clear.

Measurement of Cohesion by Use of a Shear Cell

A well known type of shear cell (Jenike Cell) is shown in Fig. 19.15. The powder is packed carefully into the two segments and a lid placed within the top segment. This lid can be loaded normally with varying loads. The force required to shear the bed can then be measured. The shear stress is found by dividing this force by the cross-sectional area of the bed and will increase as the bed is compressed by increasing the normal load. This load is therefore plotted against the corresponding value of the shear stress and the plot extrapolated back to zero normal load (Fig. 19.16). The shear stress at zero normal load is by definition equal to the cohesion of the powder.

Using this type of cell, it can be shown that the cohesion of a powder bed increases as the bed packs down and consolidates due to particle rearrangement. This happens if the bed is vibrated or tapped, and the importance of packing arrangements is discussed on page 226.

Other Methods of Estimating Cohesion

The shear cell method gives a good quantitative estimation of cohesion but there are a number of qualitative tests useful on occasions. Two of these are considered below.

1. *Rate of Sieving.* The rate of sieving is markedly influenced by cohesion due to the formation of aggregates and 'bridges' over the sieve apertures. Table 19.2 gives the rate of sieving of different sized fractions of the same granular powder through a BS 16 sieve.

Table 19.2

Arithmetic mean particle diameter (μm)	Rate of sieving g/s
306	0·603
165	0·312
90	blocked

(Quoted by Jones, 1968)

One would expect the smaller size fractions to pass more easily through the mesh but marked cohesion first impedes, and finally prevents their passage through the sieve.

2. *Mobility Test.* Since fine particles are more cohesive than coarser ones, cohesion of a bulk powder can often be reduced by adding a coarser fraction to it. The mobility test consists in finding the minimum quantity of a coarse component that is required to confer free flowing properties on a cohesive powder. The test is suitable for mildly cohesive material only, otherwise an excessive proportion of coarse fraction is needed. For a good account of these and other methods see Jones (1968).

SOME FACTORS INFLUENCING THE COHESION OF POWDERS

A great many factors influence the cohesive properties of a powder. These have been dealt with in detail by Neumann (1967), and some are mentioned briefly below.

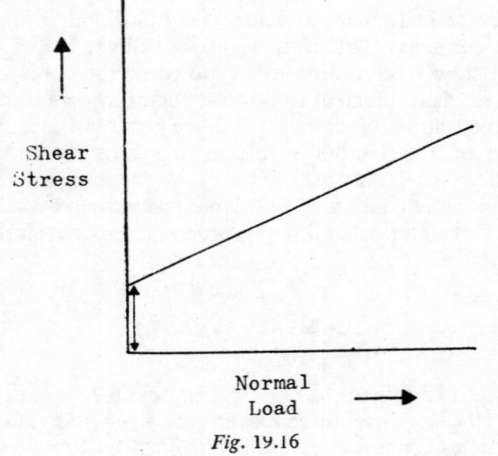

Fig. 19.16

Fig. 19.17 Angle of repose of a powder heap

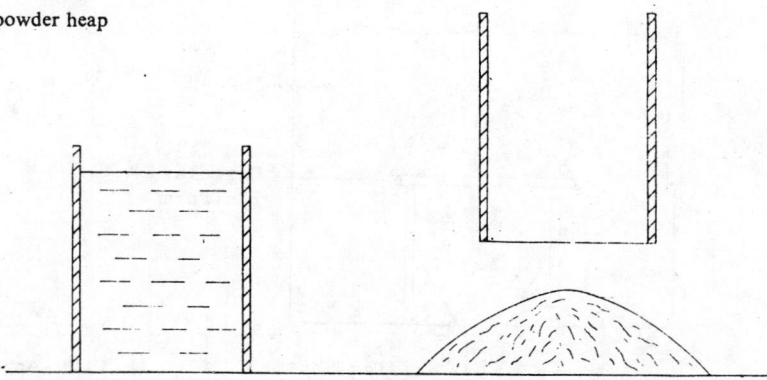

1. *Average Particle Size.* Since cohesion is a surface effect fine powders are usually more cohesive than coarser ones of the same material. Below 10 micrometres, most powders are extremely cohesive.

2. *Particle Density.* Since powders normally flow under the influence of gravity, dense substances are generally less cohesive than lighter ones, since the weight of the particles for a given volume is increased.

3. *Nature of the Surface.* The surface of any particle is associated with a surface free energy, discussed on page 33. The free energy of an uncontaminated surface is very large but is reduced by the adsorption of gases and water vapour. If it were not for this adsorption the cohesive forces would be extremely large and it is doubtful if any powder would flow under these conditions. However, a *continuous* film of moisture surrounding the particles can cause a great increase in cohesion (p. 229).

Some Other Properties Of Powder Heaps and Beds

Many attempts have been made to predict flow properties from measurements made on a static heap or bed of the powder. The measurement of cohesion has already been discussed but there are some simpler criteria that are useful.

1. *The Angle of Repose of a Powder Heap*

The student will recall from his knowledge of physics that an object resting on an inclined plane will begin to slide when the angle of inclination is increased sufficiently to overcome the frictional force between the object and the plane. In a somewhat similar way, the particles composing a conical heap of powder on a horizontal surface will slip and roll

over each other until the gravitational forces balance the interparticular forces. The sides of the heap will then form an angle with the horizontal which is known as the angle of repose. The value of this angle is high if cohesive and other forces are high, and vice versa. In general, if the angle exceeds $50°$ ($\frac{5}{18}\pi$ rad), the powder will not flow satisfactorily while materials having values near the minimum, circa $25°$ ($\frac{5}{36}\pi$ rad), flow easily and well.

Determination of Angle of Repose

The simplest way is to allow the material to flow through a funnel or orifice on to a horizontal surface beneath. The angle of the conical heap so formed can be determined from simple geometry. There are, however, some drawbacks to this simple method:

(a) it is suitable for free flowing powders only;
(b) it does not give reproducible results, since the cone shape is distorted by the impact of the falling particles.

A variation of the method overcomes these drawbacks to some extent. The powder is filled into an open-ended cylinder with the bottom resting on a horizontal surface. On withdrawing the cylinder vertically, the powder will form a heap from which the angle of repose can be found (Fig. 19.17). Even so, the angle may differ by $2°$ ($\pi/90$ rad) or $3°$ ($\pi/60$ rad) over a number of determinations on the same powder.

Train has given a comparison of some alternative methods for determining the angle of repose and stressed the need for rigidly defined conditions if reproducible results are to be obtained. His paper should be consulted for further details (Train, 1958).

Probably the best method devised to date is due to Pilpel, and the apparatus employed is sketched in Fig. 19.18. On opening the sliding shutter, the powder in the container flows out via the funnel,

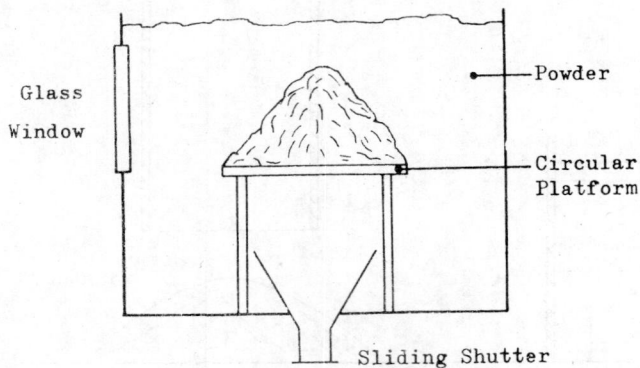

Glass
Window

Powder

Circular
Platform

Sliding Shutter

Fig. 19.18   Apparatus for measuring angle of repose

except for a conical heap remaining on the circular platform. This method avoids cone distortion due to falling particles.

A very low value for angle of repose, circa 25° ($\frac{5}{36}\pi$ rad), is indicative of monosize spherical particles with smooth surfaces, which flow extremely well. These powders also fluidise easily (*see* p. 215).

If the angle of repose is larger, between 35° ($\frac{7}{36}\pi$ rad) and 45° ($\pi/4$ rad), it is not in itself a sufficient criterion for predicting the flow properties of the powder. Most powders have angles of repose in this range. The shear angles prevalent in the flow of powder through an orifice, for example, (p. 227) are usually much greater than the static angle of repose for the same powder.

Packing of Powder Beds and Heaps

A bed or heap of powder contains a host of particles each in contact with its immediate neighbours. The fraction of a powder bed that consists of free space is known as the porosity. If the powder consists of isodiametric (same diameter) particles, the porosity

can theoretically vary from a maximum of 48 per cent for the most open (cubical) arrangement to a minimum of 26 per cent for the densest (rhombohedral) packing (Fig. 19.19). It is statistically most improbable that a 'pure' arrangement of one type of packing should exist, but it is found that the porosity of such an ideal powder (e.g. lead shot or graded sand) is constant around 39 per cent or so. This value is independent of particle size provided the particles are monosize and spherical in any given powder.

Normally a powder will have a wide range of particle size. The voids between the larger particles can then fill with smaller ones, and the porosity can vary between wide limits depending on the extent to which this has occurred.

POWDER BULK DENSITY AND PARTICLE DENSITY

The bulk density of a powder bed is simply the weight of the powder comprising it divided by the whole volume of the bed. The particle density is

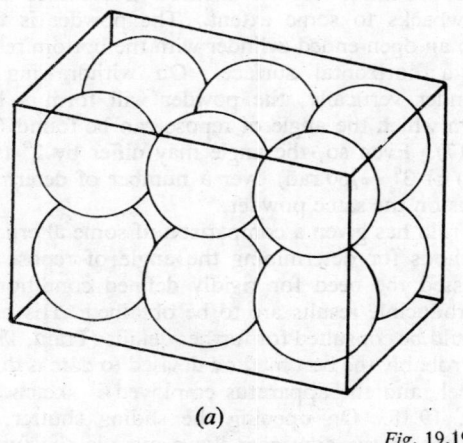

(a)

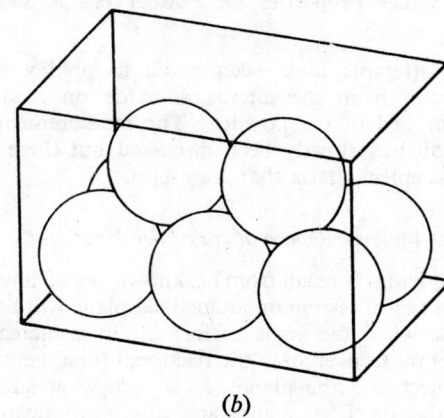

(b)

Fig. 19.19   Spheres arranged
(*a*) in cubical packing,   (*b*) in rhombohedral packing

similarly defined as the weight of the particle divided by its volume. It is always greater than the bulk density since part of the bed volume will consist of voids.

If d_B and d_p are the bulk and particle densities respectively, then these are related to the porosity of the powder bed by the expression

$$P_B = 1 - \frac{d_B}{d_p}$$

It is obvious that if there is a change from an open to a close packing within a powder bed, the bed will diminish in volume since some of the void space is eliminated. The bulk density will therefore increase. It is an easy matter to measure the bulk density of powders but it is more difficult to evaluate the true particle density.

THE PACKING DOWN OF POWDER BEDS

The change of volume occurring when void space diminishes is known as 'packing down'. It can be studied easily by using the simple apparatus devised by Neumann (1967) (Fig. 19.20). The powder contained in the measuring cylinder is mechanically tapped by means of the rotating cam run at constant speed, and diminishes from an initial volume V_0 to a final volume V_t when it has attained its most stable arrangement.

It would be expected that spherical monosize

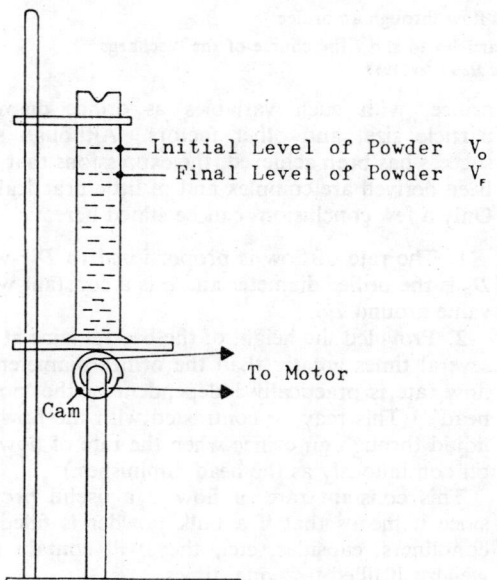

Fig. 19.20 Mechanical tapping device
(*After Neumann,* 1967)

material would quickly attain its most stable arrangement and pack down rapidly. This is in fact so, and conversely, powders composed of non-isometric particles take much longer to pack down. There are two reasons for this longer time.

1. 'Arches' and 'bridges' are formed by the interlocking of non-isometric particles. These need time to break down and disperse.
2. The smaller particles have to move into the voids between the larger particles. This considerable movement needs appreciable time to occur.

The volume change occurring for this type of powder is also very much greater than in the first case since the initial voidage is larger.

It is obvious that tablet granules, which are both monosize and spherical, will pack down rapidly. This helps to ensure uniform filling of the die and a constant tablet weight, and forms one reason for the granulation process (Table 19.1).

Flow of Powders and Granules through an Orifice

There are many examples of this type of flow to be found in pharmaceutical manufacture. It occurs when granules or powder flow via an opening in a hopper or a bin to a tablet or capsule-filling machine or other equipment. Because of its industrial importance such flow of free-flowing materials has been extensively studied, but less is known concerning the irregular flow of more cohesive material.

NATURE OF THE FLOW THROUGH AN ORIFICE

Consider a tall cylindrical container, initially full of a free flowing powder with its surface horizontal, and having a closed orifice in the base (Fig. 19.21(a)).

If the orifice is now opened, the flow patterns developed as the powder flows out are as shown in Fig. 19.21(a)–(f). They have been extensively studied, notably by Brown and Hawksley (1947). These workers used a glass-fronted two-dimensional vessel for ease of observation but similar patterns are obtained in a three-dimensional system. The observed sequence is as follows.

1. On opening the orifice there is no instantaneous movement at the surface but the particles just above the orifice fall freely through it (Fig. 19.21(b)).
2. A depression forms at the surface and spreads outwards to the sides of the container (Figs. 19.21(c)) and (d)).
3. Provided the container is tall and not too narrow, the flow pattern illustrated in Fig. 19.22 is rapidly established. Particles in zone A move

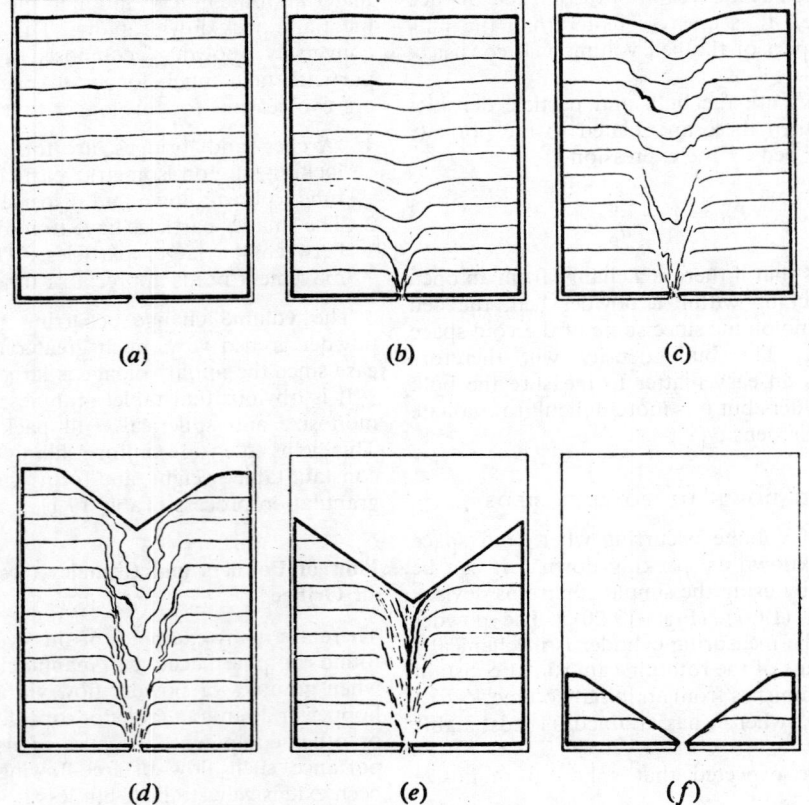

Fig. 19.21   Development of flow through an orifice
The horizontal lines are formed by indicator particles to show the course of the discharge
(After Brown and Hawksley, 1947)

rapidly over the slower moving particles in zone *B*, while those in zone *E* remain at rest. The particles in *A* feed into zone *C* where they move quickly downwards and outwards towards the orifice. The slower particles in *B* do not enter this zone.

4. Both streams *B* and *C* converge to a 'tongue' just above the orifice where the movement is quickest and the packing of the particles at its loosest. Recent work has indicated that the particles are in free fall in a zone just above the orifice.

An important practical consequence of this flow pattern lies in the fact that if the container is repeatedly refilled and partially emptied, the particles in zone *E* towards the bottom and sides of the container will never be withdrawn and may spoil.

MASS RATE OF FLOW THROUGH
AN ORIFICE

Many attempts have been made to correlate the rate at which free flowing powders will flow through an orifice, with such variables as orifice diameter, particle size, and other factors. Although some success has been achieved, the expressions that have been derived are complex and of little practical use. Only a few conclusions can be stated here.

1. The rate of flow is proportional to D_0^a where D_0 is the orifice diameter and *a* is a constant with a value around 2·6.

2. Provided the height of the bed remains at least several times greater than the orifice diameter, the flow rate is practically independent of the 'powder head'. (This may be contrasted with the flow of a liquid through an orifice when the rate of flow falls off continuously as the head diminishes.)

This constant rate of flow is a useful property since it means that if a bulk powder is filled into containers, capsules, etc., they will contain equal weights if filled for equal times.

3. Flow rate increases as the average particle size decreases. However, below about 200 μm cohesive

forces increase rapidly and the flow rate falls off once more. Figure 19.23, taken from a paper by Jones and Pilpel (1966), shows how the flow rate of granular magnesia through an orifice in a flat-based hopper varies with particle size.

Some Methods of Improving the Flow Properties of Powders

A number of such methods have been mentioned indirectly during the preceding account but are included here for the sake of completeness. Flow properties may be improved in one or more of the following ways.

1. *By Increasing the Average Particle Size.* Since large particles are less cohesive than small, and an optimum size for free flow exists, there is a distinct disadvantage in using a finer grade of powder than is necessary. It may be possible to use granules rather than a powder, and this is often essential in tablet manufacture.

The addition of a coarser fraction to a fine powder is another possible expedient for improving its flow properties (cf p. 224).

2. *By Producing the Powder in the Form of Spherical Particles.* This type of powder packs down and flows easily since the particles can 'roll over' one another. Spray drying often produces this type of powder, and spray-dried lactose is a popular diluent for tablets needing an inert material to make up bulk since it may be possible to compress such a mixture directly.

3. *By Use of Additives.* The function of glidants, such as powdered talc, to improve the flow properties of tablet granulations was referred to on page 218. It is sometimes possible to treat powders in a similar way. The cohesiveness of powders often increases with the moisture content if this is sufficient to provide a continuous moisture film between the particles. Surface tension is presumably responsible for this effect. Craik and Miller (1958) demonstrated that the angle of repose of starch, sucrose, and sodium chloride powders increased when they were exposed to air of increasing humidity. If a small proportion of very fine magnesium oxide was then added, the angle of repose was decreased. They attributed this to disruption of the water film by these particles.

The student may remember that the surface of glass containers may be rendered hydrophobic by treatment with silicones (Gunn and Carter, 1965). It is possible to treat powders by similar means and thus prevent formation of the moisture film to which cohesiveness is often due. Silicone treatment has been used to improve the flow properties of sodium bicarbonate powder in fire extinguishers. Silicone-treated talc has some advantages as a carrier in dusting powder. An article by Drake (1968) gives further details of the interesting process.

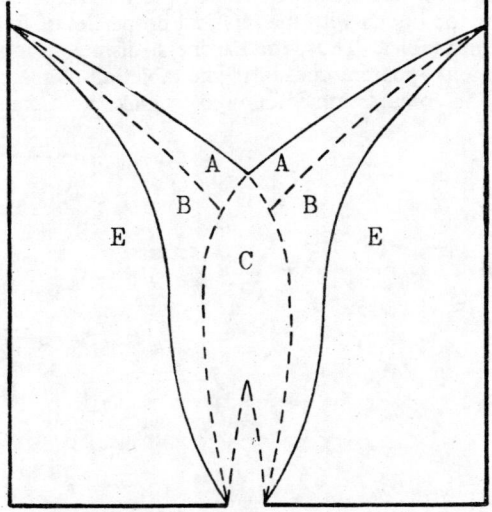

Fig. 19.22 Fully developed flow of a free-flowing powder

(*After Brown and Hawksley, 1947*)

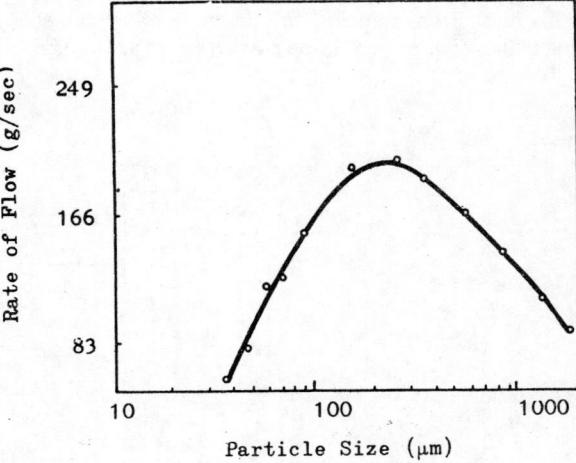

Fig. 19.23 Flow rate of magnesia through a circular orifice: the effect of particle size

(*After Jones and Pilpel, 1966*)

The Physics of Tablet Compression

Prior to 1950, little or nothing was known of the fundamentals of the compression process. About this time notable advances were made in powder metallurgy techniques (the forming of metal objects by the compression of powdered metals). This work stimulated interest in the physics of tablet compression, notably in the Schools of Pharmacy of London and Wisconsin Universities. Space precludes a consideration of all the investigations undertaken, and the discussion here will therefore be confined to those aspects that have some practical significance or application. The original papers should be consulted for further details. Kirsop (1964) has written an excellent review of the work done up to that date.

The Scope of the Investigations

The bulk of the work can be conveniently classified under one or other of the following headings:

1. Work relating the properties of compressed tablets to the force used to compress them.
2. The effect of lubricants on the transmission of forces involved in compression.
3. Pressure distribution within a granule or powder mass on compression.
4. The factors influencing the bonding of particles or granules to form the finished tablet.

Instrumentation of Tablet Machines

Many investigations have involved measurements of the force exerted by the upper punch and transmitted to the lower punch via the granule mass. This has been achieved by instrumenting tablet machines with devices known as strain gauges. The principle of their operation is easy to understand but the circuitry required is often rather complex. Single-punch machines have been largely used for this work (Higuchi *et al.*, 1954) but the rotary type has also been instrumented though this is very much more difficult (Goodhart *et al.*, 1968).

When a force is exerted via the top punch to the granules in the die the punch stem is compressed and shortened slightly (Fig. 19.24). If a strain gauge, which consists of a length of insulated alloy wire, is bonded to the punch it will also shorten and, therefore, change in resistance. If the strain gauge forms part of a suitable circuit, usually a type of Wheatstone Bridge, this resistance change can be made to cause a deflection on the trace of a cathode-ray tube or to operate a suitable recorder. The punch assembly can be calibrated by loading it, by means of a suitable press, and plotting the deflection shown by the recorder against the applied load.

Similar gauges, bonded to the lower punch, can be used to measure the transmitted force and, also, the force required to eject the finished tablet.

When the compression force is released, both punches will return to their original length since steel is perfectly elastic within the range of forces used in normal tabletting procedures.

Effect of Compression Force on Properties of Compressed Tablets

Much of the earlier work was concerned with establishing relationships between the force exerted by the top punch with the physical properties of the resulting tablet. Thus, the hardness, disintegration time, and apparent density of the tablet all increase with the compression force used to make it. Often

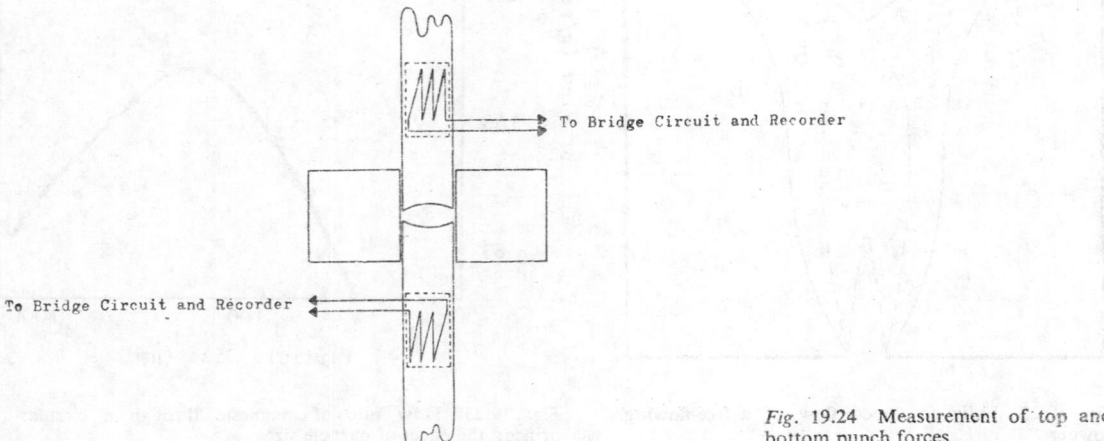

To Bridge Circuit and Recorder

To Bridge Circuit and Recorder

Fig. 19.24 Measurement of top and bottom punch forces

there is a linear relationship between the logarithm of these quantities and the compression force (Higuchi *et al.*, 1953, 1954).

An interesting curve results if the internal surface area of the tablet is plotted against the compressive force used to produce them (Fig. 19.25). The surface area may be measured by the nitrogen adsorption technique which determines the internal surface area as well as the external surface (p. 49). The initial increase is attributed to fragmentation of the granules at a fairly low compression force. When a higher force is used, rebonding occurs, reducing the free internal surface. Further evidence that tends to confirm this explanation of the process has since been obtained (p. 232).

The Effect of Lubricants

If we attempt to compress a fluid such as water in a leakproof punch and die assembly, then the force exerted by the top punch will be transmitted unchanged to the bottom punch, since a fluid exerts pressure equally in all directions. (The student should be careful not to confuse force with pressure, which is force per unit area. As both top and bottom punches have equal cross-sectional areas the force on both should also be equal, as should the pressures.)

When granules or powder are compressed, there is an attenuation of this transmitted force largely due to the friction developed between the mass and die wall. The force registered on the lower punch is therefore reduced.

Die wall friction can be minimised by adding lubricants. It makes little difference if these are added to the granules or merely used to coat the die wall (Higuchi *et al.*, 1954). The perfect lubricant,

which incidentally does not exist, would equalise the top and bottom punch forces by totally abolishing friction. In practice the ratio

$$\frac{\text{lower punch force}}{\text{upper punch force}} \quad \text{(termed } R \text{ value)}$$

is always less than one and can be used as a measure of lubricant efficiency. Magnesium stearate and other well-known lubricants have R values approaching one, but talc has a much lower value (0·6 to 0·8) confirming the statement made on page 218 that talc is a good glidant but a poor lubricant.

The efficiency of magnesium stearate and other fatty acid salts is thought to be due largely to their polar nature and they are probably adsorbed as a monolayer on the die wall (compare the surface films discussed on page 39).

Talc, on the other hand, is an example of a so-called laminar lubricant, where the action is dependent on the presence of a fairly thick film on the die wall. Train and Hersey (1960) have suggested that this type can function efficiently only if there is sufficient space between the die wall and punch for the layers to 'roll up'. In a well-fitting assembly this space is not available, hence laminar lubricants are less efficient than the polar type. It is interesting to note that the friction involved in the compression of lubricated granules is sufficient to cause an average rise in temperature of several degrees K. It is highly probable that *local* temperatures at the points of granule contact may be momentarily high enough to cause fusion and thus contribute to the bonding of the tablet.

The energy expended and the heat produced are both very much greater if unlubricated granules are compressed. Thus, lubrication permits the use of a

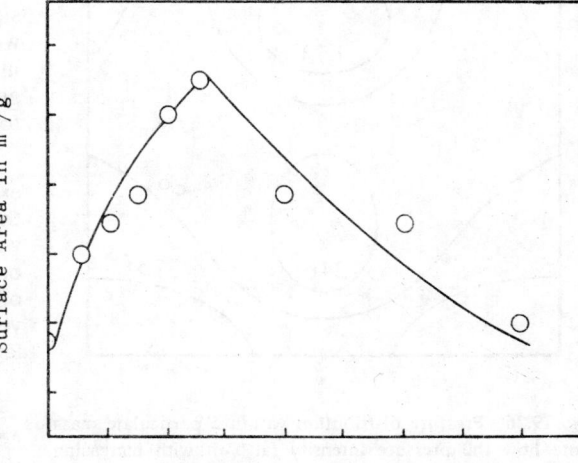

Fig. 19.25 The effect of compressional force on the specific surface area of sulphathiazole tablets

(After Higuchi et al., 1953)

low horsepower motor in the tablet machine and it may be grossly overloaded if an attempt is made to dispense with the lubricant in the tablet formulation.

Pressure Distribution in a Tablet

Since a granule mass does not behave as a fluid there can be varying pressures developed at different points. Train (1957) investigated pressure distribution during compression of magnesium carbonate. His paper should be consulted for practical details, but by means of gauges inserted into the powder mass he was able to establish the existence of pressure profiles such as are shown in Fig. 19.26. It will be noticed that high pressure areas exist near the top and centre of the compact. These have some practical significance since they may account for the common fault of tablet capping or lamination. Train suggested that the higher pressures developed near the top of the compact resulted in an elastic compression in these areas, which probably also exists in commercial tablets. When the tablet is ejected from the die, these compressed areas may relax and expand to a greater extent than the low pressure areas. The stress developed in the plane between the two areas may be sufficient to break the bonding and cause capping.

The presence of a hard, highly compressed core near the centre of the compact may account for the slow disintegration of the small portion of a tablet that is often observed in the official disintegration

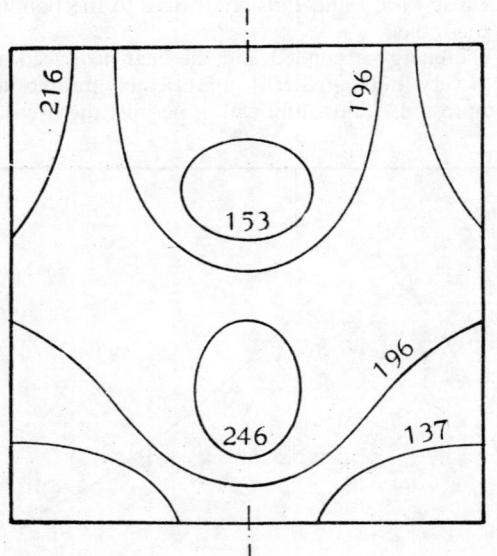

Fig. 19.26 Pressure distribution within a particulate mass Note how the pressure intensity falls off with increasing distance from the load. Contours are in N/mm²
(After Train, 1957)

test when the bulk of the tablet has fallen through the mesh (p. 222).

Bonding of Granules

The measurements made of the internal surface of compressed tablets and the deductions drawn from the results have already been mentioned. Shotton and Ganderton (1960) confirmed this mechanism by compressing granules that had been built up with a coloured outer shell in a tablet-coating pan. On compressing these granules at low compaction pressures the resulting tablet showed surface cleavage of the granules with the white inner core showing through. At higher pressures the granules broke up completely and the fragments rebonded to show coloured fragments on a white background.

Shotton and Ganderton also investigated the strength of granule bonding but their results cannot be dealt with in detail here. However, one particularly interesting result emerged concerning the capping of hexamine tablets. If these were prepared from unlubricated granules compressed hard, then capping was extensive. This was attributed to strong interparticulate bonding allowing failure to spread from grain to grain until the tablet laminated. Stearic acid, used as a lubricant, weakened the bonding and abolished the tendency to cap. If hexamine tablets were compressed in vacuo, this had no effect on capping, so it seems that entrapped air, which is often advanced as an explanation for capping, may not be the main cause of this type of fault.

Instrumented tablet machines are now becoming of practical value in the pharmaceutical industry. Since the compression force developed during tablet formation increases rapidly with slight increases in the depth of fill and vice versa, a record of compression forces during a run can replace the tedious weighing of large numbers of tablets. Wray (1969), in an instructive article, has pointed this out and given details of the use of an instrumented machine for testing alternative tablet formulations.

Tablet-making is still very much an art where experience counts for a great deal, but it is likely that the work described and new work in the future, will do much to make it less empirical. We have only been able to deal superficially with a small part of the large volume of work published in recent years but it is hoped that the student will be stimulated to read more widely on this interesting subject.

REFERENCES

ANON (1955) The coating of tablets by compression. Machines available in Great Britain. *Pharm. J.,* **174,** 362–365.

ANON (1967) High-speed film coating of tablets. *Mfg. Chem.*, **38** (3), 54.

ANON (1968) Multilayer tablet coating. *Drug. Cosmet. Ind.*, **102** (1), 84–85, 154.

BROOK, D. B. and MARSHALL, K. (1968) Crushing strength of compressed tablets. I . Comparison of testers. *J. pharm. Sci.*, **57**, 481–484.

BROWN, R. L. and HAWKSLEY, P. J. W. (1947) Internal flow of granular masses. *Fuel Sci. Pract.*, **26** (6), 159–173.

COOPER, B. F. and BRECHT, E. A. (1957) Surfactants in tablets to improve disintegration. *J. Amer. Pharm. Ass. (Sci. ed.)*, **46**, 520–524.

CRAIK, D. J. and MILLER, B. F. (1958) The flow properties of powders under humid conditions. *J. Pharm. Pharmac.*, **10**, 73–79.

DRAKE, J. (1968) Silicones as anti-caking and free flow agents. *Mfg. Chem.*, **39** (10), 38–41.

GOODHART, F. W., MAYORGA, G., MILLS, M. N., and NINGER, F. C. (1968) Instrumentation of a rotary tablet machine. *J. Pharm. Sci.*, **57**, 1770–1775.

GUNN, C. and CARTER, S. J. (1965) *Dispensing for pharmaceutical students*. 11th ed. Pitman Medical, London.

HIGUCHI, T., ARNOLD, R. D., BUSSE, L. W., and SWINTOSKY, J. V. (1953) The physics of tablet compression II. Influence of degree of compression on properties of tablets. *J. Amer. Pharm. Ass. (Sci. ed.)*, **42**, 194–199.

HIGUCHI, T., NELSON, E., and BUSSE, L. W. (1954) The physics of tablet compression, III. The design and construction of an instrumented tablet machine. *ibid.*, **43**, 344–348

JACOB, J. T. and PLEIN, E. M. (1968) Factors affecting the dissolution rates of medicaments from tablets I. In vitro dissolution rate of commercial phenobarbitone tablets. *J. pharm. Sci.*, **57**, 798–801.

JONES, T. M. (1968) Measuring cohesion in powders. *Mfg. Chem.*, **39** (3), 38–40.

JONES, T. M. and PILPEL, N. (1966) The flow properties of granular magnesia. *J. Pharm. Pharmac.*, **18**, 81–93.

KIRSOP, W. (1964) Fundamentals of tablet compression. *Australas. J. Pharm.* **45**, S73–S78

NEUMANN, B. S. (1967) The flow properties of powders. *Advances in Pharmaceutical Sciences* **2**, 181–221. London, Academic Press.

RIDGWAY, K. and SEGOVIA, E. (1966) Fluidization in pharmaceutical manufacturing. *Mfg. Chem.*, **37** (12), 39–44.

SCOTT, M. W., LIEBERMANN, H. A., RANKELL, A. S., and BATTISTA, J. V. (1964) Continuous production of tablet granulations in a fluidized bed I. Theory and design considerations. *J. pharm. Sci.*, **53**, 314–320. II. Operation and performance of equipment, *ibid.*, **53**, 320–324.

SHOTTON, E. and GANDERTON, D. (1960) The strength of compressed tablets Part I. The measurement of tablet strength and its relation to compression forces. *J. Pharm. Pharmac.*, **12**, 87–92.

SHOTTON, E. and GANDERTON, D. (1960) The strength of compressed tablets Part II. The bonding of granules during compression. *ibid.*, **12**, 93–104.

SINGISER, R. S. and LOWENTHAL, W. (1961) Enteric film coats by the air suspension coating technique. *J. pharm. Sci.*, **50**, 168–170.

SMITH, A. N. (1949) Compressed tablets. Resistance to 'wear and tear'. *Pharm. J.*, **182**, 194–195, 227–228, 477–478.

SUTARIA, R. H. (1968) Art and science of tablet coating. *Mfg. Chem.*, **39** (6), 37–41.

TRAIN, D. (1957) Transmission of forces through a powder mass during the process of pelleting. *Trans. Instn. chem. Engrs.*, **35**, 258–266.

TRAIN, D. (1958) Some aspects of the angle of repose of powders. *J. Pharm. Pharmac.*, **10**, 127–135.

TRAIN, D. (1960) Pharmaceutical aspects of mixing solids. *Pharm. J.*, **185**, 129–134.

TRAIN, D. and HERSEY, J. A. (1960) The use of laminar lubricants in compaction processes. *J. Pharm. Pharmac.*, **12**, 97T–104T.

WEBSTER, A. R. and VAN ABBÉ, N. J. (1955) Mechanical strength of compressed tablets. *ibid.*, **7**, 882–899.

WHITEHOUSE, R. C. (1954) A new method of coating tablets (press coating). *Pharm. J.*, **172**, 85.

WRAY, P. E. (1969) The instrumented rotary tablet machine. *Drug. Cosmet. Ind.*, **105**, (3), 53–56.

20

Filtration

FILTRATION may be defined as the separation of a solid from a fluid by means of a porous medium that retains the solid but allows the fluid to pass.

It will be realised that the term fluid includes liquids and gases, so that both these may be subjected to filtration, but the discussion in this chapter will be confined to liquid filtration. The principal pharmaceutical application of gas filtration is the treatment of air to produce sterile atmospheres and is considered in this context by Gunn and Carter (1965).

This chapter considers the objects of the filtration operation, the factors that affect filtration and the rate at which the process can take place, the mechanisms of filtration, and typical examples of the equipment used in practice.

For convenience in the discussion, the following terms will be used. The suspension of solid and liquid to be filtered is known as the *slurry*. The porous medium used to retain the solids is described as the *filter medium*, the accumulation of solids on the filter is referred to as the *filter cake*, while the clear liquid passing through the filter is the *filtrate*.

FACTORS AFFECTING FILTRATION

The unit operation of filtration is affected by the characteristics of the slurry, including:

The properties of the liquid, such as density, viscosity, and corrosiveness.

The properties of the solid; for example, particle shape, particle size, particle size distribution, and the rigidity or compressibility of the solid.

The proportion of solids in the slurry.

Whether the objective is to collect the solid, the liquid, or both.

Whether the solids have to be washed free from the liquid or a solute.

These characteristics will influence the choice of method of filtration, as will be seen later, and some will affect the rate of filtration.

RATE OF FILTRATION

All other things being equal, the object of the operation is to filter the slurry as quickly as possible.

The factors affecting rate of filtration were studied by Darcy in 1830 in an investigation of the flow of water through beds in the public fountains at Dijon. For this reason, the equation correlating the rate factors is known as *Darcy's law* and may be expressed as:

$$\frac{dV}{dt} = \frac{KA\,\Delta P}{\mu l} \qquad (20.1)$$

where V = volume of filtrate; t = time of filtration; K = constant for the filter medium and the filter cake; A = area of filter medium; ΔP = pressure drop across the filter medium and filter cake; μ = viscosity of the filtrate; and l = thickness of cake.

It should be noted that this represents the rate of flow through the capillaries of the filter medium and the filter cake; it is analogous to the equation for the flow through a single tube, known as Poiseuille's law (*see* Chapter 7).

Properties of the Filter Medium and Filter Cake

The constant, K, in Eqn (20.1) represents the resistance of the filter medium and filter cake. Although the resistance of the filter medium is of significance on the laboratory scale, it is relatively less important on the large scale and can usually be neglected. The magnitude of the resistance of the filter medium will change due to the early layers of solids which may block the pores or may form bridges over the entrances to the channels. For this reason, the pressure should be kept low at the start, to avoid the pores 'plugging', and increased as the cake builds up. The usual procedure is to filter at constant rate, increasing the pressure as necessary. When the normal working pressure is reached it is maintained, hence the rate of filtration decreases as the thickness of the cake increases. When the rate is uneconomically low, filtration is stopped, the filter cake removed, and filtration restarted.

The principal properties of the solid affecting the resistance of the cake are the surface area of the particles, the porosity of the cake, and rigidity or compressibility of the particles.

Although the factor is referred to as a constant in the equation, it is, of course, a constant only for a particular set of circumstances. Thus, any decrease in the resistance of the cake will show as an increased value of K, so increasing the rate of filtration. This can be done, for example, by using *filter aids* (*see* p. 237).

Area of Filter

It will be obvious that the total volume of filtrate flowing from the filter will be proportional to the area of the filter. Hence, this rate can be increased by using larger filters, but the area can also be increased by using a number of small units in parallel. This, for example, is done in the filter press (*see* p. 238).

In the rotary filter (p. 241) the filter cake is removed continuously, giving, in effect, an infinite area for filtration.

Pressure Drop

The rate of filtration is proportional to the overall pressure drop, that is, across both the filter medium and filter cake. The pressure drop can be achieved in a number of ways:

GRAVITY

A simple method of obtaining a pressure difference is by maintaining a head of slurry above the filter medium. The pressure developed will depend on the density of the slurry, but, as a rough guide, a head of 10 metres of water will create a pressure difference of about 1 bar. At one time, the method was used in pharmaceutical manufacturing, with a long tube enclosing a filter bag passing through several floors of a factory, but it is seldom used in modern practice.

REDUCED PRESSURE

The pressure below the filter medium may be reduced below atmospheric pressure by connecting the filtrate receiver to a vacuum pump and creating a pressure differential across the filter. This method has the disadvantage that the pressure difference is limited to about 1 bar, since it cannot be greater than the pressure exerted by the atmosphere on the surface of the slurry. A further disadvantage is that reduction of pressure lowers the boiling point of liquids (*see* p. 172) so that it is possible for the filtrate to boil in the receiver. Apart from the loss of liquid, which may be undesirable, the vapour may be damaging to the vacuum pump.

The use of reduced pressure has an advantage in terms of safety, since, if part of the equipment fails, it will collapse and not explode. For this reason, reduced pressure filtration is the method most commonly used in the laboratory, where the apparatus is usually made of glass. The factor is less important on the industrial scale, where the plant is usually constructed in metal and is able to withstand high pressures.

PRESSURE

Probably the commonest method in practice is to obtain a suitable difference by applying pressure to the surface of the slurry, the simplest method being to pump the slurry into the filter under pressure.

This has the advantage that greater pressure differences are possible than are obtainable with reduced pressure, and industrial plant may operate at pressures up to 15 bars.

It is important that such pressures should be used with caution, however, especially in the early stages of the process, as discussed on page 234. Otherwise the gain from the greater pressure difference will be offset by the increased resistance brought about by the pores becoming plugged or the cake compressed.

CENTRIFUGAL FORCE

In the same way that gravitational force could be replaced by centrifugal force in particle separation (*see* p. 178), so use can be made of centrifugal force in filtration processes. It is an important method in industrial practice and is considered in Chapter 21.

Viscosity of Filtrate

From fluid flow theory (*see* Chapter 11) it would be expected that an increase in the viscosity of the filtrate will increase the resistance to flow, so that the rate of filtration is inversely proportional to the viscosity of the fluid. It must be emphasised that it is the viscosity of the liquid and not of the slurry that is of importance, since the resistance to flow occurs as the filtrate flows through the filter cake.

The rate of filtration may be increased by raising the temperature of the liquid, which lowers its viscosity (*see* p. 124). This may not be practicable if thermolabile materials are involved or if the filtrate is volatile. The latter is especially true if filtration under reduced pressure is used.

Dilution is another alternative, but may not always be acceptable. In addition, it is important to ensure that there is an overall gain, that is, if the volume is doubled by diluting the filtrate with an equal volume of the liquid, the rate must be more than doubled to show any advantage.

Thickness of Filter Cake

The filtrate must flow through the filter cake formed on the filter medium as filtration progresses, hence the rate of flow will be inversely proportional to the thickness of the cake. In some slurries containing high proportions of solids, it may be advantageous to reduce the rate at which the cake accumulates. This may be done by preliminary decantation or straining, which will lower the solids content of the slurry. The filtration process is then left to remove only a smaller proportion of solids, probably those of smaller particle size.

It should be remembered that cake thickness will be affected by area of filtration, so that for a given amount of slurry, increase in area will decrease the cake thickness. Also, in the rotary filter (*see* p. 241) the filter cake is removed continuously, so that the cake thickness is minimised.

The influence of these factors will be seen when the design of various types of filters is discussed (*see* p. 237 *et seq*), apart from the resistance due to the filter medium and the filter cake, for which pages 234 and 237 should be consulted.

Mechanisms of Filtration

The mechanisms whereby particles are retained by the filter will be referred to briefly, but they are of significance only in the early stages of liquid filtration, as a rule. Once a preliminary layer of particles has been deposited, the filtration is effected by the filter cake, the filter medium serving only as a support. The precise mechanism of filtration is of greater importance where the proportion of solids is very low, as in clarification processes and, especially in air filtration.

STRAINING

The simplest filtration procedure is *straining*, in which, like sieving, the pores are smaller than the particles, so that the latter are retained on the filter medium.

IMPINGEMENT

As a flowing fluid approaches an object such as a cylinder the flow pattern is displaced, as shown diagrammatically by the streamlines in Fig. 20.1. Solids having momentum would be expected to cross the streamlines and strike the cylinder, but, in practice, some will follow the streamlines and will not be collected or will be re-entrained. Thus, particles between streamlines *A* and *B* will be collected, and the accumulation of solids will form

a ridge, roughly triangular in section, as indicated in Fig. 20.1.

The way in which this occurs will be apparent by remembering what a cylindrical object such as a telegraph pole or tree trunk look likes after a snow storm. Snow flakes impinge and accumulate in a ridge on the windward side to a width of about half the diameter of the cylinder.

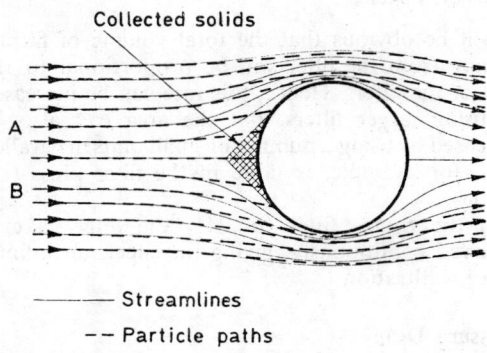

Fig. 20.1 Mechanism of filtration by impingement

ENTANGLEMENT

If the filter medium consists of a cloth with a nap or is a porous felt, then particles become entangled in the mass of fibres. Usually the particles are smaller than the pores, so that it is possible that impingement is involved.

ATTRACTIVE FORCES

In certain circumstances. particles may collect on a filter medium as a result of attractive forces. The ultimate in this method is the electrostatic precipitator, where large potential differences are used to remove particles from air streams.

In practice, the process may combine the various mechanisms, but the solids removal is effected normally by a straining mechanism once the first complete layer of solids has begun to form the cake on the filter medium.

Filter Media

As indicated in the previous section, the filter medium may be responsible for the collection of the solids, while in other cases it is no more than a support for the filter cake.

In any event, the filter medium must be strong. have a low resistance to flow, and be unaffected by the substances in the slurry.

Materials used for filter media include:

Woven materials, such as felts or cloths in wool, cotton, silk, glass, metal or synthetic fibres (rayon, nylon, etc.). Cloths may be in varying weights according to whether it is a 'light' or a 'heavy' slurry, and different weaves may be used that affect the surface and the strength. The final choice of fibre will depend on the chemical nature of the slurry.

Perforated sheet metal.

Beds of granular solids built up on a supporting medium. The solids may vary in size according to the needs of the process and, in some, a bed of graded solids may be formed to reduce the resistance to the flow of the bed. Typical examples of granular solids used for this purpose include gravel, sand, asbestos, paper pulp, and kieselguhr.

Porous solids, in which the effect is similar to the above, but which have the advantage of being pre-fabricated into single units. Sintered glass, sintered metal, earthenware and porous plastics (such as Porvic) are examples of this type.

Filter Aids

Usually, the resistance to flow due to the filter medium itself is very low, but will increase as a layer of solids builds up, blocking the pores of the medium and forming a solid, impervious cake.

Filter Leaf

The *filter leaf* is probably the simplest form of filter, consisting of a frame enclosing a drainage screen or grooved plate, the whole unit being covered with filter cloth. The outlet for the filtrate connects to the inside of the frame, so that the general arrangement is as shown in Fig. 20.2, which represents a vertical section through the leaf. The frame may be of any shape, circular, square or rectangular shapes being used in practice. In use, the filter leaf is immersed in the slurry and a receiver and vacuum system connected to the filtrate outlet. The method has the advantage that the slurry can be filtered from any vessel and the cake can be washed simply by immersing the filter in a vessel of water. Removal of the cake is facilitated by the use of reverse air flow.

An alternative method is to enclose the filter leaf in a special vessel into which the slurry is pumped under pressure. This form is commonest in filters where a number of leaves are connected to a common outlet, to provide a larger area for filtration. A typical example is the *Sweetland filter*, shown

The object of the *filter aid* is to prevent the medium from becoming blocked and to form an open, porous cake, so reducing the resistance to flow of the filtrate. Thus, the filter aid must be a light, porous, inert solid and may be used in either or both of two ways.

Firstly, by forming a *pre-coat* over the medium by filtering a suspension of the filter aid sufficient to give a coating up to 0.5 kg/m^2.

Secondly, a small proportion of the filter aid (0.1 to 0.5 per cent) is added to the slurry, ensuring that the filter cake has a porous structure. Care must be taken in the choice of the substance used as the filter aid, as materials with adsorptive properties (such as kaolin) could remove solutes from the filtrate; this may sometimes be done intentionally, for example, sugar solutions may be decolorised by means of charcoal.

Kieselguhr is a very successful filter aid and instances have been reported where as little as 0.1 per cent, added to a slurry with about 20 per cent solids, resulted in an increase in the rate of filtration of 5 times or more.

Filter aids are limited usually to clarification processes, that is, where the solids are discarded. The presence of the filter aid can sometimes be tolerated when solids are being collected, but an alternative is often to vary particle characteristics, for example, by altering the conditions of precipitation.

Industrial Filters

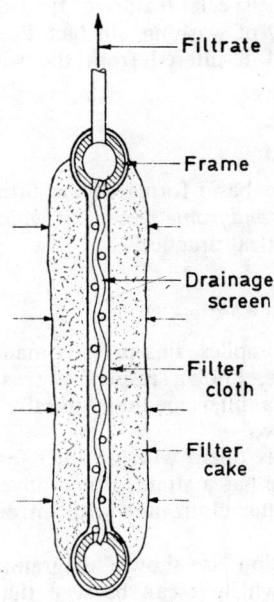

Fig. 20.2 Filter leaf

diagrammatically in Fig. 20.3, where it will be seen that the vessel is cylindrical and arranged so that it is supported by the upper part, and the lower part can be swung away. This permits the cake to be discharged by compressed air without removing the filter leaves from the vessel.

The filter leaf is a versatile piece of equipment. Area can be varied by employing a suitable number

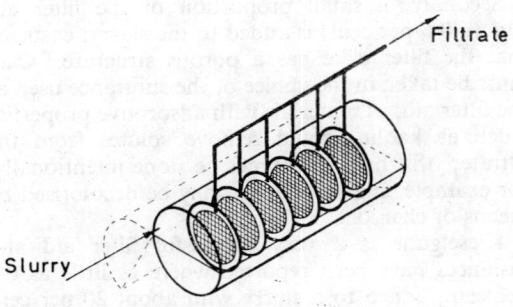

Fig. 20.3   Sweetland filter

of units, and the pressure difference may be obtained with vacuum or by using pressures up to the order of 8 bars, if suitable vessels are used. The leaf filter is most satisfactory if the solids content of the slurry is not too high, about 5 per cent being a suitable maximum. A higher proportion results in excessive non-productive time while the filter is being emptied and, provided this is observed, labour costs for operating the filter are comparatively moderate. The special feature of the leaf filter is the high efficiency of washing; in fact, the cake can be dislodged and re-filtered from the wash water if desired.

Filter Press

There are two basic forms of the filter press, but only the *plate and frame press* is of wide application in pharmaceutical practice.

PLATE AND FRAME PRESS

As the name implies, this press is made up of two types of units, known respectively as *plates* and *frames*, with a filter medium, usually filter cloth, between the two.

The frame is open, with an inlet for the slurry, while the plate has a studded or grooved surface to support the filter cloth, and with an outlet for the filtrate.

The operation is shown diagrammatically in Fig. 20.4 in which it can be seen that the slurry enters the frame (marked by 2 dots) from the feed

channel, the filtrate passes through the filter medium on to the surface of the plate (marked by 1 dot), while the solids form a filter cake in the frame. The filtrate then drains down the surface of the plate, between the projections on the surface and escapes from the outlet. Filtration is continued until the frame is filled with filter cake, when the process is stopped, the frame emptied, and the cycle re-started.

In practice, a large number of plates and frames are arranged alternately and clamped in a supporting structure. This gives a number of filtration units operating in parallel and a filtration area as large as necessary.

Channels for the slurry inlet and the filtrate outlet can be arranged by fitting *eyes* to the plates and frames (Fig. 20.5), these joining together to form a channel. In some, only the inlet channel is formed in this way, the plates having individual outlets controlled by valves. This has the advantage that the filtrate from each plate can be seen and, in the event of a broken cloth, the faulty plate can be isolated and filtration continued with one plate less. If the outlet channel is continuous, however, the process must be stopped and the press opened to find the leak. If it is essential to enclose the filtrate to avoid contamination, this can be effected by having an outlet on each plate by means of which the filtrate passes through a glass tube or *sight glass*, allowing inspection of quality, and thence through a control valve to an enclosed outlet channel.

The thickness of the cake can be varied by using frames of different thicknesses and, in general, there will be an optimum thickness of filter cake for any slurry, depending on the solids content of the slurry and the resistance of the filter cake. The reason for this is that a filter press of a particular size and number of chambers will take about the same time to dismantle, empty and refit, irrespective of the frame thickness. As filtration proceeds, the resistance of the cake increases and the filtration rate will decrease. At a certain point it will be preferable in

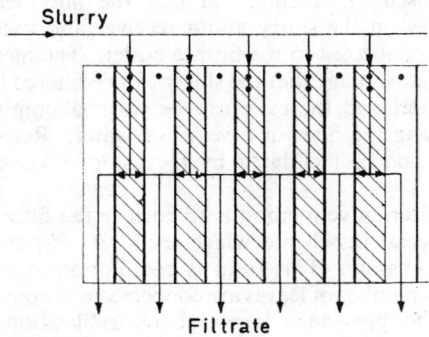

Fig. 20.4 Plate and frame filterpress: principles of operation

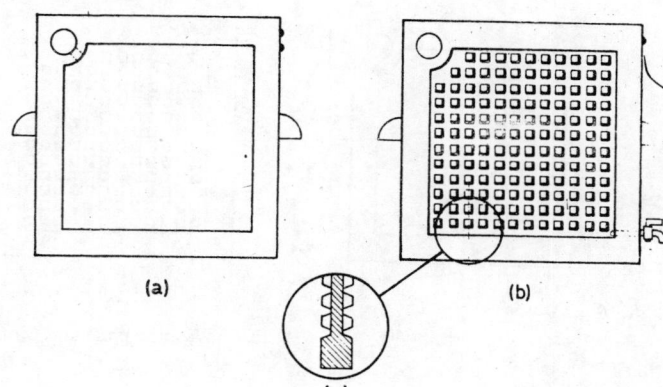

Fig. 20.5 Plate and frame filter press

(a) frame
(b) plate
(c) section through plate

terms of the overall output of the process to stop and empty the press rather than to continue filtration at a very low flow rate. As the emptying of the frames is most convenient when filled completely with filter cake, the frame thickness should be such that it is just full when the flow rate becomes uneconomic.

In this connection, it should be realised that the factor l of Darcy's expression is *half* of the frame thickness, since the filtration occurs through the filter cloths to plates on each side of the frame. Thus, two filter cakes are formed, which meet eventually in the centre of the frame.

For the control of viscosity, the plates may incorporate heating or cooling coils.

Plates and frames may be made in various metals to provide resistance to corrosion or prevent metallic contamination of the product. Non-metals avoid this problem and many have the advantage of lightness, for example, reinforced plastics. Certain varieties of wood are satisfactory materials of construction, provided the press is kept wet at all times to avoid shrinkage.

Plate and frame presses may be of considerable size, with up to 60 chambers, and plates and frames of about 1 m square. This gives a filtration area of 120 m² and, if frames 40 mm in thickness are used, the press will hold about 2·5 m³, which, in terms of average materials, represents about 1·5 Mg. Such a press will be about 6 or 7 m in length and weigh about 20 Mg.

Washing Plate and Frame Press

If it is necessary to wash the filter cake, the ordinary plate and frame press is unsatisfactory. From the description of the operation of the filter press, it will be recalled that two cakes build up in the frame, meeting eventually in the middle. This means that flow is brought virtually to a standstill, hence washing by following the filtrate through with wash water is very inefficient, if not impossible. A modification of the plate and frame press is used, therefore, if it is required to wash the filter cake, the principles of which are shown in Fig. 20.6.

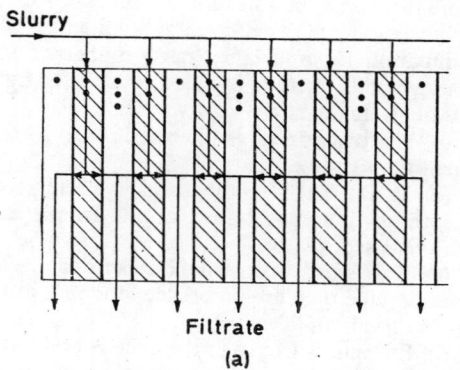

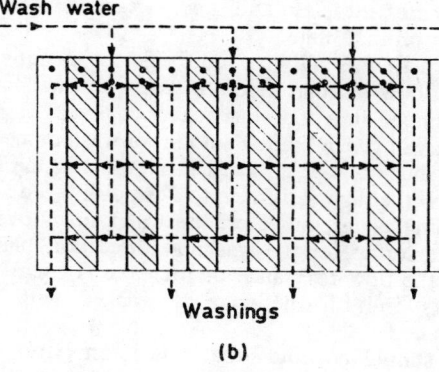

Fig. 20.6 Washing plate and frame filter press: principles of operation

(a) filtering   (b) washing

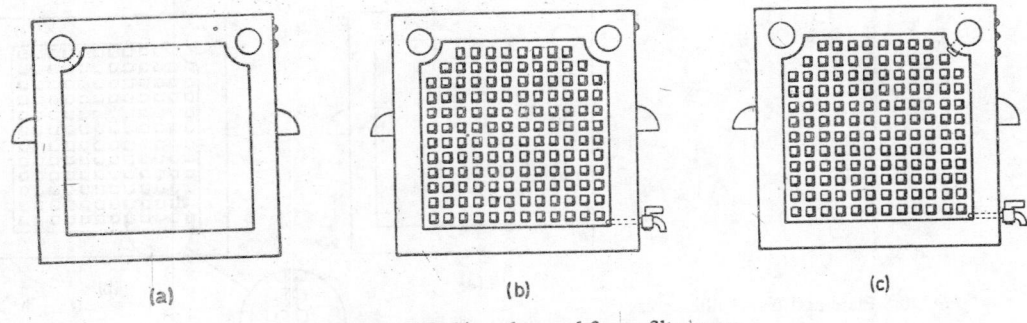

Fig. 20.7 Washing plate and frame filter press

(*a*) frame   (*b*) plate   (*c*) washing plate

The difference in design is that special plates and frames are used, having an additional channel to carry wash water (cf Figs. 20.7 and 20.5). Connections from the slurry feed channel into the frames and the filtrate outlets from the plates are identical to the ordinary press. In *half* the plates there is a connection from the wash water channel to the *surface* of the plate and these special plates are identified with three dots, compared with one dot on the ordinary plate. The two varieties of plate are used alternately, with frames between each, so that the sequence can be represented as: 1.2.3.2.1.2.3.2.1.2.3.2.1., etc.

The procedure for using the washing plate and frame press is shown diagrammatically in Fig. 20.6. Filtration proceeds in the ordinary way until the frames are filled with cake. To wash the filter cake the outlets on the washing plates (three dot) are *closed*, and wash water is pumped into the washing channel. The water enters the inlets on to the surface of the washing (three dot) plates and passes through the filter cloth on that plate from behind, through the filter cake, through the filter cloth on the ordinary (one dot) plate, down the surface of the plate and, finally, escaping from the outlet on that plate.

Clearly, this will give more efficient washing than the follow-through method, where the wash water is pumped into the slurry feed channel, since the latter will give a limited amount of washing near the inlet, but none at all at further points in the frame due to the high resistance to flow. With the special washing plates, however, the water flows over the entire surface of the washing (three dot) plate, so that the flow resistance of the cake is equal at all points and all the cake is washed with equal efficiency.

It should be noted that this is only true if the frames are *filled* with filter cake. If the solids do not fill the frame, the wash water causes the cake on the washing plate side of the frame to break, washing then being less effective. Hence, there is further emphasis on the need to use the filter press in such a way that the frames become completely filled with cake; not only is emptying of the frames facilitated, but it is essential for washing the cake correctly.

Assuming that the same pressure difference is used for washing as at the end of the filtration process, the rate of washing will be lower than the final rate of filtration. The reason for this is that half the outlets are closed, which has the effect of halving the area over which flow occurs. Also, as pointed out on page 239, the cake thickness in filtration, from the point of view of Darcy's law, is half the frame thickness. For washing, however, the water flows through the entire thickness of the frame, that is, the value of *l* is doubled. Hence, the effect of both factors is to reduce the washing rate to one quarter of the final filtration rate.

Advantages

(*a*) Construction is very simple and a wide variety of materials can be used, for example: cast iron, for handling common substances; bronze, for smaller units; stainless steel, where avoidance of contamination is important; hard rubber or plastics, where metals must be avoided; wood for lightness, although this must be kept wet.

(*b*) It provides a large filtering area in a relatively small floor space.

(*c*) It is versatile, the capacity being variable according to the thickness of the frames and the number used.

(*d*) The sturdy construction permits the use of considerable pressure difference, and it is normal to use up to about 20 bars.

(*e*) Efficient washing of the cake is possible.

(*f*) Operation and maintenance is straightforward, because there are no moving parts, filter cloths are easily renewable and, because all joints are external, any leaks are visible and do not contaminate the filtrate.

Disadvantages

(a) It is a batch filter, so that there is a good deal of 'down-time', which is non-productive.

(b) The filter press is an expensive filter, the emptying time, the labour involved, and the wear and tear on the cloths resulting in high costs.

(c) Operation is critical, as the frames should be full; otherwise washing is inefficient and the cake is difficult to remove.

(d) The filter press is used for slurries containing less than about 5 per cent solids; in view of the high labour costs, it is most suitable for expensive materials, many pharmaceutical substances coming into this category. Examples of the use of the filter press include the collection of bismuth salts, the collection of precipitated antitoxins, and the removal of precipitated proteins from insulin liquors.

Rotary Filter

Filters such as the filter leaf and filter press are batch operated and can handle dilute suspensions only, if the process is to be economic. In large-scale operation, continuous operation is sometimes desirable and it may be necessary to filter slurries containing a high proportion of solids.

The rotary filter is continuous in operation and has a system for removing the cake that is formed, hence it is suitable for use with concentrated slurries.

The operation of a rotary filter can best be understood by considering the stages a unit filter, such as a filter leaf, will follow, in a filtration cycle.

A likely sequence of events would be:

The leaf is dipped into the slurry and vacuum applied to the outlet, which is connected to the filtrate receiver.

When the cake has formed, the leaf is removed from the slurry and the cake drained by vacuum.

The leaf is dipped into wash water or is sprayed with water to wash the cake. The vacuum system is still applied to the outlet, and the liquid may be mixed with the filtrate or may be collected in a separate receiver.

Removal from the water, but retaining the vacuum connection, drains the cake and produces partial dryness.

The outlet of the leaf is connected to compressed air, which detaches the cake from the filter medium. If the cake is not completely removed, this can be effected by scraping with a knife.

The rotary filter consists of a number of filter units (usually 16 to 20) arranged so that the units are passing in continuous succession through the various stages.

One form is the *rotary disc filter* in which sector-shaped filter leaves form a disc with the outlets from each leaf connected to the vacuum system, compressed air, and the appropriate receivers, in the correct sequence, by means of a special rotating valve.

The commonest form in use in the pharmaceutical industry, however, is the *rotary drum filter*, a section of which is shown in Fig. 20.8, from which it will be seen that the filter units have the shape of longitudinal segments of the periphery of a cylinder. Thus, each filter unit is rectangular in shape with a curved profile so that a number can be joined up to form a drum. Each unit has a perforated metal surface to the outer part of the drum and is covered with filter cloth. Appropriate connections are again made from each unit through a rotating valve at the centre of the drum. In operation, the drum rotates at low speed, so that each unit passes through the various zones, shown in Fig. 20.8 and listed in Table 20.1.

Rotary filters may be up to 2 m in diameter and 3·5 m in length, giving areas of the order of 20 m².

Special attachments may be included for particular purposes; for example, if the cake shrinks and cracks as it dries out, *cake compression rollers* may be fitted. These compress the cake to a homogeneous mass to improve the efficiency of washing as the cake passes through the washing zone, or to aid drainage of wash water as the cake passes through the drying zone.

Where the solids of the slurry are such that the filter cloth becomes blocked with the particles, a *pre-coat filter* may be used. This is a variant in which a pre-coat of filter aid is deposited on the drum prior to the filtration process. The scraper knife then removes the solid filtered from the slurry together with a small amount of the pre-coat, the knife advancing slowly as the pre-coat is removed.

If removal of the cake presents problems, alternative discharge methods can be used. The *string discharge rotary filter*, for example, is especially useful for certain pharmaceutical applications, particularly for filtering the fermentation liquor in the manufacture of antibiotics where the mould is difficult to filter by ordinary methods because it forms a felt-like 'cake'. The string discharge filter is operated by means of a number of loops of string which pass round the drum, and cause the cake to form over the strings. As shown in the diagram, Fig. 20.9, the strings are in contact with the surface

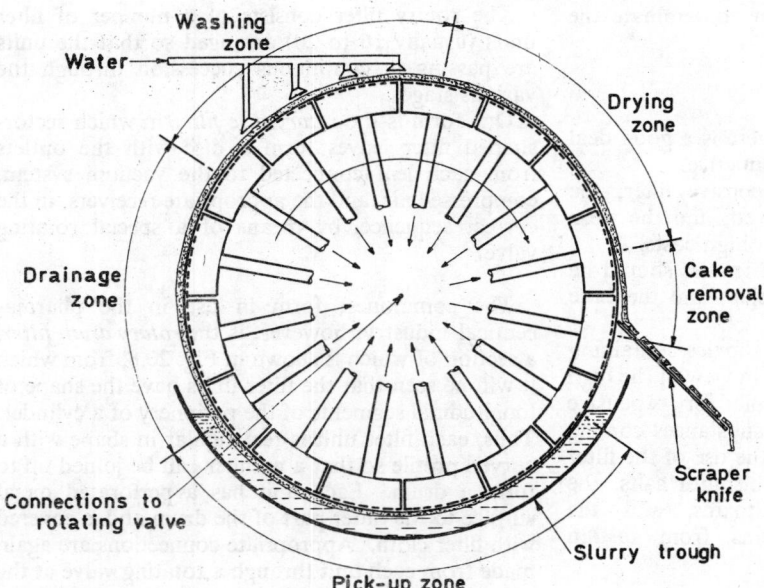

Fig. 20.8 Rotary drum filter

of the drum up to the cake removal zone, where they leave the surface and pass over additional small rollers before returning to again contact the drum. In operation, the strings lift the filter cake off the filter medium, and the cake is broken by the sharp bend over the rollers so that it is easily collected while the strings return to the drum.

Advantages

(*a*) The rotary filter is automatic and is continuous in operation, so that labour costs are very low.

Table 20.1
Rotary Filter Operation

Zone	Position	Service	Connected to:
Pick-up	Slurry trough	Vacuum	Filtrate receiver
Drainage	—	Vacuum	Filtrate receiver
Washing	Wash sprays	Vacuum	Wash water receiver
Drying	—	Vacuum	Wash receiver
Cake removal	Scraper knife	Compressed air	Filter cake conveyor

N.B. In some cases, the same receiver may be used for filtrate and for wash water

(*b*) The filter has a large capacity, in fact, the area of the filter as represented by *A* of Darcy's law is infinity.

(*c*) Variation of the speed of rotation enables the cake thickness to be controlled, and for solids that form an impenetrable cake the thickness may be limited to less than 5 mm. On the other hand, if the solids are coarse, forming a porous cake, the thickness may be 100 mm or more.

Disadvantages

(*a*) The rotary filter is a complex piece of equipment, with many moving parts, and is very expensive.

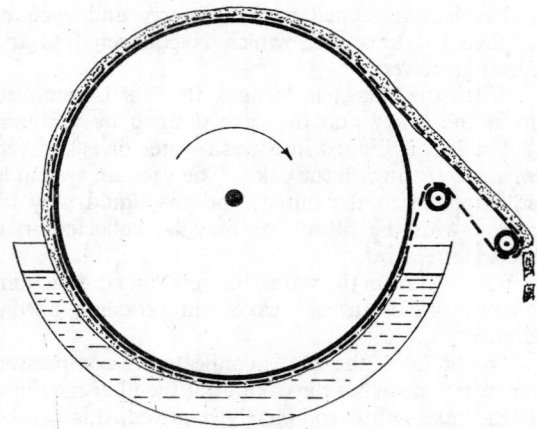

Fig. 20.9 String discharge rotary drum filter

In addition to the filter itself, ancillary equipment such as vacuum pumps, vacuum receivers and traps, slurry pumps and agitators are required.

(b) The cake tends to crack due to the air drawn through by the vacuum system, so that washing and drying are not efficient.

(c) Being a vacuum filter, the pressure difference is limited to 1 bar and hot filtrates may boil.

(d) The rotary filter is suitable only for straight-forward slurries, being less satisfactory if the solids form an impermeable cake or will not separate cleanly from the cloth.

USES OF THE ROTARY FILTER

The rotary filter is most suitable for continuous operation on large quantities of slurry, especially if the slurry contains considerable amounts of solids, that is, in the range 15 to 30 per cent.

Examples of pharmaceutical applications include the collection of calcium carbonate, magnesium carbonate, and starch, and the separation of the mycelium from the fermentation liquor in the manufacture of antibiotics.

Edge Filters

A form of filter that differs markedly from those described above is the type known generally as *edge filters*. Filters such as the leaf or press act by presenting a surface of the filter medium to the slurry. Edge filters use a pack of the filter medium, so that filtration occurs on the edges. Forms using packs of media such as filter paper can be used, but in the pharmaceutical industry greatest use is made of the *Metafilter*.

METAFILTER

The metafilter, in its simplest form, consists of a grooved drainage rod on which is packed a series of metal rings. These rings, usually of stainless steel, are about 15 mm inside diameter, 22 mm outside diameter, and 0·8 mm in thickness, with a number of semicircular projections on one surface, as shown in Fig. 20.10. The height of the projections and the shape of the section of the ring are such that when the rings are packed together, all the same way up, and tightened on the drainage rod with a nut, channels are formed that taper from about 250 μm down to 25 μm. One or more of these packs is mounted in a vessel, and the filter may be operated by pumping in the slurry under pressure or, occasionally, by the application of reduced pressure to the outlet side.

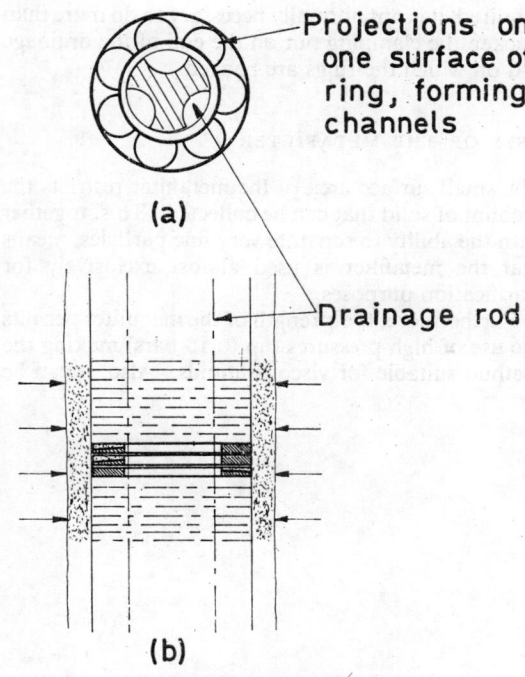

Fig. 20.10   Metafilter
(a) surface view of ring
(b) section through filter

In this form, the metafilter can be used as a strainer for coarse particles, but for finer particles a bed of a suitable material such as kieselguhr is first built up. The pack of rings, therefore, serves essentially as a base on which the true filter medium is supported.

Advantages

(a) The metafilter possesses considerable strength and high pressures can be used, with no danger of bursting the filter medium.

(b) As there is no filter medium as such, the running costs are low, and it is a very economical filter.

(c) The metafilter can be made from materials that can provide excellent resistance to corrosion and avoid contamination of the most sensitive product.

(d) By selection of a suitable grade of material to form the filter bed, it is possible to filter off very fine particles; in fact, it is claimed that some grades will sterilise a liquid by filtration. Equally well, it is possible to remove larger particles simply by building up a bed of coarse substance, or even by using the metafilter 'candle' itself if the particles are sufficiently large.

(e) Removal of the cake is effectively carried out by back-flushing with water. If further cleaning is required, it is not normally necessary to do more than slacken the clamping nut on the end of the drainage rod on which the rings are packed.

USES OF THE METAFILTER

The small surface area of the metafilter restricts the amount of solid that can be collected. This, together with the ability to separate very fine particles, means that the metafilter is used almost exclusively for clarification purposes.

Furthermore, the strength of the metafilter permits the use of high pressures (up to 15 bars) making the method suitable for viscous liquids. Also, it can be constructed in materials appropriate for corrosive substances.

Specific examples of pharmaceutical uses include the clarification of syrups, of injection solutions, and of products such as insulin liquors.

BIBLIOGRAPHY

DICKEY, G. D. (1961) *Filtration.* New York, Reinhold.
POOLE, J. B. and DOYLE, D. (Eds) (1966) *Solid/ Liquid Separation: a Review and a Bibliographical Guide.* London, H.M. Stationery Office.
SUTTLE, H. K. (Ed.) (1969) *Process Engineering Technique Evaluation: Filtration.* London, Morgan-Grampian.

21

Centrifugation

CENTRIFUGAL force is used to provide the driving force for two operations discussed earlier, that is, to create a pressure difference in the filtration process, as described by Darcy's law (*see* p. 234) and to replace gravitational force in the sedimentation process to which Stokes' law was applied (*see* p. 178). Care should be taken not to describe centrifugal processes as 'accelerated gravitational processes'. Although this is true in some cases, there are certain separations that could not be effected by gravitational force which can be brought about by centrifugal force. The separation by centrifugation of the two phases of an emulsion that is stable under the normal force of gravity is an example of this type.

Centrifugation is based on the well-known principle that an object that is rotated about a centre point at a constant radial distance from that point is acted upon by a force.

This chapter discusses the principles of centrifugation as they affect the industrial use of the operation, the equipment used, and examples of the use of the method in pharmaceutical practice.

Principles of Centrifugation

The operations using centrifugal force are described by equations including the gravitational constant (*see* Darcy's law on p. 234 and Stokes' law on p. 197). It is convenient, therefore, to measure the centrifugal force in terms of a ratio to the gravitational force, and this is known as the *centrifugal effect*, that is, the number of times the centrifugal force is greater than the gravitational force. The centrifugal effect is then inserted in the appropriate equation with the gravitational force.

The centrifugal effect is obtained as follows:

Consider a body of mass m rotating in a circular path of radius r at a velocity v (*see* Fig. 21.1). The force acting on the body in a radial direction is given by:

$$F = \frac{mv^2}{r} \qquad (21.1)$$

where F = centrifugal force; m = mass of body; v = velocity of body; and r = radius of circle of rotation.

The same body will be acted upon by a gravitational force:

$$G = mg \qquad (21.2)$$

where G = gravitational force, and g = gravitational constant.

The centrifugal effect is the ratio of the two forces, so that:

$$C = \frac{F}{G} \qquad (21.3a)$$

$$= \frac{mv^2}{mgr}$$

$$= \frac{v^2}{gr} \qquad (21.3b)$$

But:

$$v = 2\pi r n \qquad (21.4)$$

where n = speed of rotation.

$$\therefore \frac{F}{G} = \frac{(2\pi r n)^2}{gr} \qquad (21.5)$$

$$= \frac{4\pi^2 r^2 n^2}{gr}$$

$$= \frac{2\pi^2 n^2 d}{g} \qquad (21.6)$$

where d = diameter of rotation.

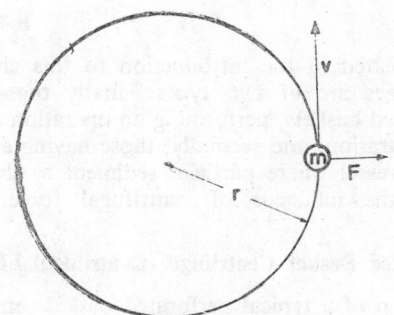

Fig. 21.1 Centrifugation principles.

The gravitational constant has a value of 9·807 m/s², so that Eqn (21.6) may be simplified to:

$$\text{centrifugal effect} = 2\cdot013n^2d \qquad (21.7)$$

provided that n is expressed in s^{-1} and d is in m.

The centrifugal effect may attain high values, as shown by the following examples.

Examples

A centrifuge with a diameter of 1 m rotates at a frequency of 15 s^{-1}:

$$\text{centrifugal effect} = 2\cdot013 \times 15^2 \times 1$$
$$= 453$$

If the same centrifuge has the frequency increased to 30 s^{-1},

$$\text{centrifugal effect} = 2\cdot013 \times 30^2 \times 1$$
$$= 1812$$

A centrifuge 100 mm in diameter is operated at a rotational frequency of 400 s^{-1}.

$$\text{Centrifugal effect} = 2\cdot013 \times 400^2 \times 0\cdot1$$
$$= 32\ 208$$

From the equations and these values, the important conclusion can be drawn that the centrifugal effect is proportional directly to the diameter, but is proportional to the *square* of the speed of rotation. Thus, if it is necessary to increase the centrifugal effect, it is of greater advantage to use a centrifuge of the same size at a higher speed, rather than use a larger centrifuge at the same speed of rotation.

It will be seen from the examples that, in the larger centrifuge, doubling the speed had the result of quadrupling the centrifugal effect, while the high speed of rotation of a small centrifuge gave a very high value to the centrifugal effect. The applications of these observations will be seen later when equipment is considered.

A further reason for using the smallest size of centrifuge that has the appropriate capacity is that the structure is subject to considerable stress in operation, largely due to the pressure of the fluid on the walls. It can be shown that the pressure is proportional to the square of the speed and to the square of the diameter. The effect of this is shown in Table 21.1, where three centrifuges are compared, with the speed varied to give the same centrifugal effect, from which it will be seen that the pressure due to water increases greatly as the centrifuge becomes larger.

It must be emphasised that a centrifuge is comparable to a pressure vessel and must be treated with

Table 21.1

Diameter (m)	Rotational frequency s^{-1}	Centrifugal effect	Pressure on wall, if filled with water (bars)
0·11	45	450	1·2
0·25	30	450	2·8
1·0	15	450	11·1

the same care as a piece of equipment such as a high pressure autoclave.

The centrifugal apparatus described later will illustrate these principles. It will be seen that for purposes requiring a low centrifugal effect on a large amount of material (that is, for filtration type processes) the centrifuge is large and operates at low speed. The centrifugal sedimentation of very small particles necessitates a high value for the centrifugal effect, and the apparatus is usually of small diameter, but operates at very high speed.

Industrial Centrifuges

As indicated in the introduction to this chapter, centrifuges are of two types: firstly those with perforated baskets, performing an operation resembling filtration, and secondly, those having a solid-walled vessel where particles sediment to the wall under the influence of centrifugal force.

Perforated Basket Centrifuge (Centrifugal Filter)

A section of a typical perforated basket centrifuge in Fig. 21.2 shows the resemblance in construction to the domestic spin dryer. A vessel, usually about 1 m in diameter on the industrial scale, has an outer wall that is perforated. It is mounted on a vertical shaft by means of which it can be rotated at a frequency of 20 to 25 s^{-1}. An outer casing with an outlet collects the liquid thrown out from the perforated basket by centrifugal force. The casing is closed by a cover which, for safety, is usually interlocked with the drive motor so that the centrifuge cannot be operated when the cover is raised.

For pharmaceutical purposes, the construction may be of stainless steel, or a metal such as mild steel may be protected by a rubber coating.

The example in the diagram has the drive motor below the centrifuge and is called *under-driven*.

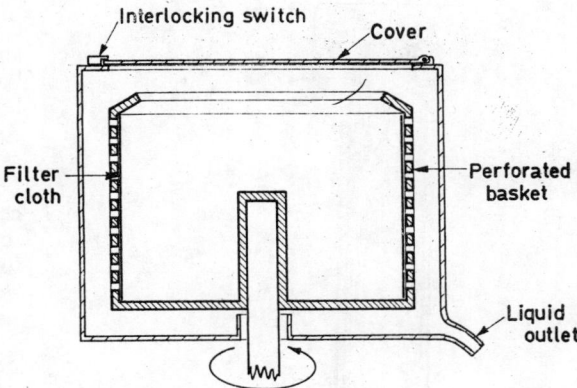

Fig. 21.2 Perforated basket centrifuge

Other forms may be *over-driven*, that is, the centrifuge is suspended by the drive system which facilitates emptying through outlets in the bottom of the basket. Other forms can be mounted horizontally, and by means of special plough devices can be made continuous in operation.

Advantages

(*a*) The centrifuge is very compact, occupying very little floor space compared with filters of similar capacity.

(*b*) Centrifugal methods can handle slurries with a high proportion of solids, even to the extent of having a paste-like consistency.

(*c*) The final product has a very low moisture content, which will be considerably less than that of a filter cake of a similar material.

(*d*) Centrifugal force removes the liquid from the cake in producing a dry product, so that dissolved solids are separated from the cake. This contrasts with the thermal drying process (*see* p. 272) where the liquid is vaporised, causing dissolved material to be deposited on the insoluble solids of the cake.

(*e*) The process is rapid. Charging, acceleration, drying washing, deceleration, and emptying takes only a short time, 300 to 600 s being typical; since a centrifuge 1 m in diameter will hold about 200 kg, this represents an hourly output of 1 to 2 Mg.

Disadvantages

(*a*) The complicated cycle of operation involves considerable labour costs, making the process expensive.

(*b*) Usually, the process is intermittent, working on the batch principle.

(*c*) If the machine is adapted for continuous operation, there is considerable wear and tear because the solids that have to be removed are in the form of a hard, abrasive cake, due to the consolidating effect of the centrifugal force.

Uses

The centrifuge can be used for removing unwanted solids from a liquid, as occurs, for example, where precipitated protein must be removed from products such as insulin. The centrifugal method permits recovery of a higher proportion of the liquid than would be removed with a filter. Hence, the cake requires little or no washing, which minimises the evaporation necessary.

The centrifuge is especially useful for separating and drying solids, particularly of crystallised substances, because of its rapidity, the avoidance of efflorescence and the removal of the mother liquor from the surface resulting in a free-flowing product. In comparison, thermal drying is much slower, is likely to remove water of crystallisation, and evaporation deposits the solute on the crystals, leading to the formation of a solid cake of product and, possibly, the retention of impurities.

Sedimentation Type Centrifuges (Centrifugal Sedimenters)

TUBULAR BOWL CENTRIFUGES

Earlier it was shown that high centrifugal effects could be obtained by using a centrifuge of small diameter rotated at high speed. This is the principle of the tubular bowl centrifuge which separates the solids of small particle size from liquids, and is illustrated in section in Fig. 21.3. A cylindrical 'bowl' about 100 mm in diameter and 1 m in length is mounted so that it can be rotated about its longitudinal axis at high frequency, usually about 300 s^{-1}, although frequencies up to 1000 s^{-1} can be used.

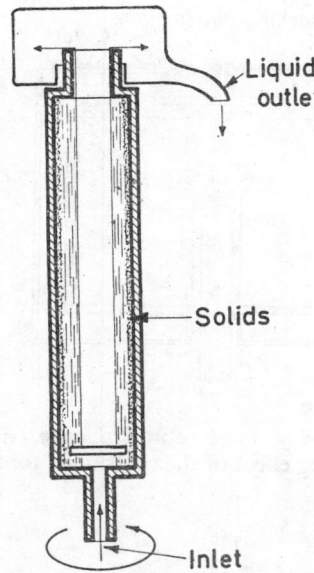

Fig. 21.3 Tubular bowl centrifuge

The inlet for the suspension is at the base, through the rotating shaft, while the clear liquid overflows from a weir at the top. Solids are deposited on the wall and are removed at intervals, as necessary.

The principles of operation of this centrifuge are compared with the sedimentation tank (*see* p. 197) in Fig. 21.4. Thus, the two processes are identical, except that centrifugal force is used instead of gravitational force. The important effect is in the increased settling velocity of particles (*see* p. 178).

The tubular bowl centrifuge can be used also for separating immiscible liquids. As a result of the centrifugal force, the liquids will form two layers, with the heavier liquid adjacent to the wall. The liquids can be collected separately by means of a

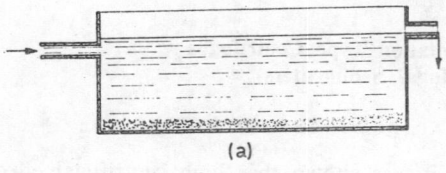

(a)

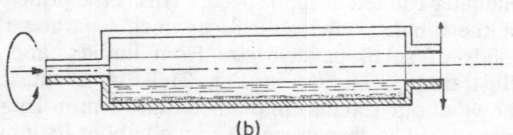

(b)

Fig. 21.4 Comparison of (*a*) sedimentation tank with (*b*) tubular bowl centrifuge

modified weir, the principle of which can be seen in Fig. 21.5, the heavier liquid passing outside the weir and overflowing from the bowl, while the lighter liquid moves inside the weir, finally escaping at a higher level to a separate collecting device. Any solids present will be thrown to the wall of the bowl, as in the ordinary tubular bowl centrifuge.

The principal difficulty with the tubular bowl centrifuge is its limited throughput, partially due to the small size of the bowl, but also to the relatively low flow rate necessary to provide sufficient time for sedimentation of the solids to the wall. This can be overcome by an alternative design.

CONICAL DISC CENTRIFUGE

The conical disc centrifuge has a larger, shallow form of bowl containing a series of conical discs

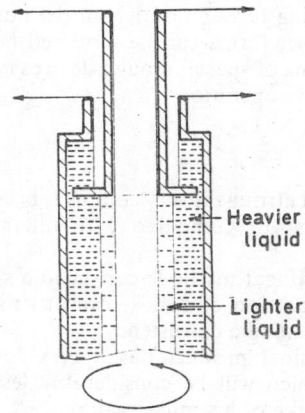

Fig. 21.5 Modified weir for liquid/liquid separation

(Fig. 21.6). The feed enters, as shown by the arrows, through a concentric tube surrounding the central drive shaft and flows into the spaces between the discs. Here, separation of the materials occurs, solids and/or heavy liquids moving to the underside, and light liquids to the upper side of the discs. These substances then move along the surfaces of the discs to the limits of the inner and outer layers, solids depositing on the wall, and liquids escaping from the outlets.

The important factor is that the separating distance is only the space between the discs, which is commonly only a few millimetres, whereas in the tubular bowl centrifuge it is at least ten times greater and often considerably more.

In view of the larger diameter and the fact that the small separating distance permits a lower value of the centrifugal effect, the disc centrifuge can operate at lower speeds than the tubular variety.

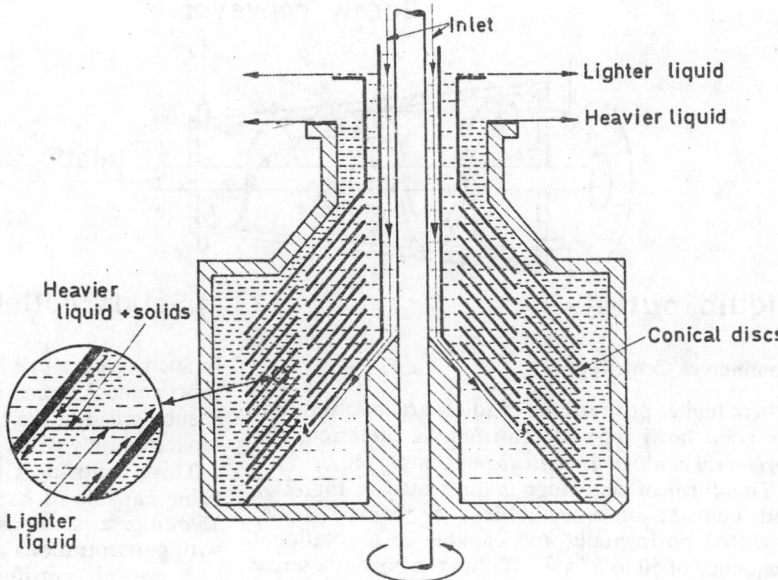

Fig. 21.6 Conical disc centrifuge

Inlet

Lighter liquid

Heavier liquid

Conical discs

Heavier
liquid + solids

Lighter
liquid

Advantages of Centrifugal Sedimenters

(*a*) These centrifuges are compact, occupying a very small space compared with filters or sedimentation tanks of similar output.

(*b*) The separating efficiency is high, so that particles are deposited very rapidly. Furthermore, particles can be sedimented that it would not be possible to separate by gravitational methods.

(*c*) Centrifugation is the ideal technique for dealing with 'difficult' solids; for example, substances that are slimy or compressible and would block a filter medium. Coagulated proteins are typical of such materials.

(*d*) Continuous separation of two immiscible liquids can be carried out, and the removal of solids also, if required.

(*e*) Classification of solids can be effected by control of the speed of rotation of the centrifuge and the flow rate, so that coarse particles are separated while finer particles remain in suspension.

Disadvantages of Centrifugal Sedimenters

(*a*) The high speed of rotation of this type of centrifuge requires special driving mechanisms, making construction complicated. Balance, for example, is extremely important to avoid dangerous vibration in operation.

(*b*) The equipment is small, and the tubular bowl in particular cannot hold a great deal of solids, so that capacity is limited. The design of the conical

disc centrifuge can be modified to permit solids that have been deposited on the wall to escape through nozzles, so that the *nozzle-discharge centrifuge* is continuous in operation and, thereby, of greater capacity.

USES OF CENTRIFUGAL SEDIMENTERS

The centrifugal sedimenter has many applications in the pharmaceutical industry, principally for liquid/liquid separation or for clarification involving small proportions of solids that are compressible or of very small particle size. These include:

The removal of dirt and water from oils; for example, in the purification of olive oil or fish liver oils.

The recovery of lanolin in the wool scouring process.

The separation of the phases in liquid/liquid extraction processes such as those used in the manufacture of antibiotics.

The removal of bacteria; in processes for making bacterial enzyme preparation, for example.

The separation of blood plasma from whole blood.

The collection of starch after the washing and purification stages.

The clarification of process liquors, such as in the manufacture of insulin, where precipitated proteins must be removed.

Using control of speed of rotation and rate of flow, to separate particles into two size fractions.

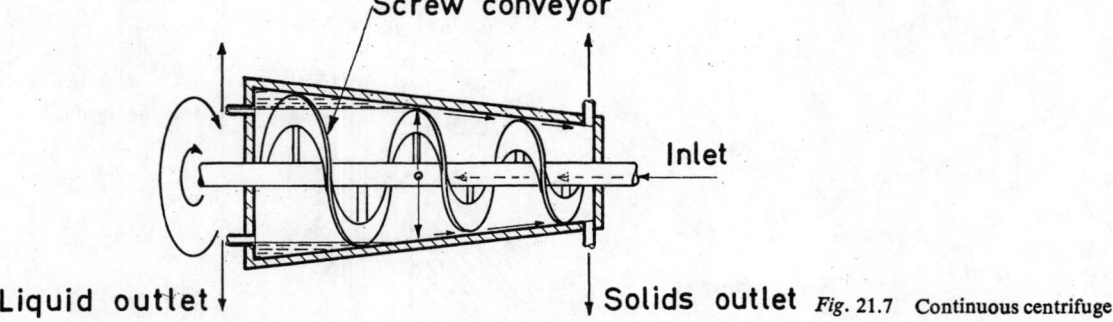

Fig. 21.7   Continuous centrifuge

Continuous Centrifuges

Where higher proportions of solids are involved, but the solid bowl type of centrifuge is preferred, the *horizontal continuous centrifuge* is employed.

This form of centrifuge is illustrated in Fig. 21.7 and consists of a cylindrical or conical bowl, mounted horizontally and capable of a rotational frequency of 50 to 65 s^{-1}. Within the bowl is a screw conveyor which rotates in the same direction as the bowl, but slightly slower. The slurry is introduced through the shaft, as shown, and the liquid separates to the wider portion of the bowl, while the solid material is carried towards the outlet by the con veyor, where it is discharged continuously through the outlets.

Apart from the continuous operation, the special feature of this centrifuge is that the solids are separated from the liquid and conveyed up the dry 'beach', so that the final discharged solid has a low moisture content, possibly 1 per cent or less. Arrangements can be made to wash the solid as it is moved between the feed point and the outlet.

The conical form in Fig. 21.7 is in common use, but some materials are difficult to convey when dry; for example, if the material is soft and compressible.

In such cases, a cylindrical bowl will be used with a short conical section near the outlet so that the solid is submerged in the liquid for most of the time and separated only when near to the discharge point.

These centrifuges are very flexible in operation, being capable of handling solids as large as 10 to 15 mm or as small as a few micrometres, in slurries with concentrations ranging from 0·5 to 50 per cent.

A typical centrifuge would have a diameter of about 0·5 m and a frequency of rotation of about 65 s^{-1}, which will give a centrifugal effect of the order of 4200.

Throughput will depend on the material, but may be up to 20 to 25 m³/h of liquid and 1 to 1·5 Mg/h solids, so that large amounts can be handled by a machine occupying only a small space.

BIBLIOGRAPHY

POOLE, J. B. and DOYLE, D. (Eds) (1966) *Solid/Liquid Separation: a Review and a Bibliographical Guide.* London, H.M. Stationery Office.

SUTTLE, H. K. (Ed.) (1969) *Process Engineering Technique Evaluation: Filtration.* London, Morgan-Grampian.

22

Extraction

ALTHOUGH many of the remedies obtained by the extraction of vegetable drugs have been replaced by synthetic medicaments, the *British Pharmacopoeia* and *British Pharmaceutical Codex* still contain a number of such preparations. Furthermore, the starting material for some products such as steroids may come from natural sources and be subjected to chemical or biochemical modification. This chapter discusses the problems and the theoretical principles involved in extraction. Large-scale production requires modification of the basic processes, and these are considered as well as factors affecting the choice of process and the means of solvent recovery. Although most of the chapter is devoted to solid/liquid extraction, the liquid/liquid extraction process has certain pharmaceutical applications and is considered briefly.

Extraction can be defined as the removal of soluble material from an insoluble residue, either liquid or solid, by treatment with a liquid solvent. It is, therefore, a solution process and depends on the mass transfer phenomena discussed in Chapter 13. The controlling factor in the rate of extraction is normally the rate of diffusion of the solute through the liquid boundary layer or layers at the interface.

LIQUID/LIQUID EXTRACTION

The small-scale use of liquid/liquid extraction will be familiar from the purification procedures used in alkaloidal assays, and large-scale processes are based on similar principles.

A solution of the substance it is desired to extract is brought into contact with another solvent for the substance that is immiscible with the first solvent. A concentration gradient is set up between the phases, and mass transfer will occur until an equilibrium is established, the distribution of the solute depending on the distribution coefficient (*see* p. 14).

As the process is controlled by mass transfer, the liquids must be thoroughly mixed to give a large enough surface area for contact, sufficient time must be allowed in the dispersed state for equilibrium to be set up and, finally, the liquids are separated. This can be achieved in stirred tanks which represent the large-scale equivalent of the separating funnel used in the laboratory. Contacting devices in the form of columns may also be used, but in pharmaceutical processes centrifugal extractors, which ensure thorough contact of the liquids in countercurrent flow, followed by rapid separation, are commonly employed. In the purification of many antibiotics multistage extraction and centrifugal extractors enable the process to be carried out with the minimum of decomposition.

Typical of these methods is the *Podbielniak Extractor*, the body of which consists of a drum mounted on a horizontal shaft, the drum containing a number of concentric perforated cylinders. The liquids enter through the shaft, the light liquid being taken to the periphery of the drum, while the heavy liquid enters at the axis of the shaft. Centrifugal action due to the rotation of the drum causes the heavy liquid to move towards the outside, so that the light liquid is displaced towards the shaft, both escaping again through the shaft.

Mass transfer coefficients are high, the perforated cylinders causing good dispersion and contact as the liquids move in countercurrent flow. In addition, liquid hold-up is low and processing time is short. A further advantage of the use of centrifugal force is the ability to deal with liquids that tend to emulsify or which have only a small difference in density.

The equipment is expensive, but is justified by the high cost of many of the medicaments, and the method is used widely in the manufacture of antibiotics.

SOLID/LIQUID EXTRACTION

The extraction of a soluble constituent from a solid by means of a solvent is commonly referred to as *leaching*, but the general term *extraction* is most frequently used in pharmaceutical practice.

Certain operations involve the extraction of a soluble substance from an insoluble mineral material, but this is subject to control by the usual factors affecting solution (*see* p. 12) and will not be considered further.

Although fewer preparations are now made by extracting the active constituents of vegetable drugs, the process is still of considerable importance and presents many more problems than the previous case.

Difficulties of Extracting Vegetable Drugs

A study elsewhere in the pharmacy syllabus will have shown that there are great variations in the characters of vegetable drugs. Thus, some are soft and spongy and can be extracted easily in the whole state, while others are very hard and tough; certain seeds, for example, remain unchanged after immersion in water for long periods. Hence, a knowledge of the botanical structure of the drug is valuable as a preliminary to extraction.

There are considerable differences in the active constituents it is desired to extract; for example, alkaloids, glycosides, tannins, resins or oils. Again, advance knowledge assists in correct selection of the extraction method.

Different forms of insoluble matter may affect the extraction process, so that, as well as the cellulose of the cell structure, there may be proteins or carbohydrates such as starch.

In many drugs the active constituent is not the only soluble material present and a drug may contain a small proportion of an alkaloid, for example, with a large proportion of sugars. In these circumstances, a solvent is chosen that is as selective as possible and, ideally, would dissolve the alkaloid only.

Wet vegetable material is an excellent medium for microbial growth and, if allowed to occur, this may lead to loss of constituents and deterioration of the product. The solvent must have, or be given, suitable preservative properties.

As a result of these difficulties, extraction methods are based to a large extent on tradition and are empirical in character. Hence, the *British Pharmacopoeia* and the *British Pharmaceutical Codex* use a number of methods, the significance of which will be appreciated if the extraction of vegetable materials is considered in general terms.

Theory of Extraction of Drugs

Examination of the extraction processes will show that all have certain stages in common:
Suitable size reduction of the drug.
Penetration of the drug by the solvent.
Solution of the soluble matter within the cells.
The escape of the dissolved material through the cell walls and through the solvent boundary layer surrounding the particles of the drug.
Finally, separation of the solution and the exhausted drug.

Each of these stages will be considered in more detail and related to the theoretical principles.

SUITABLE SIZE REDUCTION OF THE DRUG

Mass transfer theory would suggest that the maximum surface area should be obtained, which would entail reducing the drug to individual cells, but in practice this is not possible or desirable, because:
It would be very difficult to size reduce materials to this extent.
A prolonged size reduction process is likely to lead to decomposition of constituents or loss of volatile materials.
A suspension of extremely fine particles would be very difficult, if not impossible, to separate in the final stages, since particles of the size of individual cells would form an unfilterable slime.
Breakage of all cells releases the entire cell contents, including inert materials, so that dry extracts, for example, are diluted. It is preferable in practice, therefore, to keep many of the cell walls unbroken to act as a 'filter' for the retention of insoluble matter or of colloidal materials.
The degree of size reduction to be used will depend, therefore, on the botanical structure of the drug, ranging from a sliced and bruised condition for soft drugs (such as gentian) through Coarse and Moderately Coarse Powders for materials such as cascara or belladonna to Moderately Fine Powder for a hard and woody drug, of which ipecacuanha is an example.
It must be emphasised that the greatest degree of size reduction is not necessarily to be preferred. Thus, it has been shown experimentally that, if dry extracts are made from drugs such as belladonna or stramonium, it is possible to obtain a greater *total* extractive when finer grades of powder are used, but that the extract from a Moderately Coarse Powder contains a higher proportion of alkaloid.
Generally, the appropriate degree of size reduction will comply with the following requirements:
Cause some of the cells of the drug to be broken to assist penetration of the solvent and escape of soluble matter.
For similar reasons, cause some cells to be cracked or distorted.
Provide a particle size that will not result in a very long path for the solvent and the soluble matter. Otherwise, the concentration gradient will be unnecessarily long and material will be lost. This distance will be equivalent to the radius of a sphere, or the shortest distance from any point in the interior to the surface in particles of irregular shape.
Result in particles having a large enough surface area for adequate mass transfer.

PENETRATION OF THE SOLVENT INTO THE DRUG

A drug in the dry state is porous due to shrinkage, and the pores contain air that must be displaced as the solvent enters into the pores and penetrates into the cells. The process will depend on the character of the drug, and a brief outline will be given of the structure of the cells as far as it affects the extraction, a detailed discussion being beyond the scope of this book.

The cell walls consist basically of cellulose molecules in the form of ultra-microscopic, spirally-shaped fibrils running approximately parallel to the axis of the cell. These are known as *micellae* and, in the fresh material, are surrounded by a film of water. When the drug is dried, this film is lost and the micellae move together to form a continuous membrane; since most of the cells have their longest axes in the longitudinal direction, most shrinkage occurs laterally. This has been verified by experiments in drying timber, where it was found that wood showed a shrinkage of the order of 8 per cent in the tangential direction, about 5 per cent radially, but only 0.2 per cent longitudinally.

When the dry drug is moistened, the reverse occurs, the micellae take up a liquid film once more, and the tissues swell. In practice, the amount of swelling is variable, being greatest with liquids when hydroxyl groups form a great part of the molecule. Thus, water causes considerable swelling, while there is much less with ethanol. Glycerol will lead to swelling comparable to that obtained with water but, as would be expected, the greater viscosity of glycerol causes the liquid to be taken up much more slowly.

In all cases the swelling continues until the pressure caused by the liquid layers is equal to the cohesive forces between the micellae. In addition, swelling may occur due to the distension and bursting of thin-walled cells that have taken up liquid by osmosis.

Thus, swelling will be greatest when water is used to moisten a drug when the tissues consist of thin-walled cells; conversely, least swelling occurs when ethanol is the solvent for a drug with thick-walled cells.

As indicated earlier in this section, the solvent must displace air from pores in the drug and it follows that this can be aided by using a vacuum pump. If the solvent and drug are placed in a suitable vessel and the pressure reduced, air will be removed from the pores. When the vacuum is broken, the pressure of the atmosphere forces solvent into the drug, so that penetration is facilitated considerably.

SOLUTION OF CONSTITUENTS

Once the solvent has penetrated into the cells, solution of the constituents takes place and is governed by the usual factors affecting this phenomenon (*see* p. 12). The most important of these in the context of extraction is that the rate of solution (and usually the solubility also) is increased by elevation of temperature.

ESCAPE OF THE SOLUTION FROM THE CELLS

During the size reduction process, some cells are broken open, while others are damaged or distorted and, where this occurs, the escape of the solution is not impeded. Many cells remain whole, however, so that the soluble matter must pass through the walls and, although it has been suggested that phenomena such as osmosis may have an effect, diffusion is the most likely mechanism and will be assumed for this discussion.

Irrespective of the condition of the cells, dissolved material reaching the surface of the particle must pass through the boundary layer at the solid/liquid interface and the rate at which this occurs will be governed by the factors controlling mass transfer, considered on page 162. Thus, the rate of diffusion will depend on the presence of a suitable concentration gradient from the centre of the particle outwards and through the boundary layer, the thickness of the boundary layer, and the diffusion coefficients of the solutes in the solvent.

Consideration of the factors controlling mass transfer will show that the rate of extraction can be affected in the following ways.

1. Where the drug is immersed in a quantity of solvent:

(*a*) By agitating the mixture occasionally, which disperses local concentrations of the solution, thereby increasing the concentration gradient.

(*b*) By agitating the solvent and the drug continuously, which increases the concentration gradient as in the previous case, but also reduces the thickness of the boundary layer so that the concentration gradient becomes shorter and steeper. A similar effect can be achieved by using a pump to circulate the liquid.

(*c*) By suspending the drug in a cloth bag or above a perforated plate near to the surface of the liquid. As the constituents dissolve, the density of the solution increases, so that convection currents are established, leading to circulation of the solution. This, again, increases the concentration gradient through the boundary layers.

2. If the drug is positioned so that the solvent flows past the particles:

(a) The flow replaces the solution by pure solvent, causing an increase in the concentration gradient.

(b) The spaces between the particles of drug form passages through which the solvent flows; due to the small size of these capillaries, the velocity of the solvent is sufficient to reduce the boundary layers, so increasing the concentration gradient.

In both 1 and 2, the extraction can take place at elevated temperatures, if the material is thermostable and if the solvent is not affected by heating. In practice, very few drugs are sufficiently thermostable and the solvent must be a pure boiling substance or a constant boiling mixture, so that the technique is limited.

3. When elevated temperatures can be used, there are a number of advantages leading to increased extraction rates:

(a) The viscosity of the solvent is decreased, which reduces the boundary layers.

(b) Convection currents have a similar effect to agitation during extraction.

(c) The diffusion coefficient is proportional to the Absolute temperature and inversely proportional to the viscosity, so that raising the temperature influences the rate of diffusion considerably.

Commonly, the solubility of the constituents is increased as the temperature is raised.

Consideration of the factors discussed in this section will show that there is likely to be great variation in the efficiency of the extraction process.

Extraction will never be complete if the drug is simply immersed in a bulk of solvent, since an equilibrium is set up between the solution in the cells and the free solution. The efficiency will depend on the particle size; a concentration gradient exists through the particle of drug and through the boundary layer, so that a point is reached when there is insufficient driving force to continue mass transfer. Hence, the larger the particle, the longer the concentration gradient, giving rise to greater residual concentrations of soluble material in the centre of the particle.

On the other hand, extraction is virtually complete in methods where the drug forms a packed bed with the solvent flowing through it. Usually, the particles are small and fresh solvent is continually displacing the solution; although traces of soluble material will remain, the amount is negligible.

SEPARATION OF SOLUTION AND EXHAUSTED DRUG

In processes involving the immersion of the drug in a bulk of solvent, the solid material has to be strained off. Since the drug absorbs solvent and, as indicated in the previous section, there is a residue of soluble constituents in this solvent, the drug is subjected to pressure to expel as much of the solution as possible.

If the extraction process uses solvent flowing through the drug, however, the separation is part of the normal process.

Properties of Solvents Used for Extracting Drugs

The fact that many of the products made by extraction are intended for internal administration imposes considerable restrictions on the solvents that can be used. The ideal solvent would be:

1. Cheap.
2. Non-toxic.
3. Stable, that is, chemically and physically inert; this would include properties such as neutral reaction, not too volatile and non-inflammable.
4. Selective, that is, to remove the desired active constituents, with the minimum amount of the inert materials.

These characters render the majority of organic solvents unacceptable, except in certain special cases where the solvent does not remain in the product. An example is the use of petroleum ether for the removal of fat from a drug before extracting the desired active constituents.

Water and ethanol and mixtures of these two liquids are most commonly used; these two solvents are of considerable use, as the following summary of their properties shows.

WATER AS A SOLVENT

Water is a solvent of proteins, colouring matters, gums, anthraquinone derivatives, most alkaloidal salts, glycosides, sugars and tannins. In addition, water will dissolve enzymes, many organic acids, most organic salts, and small proportions of volatile oils. Waxes, fats, fixed oils and most alkaloids (that is, the free bases) are insoluble.

Advantages

(a) It is cheap.
(b) It has a wide solvent action.
(c) It is non-toxic.
(d) It is non-inflammable.

Disadvantages

(a) It is not selective; the list given above shows that it dissolves a wide range of substances, some of which are not only inert medicinally, but are also undesirable because they readily ferment or decompose.

(*b*) Moulds and bacteria grow in aqueous media. Hence, most preparations made with water must be stabilised by adding a suitable proportion of ethanol, glycerin, sugar or chloroform, or by sterilisation.

(*c*) Water promotes hydrolysis of many substances and allows enzyme action to take place.

(*d*) Concentration of an aqueous extractive involves the use of more heat than for most other solvents, due to the high latent heat of vaporisation of water.

ETHANOL AS A SOLVENT

Ethanol, known as Alcohol in the *British Pharmacopoeia*, is a solvent of alkaloids, alkaloidal salts, glycosides, volatile oils and resins, together with many forms of colouring matter (notably chlorophyll), tannins, anthraquinone derivatives, and many organic acids and salts.

Ethanol does not dissolve albuminous matter, gums, waxes, fats, and most fixed oils; sucrose is insoluble, but certain other sugars present in drugs (dextrose, for example) are soluble in ethanol.

Advantages

(*a*) It is reasonably selective; for example, in a drug containing gum, albuminous matter and a glycoside or an alkaloidal salt, ethanol in a suitable dilution with water would dissolve only the glycoside or alkaloidal salt, whereas water would usually dissolve all these constituents.

(*b*) Moulds and bacteria cannot grow in solutions containing 20 per cent or more of ethanol.

(*c*) It is non-toxic in the quantities present in medicinal doses of preparations made with it.

(*d*) It is neutral, hence preparations made with it are unlikely to be incompatible with other products.

(*e*) The presence of ethanol in preparations promotes rapid absorption of the constituents.

(*f*) The latent heat of vaporisation of ethanol is less than half of that of water, so that less heat is used in the concentration of ethanol solutions.

(*g*) Ethanol is miscible with water in all proportions; mixtures with water at different dilutions are used, giving solvents of variable properties and costs.

The principal *disadvantage* of ethanol is its cost, although the rebate of duty allowed on rectified spirit used for most medicinal preparations and the permission to use industrial methylated spirit for those preparations for internal use in which no spirit remains in the finished product, considerably reduce the cost of ethanol as a solvent.

The final selection of the solvent is based largely on the characters of the constituents, both active and inert, so that a knowledge of the pharmacognosy of the drug is of extreme importance.

Extraction Methods

In view of the foregoing factors affecting extraction, it is not surprising that a variety of methods are used, partially based on tradition, but in many cases the subject of official specification in the *British Pharmacopoeia*.

The majority of these methods are designed for small-scale use, whereas this chapter is concerned principally with large-scale processes. It is required, however, that products made by processes that have been modified for large-scale use shall be identical in character with the product of the small-scale process. The extraction procedures of the *British Pharmacopoeia* and the *British Pharmaceutical Codex* should be studied in detail and each stage examined in the light of the extraction theory. It will be found that the processes may be divided into two main groups. Maceration methods are based on the immersion of the drug in a bulk of solvent, with modification to multiple stage extraction (double or triple) to increase the yield if necessary. An alternative form of maceration is used for unorganised drugs, where the proportion of soluble matter is high. Percolation methods depend on the flow of solvent through the powdered drug, to yield products of greater concentration than the maceration methods. The standard percolation process is modified to include evaporation when concentrated liquid products or solid products are required or when the solvent is a diluted alcohol, the strength of which would be affected by evaporation. The latter method is known as the Reserve Percolate process, since the first quantity of the percolate is set on one side and forms the bulk of the liquid in the final product. Hence this portion is not subjected to evaporation and the alcohol strength is not affected.

Large-scale Extraction Procedures

Large-scale operation demands modification of many extraction processes, where the small-scale directions are inappropriate. Thus, 'shaking occasionally' presents no problems with a jar containing 500 or 1000 ml of tincture. An industrial batch is likely to be 2000 litres and may weigh 1·5 to 2 Mg in a vessel about 1 m in diameter and 2 m in height. To 'shake' such a vessel would present considerable difficulties and it is obvious that there are alternative methods of agitation that are just as effective but much simpler to put into practice.

In addition, economics become increasingly important, and one of the most important objectives is to improve the efficiency of extraction, so that less solvent is needed and evaporation requirements for concentrated products are reduced. As well as reducing the cost of evaporation, this has the further advantage of minimising the heat damage to thermolabile constituents.

CIRCULATORY EXTRACTION

The efficiency of extraction in a maceration process can be improved by arranging for the solvent to be continuously circulated through the drug, as indicated in Fig. 22.1. Solvent is pumped from the bottom of the vessel to the inlet where it is distributed through spray nozzles over the surface of the drug.

The movement of the solvent reduces boundary layers, and the uniform distribution minimises local concentrations, leading to more efficient extraction in a shorter time. Like the normal maceration process, however, extraction is incomplete, since mass transfer will cease when an equilibrium is set up. This problem can be overcome by using a multi-stage process.

MULTIPLE STAGE EXTRACTION

The equipment needed for this method is a vessel for the drug, together with a circulating pump and spray distributors, and a number of tanks to receive the extracted solution. The extractor and tanks are connected with piping and valves as shown in Fig. 22.2, so that any one of the tanks may be connected to the extractor for the transfer of solution.

The procedure is then as follows:

1. Fill extractor with drug, add solvent and circulate. Run off to receiver 1.
2. Refill extractor with solvent and circulate. Run off to receiver 2.
3. Refill extractor with solvent and circulate. Run off to receiver 3.
4. Remove drug from extractor and re-charge. Return solution from 1 to extractor. Remove for evaporation.
5. Return solution from 2 to extractor and circulate. Run off to receiver 1.
6. Return solution from 3 to extractor and circulate. Run off to receiver 2.
7. Add fresh solvent to extractor and circulate. Run off to receiver 3.
8. Remove drug from extractor and re-charge. Repeat cycle.

Examination of these procedures will show that each batch of drug is treated several times with solvent and that, once the cycle is in operation, the receivers contain solution with the strongest in receiver 1 and the weakest in receiver 3.

Advantages

The drug is extracted as many times as there are receivers—in this case, three. If more extraction stages are required, it is only necessary to have more receivers.

The last treatment of the drug before it is discharged is with fresh solvent, giving maximum extraction.

The solution is in contact with fresh drug before removal for evaporation, giving the highest possible concentration.

EXTRACTION BATTERY

In the normal percolation process, the percolate is not of the maximum concentration. Since solvent percolates through the whole of the bed, flow will occur through the upper layers even when these are exhausted and will continue until the lowest layer is

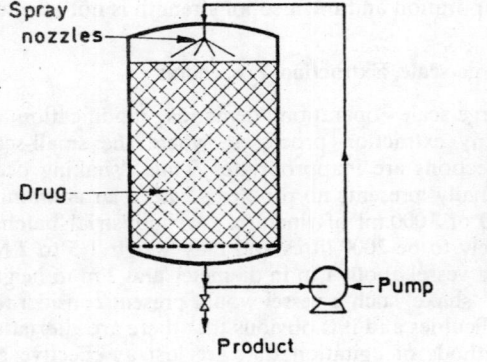

Fig. 22.1 Circulatory extraction

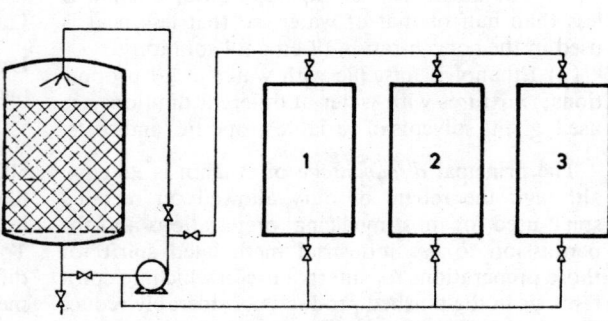

Fig. 22.2 Multiple stage extraction

also exhausted. As a result, the final runnings of the percolate are very dilute.

The ideal situation would be to have counter-current movement of the solvent and the drug whereby the drug is removed immediately after it has been treated with fresh solvent to ensure complete exhaustion, while fresh drug is added, contacting the outgoing solution to give maximum concentration.

Continuous extraction devices of this type are used in some industries where large amounts of a single material are handled; for example, the extraction of sugar from sugar beet. Pharmaceutical practice demands greater flexibility for handling various size batches of different materials and this can be achieved by treating it as a stage-wise process, so that a series of vessels is used and the extraction is semi-continuous.

The equipment is described as an *extraction battery* and consists of a number of vessels with interconnecting pipework, so arranged that solvent can be added to, and the product taken from any vessel. These vessels can, therefore, be made into a series with any one of the vessels as the first of the series. The use of the extraction battery is illustrated in Table 22.1, where the simplest arrangement of three vessels is shown.

Inspection of Table 22.1 shows that:

(*a*) One cycle of six stages uses three charges of drug, three vessels of solvent, and produces three batches of product. This represents a drug/solvent ratio of the order of 1:1, compared with the 1:4 of ordinary percolation.

(*b*) Each batch of drug is treated with five quantities of solvent, representing a drug/solvent ratio of about 1:5, ensuring efficient extraction. Depending on the character of the material, this ratio can be increased, if necessary, by using additional vessels. Thus, if N vessels are used, the drug receives $(2N - 1)$ extraction stages, without increasing the final drug/product ratio.

(*c*) The solution contacts fresh drug before discharge, giving maximum concentration.

(*d*) The drug contacts fresh solvent before dumping, ensuring exhaustion.

Thus, the use of the extraction battery gives maximum efficiency of extraction with as many stages as necessary, but with the minimum usage of solvent, so that the product is as concentrated as possible and less evaporation of the product is involved.

Continuous Extraction

The previous processes for the manufacture of concentrated preparations have involved extraction, followed by evaporation of the solvent. Continuous extraction combines the two operations, so that, immediately after contact with the drug, the solution is evaporated and the vapour taken to a condenser, whence the condensed liquid is returned to the drug to continue extraction.

One form of the apparatus is described in the *British Pharmacopoeia* for the extraction of drugs and is illustrated in Fig. 22.3. Vapour from the flask rises through the extraction chamber, passing the drug container; the vapour condenses in the reflux condenser and returns through the drug, taking the soluble constituents to the flask. The method is described as continuous *hot* extraction, since the vapour surrounds the drug container and extraction occurs at the boiling point of the solvent. In this case, extraction is a continuous percolation procedure.

Another version is the *Soxhlet apparatus* (Fig. 22.4) in which the vapour passes through the side tube and reflux returns to the extraction chamber where the solution collects. As this takes place, the liquid level will also rise in the return tube; when the liquid reaches the top of the return tube, a siphon is set up and the contents of the extraction chamber are transferred to the flask. This method is referred to as continuous *cold* extraction, since the vapour is by-passed through the side arm and does not enter the extraction chamber directly. In practice, it can be shown that the whole apparatus heats up, so that the temperature in the extraction chamber is only a degree or so lower than the vapour temperature. It will be observed, also, that the extraction is a series of short macerations, compared with the percolation of the previous method. An effect of this liquid hold-up is to demand a greater amount of solvent in the flask.

If desired, the *British Pharmacopoeia* method can be modified to a series of macerations by using a drug container with a siphon tube, instead of the perforated base.

Similar methods can be used in large-scale production; a typical industrial continuous extractor is shown in Fig. 22.5 in which the principles of operation will be seen to resemble the laboratory equipment.

Advantages

(*a*) Less solvent is needed than in the conventional method, yielding concentrated products directly.

(*b*) The drug is treated continuously with pure solvent, ensuring maximum concentration gradient and complete exhaustion.

(*c*) Extraction can be continued for as long as is necessary to exhaust the drug. Thus, depending

Table 22.1
Extraction Battery

Arrows indicate transfer of material to or from the vessels. An asterisk (*) is added after each contact stage.
Key: F = fresh drug. S = solvent. P = product. E = exhausted drug. A, B, C = extraction vessels.

Start with C empty and units A and B containing drug, with A more nearly exhausted.

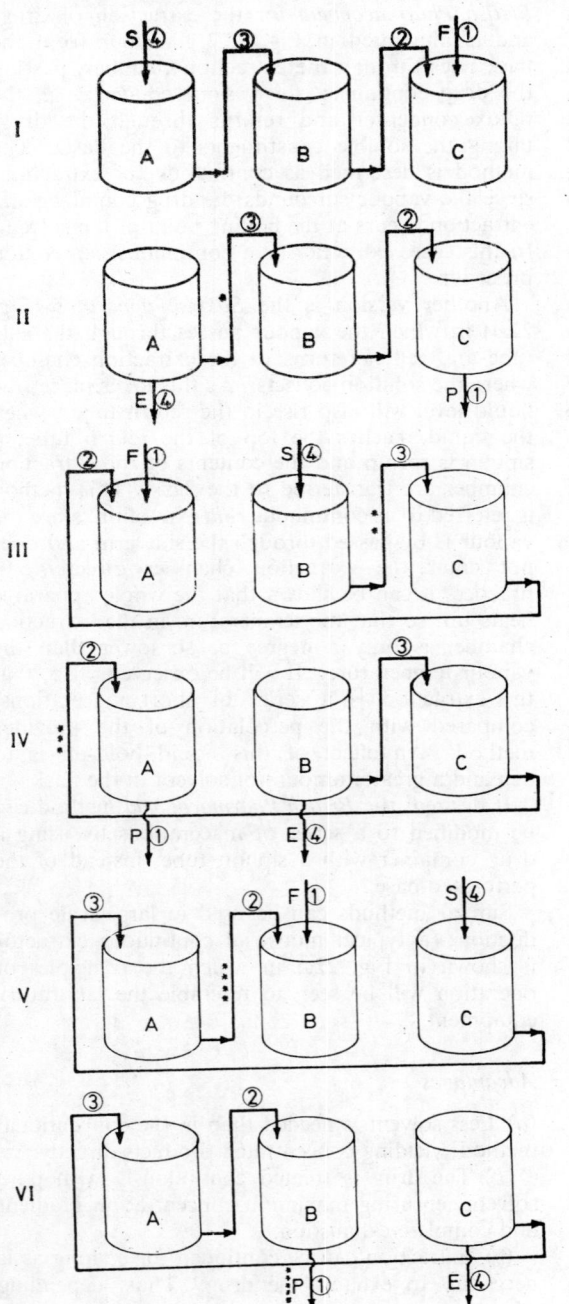

I
1. Charge fresh drug to C.
2. Transfer solution from B to C.
3. Transfer solution from A to B.
4. Add fresh solvent to A.

II
1. Remove product solution from C.
2. Transfer solution from B to C.
3. Transfer solution from A to B.
4. Dump exhausted drug from A.

III
1. Charge fresh drug to A.
2. Transfer solution from C to A.
3. Transfer solution from B to C.
4. Add fresh solvent to B.

IV
1. Remove product solution from A.
2. Transfer solution from C to A.
3. Transfer solution from B to C.
4. Dump exhausted drug from B.

V
1. Charge fresh drug to B.
2. Transfer solution from A to B.
3. Transfer solution from C to A.
4. Add fresh solvent to C.

VI
1. Remove product solution from B.
2. Transfer solution from A to B.
3. Transfer solution from C to A.
4. Dump exhausted drug from C.

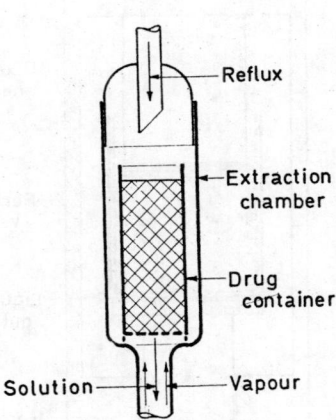

Fig 22.3 Continuous extraction:
small-scale BP apparatus

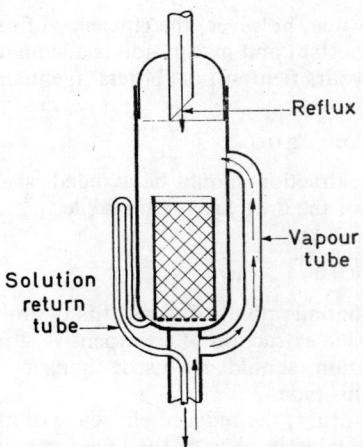

Fig. 22.4 Continuous extraction: small-scale
Soxhlet apparatus

on the character of the drug, it is possible to prolong extraction without increasing the volume of the product, corresponding to a drug/percolate ratio of any value up to infinity.

Disadvantages

(*a*) In general, the drug must be powdered, so that the method is limited in a similar manner to percolation.

(*b*) The solution is boiled continuously. This involves a considerable heat usage, as well as rendering the method unsatisfactory with drugs having thermolabile constituents. The situation can be improved by operation under vacuum.

(*c*) The solvent is boiled continuously, so that the method is restricted to pure boiling solvents (light

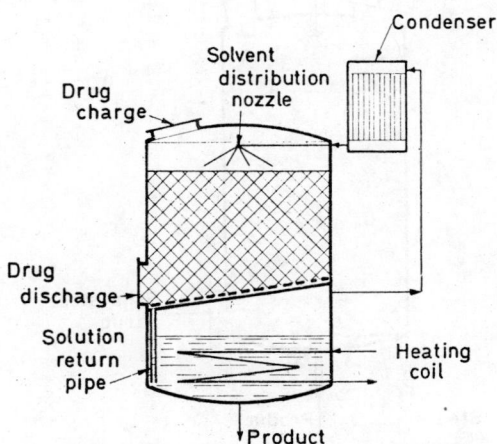

Fig. 22.5 Continuous extraction: large-scale plant

petroleum, for example) or to azeotropes. This prevents the use of continuous extraction for many products where the solvent is a dilution of ethanol in water, other than 95 per cent.

The combined effect of these factors is to limit the use of the method to very few applications, and a typical example is the extraction of fixed oils from seeds, with a solvent such as light petroleum.

Factors Affecting Choice of Extraction Process

The final choice of the process to be used for the extraction of a drug will depend on a number of factors, including:

CHARACTER OF DRUG

If hard and tough (such as nux vomica) use percolation.

If soft and parenchymatous (such as gentian) use maceration.

If 'unpowderable' (such as squill) use maceration.

If an unorganised drug (such as benzoin) use maceration.

If preferable to avoid powdering (such as senna fruits) use maceration.

Thus, a knowledge of the pharmacognosy of the drug is essential to selection of the extraction process that will give the best results.

THERAPEUTIC VALUE OF THE DRUG

When the drug has considerable therapeutic value, the maximum extraction is required, so that percolation is used, as in belladonna. If the drug has little therapeutic value, however, the efficiency of extraction is unimportant and maceration is adequate; for example, flavours (lemon), or 'bitters' (gentian).

STABILITY OF DRUG

Continuous extraction should be avoided when the constituents of the drug are thermolabile.

COST OF DRUG

From the economic point of view, it is desirable to obtain complete extraction of an expensive drug, so that percolation should be used; ginger is an example of this type.

For cheap drugs, the reduced efficiency of maceration is acceptable in view of the lower cost of the process. In particular, the cost of size reduction to a powdered state is avoided, whereas this is a significant part of the percolation process.

SOLVENT

If the desired constituents demand a solvent other than a pure boiling solvent or an azeotrope, continuous extraction should be avoided and the reserve percolate process should be used.

CONCENTRATION OF PRODUCT

Dilute products such as tinctures can be made by maceration or percolation, depending on the previous factors.

For semi-concentrated preparations (concentrated infusions, for example) the more efficient percolation process is used, unless the drug cannot be powdered or is not worth powdering, when double or triple maceration is chosen.

Concentrated preparations, of which liquid extracts or dry extracts are examples, are made exclusively by percolation, with the exception that continuous extraction can be used if the solvent is suitable and the constituents are thermostable.

Recovery of Solvent from the Marc

The residue of the drug after extraction (often known as the *marc*) is saturated with solvent and, if economic, the latter is recovered.

In some cases the drug is pressed as part of the extraction process, so that much of the liquid is removed. If not part of the process, the application of pressure is a useful preliminary recovery procedure.

A typical piece of equipment for this purpose is the *Hydraulic Press*, shown in Fig. 22.6. The marc,

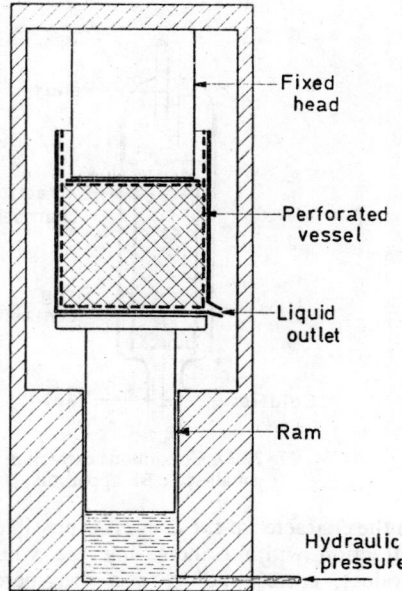

Fig. 22.6   Hydraulic press

wrapped in cloth, is placed in the perforated inner vessel, which is enclosed in another vessel having an outlet for the expressed liquid. Application of hydraulic pressure to the ram presses the marc against the fixed head, expelling residual liquid.

Recovery of the remaining solvent demands vaporisation, and special forms of distillation equipment have been devised with the object of providing

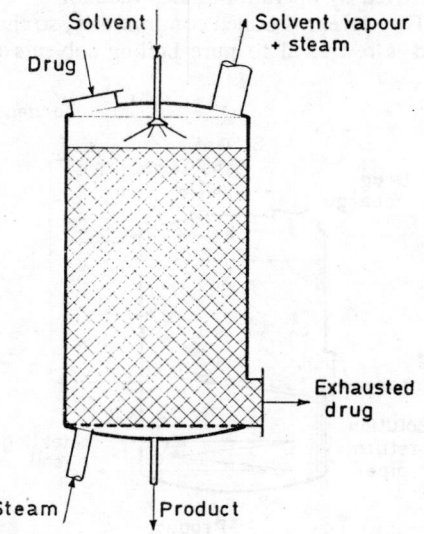

Fig. 22.7   Solvent recovery from the extraction vessel

a large area for heat transfer and an easy method of opening or closing. Such specialised apparatus now finds little use, however, and it is common to find the vacuum oven serving as a solvent recovery device (*see* p. 278).

When large quantities of drug have been processed, the transfer of the marc from the extraction vessel to a press and thence to a recovery still involves too much labour. It is preferable, therefore, to recover the solvent directly from the drug while it is still in the extraction vessel. This can be done by surrounding the vessel with a steam jacket, enabling the contents to be heated when extraction has been completed. The method is inefficient in view of the poor heat transfer properties of the marc, especially as it shrinks as it approaches dryness.

A better method is illustrated in Fig. 22.7, whereby steam is admitted to the base of the extraction vessel; heating is uniform and heat transfer is much more rapid, so that recovery of the solvent is more efficient. The vapours that pass to the condenser consist of the solvent vapour mixed with steam, however, so that a distillation stage is needed for purification (*see* p. 265).

BIBLIOGRAPHY

PECK, W. C. (1936) The Extraction of Vegetable Materials. *Quart. J. Pharm.*, 9, 401–420.
TREYBAL, R. E. (1968) *Mass Transfer Operations.* New York, McGraw-Hill.

23

Distillation

DISTILLATION may be defined as the separation of the constituents of a mixture including a liquid by partial vaporisation of the mixture and separate collection of the vapour. Such separations may include:

The separation of one liquid from non-volatile impurities.
The separation of one liquid from one or more other liquids, with which it may be miscible, partially miscible or immiscible.

As carried out in practice, it may be difficult to distinguish between evaporation, distillation, and drying. (Official monographs for dry extracts include directions such as: 'Remove the alcohol, evaporate to dryness'.)

Working definitions, which will serve to distinguish the three processes, can be based on the intention, distillation being the operation when the condensed vapour is required, evaporation when the concentrated liquid residue is needed, and drying has the dried solid residue as product.

This chapter is concerned with the operation of distillation as it is carried out on a large-scale. No theory is included; this will be found in Chapter 3. Simple distillation is considered for the treatment of single liquids, with particular reference to the purification of water and the special techniques applied to materials such as fixed oils.

Methods and plant for the separation of miscible volatile liquids are included, together with the effect of azeotropes, and illustrated by the preparation of 'Absolute Alcohol', that is, 100 per cent ethanol.

Simple Distillation

The purification of many organic liquids is carried out by the distillation process and it is necessary to use only a simple apparatus with a boiler and a condenser, so that equipment of the type described as evaporators (see p. 165) can be used. As with evaporation, the process can be carried out under reduced pressure if it is desirable to keep the temperature as low as possible (see p. 166).

PREPARATION OF PURIFIED WATER, BP AND WATER FOR INJECTIONS BP BY DISTILLATION

Purification of water by distillation is a special case, for the following reasons:

Gases dissolved in the raw water must be removed and not allowed to contaminate the distillate. Such gases include carbon dioxide, but ammonia is probably the most important gas to be avoided.

The residue of solids must not be concentrated to a point where hydrolysis occurs. Otherwise, the distillate may be contaminated by volatile materials, for example, by hydrochloric acid from the hydrolysis of chlorides.

These objectives may be achieved by using a batch distillation procedure and collecting the middle fraction only. The use of Purified Water in pharmaceutical practice is so great, however, that a continuous process is desirable.

Precautions must be taken to ensure that:

The feed water to the boiler is heated to de-gas it, since, with few minor exceptions, the solubility of gases decreases as the temperature is raised. This is usually effected by feeding the boiler through the condenser jacket, which has the added advantage of thermal economy by pre-heating the make-up water.

A constant-level device is attached to the boiler to avoid excessive concentration of salts. Since some solids will be deposited, it is necessary to de-scale the boiler periodically, the frequency depending on the hardness of the feed water.

Baffles must be included in the path of the vapour, between the boiler and the condenser, to prevent entrainment of liquid droplets by the vapour. The objective is to avoid the carry-over of soluble materials in the droplets and is especially important if the product is required to be of the quality suitable for use as Water for Injections. In this case it is contamination of the distillate by pyrogens from the feed water that must be avoided, as discussed by Gunn and Carter (1965).

A typical form of distillation unit for the continuous production of Purified Water is shown in Fig. 23.1. Note that:

The boiler may well be of cast iron, but the

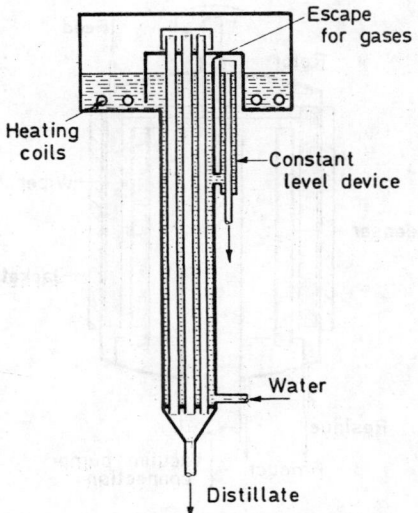

Fig. 23.1   Distillation unit for purified water

baffles and condenser tubes that contact the product are of stainless steel or monel metal.

Baffles are provided over the top of the condenser tubes to avoid the entrainment of liquid droplets with the vapour.

Cooling water enters at the bottom of the condenser and provides the supply of feed water for the boiler. This water is heated by the condensing vapour, and the flow rate is adjusted so that water enters the boiler at 90 to 95°C.

The top of the condenser jacket is open, so that gases from the water can escape to the atmosphere.

An excess of water is needed and the overflow is taken through a constant-level device from a point about a quarter of the way down the condenser. This ensures that the hottest, de-gassed water is used as make-up water for the boiler, which would not be so if a simple overflow was used at the top of the condenser.

The amount of the excess water can be calculated by a heat balance, since the condensing vapour gives up latent heat and sensible heat in cooling to the outlet temperature, while the cooling water takes up the heat as sensible heat.

From steam tables:

Heat given up by 1 kg steam at
1 bar condensing to 1 kg water
at 100°C   = 2 256·7 kJ
Heat given up by 1 kg water
cooling from 100°C to outlet
temperature (say 20°C)   =   335·2 kJ
Total heat given up   = 2 591·9 kJ/kg

Assume:
Inlet temperature of cooling water = 15°C
Outlet temperature of cooling water = 90°C
   From steam tables:
Sensible heat content of water at
   15°C   =   62·9 kJ/kg
Sensible heat content of water at
   90°C   =   376·9 kJ/kg
Heat taken up by cooling water
            = 376·9 − 62·9 =   314·0 kJ/kg

$$\therefore \quad \text{kg cooling water/kg distillate} = \frac{2591·9}{314·0} = 8·25$$

But 1 kg of water is taken into the boiler to replace 1 kg of vapour, so that 7·25 kg of cooling water will be discarded from the condenser. In practice, the ratio will be lower due to heat losses, and about 6 kg cooling water will normally go to waste for each kg of distillate. In some cases it is worth making use of this heat.

As pointed out above, the method has the advantage also of pre-heating the feed water and shows a useful thermal economy:

Sensible heat taken up/kg feed water   =   314·0 kJ
Total heat needed to vaporise water if it
   had entered at 15°C   = 2 612·9 kJ

$$\therefore \quad \text{heat saved} = \frac{314·0}{2612·9} \times 100 = 12·2 \text{ per cent.}$$

Molecular Distillation

A special application of the simple distillation process is *molecular distillation*, known also as *evaporative distillation* or *short path distillation*.

THEORY OF MOLECULAR DISTILLATION

The *mean free path* of a molecule is defined as the average distance through which a molecule can move without coming into collision with another.

The mean free path can be expressed mathematically as:

$$\lambda = \eta \sqrt{\frac{3}{p\rho}} \qquad (23.1)$$

where λ = mean free path; η = viscosity; p = pressure; ρ = density.

For materials that are of low viscosity and density, the mean free path is long, and distillation is simple. The mean free path is low for substances that are viscous and at high pressure, but can be increased if the viscosity is decreased by elevation of the temperature and the pressure is reduced. In this way, substances that are regarded as non-volatile under ordinary conditions of temperature and pressure may become volatile. As illustration, the measured paths of heavy molecules at a pressure of 0·1 N/m² (1 × 10⁻⁶ bar) is about 30 mm for butyl phthalate and 20 mm for olive oil.

Hence, under these conditions, with the evaporating surface close to the condensing surface it is possible to distil such substances.

CHARACTERISTICS OF THE MOLECULAR DISTILLATION PROCESS

Compared with the simple distillation process used for volatile liquids, molecular distillation has three characteristics:

In order to minimise collisions between molecules, the process must be operated under very high vacuum, usually of the order of 0·1 to 1 N/m² (1 to 10 × 10⁻⁶ bar). This demands efficient pumping systems, careful avoidance of leaks, and precautions such as de-gassing of the liquids prior to distillation.

The liquid area should be as large as possible; there is no boiling, and evolution of the vapour is from the surface only. This is the reason for one of the alternative titles referred to above, namely evaporative distillation.

The evaporating surface must be close to the condensing surface, accounting for the occasional use of the title, short path distillation. Usually, this distance is similar to the mean free path of the molecules to be processed, although it can be somewhat greater, as it has been shown that the molecules can withstand a number of collisions without appreciable deflection. This is the point of greatest difference when compared with the conventional distillation unit for volatile liquids where volatilisation occurs so readily that baffles must be provided to prevent entrainment, and the chances of a molecule leaving the liquid and reaching the condenser are about 1 in 1000. In the molecular still, however, the close proximity of the evaporating surfaces and the condenser makes the chances about 1 in 2.

Molecular Distillation Equipment

Industrial forms of molecular still can be divided into two main categories, according to the method of formation of the liquid film:

FALLING FILM MOLECULAR STILL

The *falling film molecular still* operates on the same principle as the falling film evaporator (*see* p. 169), so that the vaporisation occurs from a film of the liquid flowing down a heated surface. As with

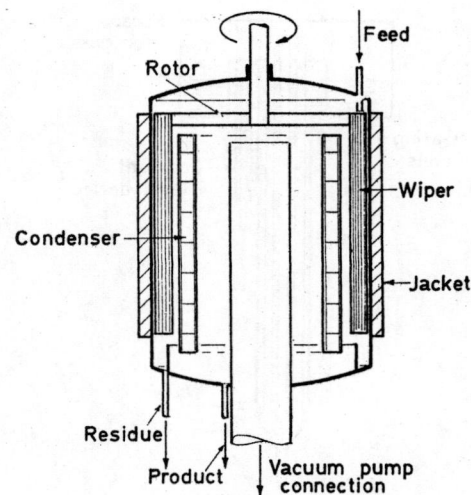

Fig. 23.2   Wiped film molecular still

evaporators, fluid flow and heat transfer can be improved by mechanical methods and a *wiped film molecular still* is shown in section in Fig. 23.2.

The vessel has a diameter of the order of 1 m and the walls are heated suitably. The distilland flows down the walls and is spread to a film by the PTFE wipers which move at about 3 m/s giving a film velocity of about 1·5 m/s; the residue collects in the bottom of the vessel and is re-circulated. Condensers are arranged as shown, and the distillate taken to a receiver. Vacuum pumps are connected by a large diameter pipe, since the residual gases occupy a large volume at the low operating pressures of such stills. Capacity of this type of still is quite large and may be about 1000 l/h.

CENTRIFUGAL MOLECULAR STILL

The alternative method of obtaining a thin liquid film is by centrifugal force. In a typical *centrifugal molecular still* (Fig. 23.3) the distilland is introduced on to the centre of a bucket-shaped vessel (1 to 1·5 m in diameter) which rotates at high speed. The film of liquid that is formed moves outwards over the surface of the vessel, heated externally by radiant heaters, while condensers and a collection device are located close to the inner surface of the rotor.

The disadvantage of the method is that the construction and operation is more complicated, due to the high speed of rotation compared with the low rotor speed of the wiped film still.

The centrifugal still has a similar throughput to the wiped film still.

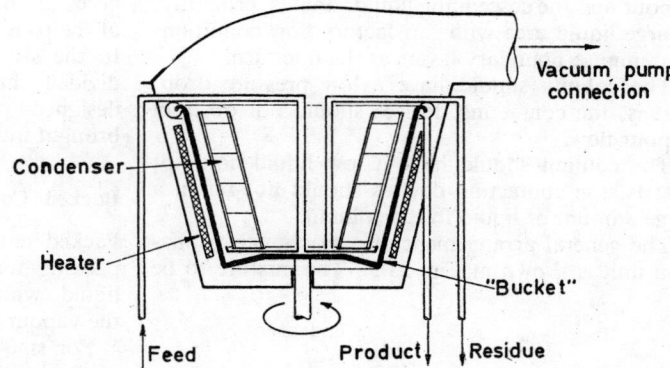

Fig. 23.3 Centrifugal molecular still

Applications of Molecular Distillation

Although molecular distillation has applications for the purification of chemicals of low vapour pressure, such as tricresyl phosphate, dibutyl phthalate and dimethyl phthalate, the most important pharmaceutical use is for refining fixed oils and separating vitamins.

The graphs in Fig. 23.4 represent the components of fixed oils that are distilled at various temperatures. The fractions collected are not 'clean', so that distillation at about 200°C, for example, will yield Vitamin A esters and triglycerides. Nevertheless, it is possible to process an oil and obtain a five-fold increase in Vitamin A potency with a 70 per cent yield of vitamin, permitting the use of a greater variety of sources of vitamin.

In general, free fatty acids are distilled off at about 100°C, vitamins and sterols between 100 and 200°C, and triglycerides from 200°C upwards. Proteins, gums and similar materials will remain as a non-volatile residue. Thus, collection of middle fractions enables a refined oil that is of low acid value and free from protein, etc. to be obtained.

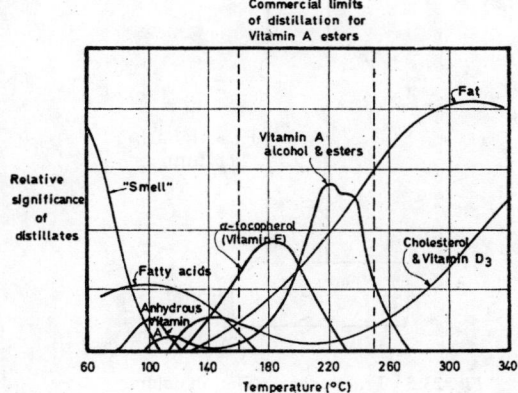

Fig. 23.4 Molecular distillation separations from oils

Fractional Distillation

The theory of fractional distillation for separating miscible liquids (discussed in Chapter 3) shows that the process depends upon heating the mixture, repeatedly condensing the vapour, and re-heating the liquid, equilibrium between liquid and vapour being set up at each stage. As indicated in connection with the theory, this can be carried out by means of a fractionating column.

From the operational point of view, fractional distillation is a mass transfer process, involving counter-current diffusion of the components at each equilibrium stage.

This can be represented diagrammatically by the concentration gradients of Fig. 13.3 (p. 163), so that the less volatile component (LVC) diffuses through the boundary layers from the vapour to the liquid phases, while the more volatile component (MVC) diffuses in the opposite direction. Counter-current diffusion occurs, therefore, with the vapour becoming richer in MVC and the liquid richer in LVC, until equilibrium is reached. This is repeated in a sufficient number of equilibrium stages until the vapour consists entirely of the MVC and the liquid is the LVC.

To meet these requirements, the fractionating column must possess certain characteristics:

Heat must be supplied to the bottom of the column to re-vaporise the liquid so that a temperature gradient is set up through the column.

A condenser is provided at the top of the column to return liquid reflux in sufficient quantity to bring about condensation of the rising vapour.

The column must contain devices to provide conditions for mass transfer between the ascending vapour and the descending liquid; that is, primarily, a large liquid area with satisfactory flow conditions to minimise boundary layers at the interface.

The column should have a low pressure drop; that is, the contacting devices should not obstruct vapour flow.

The column should have a low liquid hold-up; that is, the contacting devices should not retain a large amount of liquid in the column.

The general arrangement of a fractional distillation unit is shown in Fig. 23.5. The mixture to be

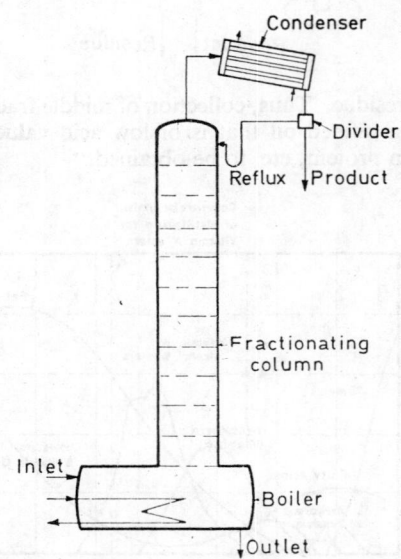

Fig. 23.5   Fractional distillation column

distilled is fed to the boiler and heated, usually by a steam coil. The broken lines across the column represent the contacting devices and there must be a sufficient number to give the appropriate 'steps' (theoretical plates) on the vapour/liquid equilibrium graph (Fig. 3.4). The vapour is taken to a condenser at the top of the column and the condensed liquid is split in a *reflux divider*, a suitable quantity being returned to the column as *reflux* and the remainder taken off as product. The ratio of reflux/product is known as the *reflux ratio*. Distillation will continue until all the MVC has been distilled off and forms the *top product*, and the LVC is left in the boiler to provide the *bottom product*.

FRACTIONATING COLUMNS

Fractionating columns may be divided into two groups: firstly, *packed columns*, where some form of packing is used within the column to effect the

necessary liquid/vapour contact and a certain height of the packing is equivalent to one theoretical plate. In the second type, *plate columns*, the column is divided into a number of sections by suitably designed 'plates', and the liquid and vapour are brought into contact on each plate.

Packed Columns

Packed columns consist of a tower containing a packing that becomes wetted with a film of the liquid, which is thereby brought into contact with the vapour in the intervening spaces.

For small-scale purposes, *Dixon gauze rings* are of high efficiency, being made from 100 mesh stainless steel gauze in the shape of cylinders $1·5 \times 1·5$ mm upwards.

For larger columns, metal or ceramic rings of various sizes can be used, including *Raschig rings* in the form of simple open-ended cylinders, and *Lessing rings* which are similar to Raschig rings but, in addition, have a septum across the diameter of the cylinder. In both cases, smaller sizes of rings are usually dumped in the column, but larger sizes are stacked. Size is important, the smaller the packing, the greater the surface area, giving a smaller column height per theoretical plate, but the pressure drop is greater.

Other forms of packing include various shapes of expanded metal, but in any case, the packing must be uniform, or flow is irregular, channelling occurs, and mass transfer is less effective.

Plate Columns

There are very many forms of plate for use in distillation columns and the two quoted below, in common use for pharmaceutical purposes, illustrate differences in design.

BUBBLE CAP PLATES

The *bubble cap plate* (Fig. 23.6) is one of the most commonly used contacting devices and consists of a plate across the column with a *weir* leading to a *downcomer*, so that a layer of liquid forms on the plate and overflows to the plate below, with the end of the downcomer sealed by the liquid on the lower plate. Vapour from below passes through the *vapour risers*, which are covered by *caps* whose edges seal into the liquid layer. Hence, the vapour can only escape by bubbling through the liquid, and the edge of the cap is usually slotted to encourage uniform bubble formation.

Small plates can be used with a single cap, but units are available that are 5 or 6 m in diameter and

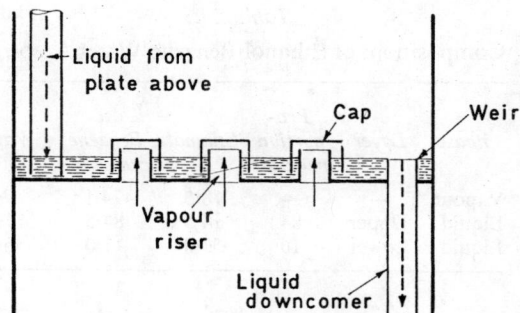

Fig. 23.6   Bubble-cap plate

fitted with upwards of 1000 caps, each about 100 mm in diameter.

Advantages

(*a*) There is excellent contact as the vapour bubbles through the liquid.

(*b*) The bubble cap plate is effective over a wide range of vapour and liquid proportions and velocities.

Disadvantages

(*a*) The layer of liquid on each plate results in a considerable hold-up of liquid over the entire column.

(*b*) The need to force the vapour out of the caps, through the liquid, leads to a large pressure drop through the column.

(*c*) The column does not drain when not in use.

(*d*) The structure is complicated, making construction and maintenance expensive.

TURBOGRID PLATE

In contrast to the complex structure of the bubble cap plate, a simpler plate can be employed. Perforations can be used, but a more recent example is the *turbogrid plate* which consists of a flat grid with parallel slots extending over the whole plate, so that there are no downcomers or vapour risers. When operating, liquid is held on the plate by vapour rising through the slots and a circulation is set up, as in Fig. 23.7, with liquid and vapour movements as shown by the arrows.

Advantages

(*a*) The construction is very simple, so the plate is very cheap to manufacture and maintain compared with forms such as the bubble cap plate.

(*b*) There is much less liquid hold-up.

(*c*) The pressure drop is low.

(*d*) The column drains when not in use.

The only important *disadvantage* is that the range of operation is limited. Too much liquid will drown the plate and an insufficient quantity will prevent contact. Similarly, an excessive vapour velocity will blow the liquid off the plate and a low vapour velocity will not maintain liquid on the plate. Thus, the proportions and velocities of liquid and vapour are critical in order to ensure the contact necessary for mass transfer.

Azeotropes

The theory of azeotropes has been discussed in Chapter 3 and the properties of these mixtures have a considerable effect on the distillation of certain pharmaceutical materials. The influence of azeotropes and the manner in which they can be used are illustrated by the methods used for the preparation of 'Absolute Alcohol'; that is, 100 per cent ethanol. The process also demonstrates the operation of distillation on a continuous basis, compared with the batch operation of page 266.

The liquor from fermentation processes is a common source of ethanol and contains approximately 8 to 10 per cent; purification is by distillation, forming an azeotrope containing 95·6 per cent ethanol and boiling at 78·15°C at atmospheric pressure.

A diagram of the plant is given in Fig. 23.8 and resembles the batch distillation unit (*see* Fig. 23.5) except that the boiler is replaced by a *reboiler*, which is smaller than the boiler and has an outlet for removing the bottom product continuously. An equilibrium is set up through the column with separate equilibria on each plate, ranging from the azeotrope as top product to water and dissolved solids as bottom product.

As the process is continuous, feed liquor must be introduced into the system and must occur at a

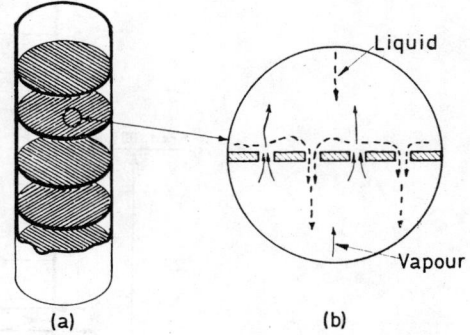

Fig. 23.7   Turbogrid plate
(*a*) general arrangement of plates in column
(*b*) liquid/vapour circulation on plate

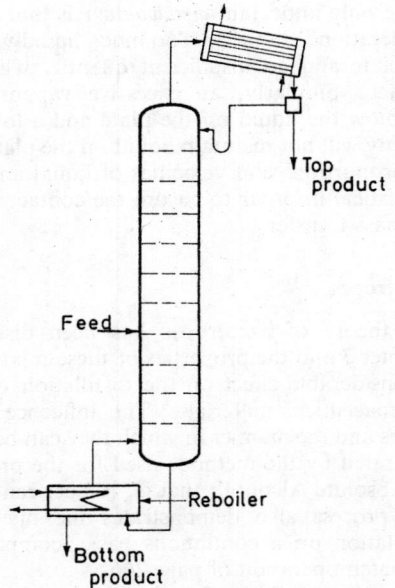

Fig. 23.8 Continuous fractional distillation

point where the equilibrium will not be disturbed. Hence, feed will take place at a plate part of the way up the column, where the equilibrium composition on the plate is similar to the feed composition. The plates below the *feed plate* form the *stripping section*

Table 23.1

Compositions of Ethanol/Benzene/Water Azeotrope

Phase	Layer	Proportion per cent	Ethanol	Benzene	Water
				per cent	
Vapour	—	—	18·5	74·1	7·4
Liquid	Upper	84	14·5	84·5	1·0
Liquid	Lower	16	53·0	11·0	36·0

(since the rising vapour 'strips' the MVC (ethanol) from the feed liquor) while the upper section is known as the *rectifying section*.

The binary azeotrope produced at this stage is freed from water by making use of the ternary azeotrope—ethanol, benzene, water.

The compositions of the vapour and liquid of the ternary azeotrope are shown in Table 23.1, bearing in mind that the liquid formed by condensation of the vapour separates into two layers.

The process requires three fractionating columns, as indicated in Fig. 23.9, which also shows the proportions of the mixtures at various stages.

The ethanol/water azeotrope, with sufficient benzene (only required at start-up) is fed to column *A* and the pure ethanol is obtained as bottom product, since the ternary azeotrope takes off the water. The azeotrope (ethanol/benzene/water) is

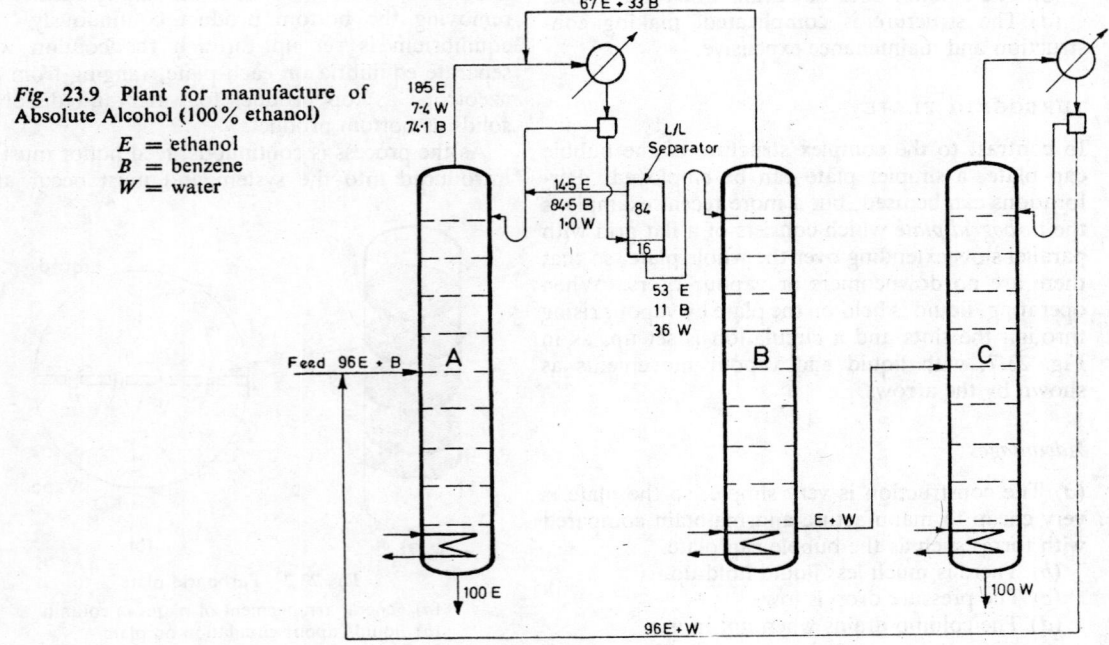

Fig. 23.9 Plant for manufacture of Absolute Alcohol (100% ethanol)

E = ethanol
B = benzene
W = water

taken from the top of the column A, condensed, and separated to the two layers, having the compositions given in Table 23.1.

The upper layer predominates and, being rich in benzene, is returned to column A. The lower layer is taken to column B, where the benzene is recovered as the ethanol/benzene binary azeotrope and is mixed with the vapour from column A. The ethanol/water residue passes to column C, where the ethanol is recovered as the ethanol/water binary azeotrope, which can be incorporated with the original feed to column A.

It should be noted that the only outgoings from the process are 100 per cent ethanol as product and water, which goes to waste; the benzene is cycled and does not leave the process.

BIBLIOGRAPHY

GARNER, J. J. and MACMURRAY, H. D. (1958) Commercial Equipment for Molecular Distillation. *Ind. Chem.*, **34**, 310–317.

GUNN, C. and CARTER, S. J. (1965) *Dispensing for Pharmaceutical Students*, 11th ed. Pitman Medical, London.

TREYBAL, R. E. (1968) *Mass Transfer Operations.* McGraw-Hill, New York.

24
Drying

DRYING is an important operation in pharmaceutical practice, since it is commonly the last stage of the process before packaging and has a considerable effect on the properties of the product. Thus, correct drying can prevent deterioration or can ensure that a product is readily soluble or is free-flowing.

This chapter is concerned with the drying of solids only, although there may be occasions when it is necessary to dry liquids or gases.

Drying may be carried out on dilute solutions, when the process resembles evaporation and is controlled by similar factors. Such cases are described as 'drying', however, through common usage of the term, but also because the plant can reduce products to lower moisture contents than evaporators.

Most drying operations are concerned with materials that are already solid and from which liquid has to be removed until the product is 'dry'. The use of inverted commas is significant, since the 'dry' condition of a solid indicates that it is in equi-librium with the atmosphere with which it is in contact. This means that it may be in a state of complete dryness or in a condition known as *air-dry*, when the solid may contain as much as 20 per cent of moisture, but this is discussed in more detail on page 272.

Just as the spin-dryer has considerable advantages for drying domestic washing, so it is worth bearing in mind that mechanical removal of the liquid from a solid by methods such as centrifuging is quicker and cheaper.

For the purposes of this chapter, drying is defined as the final removal of liquid from solids by thermal vaporisation, leaving a 'dry' solid. The discussion refers in many cases to 'water' and 'moisture', but the principles apply equally to any volatile liquid.

The chapter deals with drying from dilute solutions and the theory and methods of drying solids. Special reference is made to sublimation drying, commonly known as freeze drying, which uses slightly different principles, but is of considerable pharmaceutical importance.

Dryers for Dilute Solutions and Suspensions

The objective of these dryers is to spread the liquid to a large surface area for heat and mass transfer and to provide an effective means of collecting the dry solid. Two main types are used, the first spreading the liquid to a thin film and the second dispersing the liquid to a spray of small droplets.

Drum Dryer (Film Dryer)

Shown in section in Fig. 24.1, the *drum dryer* consists of a drum 0·75 to 1·5 m in diameter and 2 to 4 m in length, heated internally, usually by steam, and rotated on its longitudinal axis. The liquid is applied to the surface and spread to a film; this may be done in various ways, but the simplest method is that shown in the diagram, where the drum dips into a *feed pan*. Drying rate is controlled by using a suitable speed of rotation and drum temperature. The product is scraped from the surface of the drum by means of a *doctor knife*.

Advantages

(*a*) The method gives rapid drying, the thin film spread over a large area resulting in rapid heat and mass transfer.

(*b*) The equipment is compact, occupying much less space that the spray dryer, for example.

(*c*) Heating time is short, being only a few seconds.

(*d*) The drum can be enclosed in a vacuum jacket, enabling the temperature of drying to be reduced.

(*e*) The product is obtained in flake form, which is convenient for many purposes.

The only *disadvantage* is that operating conditions are critical and it is necessary to impose careful control on feed rate, film thickness, speed of rotation and temperature difference.

The drum dryer can handle a variety of materials, either as solutions or suspensions; substances that are dried by this method include milk products,

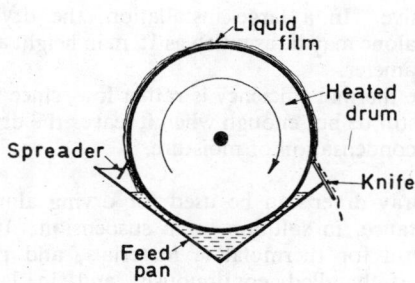

Fig. 24.1   Drum dryer

starch products, ferrous salts, and suspensions of kaolin or zinc oxide.

Spray Dryer

The *spray dryer* provides a large surface area for heat and mass transfer by atomising the liquid to small droplets. These are sprayed into a stream of hot air, so that each droplet dries to a solid particle.

There are many forms of spray dryer and Fig. 24.2 is a typical design, in which the *drying chamber* resembles the cyclone (*see* p. 198) ensuring good circulation of air, to facilitate heat and mass transfer, and that dried particles are separated by the centrifugal action.

The character of the particles is controlled by the droplet form, hence the type of atomiser is important. Jet atomisers are easily blocked and the droplet size is likely to vary, but this is not so with rotary types. One form of *rotary atomiser* is shown

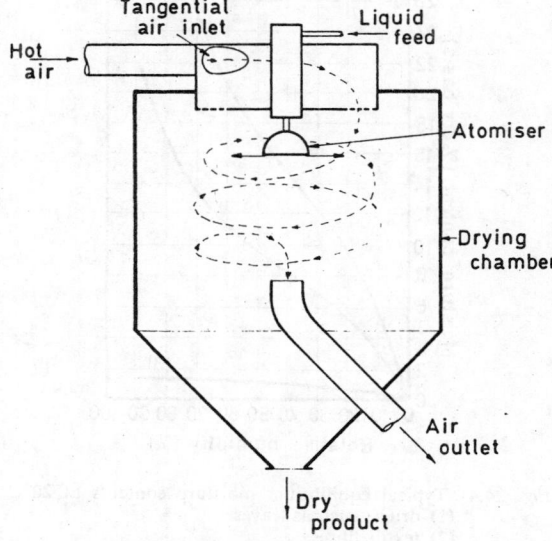

Fig. 24.2   Spray dryer

in Fig. 24.3. Liquid is fed on to the disc, which is rotated at high speed (up to 20 000 rev/min); a film is formed and spreads from the small disc to a larger, inverted, hemi-spherical bowl, becoming thinner, and eventually being dispersed from the edge in a fine, uniform spray. In addition, the rotary atomiser has the advantage of being equally effective with suspensions of solids and it can operate efficiently at various feed rates.

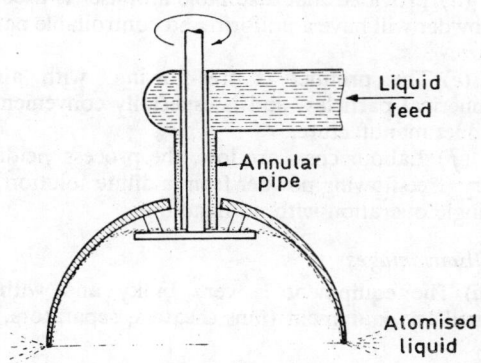

Fig. 24.3   Rotary atomiser

For crude products, drying can be effected by direct use of furnace gases, but for pharmaceutical purposes it is usual to filter the air and to heat it indirectly by means of a heat exchanger. Dust carried over in the air stream may be recovered by a cyclone separator or filter bag; in some cases the air may be scrubbed in a tower by means of the feed liquid. This has the advantage that undersize particles are dissolved and cycled back to the dryer and that the feed is pre-heated reducing the heat requirements.

Spray dried products are easily recognisable, being uniform in appearance and, if examined by means of a hand lens, the particles have a characteristic shape, in the form of hollow spheres with a small hole. This arises from the drying process, since the droplet enters the hot air stream, and dries on the outside to form an outer crust with liquid still in the centre. This liquid then vaporises, the vapour escaping by blowing a hole in the sphere.

It has been suggested that this method of drying allows a dry product to retain some properties of the feed; for example, a droplet from an emulsion dries with the disperse phase inside and a layer of the continuous phase on the outside. When reconstituted, the emulsion is easily re-formed.

Advantages of the Spray Drying Process

(a) The droplets are small, giving a large surface area for heat and mass transfer, so that evaporation is very rapid. The actual drying time of a droplet is only a fraction of a second, and the overall time in the dryer only a few seconds.

(b) Because evaporation is very rapid, the droplets do not attain a high temperature, most of the heat being used as latent heat of vaporisation.

(c) The characteristic particle form gives the product a high bulk density and, in turn, ready solubility.

(d) Provided that a suitable atomiser is used, the powder will have a uniform and controllable particle size.

(e) The product is free-flowing, with almost spherical particles, and is especially convenient for tablet manufacture.

(f) Labour costs are low, the process yielding a dry, free-flowing powder from a dilute solution, in a single operation with no handling.

Disadvantages

(a) The equipment is very bulky and with the ancillary equipment (fans, heaters, separators, etc.)

is expensive. In a large installation, the drying chamber alone may be as much as 15 m in height and 6 m in diameter.

(b) The thermal efficiency is rather low, since the air must still be hot enough when it leaves the dryer to avoid condensation of moisture.

The spray dryer can be used for drying almost any substance, in solution or in suspension. It is most useful for thermolabile materials, and particularly if handled continuously and in large quantities; outputs of 2000 kg/h can be attained, although pharmaceutical plants are usually somewhat smaller.

Examples of substances that are spray dried include borax, citric acid, hexamine, sodium phosphate, gelatin, acacia and extracts, while starch, barium sulphate and calcium phosphate are typical of insoluble materials. In addition, the method is widely used for products of indirect pharmaceutical interest, such as milk, soap, and detergents.

Dryers for Solid Materials

The treatment of solid materials, as distinct from solutions, is drying in the usual sense of the term.

GENERAL PRINCIPLES

Equilibrium Moisture Content

An understanding of the theory and practice of the operation demands an appreciation of the behaviour of different substances at particular temperatures and humidities.

Exposure to air at a definite temperature and humidity will cause a material to lose or gain moisture until an *equilibrium moisture content* is attained. The values will vary, depending on the temperature and humidity of the air and on the properties of the material, being low with non-porous solids, but higher and variable with fibrous or colloidal organic substances.

Equilibrium moisture contents can be represented as curves (Fig. 24.4) in which, for a stated temperature, moisture content is plotted against relative humidity. Ordinary atmospheric conditions are of the order of 20°C and 70 to 75 per cent relative humidity, so that, if exposed to the atmosphere, a substance such as kaolin will contain about 1 per cent moisture; textile fibres, as in surgical dressings, will contain about 15 per cent, while drugs, such as leaves, may have as much as 25 to 30 per cent.

The effect of this variation of equilibrium moisture content is that:

When a material leaves a dryer it may or may not be *bone dry*, that is, completely free from moisture, depending on the temperature and humidity of the air at the dryer outlet.

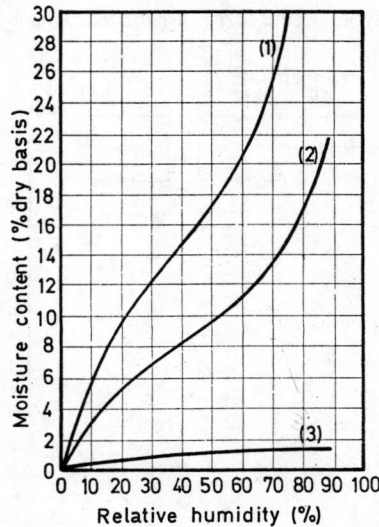

Fig. 24.4 Typical equilibrium moisture contents at 20°C
(1) drugs, such as leaves
(2) textile fibres
(3) inorganic substance, such as kaolin

Even if a material is reduced to the bone-dry state, there will be a *moisture regain* if it is exposed to the atmosphere.

'Over-drying' should be avoided; that is, drying should be stopped when the moisture content has reached a level equivalent to the equilibrium moisture content under the conditions to which the material is to be exposed. This precaution is advantageous from the economic point of view, as the drying time is thereby reduced, and the heating of thermolabile materials minimised. This is especially true as the final stages of drying are the slowest.

It is worth bearing in mind that some materials used in tablet manufacture have substantial equilibrium moisture contents under normal atmospheric conditions; for example, starches have an equilibrium moisture content of about 8 to 10 per cent at 20°C and 75 per cent relative humidity. This behaviour should be taken into account in selecting raw materials and drying and storing tablets.

Moisture Content

The moisture present in a solid may exist in more than one physical condition:

BOUND MOISTURE

Bound moisture in a solid is liquid that exerts a vapour pressure less than that of the pure liquid at the same temperature. This reduction of vapour pressure may be because the liquid is in small capillaries, in solutions, in cells or is combined, for example, by adsorption to a surface.

Conversely, *unbound moisture* exerts a vapour pressure equivalent to that of the free liquid. Thus, in a non-hygroscopic material all the liquid is unbound, and in a hygroscopic material the unbound moisture is the liquid in excess of the equilibrium moisture content, corresponding to saturation humidity.

FREE MOISTURE

Free moisture at a particular temperature and humidity is the liquid in excess of the equilibrium moisture content. Thus, under conditions of saturation humidity, the free moisture is the same as the unbound moisture, but in other circumstances the free moisture may consist of both unbound and bound moisture.

EXPRESSION OF MOISTURE CONTENT

For the purposes of drying, the moisture content is expressed as *percentage moisture content, dry basis*, that is, the number of parts by weight of moisture per hundred parts of *bone dry solid*. Thus, 50 per cent moisture content, dry basis, represents 50 kg moisture per 100 kg dry solid. Alternatively, the statement may be made as parts per part and the previous quantity would be expressed as 0·5 kg/kg.

The usual method of describing percentages is not used, since to give the moisture as a percentage of the total weight would mean that comparisons would be made on a continually changing basis. Use of the dry weight of the solid gives a constant basis for comparison.

All references to moisture contents in this book are made on dry basis, unless otherwise stated.

Rate of Drying

The rate at which drying occurs has been found to show certain phases, which are illustrated in Fig. 24.5, where the change in moisture content is plotted against time. From A to B the relationship is linear, which is known as the *constant rate period*, while from B to C the rate of loss of moisture decreases and is known as the *falling rate period*. The end of the constant rate period, B, is referred to as the *critical moisture content*.

An alternative method of representing the drying process is given in Fig. 24.6 which shows the variation of drying rate as the moisture content changes. From the graphs it can be seen that there is considerable variation in the behaviour of different materials. The critical moisture content may vary also, being low with non-porous materials (sand has a value of less than 10 per cent) while colloidal organic substances may have a critical moisture content in excess of 100 per cent.

The curves for the falling rate period may have different shapes, so that for a material such as soap

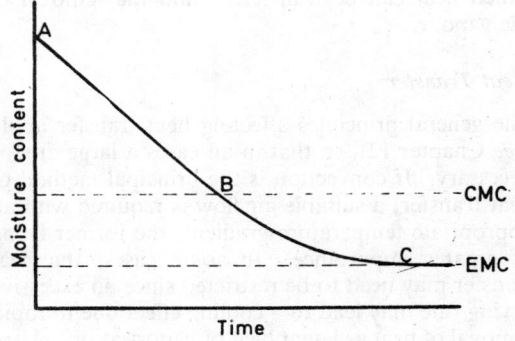

Fig. 24.5 Drying curve
CMC = critical moisture content
EMC = equilibrium moisture content

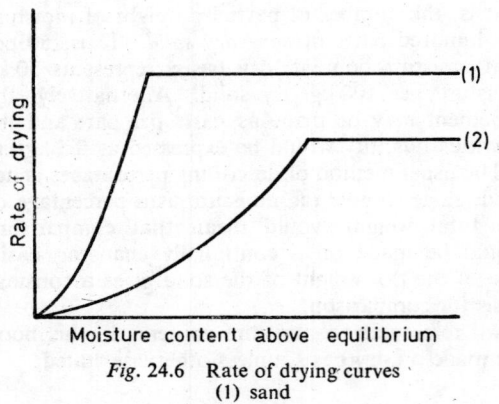

Fig. 24.6   Rate of drying curves
(1) sand
(2) soap

(curve 2) the falling rate of drying shows a continuous decrease. In other substances, sand is a typical example, the falling rate period shows two phases. The *first falling rate period* has a linear relationship, that is, the decrease in rate is uniform, while in the *second falling rate period* there is a continuous decrease until the equilibrium moisture content is reached.

Each of these periods will be considered in more detail.

CONSTANT RATE PERIOD

For given conditions of temperature and humidity, most substances dry at a similar rate in the constant rate period. It is found that the evaporation rate is similar to that from a free liquid surface under the same conditions, indicating that the evaporation takes place from the wet surface of the solid and that the liquid is replaced from below as fast as it is vaporised.

Controlling factors in this period are the rate at which heat can be transferred and the removal of the vapour.

Heat Transfer

The general principles affecting heat transfer apply (*see* Chapter 12), so that in all cases a large area is necessary. If convection is the principal method of heat transfer, a suitable air flow is required with an appropriate temperature gradient, the former being of greater importance. In some cases, the heat transfer may need to be restricted since an excessive drying rate may lead to a cooling effect due to rapid removal of heat as latent heat of vaporisation. Also, rapid drying may lead to the formation of a surface 'skin' that will hinder mass transfer and so reduce the drying rate.

Conduction dryers demand good contact between the heating surface and the solid. With radiant heat transfer, the efficiency is very high and, provided the emitters can 'see' the surface of the solid, the heat transfer occurs at the surface where the drying is taking place. In all cases, but particularly with radiation, there is a danger of overheating the surface at the end of the constant rate period.

Removal of Vapour

Drying in the constant rate period depends on mass transfer through the air boundary layers. Application of the theory of Chapter 13 will show that turbulent flow conditions are required, which will lower the partial vapour pressure in the atmosphere and reduce the thickness of the air boundary layers. The effect of both of these factors is to increase the partial pressure gradient, leading, in turn, to a higher mass transfer coefficient.

FIRST FALLING RATE PERIOD

As moisture is removed from the surface, a point will be reached when the rate of vaporisation is insufficient to *saturate* the air in contact with the surface. Under these conditions, the rate of drying will be limited by the transfer of liquid to the surface and, since this becomes increasingly difficult, the rate decreases continuously.

For some substances with a complex structure such as gels or vegetable drugs, the rate of movement can be described by expressions resembling the diffusion equation, so that it is dependent on a moisture concentration gradient.

In packed beds of particulate materials, other factors are involved and capillary forces have a controlling effect. The liquid in the pores exerts a *suction potential* (due principally to the surface tension of the liquid) and the value of the suction potential increases as pore size decreases. Pore size will vary according to particle size and the packing of the particle (*see* Chapter 19), cubical pores being larger than rhombohedral pores. Higher values of the suction potential make removal of the water from the pore more difficult, so that larger pores near the surface open first, followed by smaller pores. During drying, moisture will be drawn from the lower pores, moving to smaller pores near the surface that have been emptied, or to the surface, according to the relative values of the suction potential. This movement of the moisture is important in connection with the migration of dissolved solids; thus a potent medicament dissolved in the granulating liquid may be uniformly dispersed at the start of the drying process, but not when the granules are finally dry.

Eventually, the suction potential of the pores still containing moisture is so great that movement cannot occur and drying at the surface will end. As the drying rate decreases, less heat is used as latent heat of vaporisation, so that the heat transfer coefficient should be reduced.

SECOND FALLING RATE PERIOD

Any moisture that remains at the end of the first falling rate period is unable to move, so that drying cannot take place on the surface. Hence, the plane of vaporisation retreats from the surface into the body of the solid, and the drying rate depends on the movement of the vapour through the pores to the surface, in general, by molecular diffusion.

In both cases, minimum humidity of the atmosphere above the solid will assist in maintaining the maximum vapour pressure gradient. In addition, the thermal conductivity of the solid decreases as it becomes dry; if thermostable it is safe to allow temperature gradients to increase to maintain the rate of heat transfer, but if the material is thermolabile the heating must be decreased.

Types of Dryer

A number of methods have been suggested for the classification of dryers and, while sub-division according to uses, for example, has advantages, it is logical to group dryers according to the form of heating. Hence, dryers will be considered in classes according to the *principal* method of heat transfer: convection, conduction, or radiation. It must be emphasised that a piece of equipment may be designed to utilise a particular method of heat transfer, but other forms are also involved. Thus, a hot-air oven has convection as the predominant source of heat, but an object on a shelf receives heat by conduction and by radiation from the walls.

The following dryers are typical examples of the various classes used for pharmaceutical materials.

CONVECTION DRYERS

Compartment (or Tray or Shelf) Dryers

The simplest form of dryer in this category is a cabinet with a heater, usually at the bottom to assist convection, but it is of limited value, giving virtually no control of heat transfer or humidity. The situation can be improved by including a fan, so that forced convection takes place, with increased heat transfer and reduced local vapour concentrations, but control is still inadequate.

The best type in this category is the *directed circulation* form, in which air is heated and is directed across the material in a controlled flow. Figure 24.7 is an example in which the alternate arrangement of the shelves causes air flows in the directions shown by the arrows. Heaters are positioned as shown, so that the air is re-heated before passing over each shelf, which is an advantage since the air temperature is minimised. As the air passes over each shelf, a certain amount of heat is given up to provide latent heat of vaporisation. To carry out the heating in one stage it would be necessary to heat the air to a very high temperature. By using the re-heating method, however, the maximum air temperature is much lower and less air is needed to carry the same amount of moisture.

A further economy of heat can be effected by re-circulating a portion of the air through the duct connecting the outlet back to the inlet. This also enables the humidity to be controlled for materials that crack or case-harden (that is, form a surface skin, *see* p. 274).

The compartment dryer is very flexible and versatile, with good control of heat and humidity, if designed correctly. The output, however, is limited due to size and to batch operation. Further, unless the material is moved, that nearest to the inlet will dry first, but the process must continue until all is dry, so that drying capacity is wasted. This difficulty can be overcome in a simple manner if the material is on trays; at intervals, the tray nearest to the air inlet is removed, all others moved one position nearer to the inlet, and a fresh tray of moist material inserted into the last position before the air outlet. The effect is to obtain semi-continuous operation with greater efficiency by having counter-current movement of air and drying solid.

Uses of the compartment dryer are very varied because of the versatility of the method, and include

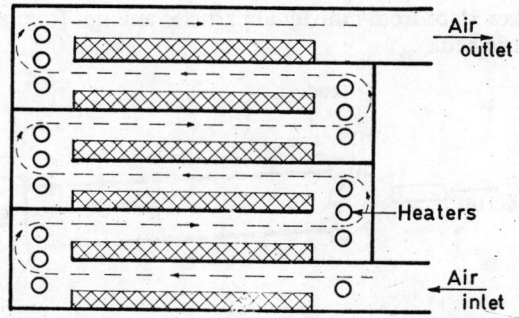

Fig. 24.7   Directed-circulation compartment dryer

the drying of crude drugs, chemicals, powders, tablet granules, or items of equipment.

Tunnel Dryers

The previous section referred to the improved drying efficiency that could be obtained by moving material so that the outgoing material met the incoming air to ensure maximum drying, and the outgoing air contacted the wettest material so that the air was as nearly saturated as possible.

Such counter-current movement of air and drying solids is arranged much more conveniently in the *tunnel dryer*, where the drying method resembles the compartment dryer, but takes the form of a long tunnel, with heated air entering at one end and some means of moving the material to be dried at the opposite end. The tunnel dryer can be of any size, and the movement can be effected in a very simple manner; for example, the solids may be placed on trays on rails and, at suitable intervals, a tray may be pushed into the inlet, thereby displacing a tray from the dry end. On the other hand, a more sophisticated arrangement is a mechanical conveyor that has an automatic speed control and temperature and humidity control, including re-heaters if necessary.

Compared with the compartment dryer, the tunnel dryer has the advantage of being semi-continuous or continuous in operation; applications are similar, but more suitable for large-scale production.

Rotary Dryer

If powdered or granular substances are dried in the tunnel dryer (see above) on the usual form of conveyor, the drying takes place from a static bed of the solid. The *rotary dryer* is a modified form of the tunnel dryer in which the particles are passed through a rotating cylinder, counter-current to a stream of heated air. Due to the rotation of the cylinder, the material is turned over and drying takes place from individual particles and not from a static bed.

As indicated in the section in Fig. 24.8, the cylindrical shell (which may be as much as 10 m in length) is mounted with a slight slope, of the order of 1 in 20, so that the material will move through the shell as it is slowly rotated at about 10 rev/min. To improve contact, the shell contains baffles or *flights* which lift the solids and spill the particles through the air stream. This gives rapid drying, so that outputs of 4 Mg/h can be obtained with larger versions.

The rotary dryer is used for continuous drying on a large-scale of any powdered or granular solid.

Fluidised Bed Dryer

Another method of obtaining good contact between hot air and particles is used in the *fluidised bed dryer;* the technique of *fluidisation* is used widely for fluid/solid contacting operations of all types and the general principles will be summarised before the applications to drying.

Consider the situation in which particulate matter is contained in a vessel, the base of which is perforated, enabling a fluid to pass through the bed of solids from below. The fluid can be liquid or gas, but air will be assumed for the purposes of this description, as it is most relevant to the drying process.

If the air velocity through the bed is increased gradually and the pressure drop through the bed is measured, a graph of the operation shows several distinct regions, as indicated in Fig. 24.9. At first, when the air velocity is low, A, flow takes place between the particles without causing disturbance, but, as the velocity is increased a point is reached, B, when the pressure drop has attained a value where the frictional drag on the particle is equal to the force of gravity on the particle. Rearrangement of the particles occurs to offer least resistance, C, and eventually they are suspended in the air and can move; pressure drop through the bed decreases slightly because of the greater porosity, D. Further increase in the air velocity causes the particles to separate and move freely, and the bed is fully

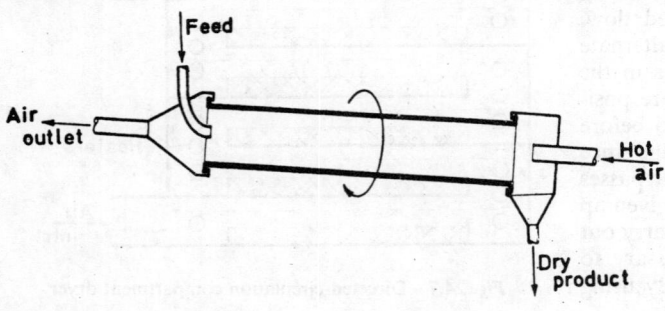

Fig. 24.8 Rotary dryer

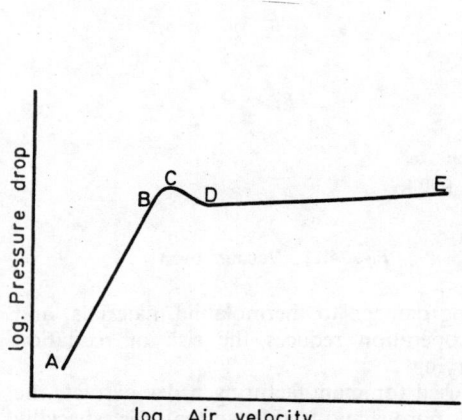

Fig. 24.9 Effect of air velocity on pressure drop through a fluidised bed

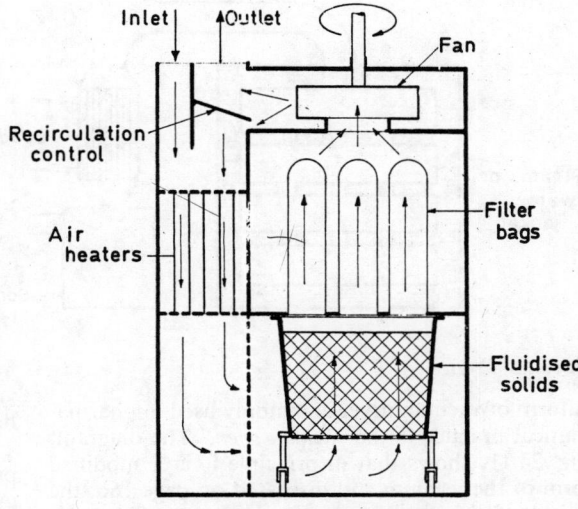

Fig. 24.10 Fluidised bed dryer

fluidised. Any additional increase in velocity separates the particles further, that is, the bed expands, without appreciable change in the pressure drop, until *E* when the velocity is sufficient to entrain the solids and cause transport of the particles.

In the region *D-E*, fluidisation is irregular, much of the air flowing through in bubbles, the term *boiling bed* being commonly used to describe it. The important factor is that it produces conditions of great turbulence, the particles mixing, with good contact between air and particles.

Hence, if hot air is used, the turbulent conditions lead to high heat and mass transfer rates, the fluidised bed technique therefore offering a means of rapid drying. The arrangement of such a dryer is shown in Fig. 24.10 and sizes are available with capacities up to 100 kg.

Advantages

(*a*) Efficient heat and mass transfer give high drying rates, so that drying times are shorter than static bed convection dryers. A batch of tablet granules, for example, can be dried in 20 to 30 minutes, whereas a compartment dryer would require several hours. Apart from obvious economic advantages, the heating time of thermolabile materials is minimised.

(*b*) The fluidised state of the bed gives drying from individual particles and not from the entire bed. Hence, most of the drying will be at constant rate and the falling rate period (when the danger of overheating is greatest) is very short.

(*c*) The temperature of a fluidised bed is uniform and can be controlled precisely.

(*d*) The fluidised state produces a free-flowing product.

(*e*) The free movement of individual particles eliminates the risk of soluble materials migrating, as may occur in static beds (*see* p. 274).

(*f*) The containers can be mobile, making handling simple, and reducing labour costs.

(*g*) Short drying times mean that the unit has a high output from a small floor space.

Disadvantages

(*a*) The turbulence of the fluidised state may cause attrition of some materials, with the production of fines.

(*b*) Fine particles may become entrained and must be collected by bag filters, with care to avoid segregation and loss of fines.

(*c*) The vigorous movement of particles in hot dry air can lead to the generation of charges of static electricity, and suitable precautions must be taken.

The fluidised bed dryer can be used for drying any powdered material; a special application is the drying of tablet granules, for which it is an excellent method (*see* p. 215).

CONDUCTION DRYERS

Conduction is used as the principal method of heat transfer in dryers that are operated under vacuum; obviously convection cannot occur when air is virtually absent.

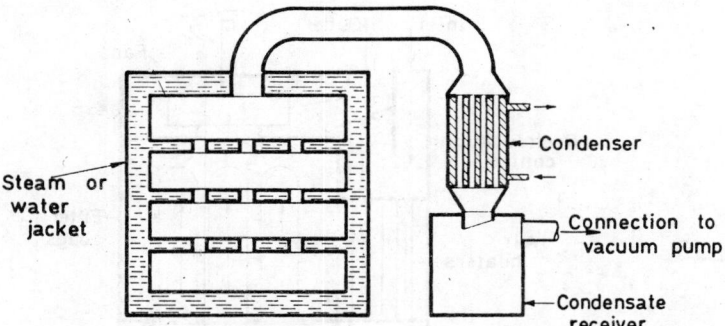

Fig. 24.11   Vacuum oven

Vacuum Oven

A form of vacuum dryer commonly used in pharmaceutical practice is the *vacuum oven*. The diagram, Fig. 24.11, shows that in principle it is a modified form of the vacuum still discussed on page 166, the object of the modifications being to provide easy opening and closing and a large area for heat transfer, so that trays of solid materials can be processed.

The vacuum oven is essentially a jacketed vessel, sufficiently stout in construction to withstand vacuum within the oven and steam pressure in the jacket. In addition, the supports for the shelves form part of the jacket, giving a larger area for conduction heat transfer. The oven can be closed by a door that can be locked tightly to give an air-tight seal. The oven is connected through a condenser and receiver to a vacuum pump, although if the liquid to be removed is water and the pump is of the ejector type that can handle water vapour, the pump can be connected directly to the oven.

Operating pressure is usually about 0·03 to 0·06 bar, at which pressures water boils at 25 to 35°C. Some ovens may be large, and continuous forms have been devised, but for pharmaceutical purposes an oven of about 1·5 m cube and with 20 shelves is commonly used, this giving an area of about 45 to 50 m² for heating.

In an alternative design there are a number of small compartments rather than one large one. This simplifies construction and operation by avoiding the need for one large and heavy door, which is replaced by small doors to each compartment. If the compartments are used in sequence, the pumping load is spread and semi-continuous operation is achieved.

Advantages

(*a*) The method is especially suitable for unstable materials; drying takes place at low temperature, minimising damage to thermolabile materials, and vacuum operation reduces the risk of oxidation during drying.

(*b*) If used for manufacturing a dry extract, the product is porous and friable, so that it is especially useful for tabletting. The product is porous because the extract goes through a viscous liquid stage, the reduced pressure encourages the formation of vapour bubbles, and the product eventually solidifies in this form.

(*c*) The use of a condenser enables solvents to be recovered, which is useful with expensive or inflammable solvents. The equipment can also be used for solvent recovery from exhausted marcs (*see* p. 260) as well as for drying extracts, which is economically advantageous in smaller plants.

Disadvantages

(*a*) Heat transfer coefficients are low. Most of the heating is by conduction, although some is by radiation from the walls and from the shelf above. It is important to ensure close contact between shelf and tray, otherwise conduction heat transfer is reduced and only radiation can occur across the gaps.

(*b*) The vacuum oven is of limited capacity. For larger amounts of material the *agitated vacuum dryer* is to be preferred. This may take a form resembling the vacuum evaporating pan (*see* p. 166) but with the addition of an agitator, or it may be a jacketed cylindrical vessel that can be agitated. This method gives larger capacity and improved heat transfer as the solids dry, but is not suitable for substances that become 'sticky' or 'ball'.

(*c*) Labour and running costs are high.

(*d*) There is a danger of an excessive temperature gradient, especially as the coefficient of thermal conductivity of the material will decrease as it dries, leading to over-heating and to decomposition. It is sometimes overlooked that, although the vacuum gives a low evaporating temperature, contact with a steam-heated surface can give as much heat damage as under atmospheric pressure.

The above factors mean that vacuum drying is of specialised application and its uses include the drying of: thermolabile materials, such as penicillin; products where the porous form is useful, such as dry extracts; and removal of liquids other than water, where the solvent recovery is advantageous, ethanol extractives, for example.

Freeze Drying

Although the process is commonly known as *freeze drying*, the alternative title *sublimation drying* is strictly more accurate as it is descriptive of the mechanism of drying, whereas the former title is simply derived from the physical state of the material.

The principles of sublimation are discussed in Chapter 3; sublimation drying consists simply of reducing the temperature and pressure to values below the triple point. Under these conditions, any heat transferred is used as latent heat and the ice sublimes directly to the vapour state.

Figure 3.1 (p. 18) represents the ice-water-water vapour system and shows the triple point at 610 N/m^2 and at a temperature of $0.0098°C$. In principle, therefore, the freeze drying process is simple, but the practice is more complicated and the following aspects must be taken into account:

The temperature must be kept well below the triple point temperature, and it is usual to work in the range -10 to $-30°C$.

Similarly, the pressure must be below the triple point and pressures between 10 and 30 N/m^2 are used. This presents greater difficulties, as vapour must be removed, otherwise the vapour pressure would exceed this value very rapidly.

The material is frozen and vapour sublimes from the surface, the ice front receding into the solid in a similar manner to drying during the second falling rate period in the ordinary process (*see* p. 275). It follows that a large area is required.

For the same reason, a thin layer should be used to reduce the distance over which the ice front must retreat through the solid.

The final product has a very low moisture content and contact with the atmosphere must be avoided. It is usual to dry the product in the final containers, which can be sealed quickly, sometimes without removing from the dryer.

STAGES OF THE DRYING PROCESS

Usually, the material is frozen before application of vacuum, to avoid foaming; under these conditions the primary drying stage by sublimation can reduce the moisture content to 0.5 to 1 per cent. If it is necessary to remove the final traces, the temperature is raised or a desiccant used, so that secondary drying is an ordinary vacuum drying process.

FREEZING

A number of methods are used to effect freezing, while ensuring that a large surface is produced.

Pre-freezing

The solution can be pre-frozen, that is, before the start of the drying process, and this is usually applied to larger containers such as blood bottles.

In *shell freezing* the bottle is used only part filled with product and is rotated slowly, almost horizontally, in a refrigerated bath. The material freezes in a shell round the walls of the bottle in a similar manner to the formation of the roll-tube used in microbiology.

This gives a thin layer, a large area for sublimation (in fact, the area increases as drying occurs), and the maximum area for heat transfer, as shown in Fig. 24.12. The freezing is slow, however, so that large ice crystals, which may have an adverse effect on some biological products, form.

The *vertical spin freezing* method produces small crystals of ice. The bottles are first chilled and then spun individually in a vertical position in a stream of very cold air. The liquid becomes supercooled and freezing occurs with great rapidity. Small ice crystals are preferred for products such as blood and blood plasma.

Shelf Freezing

The solution can be frozen in the dryer itself and is used with trays of bulk material or for small containers such as antibiotic vials. The method is

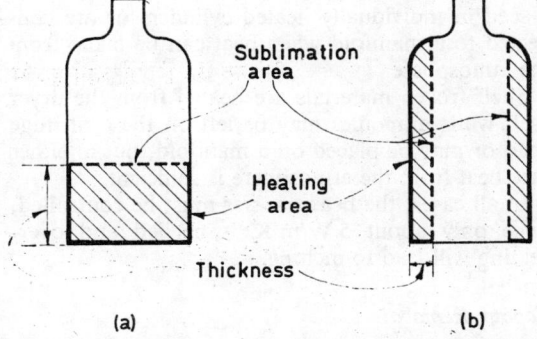

Fig. 24.12 Comparison of (*a*) ordinary and (*b*) shell frozen layers in a container

convenient and reduces handling, while the squat design of the vials gives a reasonable surface area and thin layer (*see* p. 138).

CENTRIFUGAL EVAPORATIVE FREEZING

The *centrifugal evaporative freezing* method makes it possible to freeze liquids in small containers, without refrigeration. Vacuum is applied to the liquid system, when boiling occurs, but foaming is prevented by spinning the containers in a centrifuge. Rapid vaporisation under the low pressure removes so much heat as latent heat of vaporisation that the liquid freezes, and about 20 per cent of the water is removed before freeze drying, as such, begins. The advantage of the method is that it shortens the primary drying stage, as well as obviating the need for refrigeration. Ampoules are usually frozen in this way, a number being spun in a vertical position in a special centrifuge head so that the liquid is thrown outwards and freezes in a wedge shape.

VACUUM

To reduce the pressure sufficiently it is necessary to use efficient vacuum pumps, usually two-stage rotary pumps on the small-scale, and ejector pumps on the large-scale.

PRIMARY DRYING

During the primary drying, the latent heat of sublimation must be provided and the vapour removed. The apparatus may resemble the vacuum oven (*see* p. 278) or containers may be attached to individual outlets on a manifold.

Heat Transfer

Heat transfer is critical; insufficient heat prolongs the process, which is already slow, and excess heat will cause melting.

Pre-frozen bottles, of blood for example, are placed in individually heated cylinders or are connected to a manifold when heat can be taken from the atmosphere.

Shelf frozen materials are heated from the dryer shelf while ampoules may be left on the centrifuge head or may be placed on a manifold, but in either case heat from the atmosphere is sufficient.

In all cases, the heat transfer must be controlled, since only about 5 W/m²K is needed and overheating will lead to melting.

Vapour Removal

The vapour formed must be removed continually to avoid a pressure rise that would stop sublimation.

On the small-scale, vapour is absorbed by a desiccant such as phosphorus pentoxide, or is cooled on a small condenser with solid carbon dioxide.

Condensation may be used on the large-scale, but mechanically refrigerated condensers are used. Accumulation of ice decreases heat transfer, and for very large installations the condenser can be scraped, the ice compressed to a solid block and ejected through a special pressure lock.

On the large-scale, vapour is commonly removed by pumping but the pumps must be of large capacity and must not be affected by moisture. The extent of the pumping capacity needed will be realised from the fact that, under the pressure conditions used during primary drying, 1 g of ice will form 1000 litres of vapour. Ejector pumps are most satisfactory for this purpose.

Rate of Drying

The rate of drying in freeze drying is very low, the ice being removed at a rate of about 1 mm depth per hour. The drying rate curve illustrated in Fig. 24.13 shows a similar shape to the normal drying

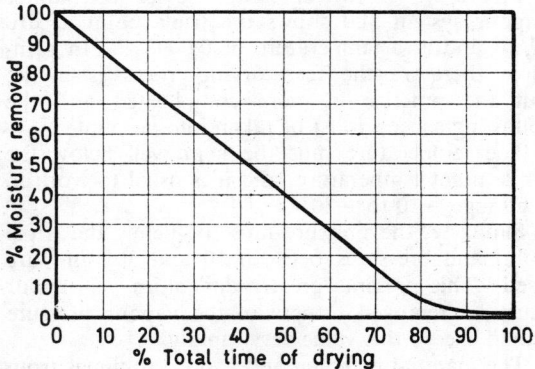

Fig. 24.13 Sublimation drying: rate of drying curve

curve, the drying being at constant rate during most of the time. The two curves are not really comparable, however, since the mechanism of freeze drying resembles the falling rate period of the normal drying process. A constant rate is shown because the rate of sublimation is so slow that it is the controlling factor, whereas in the normal drying process the rate is limited by vapour diffusing through the pores. Any attempt to increase sublimation involves raising the heat transfer coefficient and would only lead to melting.

SECONDARY DRYING

The primary drying process leaves products with about 0·5 per cent moisture in the solid and this is removed in the secondary drying process. The usual method is to raise the temperature, often as high as 50 to 60°C. The use of such a high temperature may seem surprising in view of the remarks in the previous section, but the secondary drying period is ordinary vacuum drying, the product is virtually free from moisture, and the risk of hydrolysis is negligible.

Frequently, because of the drop in the rate of drying at the end of primary drying, the secondary drying stage may be started at a higher moisture content, often 5 to 2 per cent.

PACKAGING

Attention must be paid to packaging freeze dried products to ensure protection from moisture. Containers should be closed without contacting the atmosphere, if possible, and ampoules, for example, are sealed on the manifold while still under vacuum. Otherwise, the closing must be carried out under controlled atmospheric conditions.

Advantages

Freeze drying, as a result of the character of the process, has certain special advantages:

(*a*) Drying takes place at very low temperatures, so that enzyme action is inhibited, and decomposition, particularly hydrolysis, is minimised.

(*b*) The solution is frozen, so that the final dry product is a network of solid occupying the same volume as the original solution. Thus, there is no case-hardening and the product is light and porous.

(*c*) The porous form of the product gives ready solubility.

(*d*) There is no concentration of the solution prior to drying. Hence, salts do not concentrate and denature proteins as occurs with other drying methods.

(*e*) Under high vacuum, there is no contact with the air, and oxidation is minimised.

Disadvantages

There are two main disadvantages of freeze drying:

(*a*) The porosity, ready solubility, and complete dryness yield a very hygroscopic product. Unless dried in the final container and sealed *in situ*, packaging requires special conditions.

(*b*) The process is very slow and uses complicated plant, which is very expensive. It is not a general method of drying, therefore, but is limited to certain types of valuable products that cannot be dried by any other means.

Uses of Freeze Drying

The method is applied only to biological products; for example, antibiotics (other than penicillin),

blood products, vaccines (such as BCG, yellow fever, smallpox), enzyme preparations (such as hyaluronidase) and microbiological cultures.

RADIANT HEAT DRYERS

In general, radiant heat dryers are not specially designed, but are modifications of the dryers already discussed; for example, drum, compartment, or tunnel dryers.

Sources of the radiant energy may be:

Lamps—so called *infra-red lamps*; usually the operating temperature is too high, giving a total emission of energy that is too great and that causes overheating.

Low temperature sources—electric rods or electric or gas-heated panels are used. They may operate at red heat or down to 'black' heat (to about 500°C). Such sources give better heating control and are to be preferred.

Uses of Radiant Heat Drying

Dryers adapted for radiant heat transfer may be used for most materials, solid or liquid in thin layers. The method is very effective for thin liquid films, as on drum dryers, and powders or granules may be dried quicker by radiant heat than by convection heating. Care must be taken to avoid surface overheating, however.

BIBLIOGRAPHY

CROSBY, E. J. and MARSHALL, W. R. (1958) Effect of Drying Conditions on the Properties of Spray-dried Particles. *Chem. Eng. Progr.*, **54** (7), 56–63.

FOWLER, H. W. (1952) The Application of Infra-red Heating to Pharmaceutical Products. *J. Pharm. Pharmac.*, **4**, 932–943.

OLIVER, T. R. and NEWITT, D. M. (1949) The Mechanism of Drying of Solids: Part II, The Measurement of Suction Potentials and Moisture Distribution in Drying Granular Solids. *Trans. Instn. Chem. Engrs.*, **27**, 9–18.

PEARSE, J. F., OLIVER, T. R., and NEWITT, D. M. (1949) The Mechanism of the Drying of Solids: Part I, The Forces Giving Rise to Movement of Water in Granular Beds, During Drying. *Trans. Instn. Chem. Engrs.*, **27**, 1–8.

SCOTT, M. W., LIEBERMAN, H. A., RANKELL, A. S., CHOW, F. S., and JOHNSTON, G. W. (1963) Drying as a Unit Operation in the Pharmaceutical Industry I: Drying of Tablet Granulations in Fluidised Beds. *J. pharm. Sci.*, **52**, 284–291.

STRATTON, R. A. (1965) Batch Drying in Industry. *Chem. and Ind.*, 67–80.

25

Materials of Pharmaceutical Plant Construction

In selecting materials for the construction of satisfactory plant the pharmaceutical engineer encounters problems involving chemical, physical, and economic factors. The following brief outline of these factors indicates something of the scope and limitations of his choice.

CHEMICAL FACTORS

Two aspects of chemical action must be considered under this heading, namely—

The possible contamination of the *product* by the material of the plant.

The effect on the *material of the plant* by the drugs and chemicals being processed.

The importance of the first of these becomes evident when it is realised that impurities often have considerable physiological effects and, also, that impurities, even in traces, may cause the product to decompose. An example of the latter is the inactivating effect of heavy metals on penicillin. The appearance of a product may also be affected by changes in colour due to contamination from the material of the plant.

It should be remembered that contamination from some materials may be innocuous, the products being non-toxic.

Our increasing knowledge of materials of plant construction is assisting greatly in providing plant that will be resistant to attack and deterioration in use from the effects of acids, alkalis, oxidising agents, tannins, etc. New alloys, having special physical and chemical properties, have been developed and quite new materials such as plastics have been introduced to meet the problems encountered.

PHYSICAL FACTORS

These include strength, weight, wearing qualities, ease of fabrication, thermal conductivity and expansion and electrical conductivity. Subsidiary factors, of importance in certain cases, include ease of cleaning and sterilising and transparency.

Strength. Sufficient mechanical strength is an obvious necessity and will be suited to the size of the plant and the stresses to which it will be subjected.

Weight. In most cases weight will be reduced to a minimum, other factors being satisfactory, and especially in plant that may have to be moved about from place to place.

Wearing Qualities. These are particularly important where there is a possibility of friction between moving parts, an extreme case in point being the material used for the grinding surfaces of mills.

Ease of Fabrication. It must be possible to process the material in order to fabricate the various units of the plant. Properties that enable materials to be cast, welded, forged, or machined, are of prime importance.

Thermal Expansion. The design of plant may be greatly complicated by the use of material that has a high coefficient of expansion. This increases the stresses and the risk of fracture with temperature changes, and the temperature range over which the plant will be operated is likely to be considerably restricted.

Thermal Conductivity. In plant such as stills and evaporators, a good thermal conductivity is desirable. It must be remembered, however, that resistant films greatly modify heat transference (*see* p. 152).

Cleansing. Smooth polished surfaces simplify cleansing processes, and materials that can be 'finished' with such surfaces are ideal when scrupulous cleanliness is necessary.

Sterilisation. Where sterility is essential the material should be capable of withstanding the necessary treatment, usually steam under pressure. This factor is to some extent bound up with the previous one since cleansing is a normal preliminary to the sterilisation of apparatus and plant.

Transparency. This may be a useful property where it is possible, and is one reason for the increasing use of borosilicate glass in the construction of pharmaceutical plant.

Economic Factors. Cost and maintenance of plant must, of course, be economic. Here the main concern is not simply to obtain the least costly material. Better wearing qualities and lower maintenance may well mean that a higher initial cost is more economical in the long run.

A brief description of the common materials of construction is given below under the following simple classification—

Metals {Ferrous
{Non-ferrous

Non-metals {Inorganic
{Organic

Metals

FERROUS METALS

Cast Iron. This consists of iron with a proportion of carbon. The amount of carbon varies, giving products with different properties. Its characteristics may also be altered by alloying with other elements such as silicon, nickel, chromium. Silicon alloys have found considerable application in chemical engineering processes since they are more resistant to acids. They are very hard and brittle, however, and cannot be machined.

Cast iron is resistant to concentrated sulphuric and nitric acids and to dilute alkalis. It is attacked by dilute sulphuric and nitric acids and by both dilute and concentrated hydrochloric acid. At high temperatures it is attacked by ammonium salts and, important in pharmacy, it reacts with tannins.

It is commonly used as the supports for plant, for the jackets of steam pans etc. It is cheap and is, therefore, often used in place of more expensive and more resistant materials by coating with enamel, plastic or other protective substance.

Steels. Mild steel is an iron alloy that contains only a small percentage of carbon and, unlike cast iron, it can be worked by welding, machining and so on. It has much greater mechanical strength than cast iron and is much less brittle.

Its resistance to attack by chemicals is similar to that of cast iron but varies according to the composition.

A greater tonnage of mild steel is used in the chemical and pharmaceutical industries than any other material of construction. It is used for supporting structures such as girders and bases for plant vessels and for much machinery, vessels, pipe lines and smaller accessories such as nuts and bolts.

As in cast iron it may be used for vessels and pans if the surface is protected with a non-corroding lining.

Stainless Steels. These are steel alloys, usually with nickel and chromium, and are characterised by their high resistance to corrosion. Steels containing 18 per cent of chromium and 8 per cent of nickel and known as '18/8 stainless steel', have considerable use in the pharmaceutical industry. Plant of various shapes and size can be made from this material since it can be worked like mild steel, but considerable skill and knowledge is necessary to avoid altering its corrosion-resistant properties during heating processes such as welding, due to carbide precipitation at the crystal-grain boundaries. Reduction of carbon content or the inclusion of stabilisers such as titanium, molybdenum or niobium may prevent this.

Stainless steels can be used for most pharmaceutical plant, including storage and extraction vessels, evaporators and fermenting vessels. Small apparatus commonly made from stainless steel includes, funnels, buckets, measuring vessels, and shovels. Sinks and bench tops are also made of stainless steel where a good surface with high corrosion-resisting qualities is necessary.

The high cost often excludes its use but often the cost may be justified even on a very large scale. For example, a great deal of the plant used in the production of penicillin is of this material since it is by far the most satisfactory, being strong, corrosion-resistant, non-contaminating and readily cleansed and sterilised.

NON-FERROUS METALS

Copper. Copper is malleable and ductile and is, therefore, easily fabricated. It has a thermal conductivity 8 times greater than steel but is corroded by a number of substances, particularly oxidising agents. It is attacked by nitric acid in all concentrations, by hot concentrated hydrochloric and sulphuric acids, and by some organic acids. Ammonia reacts with it readily to form blue cupro-ammonium compounds. Many drug constituents react with it, and for this reason copper is usually protected by a lining of tin when used for pharmaceutical plant.

It is used for evaporators, pans of various kinds, stills, fractionating columns, and so on, and was most popular in the past because of its malleability, which ensured ease of fabrication and good thermal conductivity. Because of its susceptibility to attack by pharmaceutical materials there is a tendency to-day to replace it by stainless steel where corrosion is likely.

Copper piping is easy to make because of the ductility of the metal and it is used extensively for services such as cold water, gas, vacuum, and low-pressure steam. Where necessary, copper piping may be tinned, e.g. for distilled water.

Copper Alloys. These include alloys with zinc, tin, aluminium, silicon and nickel, all of which have their special uses.

Copper–Zinc Alloys (Brasses). The output of brasses exceeds that of any other copper alloy although their use is restricted in pharmaceutical plant since their corrosion resistance is less than that of copper. They are easily worked and their tensile strength is greater than copper. Like copper, brass is often used where rusting is to be avoided.

Brasses are used for tube plates in evaporators and condensers, for tubes and valves, and extensively in making nuts, bolts, rods, etc.

Copper–Tin Alloys (Bronzes). These usually contain 2 to 13 per cent of tin with a small amount of phosphorus and often traces of other elements. Harder and more durable than brass they are used for filter gauzes, stirrers, valves, pumps, high pressure pipes, autoclaves, and special tablet punches and dies.

Aluminium. Aluminium has good corrosion resistance to many substances although it is attacked by mineral acids (it is resistant to strong nitric acid), caustic alkalis, mercury and its salts. Its resistance is often due to the formation of a film on the surface. For example, acetic acid forms a film of gelatinous aluminium subacetate which is then resistant to acetic acid, and pure strong ammonia solutions form a resistant film of aluminium hydroxide. It is also highly resistant to oxidising conditions since it forms a compact oxide film.

Pure aluminium is soft but more corrosion-resistant than most of its alloys such as Duralumin. Alloys combining corrosion resistance with strength are formed with small percentages of manganese, magnesium, or silicon. Plant is easily fabricated and has excellent thermal conductivity.

For plant producing medicinal substances its most valuable property is probably the non-toxicity of its salts which are, moreover, colourless. As it is also non-toxic to micro-organisms it has considerable use in biosynthetic processes such as the production of citric and gluconic acids, and of streptomycin by deep culture methods. The metal is also suitable for plant used for preparing culture media and for absorption and extraction vessels used in preparing

antibiotics. Because of the formation of resistant films it is used for acetic acid plant and storage vessels for ammonia. The use of welded aluminium vessels, it has been claimed, made the nitric acid industry possible. Because of its low density it is most useful for transport containers such as drums and barrels, road and rail tankers.

Lead. Much lead is used in the chemical industry because of its remarkable resistance to corrosion and the great ease with which it can be made into complicated shapes. The lead chamber process for manufacturing sulphuric acid is one example from many in the heavy chemical industry. It is little used, however, in pharmaceutical practice because of the risk of contamination by traces of poisonous lead salts. It is used for cold water pipes, waste pipes and dilution tanks for laboratories.

Tin. Tin has a high resistance to a great variety of substances and, since its salts are non-toxic, it has a wide use throughout the food industry. It is, however, weak, its main use being to provide a protective coating for steel, copper, brass, etc. The coating of other metals with tin has been known for over 2000 years and today more than half the output of the metal is used for this purpose.

'Tin plate'—sheet steel coated with tin—is used for containers. Condenser tubes are often coated or 'tinned'.

Silver. Because of its high cost, silver is used only as a material of plant construction in special cases and usually silver-coated material is used rather than solid silver. It is not resistant to concentrated hydrochloric or sulphuric acids, any strength of nitric acid, and sulphur and sulphur compounds. It is resistant to organic acids and their salts.

It is even more malleable and ductile than copper and, therefore, capable of being readily worked. It has a higher thermal conductivity than all other metals.

A few examples of its special uses are—plant for the manufacture of salicylates and acetic acid; a silver-plated basket for a hydroextracter used in vitamin crystallisation; a solid silver vessel in a cast-iron jacket for bromination.

Nickel. Nickel is resistant to oxidation and alkalis but is attacked slowly by dilute mineral acids and rapidly by concentrated acids. It is resistant to the weak organic acids occurring in pharmaceutical preparations, e.g. citric, tartaric, and stearic. It is also resistant to phenols. Its salts are non-toxic.

It is useful for such plant as pans, vats, tanks, mixers, valves, and pumps, and nickel wire may be woven to form filter cloths.

Monel metal, an alloy of nickel (2/3), and copper (1/3), which is harder and more resistant than nickel, can replace steel where corrosion resistance is essential.

Chromium. Although hard and resistant to corrosion, chromium is not normally used as a material of plant construction. It forms resistant alloys with nickel and, probably, its most important use is in the manufacture of stainless steel.

It is also, of course, used as a plating to protect steel.

Non-metals

INORGANIC

Glass. Glass is very resistant to attack and is widely used for small-scale apparatus. Only recently has it been developed as a material of construction for use on a larger scale.

Ordinary soda glass is used for bottles and other cheap articles but is not satisfactory for large-scale plant or for containers where alkali contamination might be a serious drawback. For these purposes borosilicate glass is used. Such glass has several advantages over soda glass. It is, for example, less brittle. It has a low thermal expansion and can be used with safety over wide temperature ranges. However, its thermal conductivity is low and therefore it should be heated gradually to avoid fracturing. Pipe line may be used with pressures up to 8 bars if the pipe diameter is less than 50 mm and pipe lines with larger diameters are used with pressures up to 4 bars.

Special advantages of glass are that it can be easily cleaned and sterilised and, also, that the contents of vessels can be readily examined for colour and clarity.

A disadvantage is the difficulty of joining sections of glass plant together. Ground-glass joints are sometimes satisfactory, especially in small-scale apparatus, but are rigid. Gaskets of rubber, plastics, fibre, and asbestos are used to form a more flexible jointing but these must be chosen with care as they are normally less resistant to attack than glass.

Glass pipe line is useful for transporting liquids from stage to stage in various operations. Such pipe line is available from 15 mm to 0·3 m in diameter with fittings for the assembly of complete systems.

All-glass stills are used for preparing Water for Injections and other distilled preparations. Vessels up to 100 l are used and larger tanks can be made by clamping glass plates in frames.

Glass fibres are excellent for heat insulation or refrigeration plant. Such fibre, treated with oil, is used for filtering air for asepsis rooms. Woven fibre may be used for filter cloths and glass may be sintered in the preparation of filters.

Glass Linings and Coatings. Metal may be coated with glass to give a protective lining. The dangers of such apparatus are those of uneven expansion of metal and glass, and of the glass surface accidentally chipping. Great care must therefore be taken in heating and cooling and in protecting the glass lining from accidental damage.

Vessels of up to 50000 l capacity, pipe line and fittings, valves, condensers, columns, pumps, stirrers and mixers are among the many glass-coated items in use.

High resistance to corrosion and ease of cleaning make it valuable for pharmaceutical use.

Stone Ware. Ceramics are reasonably cheap, but weight, low thermal conductivity, and fragility give only a low resistance to mechanical and thermal shock. Corrosion resistance is usually due to a surface glaze which may become chipped.

Ceramics are used widely on a small scale but only to a limited extent on a large scale. Pipe line, tanks, vessels and filters are among the items made from it. Of special interest among ceramic products are bacteria-proof filters.

Stone, Slate, Brick, and Concrete. These have their particular uses, among which are granite for certain types of mill, vitrefied acid-resisting bricks for tanks, drains, culverts, etc., and concrete for structural purposes and sometimes for tanks.

Asbestos. Being a poor conductor of heat, asbestos is used for heat insulation. Since it is extremely inert it is used for pipe lining and for pipe jointing. It is fibrous material and may be woven into cloth for filters.

ORGANIC

Plastics. It will be convenient for the purpose of this brief account to group plastics under the following headings—

Rigid material.
Flexible material.
Coatings and linings.
Cements and fillers.
Special cases.

'Keebush' is an example of a rigid material. It is a phenolic resin with various inert fillers selected for their particular purpose. It may be machined, welded, and worked in other ways and is resistant to such an extent that it can be used for gears, bearings, and similar items with a noise reduction of two thirds compared with iron. Its weight is about one quarter that of iron.

It is resistant to corrosion except that of oxidising substances and strong alkalis.

Any item may be made from this material—vessels, pipes, fittings, valves, pumps, fans, ducts, filter presses and many others.

Polyethylene and polyvinyl chloride (PVC) are similar materials and are rigid or flexible, depending upon the amount of plasticiser added.

These do not withstand high temperatures but are non-resistant only to strong oxidising acids, halogens, and organic solvents.

Rigid or semi-rigid mouldings may be used for tanks, pipes, ducts, and other similar items and slightly flexible funnels, buckets and jugs are made which are almost unbreakable.

Metallic surfaces may be protected from corrosion by plastics of the polyethylene or PVC types prepared for coating with suitable plasticisers. Perfect adhesion of plastic to metal is sometimes difficult, and disadvantages are the differences in thermal expansion of plastic and metal and the danger of the coating accidentally chipping.

Uses of these materials include the lining of tanks and vessels and the coatings on stirrers and fans.

Plastic cements are used for spaces between acid-resistant tiles and bricks, and for similar purposes.

Special cases include transparent plastic guards for moving parts of machinery and asepsis screens. Nylon and PVC fibres may be woven into filter cloths.

Rubber. Hard rubber may be used for purposes similar to those mentioned under plastics. Soft rubber may be used for linings and coatings. Rubber swells in contact with oils; it is subject to oxidation and is attacked by some organic solvents. Synthetic rubbers that have greater resistance have been developed.

Timber. The use of wood for tanks and vats has greatly diminished since it has the disadvantage of absorbing the contents. Its lightness is an advantage where parts have to be handled, and filter presses are sometimes made of wood for this reason.

BIBLIOGRAPHY

GACKENBACH, R. E. (1960) *Materials Selection for Process Plants.* New York, Reinhold.

HEPNER, I. L. (Ed.) (1962) *Materials of Construction for Chemical Plant.* London, Leonard Hill.

RUMFORD, F. (1960) *Chemical Engineering Materials.* 2nd ed. London, Constable.

PART THREE

Biological Pharmacy

26

Outline of the Development of Microbiology

THE following brief survey of the development of microbiology, and of advances in pharmacy that were influenced by this development, is intended to provide students with a background knowledge that will help them to understand the present relationship between pharmacy and microbiology.

INFECTION AND ISOLATION

The idea that disease could be transmitted by contact was not conceived until the early part of the christian era. Leprosy was a scourge of the Middle East and in biblical times isolation of lepers was the only means of preventing the disease spreading in the community. It was rigidly practised, and in consequence leprosy has become rare in Europe. At various times in history it was found that isolation of sufferers from bubonic plague prevented rapid spread of the disease. Isolation hospitals were set up so that patients who had diseases that could spread rapidly through a community could be confined and, as recently as the nineteen forties, this form of control was practised for diseases such as scarlet fever, diphtheria, and poliomyelitis. Nowadays, the advent of antibiotics and other chemotherapeutic agents has made isolation unnecessary except for typhoid fever, smallpox and tuberculosis. The term quarantine is derived from the latin word *quarantina* meaning a period of forty days, which was the period of isolation imposed during the middle ages on incoming travellers arriving at the Republic of Ragusa (now a port in Yugoslavia). Quarantine is still used to protect communities from infection, though it is adjusted to a period of time that will ensure freedom from the suspected infection. The common example of this is the quarantine of dogs coming into the United Kingdom and a dramatic recent application was the isolation of the astronauts after their return from the moon.

A form of permanent quarantine is practised in the food industry where passive carriers of *Salmonella typhi* are excluded from jobs because this organism is transmitted by food infection.

INFECTION

Smallpox was one of the most serious epidemic diseases in England up to the nineteenth century.

Sometimes outbreaks of the disease were mild in character but often it was very malignant, and the death rate was very high. It was observed that persons who suffered a mild attack seldom succumbed in a subsequent grave epidemic. Although the mechanism of protection was not understood at the time, this fact became the basis of a protective measure that had originated in the East and was introduced into England in the first half of the eighteenth century. The method was arm-to-arm infection, the person desiring protection being inoculated by scarification with material from the pustules of a person suffering from a mild attack of smallpox. A similar mild attack ensued in the inoculated person, thus providing protection from a grave one for a number of years, sometimes for life. In 1796 Edward Jenner, a medical practitioner in Gloucestershire, discovered that a similar protection could be obtained by infecting patients with cowpox, which was less dangerous than smallpox infection. He was familiar with smallpox and had also been called upon to treat cowpox on the fingers of dairy workers. He noticed the similarity between the pustules produced by both diseases, and that patients who had been infected by cowpox did not contract serious infection even in grave epidemics of smallpox. He believed that this relationship between the two diseases could be applied to produce immunity to smallpox. To test his theory he infected a boy with cowpox from a pustule on the arm of a dairymaid. The boy developed cowpox, and when he recovered Jenner inoculated him with matter from a smallpox pustule, and the boy did not develop smallpox. Encouraged by this success Jenner continued to experiment, developing the system of vaccination for which he became famous. The word vaccine arises from the name *vaccinia*, the scientific name of cowpox.

RECOGNITION OF ORGANISMS AS CAUSATIVE AGENTS OF DISEASE

The idea that disease may be caused and transmitted by living matter was first advanced by Fracastoro of Verona (1483 to 1553) but without any experimental or observational evidence (microscopes were not then available). The first attempt at direct observation is credited to Kircher (1659) who reported minute worm-like structures in the blood of patients suffering from plague, but it seems improbable that any bacteria could have been seen with the crude lenses then available.

Antony Leeuwenhoek (1632–1723)

Leeuwenhoek lived in Delft in the Netherlands. As a hobby he learned the rudiments of lens grinding from spectacle makers and, also, acquired skill in metal working. He became very interested in the things he could see through the lenses he produced and patiently worked on the production of better lenses. In 1672, a neighbour, Regnier de Graaf, a corresponding member of the Royal Society, was allowed to examine various objects through the lenses. He was so impressed that he wrote to the Royal Society suggesting that Leeuwenhoek should be invited to report his discoveries to it. Leeuwenhoek replied at length to its letter and contributed regularly to its proceedings, being made a Fellow of the Royal Society in 1680. It was in 1677 that he first saw 'animalcules', as he called them. While examining a drop of rain water he saw minute organisms swimming about, and thus a new, hitherto invisible, world was discovered and the science now called microbiology was born. Being of a careful disposition, Leeuwenhoek examined water from many different sources and found the minute organisms which, 'compared with a cheese mite (thought to be the smallest organism), were as a bee to a horse'. He also thought that the sharp taste of pepper was due to fine points on the particles of pepper. He found that ground pepper was too coarse for observation with his microscopes so he put some pepper in water to soften it. Some weeks later when the pepper was soft enough to dissect with needles, Leeuwenhoek examined some of the material in a drop of water and discovered, not the fine points he expected but a very large number of minute organisms. This discovery was then reported to the Royal Society, with descriptions and drawings, together with an indication of their dimensions. The report was greeted with disbelief, the Fellows asking for details of how the measurements were done and how the microscope was made. They received a full reply to the first part, but the means of making the microscope remained Leeuwenhoek's secret. To follow up this discovery the Royal Society commissioned new microscopes, prepared a sample of pepper water and on 15th November 1677 saw for themselves the organisms that had been described so accurately by Leeuwenhoek. The connection between the organisms and disease was not suspected at that time.

Louis Pasteur (1822–1895)

It was not until the latter part of the nineteenth century that special organisms were recognised as the causative agents in contagious diseases, the credit for establishing this fact belonging to Pasteur, a French chemist. Pasteur's early chemical researches were into problems of optical activity and molecular asymmetry, as exhibited by the tartrates. He was the first chemist to separate the two optical isomers of the tartrates. His studies led Pasteur to the belief that optically active substances could be produced only by living things, and it was this belief that influenced his studies on fermentation. It had already been noted that lactic fermentation of a solution of sugar gave rise to a proportion of amyl alcohol, both sugar and amyl alcohol being optically active. Pasteur considered that it was impossible for amyl alcohol to be formed from sugar by a simple breakdown process and assumed that the optically active molecules of sugar were first split into simple substances without optical activity, from which the optically active amyl alcohol was built up. The synthesis of an optically active substance from inactive substances could, in Pasteur's view, be effected only by living things; consequently he suggested that the yeast cells known to be present in fermenting sugar solutions were living organisms.

The two most important general conclusions from Pasteur's investigation into fermentation were—

(a) That fermentation was due to living organisms capable of reproduction and multiplication.
(b) That different ferments produced different effects, each type of ferment producing only one type of fermentation, i.e. each kind of organism produced specific effects.

When Pasteur subsequently turned his attention to disease, he applied to it the general concepts gained from his studies of fermentation and suggested that infection was due to organisms that multiplied in the host, producing disease, and that each disease was caused by a particular organism. These ideas were established by his subsequent researches into the infective processes.

VARIATION IN SUSCEPTIBILITY AND VIRULENCE

Variation in susceptibility to disease, and variation in virulence, were two important discoveries made by Pasteur. In connection with his investigation of anthrax, he found that birds were relatively more resistant than men or sheep to infection by the anthrax bacillus. This resistance arises from the higher body temperature of the birds, which does not favour vigorous growth of the bacillus. From this observation arose the concept of variation of resistance to disease from one species of animal to another. Pasteur also showed that repeated cultivation of bacteria in a test-tube reduced the virulence of anthrax, when incubation temperatures were higher than the body temperature of man. When cultures of a virulent strain were grown in broth at higher temperatures and then injected into sheep, they produced only a mild form of anthrax. He also showed that sheep subjected to infection by the 'weakened' (attenuated) bacteria, became immune to subsequent attacks by the virulent strains.

Pasteur also showed that the organism producing chicken cholera could be attenuated by similar treatment and still protect chickens against invasion by virulent organisms. From these findings Pasteur formulated concepts of virulence and attenuation and demonstrated that attenuated cells will induce immunity to infection by a virulent strain of the same species of organism.

The term vaccine, already in use to designate the infective material from pustules induced by cowpox, was widened by Pasteur to include all preparations containing attenuated living bacteria.

Robert Koch (1843–1910)

Koch's interest in the microbial origin of disease began with the gift from his wife of a microscope on his twenty eighth birthday, when he was a medical practitioner at Wollstein hopelessly attempting to cure diseases about which little was known. In the blood of animals that had died of anthrax he found small rod-like structures not present in the blood of healthy animals. After exhaustive experiments he proved that these were the cause of anthrax. Koch discovered that under certain conditions, small oval bodies appeared inside the anthrax organisms. Even after drying and storage, these structures, or spores as he named them, when transferred to a suitable medium, developed into the ordinary cells which then multiplied rapidly. He also found that—

1. Spores were never present in the body of an infected animal during life, but developed shortly after its death while the body was still warm; the spores were viable after storage in an ice chest.

2. Spores did not form if the organs from the dead animal were immediately placed in an ice chest, because the ordinary form of the bacterium was killed by the low temperature. These facts—

(a) Explained the latency of anthrax. Outbreaks of the disease in sheep grazing in pastures from which infected animals had been excluded for long periods had hitherto been inexplicable, but Koch's work showed that the spores from dead carcases remained viable in the soil for months, ready to germinate when they gained access to animals.

(b) Indicated a new method of fighting epidemics when it was impossible to burn the carcases immediately after death; namely, immediate burial deep in the soil, where the temperature would be low enough to kill the ordinary form of the bacterium before the formation of resistant spores could take place.

This contribution to the new science of bacteriology was followed by equally painstaking researches into other contagious diseases, notably tuberculosis (the causative organism of which is sometimes called 'Koch's bacillus'). It was Koch's good fortune to discover accidentally a method of producing pure cultures, i.e. a growth of one kind of germ only, with no contamination by others. Many attempts had been made to devise apparatus for this purpose but they were unsuccessful because, at that time, only fluid media or animal tissues were used for artificially cultivating bacteria. In spite of attempts to exclude other organisms, these often gained access, or were present in the original tissues undergoing examination, and contaminated the culture producing effects that obscured or vitiated the results of the experiment.

Half a boiled potato had been left lying on a laboratory table and Koch noticed differently coloured specks on its surface. He examined each speck, in turn, and found that although the specks consisted of different bacteria, all the bacteria from one speck were alike. He immediately saw the reason for this: each speck (colony) had been formed from a single bacterium which, falling on the surface of the potato, had to remain exactly where it fell. Koch realised that growth on solid food offered a means of separating mixtures of bacteria; he mixed different organisms with water, spread a drop of the suspension on the cut surfaces of boiled potatoes and obtained colonies, each consisting of millions of the same kind of bacteria. The discovery revolutionised bacteriology by providing a means of growing one kind of bacteria unmixed with others. Subsequently, Koch invented other solid media by solidifying beef broth with gelatin. In his researches into tuberculosis, failing to obtain growth of the tubercle bacillus on his synthetic media, though he knew they were present from microscopic examination of tissues, Koch realised that media prepared from body fluids were essential for the growth of certain delicate organisms and succeeded in growing the tubercle organisms on blood serum coagulated by sufficient heat to form a jelly.

ELABORATION OF THERAPEUTIC PRODUCTS

Koch and, particularly, Pasteur attempted to find curative or preventive measures against the various microbial diseases they studied. Koch showed how infection was spread (e.g. in anthrax, by the formation of resistant spores soon after the death of the animal; in the case of cholera, from water polluted by faecal matter), thus indicating means by which these diseases could be checked. Pasteur showed that immunity could be obtained to certain diseases by the injection of the causative organism in an attenuated form. It remained for their followers to discover safer means of acquiring immunity and methods of combating disease already present in a host.

Friedrich Loeffler (1852–1916)

Loeffler, working with Koch, discovered the causative organism of diphtheria but just failed to realise the significance of his discoveries. Two points that baffled him were—

(a) The presence of the diphtheria bacillus detected in the throat of a child with no symptoms of diphtheria; now recognised as an immune diphtheria carrier.

(b) Diphtheria bacilli were confined to the throat, often in relatively small numbers, yet the patient died of the disease. In other bacterial diseases then known, the progress of the disease was accompanied by great increase in the number of bacteria that could be isolated from the patient.

To account for this phenomenon Loeffler advanced the hypothesis that the diphtheria organisms, though localised in the throat, made a poison that escaped from the cells and diffused to other parts of the body, there producing effects that caused death.

Roux and Yersin

Soon after publication of Loeffler's work, two of Pasteur's assistants, Roux and Yersin, took up the study of diphtheria. In 1889 a grave epidemic of the disease was sweeping Paris; they isolated the bacteria implicated in the outbreak, grew them in broth and then injected the liquid culture into rabbits. The rabbits developed typical symptoms and died, but on autopsy, no diphtheria organisms could be found. Roux remembered Loeffler's hypothesis that diphtheria was due to a poison released by the bacteria into the blood stream and realised that the poison in the broth and not the organisms had caused the death of the rabbits. To test this theory, diphtheria bacilli were grown in broth and the culture was filtered through a bacteria proof filter to produce a cell free filtrate, which was injected into rabbits. At the first attempt the experiment failed because insufficient time had been allowed for the poison (toxin) to be formed. Further tests, allowing a longer incubation time, produced very potent filtrates; minute doses proved fatal to rabbits which died with typical diphtheria symptoms. In this way Roux and Yersin proved that Loeffler's theory was right. They demonstrated two stages in the progress of the disease: the local growth of the organisms in the throat, followed by poisoning by the toxin released into the blood by the organisms. The latter is known as toxaemia or intoxication.

Emil Augustus Behring (1854–1917)

The next step was taken by Behring, one of Koch's assistants. Behring attempted a chemical cure of diphtheria, which consisted of injecting the toxin-containing filtrate and the chemical under test into a group of guinea-pigs, and toxin only into a control group. The tests were a failure except for one drug, iodine trichloride; even in this case the success was only partial because some of the animals that received it died. Behring decided to test the guinea-pigs that had recovered to see if they had developed immunity to diphtheria, so he injected some with toxin, leaving the rest as controls. He also injected toxin into fresh guinea-pigs to ensure that the toxin was still potent. The result was that the uninjected survivors and those receiving toxin all lived whereas the fresh guinea-pigs given toxin all died.

Behring concluded that the blood of the immune animals must contain a substance that rendered the toxin harmless; he made two experiments to test this idea—

1. He withdrew blood from an immune animal, separated the serum, mixed it with toxin and injected the mixture into fresh guinea-pigs.

2. He withdrew blood from a non-immune animal, separated the serum, mixed it with toxin and then injected it as in experiment 1 above.

The injected animals from experiment 1 survived, but those from experiment 2 died, thus showing that only the immune serum contained the agent that neutralised the toxin.

It was hoped that this immune serum would be a preventive for diphtheria, but when the interval between administering the serum and the toxin was increased the protective effect was decreased until the point where there was a three-weeks interval before administering the toxin, when the serum afforded no protection. Because protection was too transient Behring gave up the idea of using the serum to *protect* against diphtheria, but he decided to test the ability of the serum to *cure* diphtheria. He injected several guinea-pigs with diphtheria bacilli, allowed the disease to become well advanced, then injected half the group with the immune serum. The animals receiving serum quickly recovered, while the other group died.

The first attempt at clinical treatment with serum occurred on Christmas Day 1891; a child in Berlin was dying of the disease, immune serum was injected and the child recovered. The manufacture of this 'antidiphtheritic' serum was begun soon afterwards and within three years more than 20 000 cases of diphtheria had been treated and 'miracle cures' obtained. The use of this antitoxic serum soon became a routine treatment for cases of diphtheria. From this beginning the production of antitoxic sera for several diseases was developed.

VIRUS VACCINES

Two virus vaccines, smallpox and rabies, were developed early but most of the work in the late nineteenth century was aimed at controlling bacterial diseases, largely because techniques for isolating and characterising viruses were not yet available.

Influenza and the Common Cold

The major problems involved in the production of protective vaccines for these two diseases are—

(a) There are many strains of these viruses and cross-immunisation between the strains does not occur.

(b) Any immunity produced is very short lived. Despite these difficulties vaccines have been produced (p. 395) and these have reduced the infection and mortality rate in influenza, but their value for the common cold is not yet fully established.

Yellow Fever

In 1900, an American army was fighting in Cuba and deaths were greater from yellow fever than from wounds. Scientists were sent out to investigate this disease. One contracted the fever after allowing himself to be bitten by an infected mosquito; the disease was fairly severe but the patient recovered and his blood was found to contain antibodies to yellow fever. No organisms could be found in the body tissues and fluids but filtered blood from infected patients, when injected into monkeys, caused the disease which, therefore, was thought to be due to a 'filterable virus'. Immunisation of monkeys was achieved in 1929, and in 1937 an attenuated strain, 17D, derived from a virulent West African strain was tested. It proved to be non-lethal to humans but still retained its antigenicity and, later, was found to be suitable for cultivation in chick embryo from which a vaccine was developed by 1939. This was used in large quantities by allied troops in tropical theatres of war from 1939 to 1945.

Poliomyelitis

This disease produced a large number of deaths and many cases of paralysis as recently as the late nineteen fifties. Kolmer (1934) prepared a vaccine from the spinal cords of monkeys previously injected with live virus attenuated by serial passage through monkeys. In 1949 Enders and others perfected a technique for cultivating the virus in sheets of cells grown artificially from cells obtained from monkey kidneys or testicles. Three groups of antigenic strains were recognised and it was shown that virus inactivated by formalin treatment could be used to produce immunity in humans. Large-scale trials of this material were carried out in 1954, and several batches were used to immunise children. One batch of this vaccine was implicated in an outbreak of the disease, with a number of fatalities. It was shown that the inactivation was minimal and some batches could be issued while still infective. More rigorous testing has overcome this problem but after considerable use of the vaccine it was discovered that the immunity was somewhat transitory, so this type of vaccine (the Salk vaccine) was eventually superseded.

Because large numbers of children were involved, it was felt that an oral vaccine would be more satisfactory provided its antigenicity could be assured. Living attenuated viruses are given by mouth; they colonise the gut and, because they multiply there, a much stronger and longer stimulus to antibody production is provided than when inactivated (Salk) vaccine is used. Some of the virus particles are voided in the faeces, so this reservoir may accidentally vaccinate other hosts. The first vaccine of this type was produced by Koprowski in America in 1946, but it was discovered that one of the strains of virus was genetically unstable; because of the transmitted infection and the chance of the virus recovering its virulence this vaccine was abandoned. Later Sabin, in Cincinatti, produced an oral vaccine which he proved, by extensive tests on animals and human volunteers, was safe in use and genetically stable. He received permission to carry out a large-scale trial on millions of people in Russia in 1957. In 1958 a type-2 vaccine successfully controlled an epidemic of type-1 virus because the colonisation of the gut prevented invasion by the other type. However, development continued towards the production of a trivalent vaccine, actively immunising against all three strains, and this vaccine came into general use in 1960. Experience has confirmed that this vaccine produces an initial immunity adequate to cope with normal epidemics and that this immunity is maintained by the resident flora of virus in the gut.

ADVANCES INFLUENCED BY BACTERIOLOGY

Joseph Lister (1872–1912)

Before Pasteur's discovery that disease was caused by microbes, surgery had been performed without precautions to prevent infection, because the importance of these was not fully appreciated. This was despite the fact that Collins in Dublin and Semmelweiss in Vienna had shown that puerperal fever could be transferred by midwives and obstetricians and controlled by cleaning the hands with bleach between examinations of patients. Conditions that often killed patients after surgery were septicaemia, gas-gangrene, and tetanus. It is recorded that Lister who was professor of surgery at Glasgow, lost 43 per cent of his patients before he used phenol. He became acquainted with Pasteur's work and came to the conclusion that gas-gangrene was a fermentation caused by airborne microbes gaining access to wounds. Pasteur had shown that to eliminate the effects of these microbes everything must be sterilised. At first Lister applied phenol directly to tissues, but this caused necrosis so he changed to spraying weak solutions around the area of the operation. He realised the importance of sterilising everything in contact with the wound and used phenol to sterilise bedding, clothing, instruments, and dressings. The system he developed became known as the Listerian system of antiseptic surgery. His efforts were at first ridiculed by other surgeons but when mortality following operations dropped considerably they began to apply his principles to their own work. Some years later antiseptic surgery gave way to aseptic techniques in which all equipment that can be subjected to heat safely is sterilised by wet heat in an autoclave or dry heat in an oven, and only the skin of the patient, surgeons and nurses is sterilised by chemical means.

Specific Remedies—Chemotherapy

Paul Ehrlich (1854–1915)

Though great advances were made in the new science of bacteriology, it was found that some infections could not be attacked by the methods that had proved so successful with diphtheria and many other diseases. For example, satisfactory antisera against protozoa, such as malaria, and some bacteria, e.g. tuberculosis and syphilis, could not be produced. Other methods of treating these diseases were sought. Ehrlich was the first to make progress, largely because he had developed a theory known as the side-chain theory to explain the specific antigen-antibody reaction. The crux of the theory was that toxins produce their poisonous effects by combining with the complex components of particular cells of the body which are then unable to function in the normal manner. Antibodies, when present, unite with the toxin and prevent its binding with the cell component, i.e. it is no longer toxic to the body. Ehrlich recognised that antibodies were perfect specific remedies, in that they are harmless to the host but antagonistic to the bacteria or toxins that induced their formation. Ehrlich likened them to magic bullets drawn by an irresistible urge to strike their particular objective and to harm no other. He was determined to find synthetic chemical substances which, like antibodies, would destroy organisms and yet be comparatively non-toxic to the host. He experimented with dyes because they had already been successfully used to stain bacteria, which suggested affinity for bacterial protoplasm. Ehrlich modified the chemical structure of the dyes in an attempt to modify the affinity of the dye to favour fixation by the bacteria but not by the host. He obtained slight success with this work in that trypan red could be used to kill the trypanosomes responsible for sleeping sickness. Ehrlich next turned his attention to arsenical compounds and found that Atoxyl would kill the trypanosomes of sleeping sickness, but in vivo, remission of the disease occurred only rarely and the patient went blind. In an effort to find an effective and safe arsenical a large number of organic compounds were prepared and tested. In 1909 Bertheim prepared compound number 606 in the series and when tests proved to be satisfactory it was called Salvarsan. Syphilis had been found to be bacterial in origin and though there was no close relationship between this organism and trypanosomes Ehrlich decided to try the effect of Salvarsan on the disease. It proved to be successful, but because the drug was strongly alkaline when dissolved in water a very dilute solution had to be injected. Later a less alkaline derivative came into general use and was named Neosalvarsan (official name neoarsphenamine). Some 6000 organic arsenical compounds have been synthesised in attempts to find a 'magic bullet' but only a few have been useful in medicine; e.g. neoarsphenamine, sulpharsphenamine, tryparsamide, carbarsone, and acetarsol. Ehrlich's work led to intensive efforts to find chemotherapeutic agents for other diseases. For example—

Organic derivatives of antimony, e.g. stibophen, used for kala-azar caused by a trypanosome.

Dyestuffs and their derivatives

The pararosaniline group—the native dye was gentian violet but pure samples of crystal violet, brilliant green and other derivatives have been used to prevent the development of pyogenic cocci in wounds and in burns, and for treating fungus diseases such as tinea pedis.

The acridine group—these are dyes with a large cation which act at low concentrations against a large variety of organisms; they were used mainly in the treatment of wounds and burns to prevent the growth of pyogenic cocci and the clostridia responsible for gas gangrene.

Derivatives of quinoline—these are used to treat amoebic dysentery. Clioquinol or 'Vioform', active against amoebae, is also recommended as a prophylactic against sundry stomach upsets often encountered in countries in which the standards of hygiene are not as high as in the United Kingdom.

The sulphonamides—these are the most important derivatives of a dyestuff to be used in chemotherapy. Domagk in 1935 reported that the diazo dye Prontosil Rubrum was capable of destroying haemolytic streptococci in mice. It was later shown that this activity was due to part of the molecule— the sulphanilamide moiety. There were some side effects, but the chief disadvantage was the frequency of dosage, which was every four hours. A number of drug companies started research to find more effective and more satisfactory 'sulphonamides' by substituting various chemical groups for one of the hydrogen atoms in the amide grouping of the parent drug. Over 5000 of these compounds are reputed to have been made, one of the most famous being sulphapyridine or M & B 693. It was found that the drugs were effective against staphylococci and a number of other pathogenic bacteria and were well tolerated by humans and mammals. Prolonged dosage, however, did not continue to produce improvement in the condition of the patient and it was realised that organisms not killed in the early part of a treatment could become resistant to the drug. Woods, Fildes, and others found that the action of sulphanilamide could be prevented by yeast extract; the antagonistic substance proved to be para-aminobenzoic acid, an essential metabolite for the susceptible organisms but not required by organisms insensitive to the drug.

Antimalarial drugs. Some chemotherapeutic agents are the active principles of drugs that have arisen from folk medicine. When the mode of action of these principles is fully or partly understood, synthetic analogues can be prepared to find more potent or less toxic substitutes. The best example of this type of development is quinine, which is used for the treatment of malaria because of the use of cinchona bark by the natives of South America. During the 1939–45 war there was a shortage of quinine in the United Kingdom and so it was necessary to find drugs to replace it as a prophylactic measure for soldiers in malarial areas. The German drug Atebrin was copied, under the name of mepacrine, and was reasonably successful. Nowadays, quinine is not commonly used because it is fairly toxic when administered over a long period and there are several substitutes in use.

Discovery and Development of Antibiotics

Antibiosis is a term used to describe a mechanism in nature whereby one organism produces a chemical substance (an antibiotic) which inhibits the ability of other organisms to compete with it in a given environment. However, the term antibiotic is usually used in the specialised sense of: 'a substance produced by an organism (usually a microbe), or a similar substance produced by other means, used for the treatment of disease in man, animals or plants.'

There have been two major pathways for the development of antibiotics since their existence was first reported by Pasteur and his co-workers in 1877. One arose from the discovery by Emmerich and Loew, in 1889, that *Pseudomonas aeruginosa* produces a substance that inhibits the growth of a number of organisms; because this organism is also known as *Ps. pyocyanea* the chemical was named pyocyanase, and it subsequently proved to be an enzyme. Later it was found that in some circumstances a fungus of the genus *Aspergillus* produces a substance that inhibits the growth of the anthrax bacillus. As these organisms are indigenous to soil it was considered that a substance antagonistic to a particular species of organism might be obtained by adding the organism to growing cultures of soil organisms, one or more of which might produce an inhibitory substance. The most outstanding research in this field was carried out in America by Dubos who, in 1939, isolated gramicidin which was active against Gram-positive organisms but on chemical analysis proved to be a mixture of two polypeptides, tyrocidin and tyrothricin, which produced lysis of red blood cells if administered by injection. This antibiotic was very useful topically for the prevention of sepsis in wounds and was used by the German army during the 1939–45 war. Subsequently, soil samples were taken from many habitats and tested for antibiotic substances; potentially useful organisms were identified, and the antibiotic was isolated, purified and characterised. It was then tested against microbes and, if successful, toxicity tests were carried out. Few chemicals suitable for clinical use came from this activity but it has been the chief source of new antibiotics.

The second route arose from a chance discovery by Fleming that a fungus produced a substance that inhibited the growth of streptococci. This property had been reported in 1897 by Duchesne, but no practical use was made of it. In 1928 Fleming was investigating the effect of lysozyme from amniotic fluid; lysozyme is also found in tears and other body fluids and is a natural antibiotic, secreted by mammals, that inhibits the growth of Gram-positive organisms by breaking down the structure of their cell walls. Consequently Fleming was looking for lysis of cells. One of his plates became contaminated with a fungus, and on incubation none of the streptococci in the region immediately around the fungal colony had grown. The mould, which was greenish in colour and produced a characteristic colony, was found to be *Penicillium notatum*. Liquid cultures were then prepared, filtered to remove the mycelium and the filtrate was tested against the streptococci and found to produce inhibition of growth. It also inhibited other Gram-positive organisms notably those causing pneumonia. Fleming called the active substance in the filtrate, penicillin. Unfortunately it was very unstable and none of the extraction methods available at the time would produce the pure substance. One problem was that the filtrate contained protein that produced anaphylactic reactions if the material was injected into man. The Second World War stimulated interest in penicillin and a team of scientists, including Florey, Chain, Abraham, and Heatley, were brought together at Oxford to find a solution to the extraction problem. Concurrently, experiments were being carried out to find a way to dry blood plasma and freeze-drying (*see* p. 279) was found to be the answer. This method was also successful for obtaining dry concentrates of purified penicillin. When manufacture started the method of growing the cultures was in long rows of milk bottles; yields were low, and the space involved was very large. Because in war-time Britain resources were inadequate the work was continued in America, and eventually a deep culture technique was developed. The organism most suited to this mode of growth was *Penicillium chrysogenum*. Genetic variation of the culture was shown to be possible, and chemical and ultra-violet methods were tried as mutagenic agents; mutants were selected on the basis of their yields of benzylpenicillin. Rapid progress was made and penicillin was released for use in general practice in 1946. This substance, more than any other, has gone much of the way towards fulfilling Ehrlich's dream of a magic bullet, for the following reasons—

(*a*) Its toxicity to humans is very low.

(*b*) There is no destruction of red or white blood cells.

(*c*) Its action is not unduly impaired by the presence of blood or pus.

(*d*) It is active against Gram-positive organisms at concentrations that can be achieved readily in blood.

(*e*) Water or normal saline can be used as solvent.

(*f*) The dry material is stable provided care is taken to exclude water and to keep the temperature at a low level, though refrigeration is not necessary.

Against these must be set the disadvantages, namely—

(*a*) The range of organisms against which it is effective is limited.

(*b*) Because it is not active in the presence of acid, oral administration presents problems.

(*c*) Excretion of the drug is rapid, and therefore the dose must be repeated frequently.

(*d*) Because some organisms can produce penicillinase which destroys the drug, aseptic processing is necessary.

Further research into the production of penicillin led to the discovery that under suitable conditions a culture could be induced to synthesise 6-aminopenicillanic acid, the basic structural unit of penicillin. This was of great importance because it was desirable to produce penicillins that would resist decomposition in acid conditions and hydrolysis by the enzyme penicillinase. It became possible to add various groups to the amide part of the basic molecule and thus to vary the properties of the compound. The results of this type of development have been fairly satisfactory; oral preparations of penicillin have almost completely replaced injectable preparations; there are penicillins available for the treatment of diseases resistant to benzylpenicillin; and at least one of the modern penicillins has a broad spectrum of activity.

The development of other antibiotics proceeded alongside the development of penicillin. The introduction, in 1943, of streptomycin for the treatment of tuberculosis, produced a considerable change in the prognosis of this disease. Chloramphenicol was introduced in 1947; this antibiotic was active against a new range of organisms, particularly the typhoid organisms, and had some value in the treatment of whooping cough. Unfortunately, prolonged administration of this drug gave rise to irreversible changes in white blood cells and it is reserved for treating typhoid and for cases where other antibiotics have failed. Subsequent antibiotic introductions were, aureomycin (1948), oxytetracycline (1950), and tetracycline (1952). These are wide spectrum antibiotics, active against a very wide range of bacteria, plus some rickettsia and a few viruses, though the usefulness against the latter is very limited. Most antibiotics are more toxic than penicillin and, after prolonged administration, there is a danger of micro-organisms becoming resistant to their action. The continuing search for new antibiotics aims to provide alternatives for use against strains resistant to older types and to produce substances with activity against viruses and cancer.

The problem of resistance to antibiotics has resulted in great advances in the study of bacterial genetics. Recent findings have shown that some of the colon bacteria have a recognisable chromosome, and that characteristics can be transferred by soluble factors. One of the most depressing aspects of this is that one of these soluble factors carries the ability to resist the action of a number of antibiotics (multiple antibiotic resistance factor). In the laboratory this factor has been transferred to non-resistant strains from resistant strains of the same organism and also from one resistant species to a non-resistant species in the same culture or in the same environment.

BIBLIOGRAPHY

BROCK, T. D. (Ed.) (1961) *Milestones in Microbiology*. Prentice Hall: London.

BURNET, F. M. (1962) *The Natural History of Infectious Disease*. University Press: Cambridge.

GRAINGER, T. H. (1958) *A Guide to the History of Bacteriology*. Ronald Press: New York.

LUDOVICI, L. J. (1952) *Alexander Fleming, the Discoverer of Penicillin*. Dakers: London.

MAUROIS, A. (1959) *The Life of Alexander Fleming*. Wiedenfeld and Nicholson: London.

PHARMACEUTICAL SOCIETY (1962) *Antibiotics*. Pharmaceutical Press: London.

PARISH, H. J. (1965) *History of Immunisation*. Livingstone: Edinburgh.

PARISH, H. J. (1968) *Victory with Vaccines*. Livingstone: Edinburgh.

POSTGATE, J. (1969) *Microbes and Man*. Penguin Books: London.

VALLERY-RADOT, R. (1948) *The Life of Pasteur*. Constable: London.

REFERENCE

WOODS, D. D. (1962) The biochemical mode of action of the sulphonamides. *J. gen. Microbiol.*, **29**, 687–702.

27

Fundamentals of Microbiology

A. Bacteria

BACTERIA occur very widely in nature and in very large numbers. They are found in animals, plants, soil, water and the atmosphere. The majority do not produce disease but serve as useful scavengers in the breakdown of organic matter and its re-synthesis into living organisms; they are essential in the cycle of life. The power to invade tissues and produce disease in higher animals and plants is regarded by most bacteriologists as a form of aberration because it is self-defeating; i.e. the host is destroyed by the invasion.

PATHOGENICITY

The phenomenon of invasion and destruction of tissues is known as pathogenicity. This includes the whole sequence of events by which invading organisms enter the host, establish growth within its tissues, and eventually give rise to symptoms that are recognised as disease. Most bacteria do not have powerful means of movement and so the mode of invasion is often complicated (*see* p. 375).

Morphology

THE INDIVIDUAL CELL (Fig. 27.1)

Slime Layer

This is the outer layer of a bacterium. Often it is rather ill-defined but when it has a distinct edge it is known as a *capsule*. It may be demonstrated by direct staining but generally it is more effectively displayed by staining the organism and then covering the slide with a film of a dark particulate dye (e.g. Indian ink) that is too thin to cover the cells, when the capsule is seen as a clear space between the bacterium and the surrounding film. Chemically it consists of polysaccharide (usually) or polypeptide. It is of significance in immunity and in the manufacture of dextran, but its physiological function seems to be protection of the organism against changes of environment, though it may also be an excretory product.

Cell Wall

In most bacteria the cell wall is a rigid structure that renders the cell capable of survival even when there are great differences of osmotic pressure between cell and environment. In some species of soil bacteria and in the mycoplasmas the cell wall is flexible; in others it is very rigid and consists of chitin-like material; but in the majority of bacteria

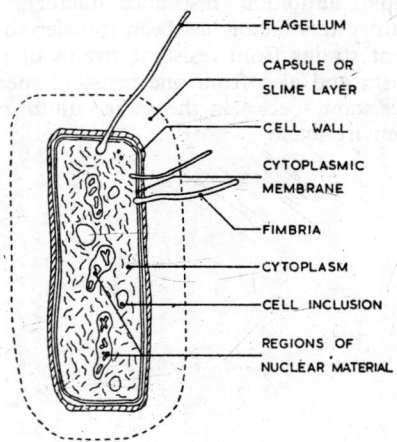

FLAGELLUM

CAPSULE OR
SLIME LAYER

CELL WALL

CYTOPLASMIC
MEMBRANE

FIMBRIA

CYTOPLASM

CELL INCLUSION

REGIONS OF
NUCLEAR MATERIAL

Fig. 27.1   A typical bacterial cell

of interest in pharmacy the cell wall consists of protein and polypeptide with mucin, polysaccharide, or phospholipid components. Polypeptide and muramic acid form a matrix while the other components are in semi-liquid or liquid form filling the interstices. An uncommon amino-acid, di-aminopimelic acid, is also present. The protein-like matrix is more highly developed in Gram-positive organisms (q.v.). Lysozyme destroys the chemical structure of the cell wall and causes the contents to leak away and the organism to die unless the medium in which the cell is suspended has an osmotic pressure that prevents rupture of the underlying membrane.

Flagella and Fimbria

These are outgrowths of the protoplasm protruding through the cell wall. *Flagella* are whip-like processes about 0·01 μm in diameter and of varying length. To make them visible under the light microscope they are treated to cause swelling and then stained. They are uncommon in spherical bacteria but occur on about 50 per cent of rods. They are responsible for movement in most types of motile bacteria and are useful in identification (Fig. 27.2) and important in immunology.

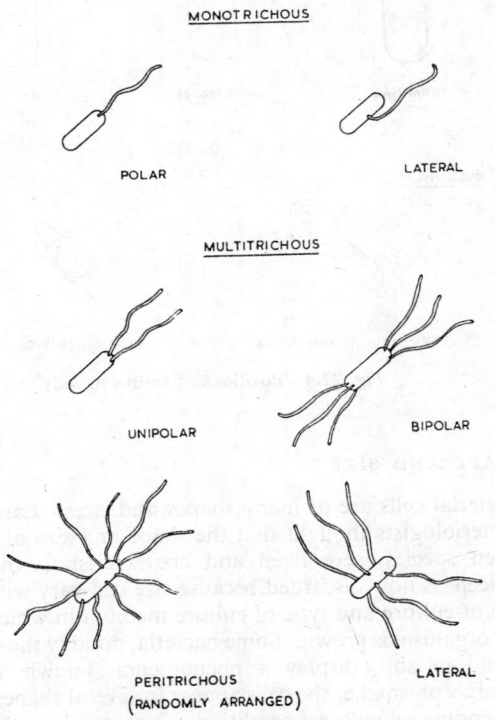

Fig. 27.2 The arrangement of flagella

Fimbria form a fringe of short hair-like processes and are very similar to flagella but usually shorter and stiffer. One of their functions is attachment but in some organisms they are involved in the transfer of genetic material from the donor (male) cell to the recipient (female) cell.

Cytoplasmic Membrane

The existence of a limiting membrane within the cell wall has been demonstrated by special staining techniques and confirmed by electron microscopy. Mitchell and Moyle (1956) describe it as a closely packed lipoprotein sheet, two to four molecules thick, having a low affinity for water but with a limited number of water-filled pores passing through it. It is the semi-permeable membrane of the cell and the site of considerable physiological activity (Mitchell, 1958).

Cytoplasmic Constituents

There are a number of recognisable inclusions within the cytoplasm.

Nuclear Material. The bacterial cell does not have a defined nucleus bounded by a nuclear membrane, as in plant and animal cells, but it does contain genetic material. A circular chromosome has been postulated for *Salmonellae* and possibly other *Enterobacteriaceae*.

Endospores. Under conditions unfavourable to continued growth of the cell, certain bacteria can produce a resting body (spore) within the cell wall. Spores are 1 to 3 μm in diameter, ovoid in shape and may be found free or enclosed in the remnants of the bacterium (mother cell). Under a light microscope they are seen as highly refractile bodies; they are resistant to a wide range of chemical and physical agents. The outer coat is water repellant and the whole structure contains much less water than the vegetative bacterium from which it was formed. In the *Bacilli*, in which the genetic material is rod-like, spores are formed by this rod breaking into four equal segments, three of which disintegrate; the fourth remains and the spore body is built up around it. This means that there are two origins for spores, terminal or sub-terminal; the term 'equatorial', found in the literature, refers to a sub-terminal spore that has become centralised during the later stages of its development (Fig. 27.3). Spores may cause the mother cell to bulge. Central, bulging spores with small tapered parts of the vegetative cell at each end have the appearance of a boat (navicular), while cells with a terminal, bulging spore look like a drumstick (Fig. 27.4).

Ribosomes. By gravity gradient centrifugation and other techniques, structures known as ribosomes can be obtained from disintegrated bacteria. These are sites of protein synthesis.

Mitochondria. Bacteria do not contain structures recognisable as mitochondria but parts of the cytoplasmic membrane fulfil the same functions.

Vacuoles. Under special cultural conditions, clear areas may appear in the cytoplasm of bacterial cells. These are thought to be analogous to the

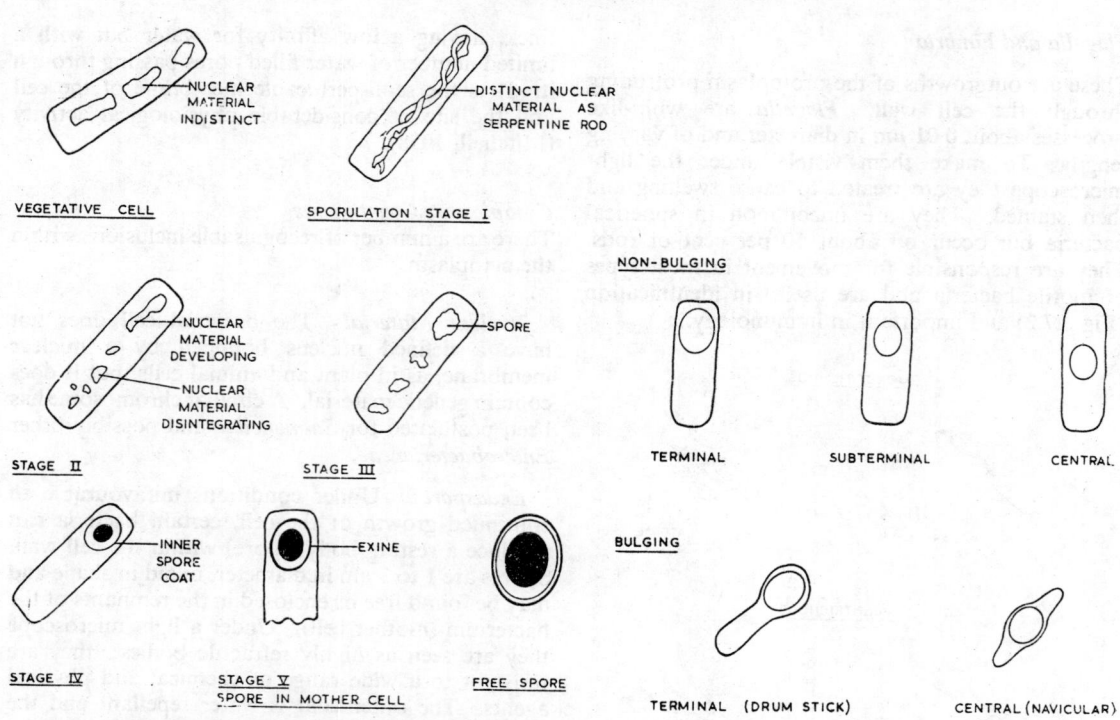

Fig. 27.3 The mode of formation of a bacterial spore

Fig. 27.4 Positions of spores in cells

vacuoles of other cells and are given the same name. Their presence in cells grown on glucose agar is used to differentiate species of the genus *Bacillus*.

Oil and Wax Droplets or Crystals. In certain media, e.g. one containing glycerol, some bacteria synthesise excess fatty material which appears as globules within the cell; this material is important because it influences the partition of certain chemicals between the cell and the aqueous environment, and thus its susceptibility to chemicals. Waxes have a similar influence and may make the cells less permeable to aqueous solutions.

Other Crystalline Material. Occasionally other material is present as crystals. The classical example is the large crystal of protein material accompanying the spore of *Bacillus thuringiensis*, which consists of crystalline enzymes. It is diagnostic for this organism, and the nature of the protein differs between strains, a feature that is useful in tracing the spread of disease due to this species in insect colonies. The protein is toxic to the larvae of certain species and might be useful in developing a highly specific insecticide.

SHAPE AND SIZE

Bacterial cells are of many shapes and sizes. Early bacteriologists thought that the shape and size of a given species were fixed and characteristic; this concept is now discarded because size can vary with age of culture and type of culture medium in which the organism is grown. Some bacteria, notably those found in soil, display a phenomenon known as pleomorphism, i.e. the cells appear in several shapes, depending on cultural conditions. Nevertheless, the shapes of bacterial cells are classified as follows—

Cocci. Spherical bodies with a smooth outline and diameters in the range 0.75 to 3.0 μm.

Rods (bacilli). Approximately cylindrical in shape and varying greatly in length and diameter (length 0.75 to 10 μm; diameter 0.75 to 3 μm). The ratio of length to diameter is often diagnostic. Some rods are almost ovoid (cocco-bacilli), others are comma shaped (vibrios) or in the form of partial spirals (spirillae).

Spirochaetes. When an organism has a number of turns (a true spiral) and is flexuous, it is known as a spirochaete.

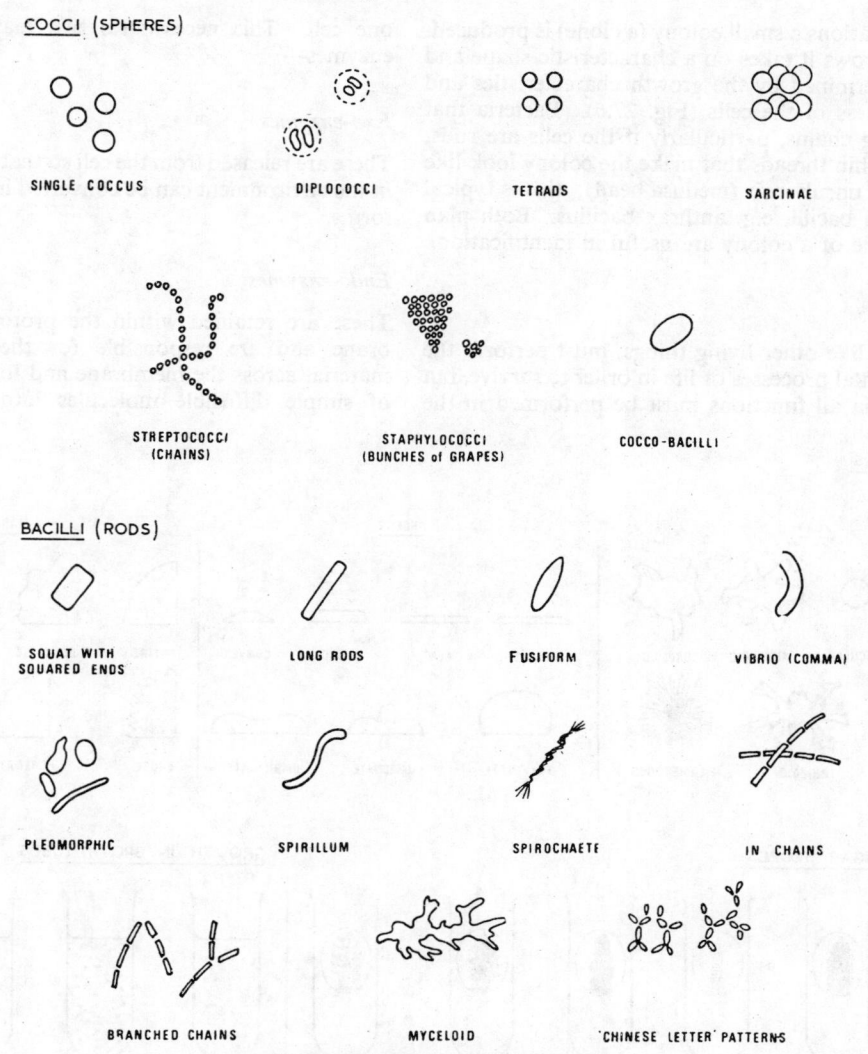

Fig. 27.5 Bacterial shapes and arrangements

Branching rods. Some bacteria form true branches and remain adherent in chains, giving a formation that resembles fungal mycelia; hence they are sometimes known as ray fungi. Examples are the genera *Actinomyces* and *Streptomyces*.

Amoeboid. The pleuropneumonia-like organisms (**PPLO** or **Mycoplasmas**) are very small, non-motile, amoeba-like cells with no defined shape and no cell wall but with a cell membrane corresponding to the cytoplasmic membrane of other bacteria.

CELL AGGREGATION

Many bacteria are aggregated to varying degrees. The form of aggregation is controlled to some extent by the method of cell division. If successive divisions take place in the same plane and the cells do not separate, a chain of cells develops. The chain length depends on the adhesiveness of the cells and the rate of division, but mechanical factors, such as shaking, also have an effect in artificial cultures. If two generations of a single bacterium first divide in one plane and then in another at right angles to the first, tetrads are formed; a further division, again at right angles, produces cubical packets of eight cells (Sarcina). Uneven division results in random groups, e.g. staphylococci (Fig. 27.5).

COLONY FORMATION

Bacteria grown on the surface of a solid medium divide according to their normal habit and after a few generations a small colony (a clone) is produced. As this grows it takes on a characteristic shape and form determined by the growth characteristics and adhesiveness of the cells (Fig. 27.6). Bacteria that form long chains, particularly if the cells are rods, produce thin threads that make the colony look like a head of unruly hair (medusa head); this is typical of certain bacilli, e.g. anthrax bacillus. Both plan and profile of a colony are useful in identification.

Physiology

Bacteria, like other living things, must perform the fundamental processes of life in order to survive, but in bacteria all functions must be performed in the one cell. This necessitates two major groups of enzymes—

Exo-enzymes

These are released from the cell so that food materials in the environment can be converted into assimilable forms.

Endo-enzymes

These are retained within the protoplasmic membrane and are responsible for the transport of material across the membrane and for the synthesis of simple diffusible molecules into the complex

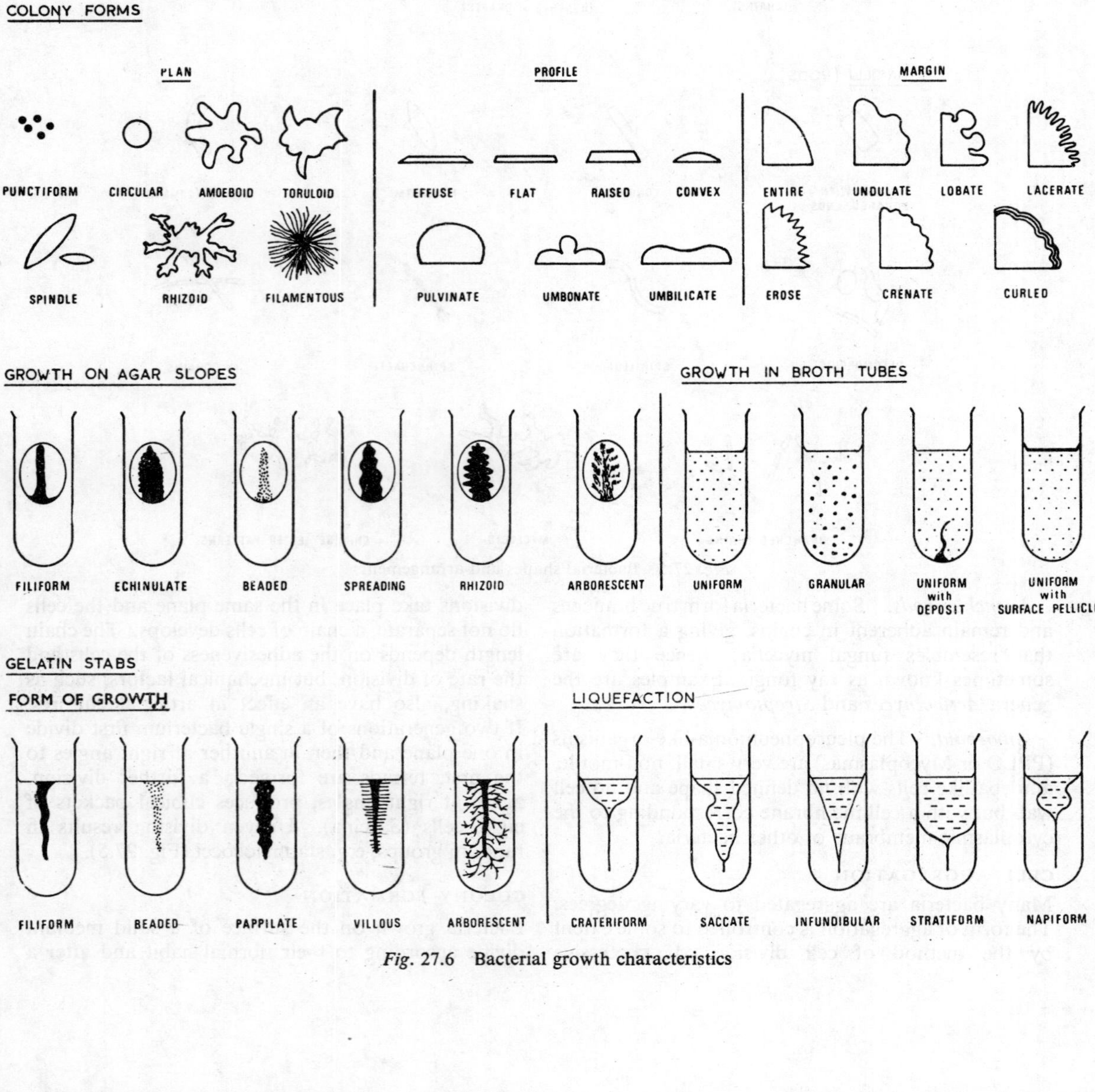

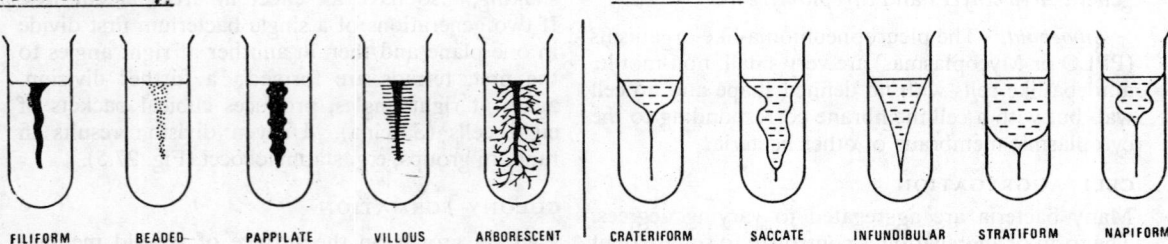

Fig. 27.6　Bacterial growth characteristics

molecular components of the cell. Some are involved in the production of energy for other synthetic activities.

NUTRITIONAL REQUIREMENTS

For survival, bacteria require the following elements: carbon, nitrogen, oxygen, phosphorus and sulphur, in fairly large amounts; iron, calcium, magnesium, potassium and sodium, in smaller quantities; and manganese, zinc, copper, silica, bromine and iodine in trace quantities, depending on species. One system of classifying bacteria is to group them according to the way they use certain elements and to their sources of energy.

1. *Autotrophic bacteria*. These are bacteria that can synthesise carbohydrates and obtain energy from simple inorganic sources of carbon such as carbon dioxide or carbonates. Many can do this without the use of light. (Those that require light are called photosynthetic bacteria and have pigments allied to chlorophyll, either in plastids or in solution in the cytoplasm.) Most cannot elaborate complex nitrogenous compounds from inorganic sources but a few can utilise nitrates and ammonia as sole sources of nitrogen. To carry out these complex syntheses such organisms possess a very complete set of enzymes. Autotrophs are of interest in pharmacy because they cause deterioration of products and packaging materials.

2. *Heterotrophic bacteria*. This group comprises the so-called higher bacteria. They are unable to grow without elaborated sources of carbon and many require complex sources of nitrogen. Sugars are the usual carbon sources, but amino-acids can be utilised by some organisms for energy production. Requirements vary between species; for instance, *Salmonella typhi* needs the amino-acid tryptophan. Heterotrophs are often subdivided into two classes—

(*a*) *Parasites*. In nature these require the environment of living cells. A number can be grown under artificial conditions, using highly specialised media; one that cannot be grown in this way is *Mycobacterium leprae*.

(*b*) *Saprophytes*. These are organisms that can grow on organic matter from dead plants or animals. They are the scavengers of the bacterial world and, because they are responsible for the decay of dead material, are of supreme importance in nature. Normally, they are not pathogenic, but some, if they gain access to diseased or damaged tissues, may produce harmful toxins. In some circumstances, they are capable of invading the body giving rise to diseases that are difficult to treat.

Growth and Multiplication

Usually the term growth is applied to increase in size but for bacteria it is commonly used to describe increase in numbers. Bacteria of one species are not all the same size and this causes difficulties when optical properties are used to estimate numbers of cells in a culture. Cells grow until they reach a limiting size at which point they divide into two cells and the cycle is repeated. If an optical density measurement is being made, the light cut off is proportional to the total quantity of protoplasm; thus, if there is a marked difference in size or density of the cells, optical density ceases to be an accurate indication of the number of organisms. When cell division in a culture is not synchronous (as is often the case) this effect is less important provided calibration and readings are based on the same period of incubation. Bacterial growth curves are discussed by Gunn and Carter (1965) and a kinetic approach to growth and death of bacterial cultures is presented by Dean and Hinshelwood (1961).

Heat Relationships

Bacteria may be classified by their heat characteristics which are of two kinds—

GROWTH CHARACTERISTICS

Psychrotrophs

Usually, organisms that will grow below 25°C are known as psychrotrophs although the term psychrophils is often found in the literature. Psychrotrophs is preferable because, although these bacteria will grow at low temperatures, their optimum is above 25°C. Because they can grow slightly at 0 to 4°C they may cause spoilage of blood and unsterilised pharmaceutical preparations in refrigerators.

Mesophils

These like a temperature range of 25 to 45°C which includes the body temperatures of most animals. Most organisms pathogenic to man and animals are found in this group.

Thermophils

Bacteria in this group will not grow well below 45°C and their optimum temperatures lie between 55 and 65°C. In tropical climates they cause spoilage in sealed containers of food. Dried milk products often contain thermophils that can be troublesome if these products are used in formulations.

TOLERANCE CHARACTERISTICS

Organisms that are very resistant to heat treatments are said to be thermoduric. This resistance is of two types: firstly, many soil organisms form spores that, because of their low water content, resist heat treatments, even surviving 121°C for 20 minutes or more in an autoclave, and up to three hours at 160°C in a hot air oven; secondly, some vegetative bacteria can survive abnormally long periods at above 60°C. Some bacteria associated with meat products fall into the latter category; hence, in cookery, meat preparations, such as stocks, should be given adequate heat treatment. The majority of pathogens in vegetative form will not survive 55°C for more than about 15 minutes. Heating a suspension of spore-forming bacteria at 80°C for 10 minutes is used to ensure that the suspension consists entirely of spores.

Oxygen Requirements

Bacteria can be classified according to their oxygen requirements—

AEROBES

These must have atmospheric oxygen in order to grow.

ANAEROBES

These do not employ molecular oxygen as a hydrogen acceptor. If the organism is an obligate anaerobe oxygen produces death in a few minutes and such organisms survive only if they can form spores. Various devices are used to cultivate anaerobes—

Anaerobe Jar

The merit of this method is that it can be used for incubating liquid and solid media. Cultures are put into the jar (Fig. 27.7) and the lid is placed on top and screwed down tightly. The lid has two taps: one is connected to a good vacuum system by which means as much air as possible is removed, then the tap is closed; next the other tap is connected to a hydrogen cylinder and the jar filled with the gas; finally both taps are closed and the jar is placed in the incubator. The hydrogen in the jar combines with residual oxygen under the influence of a catalyst attached to the lid. A side tube containing an appropriate indicator is used to show that the jar is suitable for anaerobic culture. In a modified version a sachet is placed in the jar; when broken this generates gas which drives out residual oxygen.

Sodium Pyrogallate Tube

There are several variations of this, of which some are shown in Fig. 27.8.

Solid Anaerobic Media

Use of an anaerobe jar is not entirely satisfactory because of oxygen dissolved in the culture media. To overcome this, reducing substances are added to both liquid and solid media. Suitable non-toxic chemicals are glucose and other reducing sugars, SH-containing amino-acids such as cystine, and simple reducing agents, e.g. sodium thioglycollate. The most common solid anaerobic medium is

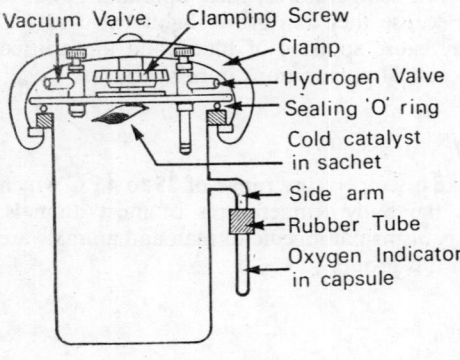

Modified McIntosh and Fildes jar

Vacuum Valve.
Clamping Screw
Clamp
Hydrogen Valve
Sealing 'O' ring
Cold catalyst in sachet
Side arm
Rubber Tube
Oxygen Indicator in capsule

a

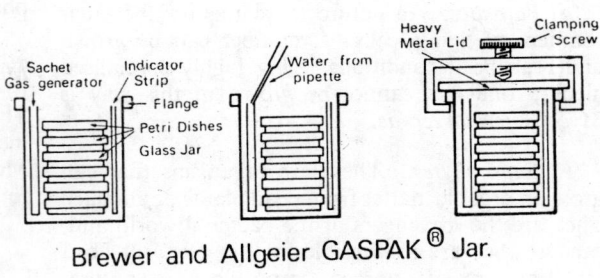

Sachet
Gas generator
Indicator Strip
Flange
Petri Dishes
Glass Jar
Water from pipette
Heavy Metal Lid
Clamping Screw

Brewer and Allgeier GASPAK® Jar.

b

Fig. 27.7   (*a*) Anaerobic culture jar, (*b*) Anaerobic culture jar (*Courtesy Becton, Dickinson Ltd*)

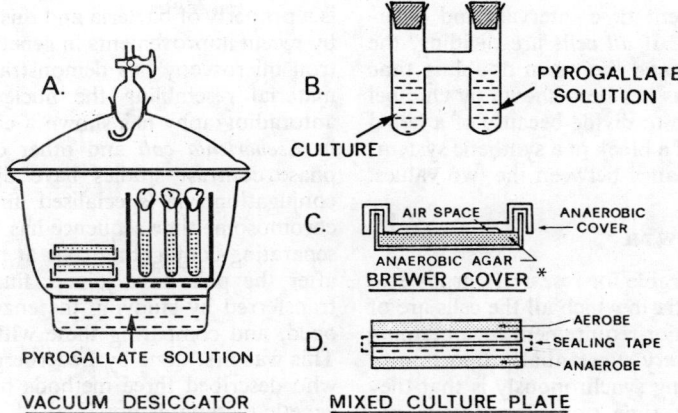

A. VACUUM DESICCATOR   PYROGALLATE SOLUTION

B. PYROGALLATE SOLUTION   CULTURE

C. AIR SPACE   ANAEROBIC COVER   ANAEROBIC AGAR   BREWER COVER *

D. AEROBE   SEALING TAPE   ANAEROBE   MIXED CULTURE PLATE

Fig. 27.8   Pyrogallate and other anaerobic techniques

*(Courtesy Becton, Dickinson Ltd)

Reinforced Clostridial Medium (Difco Laboratories, 1953, and Oxoid Laboratories, 1965).

Liquid Anaerobic Media

Liquid media are more useful, particularly if it is necessary to detect the presence of small numbers of organisms, as in sterility or disinfectant testing. For these purposes aerobic culture media have been modified by adding reducing substances of the types already mentioned. Such media are stored in screw-capped bottles which should be nearly full to reduce the air space. Some are designed to test for aerobes and anaerobes but are unsatisfactory for exacting species at either end of the scale. A full account of anaerobic media is given by Gunn and Carter (1965) but short descriptions of two of the most important will be given here—

Robertson's Cooked Meat Medium is a nutrient broth with not less than 1 cm depth of diced lean heart meat in the bottom. It should be used fresh or recently heated to 100°C to expel oxygen and allowed to cool with the top tightly closed.

Thioglycollate Medium. There are several media of this type. As well as reducing agents they usually contain agar to reduce the rate of diffusion of oxygen into the medium. An oxygen-reduction indicator is often included and this should not be coloured to more than one third of the depth of the medium.

Inoculation should be into the bottom of the tube and should be performed in such a way that the minimum of oxygen is introduced with the inoculum.

MICROAEROPHILS

These can grow satisfactorily at very low oxygen levels. However, growth is more prolific if a good supply of the gas is available. No growth takes place if oxygen is absent. In agar-containing thioglycollate media such organisms grow as slender, beaded streaks downwards from the coloured layer.

FACULTATIVES

These can grow well under aerobic and anaerobic conditions. There is usually an oxygen tension at which individual species will grow more readily, e.g. *Escherichia coli* is normally aerobic, while *Clostridium sporogenes* is normally anaerobic.

Reproduction

Bacteria belong to the Schizomycetes, i.e. organisms that multiply by binary fission. The protoplasm enlarges to a limiting size, the genetic material forms into two units, cross walls are laid down, and the cells separate. Some bacteria are capable of very rapid division, e.g. *Escherichia coli* divides about every twenty minutes under ideal conditions while *Mycobacterium tuberculosis* probably takes up to a day to make its first division after transfer to a synthetic medium, subsequently dividing every five hours or so. Once the culture has settled down to a steady state the interval between successive divisions remains substantially constant. This interval is known as the *mean generation time*. Another parameter of growth of more practical value is the *mean doubling time*. This can be found by making total counts at fairly frequent time intervals and determining a mean value. If *all* cells are dividing, the mean generation time and the mean doubling time will be the same but, as has been shown by Quesnel (1960) some cells cease to divide because of a lethal mutation or because of a block in a synthetic system; then there is a discrepancy between the two values.

SYNCHRONOUS GROWTH

It has been found desirable for research purposes to have cultures of bacteria in which all the cells are of the same age. The major requirement for obtaining a culture in which a very substantial proportion of the bacteria are dividing synchronously is that they should be held for a time under conditions unfavourable to growth; then, when the cells are removed to an ideal environment, they will grow and divide with reasonable synchrony for the first few

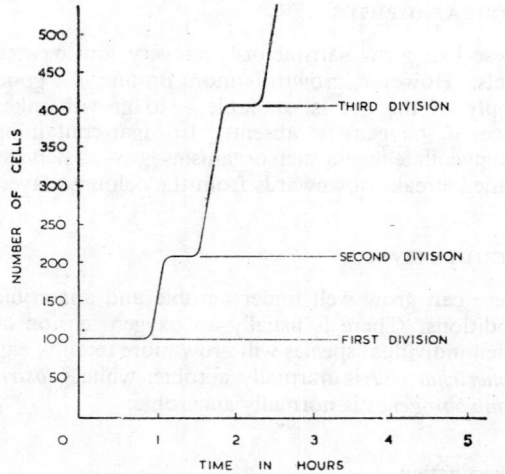

Fig. 27.9 Synchronous growth curve

generations. A popular way of doing this is to grow the culture until it is in the early logarithmic phase of growth, then to cool it fairly rapidly to below 10°C and hold it at that temperature for a few hours; on removal to an incubator at the optimal growth temperature for the organism, nearly all the cells will, after an interval, divide together for three or four generations (Fig. 27.9).

SEXUAL REPRODUCTION

Because bacteria are so small it has been difficult to decide if sexual reproduction takes place. Marked variation in characteristics and changes in genetic patterns have indicated for some time that sexuality

is a property of bacteria and this has been confirmed by recent improvements in genetic techniques. Electron microscopy has demonstrated the presence of material resembling the nucleus of higher cells, autoradiography has shown a circular chromosome in *Escherichia coli* and other colon bacteria, and phase contrast studies have disclosed a form of conjugation via specialised fimbrial threads. A chromosome time sequence has been worked out by separating conjugating cells at predetermined times after the pair have joined, finding the characters transferred by studying the enzyme patterns developed, and comparing these with the original cells. This was first done by Lederberg and Tatum (1946) who described three methods by which transfer of genetic material is possible—

Recombination (*Conjugation*), which occurs in the manner described above.

Transformation, which takes place by the transference of water-soluble genetic material (fragments of DNA) via an aqueous medium. These fragments may come from the breakdown of the main genetic material as a result of invasion by bacteriophages (bacterial viruses). In colon bacteria, virulence, multiple antibiotic resistance and ability to ferment certain substrates can be inherited by this mechanism.

Transduction, which is a result of small portions of DNA being introduced into the nuclear material as a result of invasion by temperate phages (q.v.). One, or at most two, characters can be transferred in this way and the statistical probability of occurrence is related to the number of phage particles per unit volume of culture.

For further information on the transfer of genetic material in bacteria see Symposium of the Society for General Microbiology (1965).

Variation

There are two distinct types of bacterial variation—

1. INDUCED VARIATION

This type of variation is reflected in the synthetic ability of a cell and results from exposure to a new substrate or some other environmental factor. It may arise from one of two mechanisms. First, the new substrate or factor may select from within the population accidental mutants that can ferment that substrate or survive in the new environment. These will multiply and become the majority of cells within the culture. Secondly, there may be a 'controller' in the genetic make-up of the bacterium which, while the original substrate is available, suppresses the production of enzymes capable of using a second substrate. When the first substrate is absent or its concentration is below a certain level, suppression no longer occurs and the organism synthesises the enzymes necessary to utilise the second substrate. For example, when *Leuconostoc mesenteroides* is grown in a glucose medium and then transferred to one containing lactose only, growth is arrested, at least for a period. If, however, the cells are grown on lactose medium, on transfer to a glucose medium it is found that both glucose and lactose utilising systems are functional. This demonstrates that glucose suppresses the lactose utilising enzyme but lactose does not suppress the glucose enzyme.

2. MUTATION

This is a permanent change brought about by a complete change in the DNA of the genetic material of a bacterium. Such a change is inherited by progeny and will continue for many generations. It is caused by material being transferred in one or more of the modes described on page 306 or by the action of certain radiations (e.g. X or gamma rays) or chemicals (e.g. nitrogen mustard or colchicine) that induce genetic changes. Artificially induced mutation may be used by man to obtain mutants with desired characteristics such as ability to produce higher yields of antibiotics.

MANIFESTATIONS OF VARIATION

Physiological Changes

1. Virulence.
2. Antigenic properties of the cells.
3. Response to noxious stimuli such as heat, chemicals or bacteriophages.
4. Metabolic activities of the cell in respect of growth requirements, oxygen requirements, ability to ferment carbohydrates, toxin production or pigment production.

Changes in Cell Morphology

1. Size; giant forms and other variations.
2. Shape; L-forms (where cross walls are not laid down) and pleomorphism.
3. Ability to form spores.
4. Ability to form capsules or slime.
5. Reaction to specific stains.
6. Loss of motility; usually associated with loss of flagella and the flagella antigens (*see* opposite).

Colony Variations

The appearance of colonies on a given medium may show variation in respect of shape, size, colour, margin and surface appearance. The S—R and H—O transformations (*see* below) are particularly important examples of variations in which changes of colony features are found.

Phase Variation

The antigenic structure of a micro-organism varies according to the constituents of the medium in/on which the culture is grown, the time for, and temperature at which the culture is incubated, and the oxygen supply. The loss of activity of a culture as an antigen (*see* p. 308) occurs in a series of recognisable steps or phases—

Phase I is a fully virulent organism with a full complement of antigens.

Phases II and III are intermediate, with graded decreases of antigenic ability.

Phase IV is non-toxic, non-virulent and non-antigenic.

ANTIGENS

These are substances in the bacterial cell that induce the production of specific antibodies in the host when the bacteria invade. A single bacterium may carry several antigens (Fig. 27.10) which are often classified according to the position they occupy.

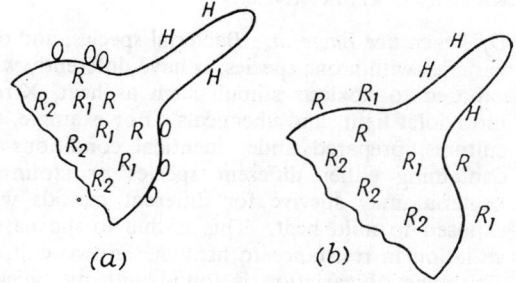

Fig. 27.10

H = flagella antigens
O = surface antigens
R, R₁, R₂ = deeply situated antigens

Flagellar (H) antigens are associated with the flagella. The letter H is derived from the German word Hauch (film) because the colony of the non-variant strain is spreading and film-like. Under unfavourable cultural conditions the flagella and, therefore, the H antigens are lost. The resulting variant is known as the O form, the O standing for *ohne Hauche* (without film), because the non-motile cells produce a compact colony.

Surface (S) antigens are associated with structures at the surface of the cell; e.g. the capsule or cell wall.

Somatic (O) antigens are associated with the body of the bacterium and may occur in several layers within the cell (*see* Fig. 27.10).

The S—R (smooth to rough) transformation is associated with loss of the surface antigen. A smooth, round, glistening colony becomes rough, dull and irregular. This change is sometimes accompanied by an H—O change and/or loss of one or more of the somatic antigens.

Variation and Official Immunological Products

S and H forms of disease-causing bacteria are more virulent than R and O forms. If variant forms, with their reduced complement of antigens, are used in the preparations of vaccines, antibody production in the body may be inadequate to cope with an invasion by the non-variant form.

Resistance

A further property of bacteria that is subject to variation is resistance to noxious stimuli.

NATURAL RESISTANCE

Of Vegetative Bacteria. Bacterial species, and even varieties within one species, behave differently when exposed to noxious stimuli such as heat, X-rays, ultraviolet light, and chemicals. For example, two cultures, prepared under identical conditions but containing either different species or strains of bacteria, may survive for different periods when exposed to mild heat. This is due to the natural variation in resistance to heat of the two cultures. This type of variation is found with all types of stimuli but the order of resistance of a given set of organisms to one stimulus (e.g. heat) will not be the same as that to another (e.g. phenol). Due allowance for this variation must be made in the heat sterilisation of pharmaceuticals; in deciding the concentration of a disinfectant appropriate to a given situation; in determining the dose of radiation required to destroy bacterial spores; and in judging the level of an antibiotic necessary to control an infection.

Of Resting Bacteria. Bacterial spores can survive greater exposures to unfavourable conditions than vegetative cells. Some show extremes of resistance; e.g. strains of *Bacillus anthracis* survive boiling water for three hours or exposure to 5 per cent phenol for one day. The order of resistance for the spores of different bacterial species varies in much the same way as for vegetative cells but the level of stimulus required to produce a given effect is higher for spores. The problems consequent on the presence of spores in pharmaceutical materials are much more difficult to solve than those for vegetative cells.

ACQUIRED RESISTANCE

An organism, originally sensitive to a noxious stimulus, may, if subjected to a level of stimulus below the effective level, develop tolerance or resistance. If the intensity or duration of the stimulus is gradually increased with successive serial cultures of the organism it is possible, in some cases, for that organism, after many subcultures, to become resistant to stimuli many times greater than the maximum it could tolerate at the beginning of the experiment. This technique is sometimes called training and a number of explanations have been put forward—

1. In the presence of the stimulus a specific enzyme system is inactivated but an alternative synthetic pathway, which allows the bacterium to grow, is activated. As the stimulus is increased, the action of the alternative pathway compensates for the inhibition and the bacterium is able to survive high levels of the inhibitor. In some cases a state is reached where growth of the cells is dependent on the presence of the stimulus. This has been shown with a strain of *Escherichia coli* that requires streptomycin in order to grow.

2. The stimulus acts as a selector, killing off all sensitive cells but allowing resistant forms to grow. This process of selection eventually produces a new population of cells resistant to the stimulus.

Where resistance results from the application of a stimulus it is termed acquired resistance. The resistance of trained cultures is often transitory and after a few generations in the normal medium, without the stimulus, the resistance of the culture returns to normal. When resistance is due to a genetic change it is more permanent and, therefore, more serious. An example is the resistance of streptococci to penicillin, which is due to acquisition of inherited ability to synthesise the penicillin-destroying enzyme, penicillinase.

B. Rickettsiae

This is a group of tiny micro-organisms that, because of their inability to grow outside living cells, were originally believed to be closely related to the viruses.

Better knowledge of their properties has shown much closer relationship to bacteria; for example—

1. they are retained by bacteria-proof filters;
2. they are visible under the light microscope;
3. they can be stained (e.g. they are Gram-negative);
4. they reproduce by binary fission;
5. they have a cell wall containing muramic acid, a constituent of the cell walls of bacteria;
6. they produce metabolic enzymes;
7. they contain both DNA and RNA;
8. they are sensitive to wide-spectrum antibiotics.

Separate grouping is justified by their growth requirements and the similarity of the diseases they produce. Their other important properties are—

(a) They are small rods or cocci about 300 μm in size but they exhibit pleomorphism, producing chains and longer rods.

(b) Most are destroyed easily by low heat, formaldehyde (p. 398) and phenols but they resist freeze-drying and treatment with ether (p. 399). Their growth is stimulated by the sulphonamides.

(c) In the laboratory they are grown most successfully in small rodents or in the yolk sac of the living chick embryo.

(d) They produce a soluble antigen that diffuses into the surrounding medium (p. 399).

(e) They are primarily parasites of arthropods (fleas, lice, mites, and ticks) from which the disease is transmitted to man. The arthropods frequently infect animals, such as rodents, which then serve as reservoirs of infection.

Some of the rickettsial diseases are given in Table 27.1, together with the names of the causative organisms and the normal vectors and reservoirs.

Table 27.1

Disease	Organism	Arthropod vector	Reservoir
Epidemic typhus	*Rickettsia prowazeki*	Louse	Man
Murine typhus	*R. typhus*	Flea	Rats
Scrub typhus	*R. tsutsugamushi*	Red mite	Wild rodents
Trench fever	*R. quintana*	Louse	Man
Rocky mountain spotted fever	*R. rickettsi*	Tick	Wild rodents

C. Viruses

Viruses are different from bacteria in the following respects—

1. They are much smaller.
2. They are obligate intracellular parasites.
3. They contain only one type of nucleic acid.
4. They do not reproduce by binary fission.
5. Most are insensitive to antibiotics.

Size

Animal viruses range in size from about 10 μm (foot and mouth virus) to about 250 μm (vaccinia virus). All but the very largest are invisible under the light microscope and will pass through conventional bacteria-proof filters.

Their sizes can be determined by the following methods—

(a) Thin membranes made from cellulose esters in a range of very fine and accurate porosities are available. An estimate of the size of a virus can be obtained from knowledge of the pore size of the membrane through which it will just pass.

(b) From calculations based on the rate at which the virus is deposited in an ultracentrifuge.

(c) The electron microscope can resolve particles as small as 1 μm and, therefore, can be used to examine and photograph viruses. Sizes can be measured directly on the electronmicrographs.

Parasitism

Since viruses will grow only within living cells they cannot be cultivated in ordinary bacteriological culture media. A living system is necessary. Suitable systems are—

1. Whole organisms, i.e. free-living animals.
2. Fertile eggs.
3. Tissue cultures, i.e. small fragments of tissue kept alive in a suitable nutritive medium.

Because all of these are used in the preparation of viral vaccines they are discussed in detail in Chapter 33.

Structure

Viruses consist of a central core, containing a single nucleic acid, surrounded by a protein shell. The nucleic acid may be either DNA, as in vaccinia virus, or RNA, as in poliomyelitis virus.

The shell, known as the capsid, is built up of a large number of small units (capsomeres) arranged symmetrically around the core. This subunit structure is believed to be due to inability of the necessarily small, nucleic acid core to synthesise more complex protein molecules.

There are three types of symmetry—

1. Helical, in which the subunits are in helical arrangement around the core (Fig. 27.11), e.g. influenza virus.
2. Icosahedral, which is a special form of ·cubic symmetry in which the subunits are arranged at the edges or over the surfaces of an icosahedron (a polygon with 20 faces) (Fig. 27.12), e.g. poliomyelitis virus and the adenovirus. Superficially, icosahedral viruses appear to be spherical while helical viruses are often rod-shaped or, like influenza, can have rod-shaped forms.
3. Complex, in which the subunit arrangement is

less easy to distinguish because of the relatively advanced structure of the virus. Larger viruses (e.g. vaccinia) and bacteriophages are of this type.

Some viruses (e.g. influenza and measles) are surrounded by a lipid envelope. This is usually soluble in organic solvents and the viruses that have such a covering are very sensitive to ether and alcohol (see Measles Vaccine, p. 397).

Occasionally there are spikes projecting from the surface, which probably assist adsorption on to the host cell. They may contain specific antigens such as the haemagglutinin of influenza virus.

Reproduction

The life cycle of a virus involves the following sequence of events—

1. ADSORPTION ON TO THE HOST CELL MEMBRANE

The virus first attaches itself, by means of structures such as the haemagglutinin-containing spikes of influenza virus, to chemically complementary receptors on a host cell.

2. PENETRATION OF THE HOST CELL

It seems that the host cell behaves like an amoeba and engulfs the complete virus.

3. THE ECLIPSE PHASE

During the first few hours after penetration infective virus cannot be detected within the cell and, therefore, this period is known as the eclipse phase.

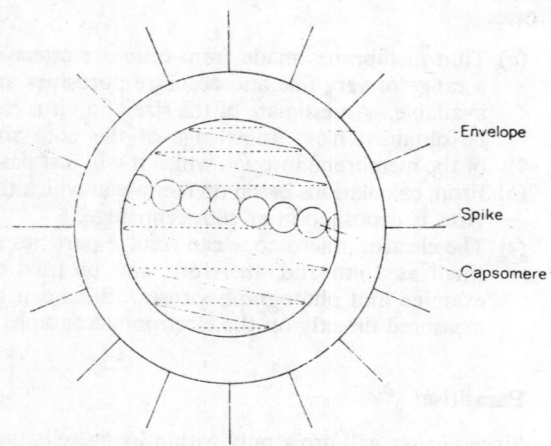

Fig. 27.11 Helical virus (capsomeres shown on part of helix only)

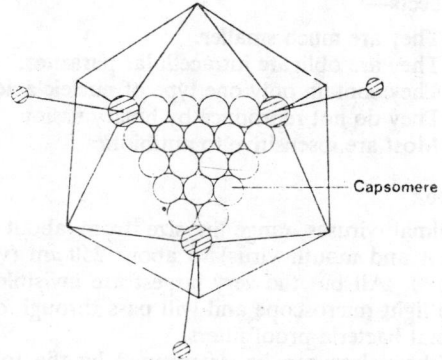

Fig. 27.12 Icosahedral virus (capsomeres shown on one face only)

Meanwhile the capsid of the virus disintegrates, freeing the nucleic acid core which inhibits the functioning of the host nucleic acid and then takes over the cell's metabolic activity and directs it to the synthesis of virus protein and nucleic acid.

4. VIRUS REPLICATION

The virus nucleic acid can both replicate itself and synthesise protein. As the new molecules become available the protein components are gradually built up around the nucleic acid in the geometric arrangement characteristic of the virus type.

If the virus has an envelope this is contributed by the cell-membrane of the host cell as the virus is 'budded out', in a reversal of the penetration mechanism, and freed.

5. LIBERATION FROM THE CELL

In some cases, such as the enveloped viruses, the release of virus does not damage the host cell immediately although deleterious changes may occur later. The organisms leave gradually and the release is often exponential.

On the other hand, certain classes of virus, including the pox group (containing smallpox) and the enteroviruses (of which poliomyelitis virus is an example) cause the cell to disintegrate completely, releasing the viruses in a burst.

Resistance to Chemical and Physical Agents

Viruses are more resistant than bacteria to many disinfectants and antiseptics. Chemical inhibition and destruction of bacteria are often the result of damage to metabolic enzymes and as these are lacking in viruses the latter are insensitive to this type of antimicrobial attack. The most useful virucides are the halogens and formaldehyde.

Antibiotics are ineffective against all but the largest viruses, possibly because by the time infection is recognised the multiplication stage, at which attack is likely to be most effective, is virtually over.

The development of antiviral drugs is limited by the fact that the intracellular growth of viruses is so intimately linked with the host cell. Consequently, substances toxic to the former usually harm the latter.

Most viruses are easily destroyed by heat. They are about as susceptible as vegetative bacteria and only a few, e.g. the virus of homologous serum jaundice, have a resistance approaching that of bacterial spores.

When exposed to ultra-violet light under conditions that avoid wastage of radiation in the surrounding medium (*see* Gunn and Carter, 1965) viruses are inactivated and this method has been used in the preparation of dead vaccines and to destroy the virus of homologous serum jaundice in blood plasma.

Detection and Identification of Viruses

As most viruses are invisible in the light microscope and, unlike bacteria, do not produce visible colonies, special methods are used to detect their presence—

1. LESIONS ON THE CHORIOALLANTOIC MEMBRANE

Immediately under the shell of a hen's egg is the tough, thin, shell membrane, and below this is a layer known as the chorioallantoic membrane. By a special technique (p. 394) viruses can be inoculated on to this layer, and if the suspension is dilute enough each virus will produce a separate lesion. These lesions (pocks) are areas of damaged tissue and their appearance is often distinctive. This is a useful method for identification and counting if the virus will grow on the chorioallantoic membrane.

2. CYTOPATHOGENIC EFFECTS IN TISSUE CULTURES

The degenerative changes caused in living cells by virus infection can be seen under the light microscope.

The virus is added to a small fixed-cell tissue culture, i.e. one grown as a layer, one cell thick, on the side of a test-tube. After incubation, the tube is examined under a microscope and the presence of virus is detected by cytopathogenic changes such as rounding, shrinking, granulation, and separation of the cells.

Because large numbers of tests are necessary in diagnostic virology, the tubes are mounted for incubation in large horizontal drums (Fig. 27.13) which are slowly rotated (e.g. 10 revolutions per hour) to ensure that the tissue cells are well aerated.

The method can be used to detect the presence of a suspected virus and, where a virus causes characteristic changes in the cells, for identification. The fact that some viruses will grow in certain types of tissue and not in others can also be of diagnostic value.

3. PLAQUES IN AGAR-COVERED TISSUE CULTURES

If a fixed-cell tissue culture is prepared on one side of a flat-sided bottle, inoculated with virus, and then layered with a thin film of the nutrient medium solidified with agar, the cytopathogenic effects are more localised because the spread of the virus is limited. As a result, the areas of disintegration are seen as clear zones in the otherwise opaque or

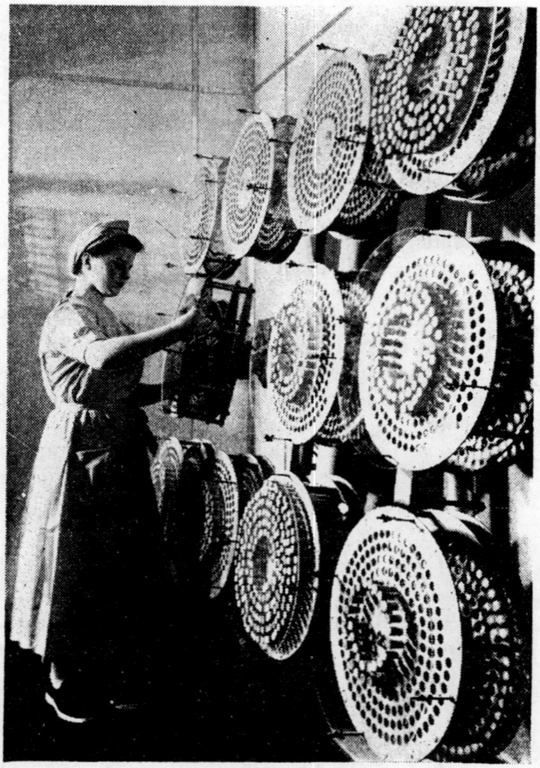

Fig. 27.13   Roller tube tissue cultures

(Courtesy Glaxo Laboratories Ltd)

coloured (if the cells have been stained with a harmless dye) monolayer. This technique is of particular value for counting and purifying virus suspensions.

4. HAEMAGGLUTINATION

Certain viruses, e.g. influenza, have surface haemagglutinins by which they can attach themselves to red blood cells. Since each virus can link two erythrocytes and each of the latter can adsorb a number of viruses, clumps are produced which, if the test is performed in a tube, adhere irregularly to the glass. In the absence of virus the cells settle to a button

on the base of the tube. This is a useful method for certain viruses that are not cytopathogenic.

5. VIRUS INTERFERENCE

This is an alternative technique to haemagglutination when a virus does not cause cytopathogenic changes in tissue cultures.

The preparation under test is inoculated into a tissue culture and incubated to allow the virus, if present, to establish itself in the cells. Then a cytopathogenic virus is added and if this fails to damage the cells it is concluded that the test material contained viruses that have prevented the establishment of a second infection. For a fuller explanation see the section on 'Interferon' (p. 313).

6. STAINING WITH FLUORESCENT ANTIBODY

This method, now widely used for identifying bacteria, is also a valuable aid in detecting viruses.

Counting Viruses

1. TOTAL COUNT

Viruses can be counted directly under the electron microscope. A known volume of the suspension is mixed with a known volume of a suspension of polystyrene latex particles. The latter are perfect spheres, easily distinguishable from viruses, and the concentration of a suspension can be determined accurately by physical measurements. The latex particles and viruses are counted in a suitable number of fields, and from knowledge of the concentration of the latex particles and the proportions in which the two suspensions were mixed the number of viruses in the original preparation can be calculated.

2. VIRUS TITRE

Virus titre is the virologist's equivalent to the bacteriologist's viable count. It involves determining the number of infective units in the virus suspension by methods resembling the fluid media (limiting dilution) techniques used for counting bacteria (p. 330).

The titre, or unit of activity, is the highest dilution of the virus suspension that will cause infection. To improve the accuracy of the determination many replicates are performed and the highest dilution that infects 50 per cent of the tests is taken as the titre. A 50 per cent, rather than a 100 per cent, end point is chosen because infection curves are often sigmoidal, i.e. flat at the beginning and end (Fig.

29.2) and, therefore, the end point can be found more precisely in the central portion. As an example, if 1 in 100 000 was the highest dilution of the suspension to cause infection in 50 per cent of the tests the titre would be 10^{-5}.

The highest dilution causing 50 per cent infection is also known as the ID 50 (infective dose for 50 per cent) or, if death is the effect produced, the LD (lethal dose) 50. The number of ID 50 doses in the suspension is the reciprocal of the titre, i.e. 10^5 in the above case.

The determinations involve preparing replicates of a series of ten-fold dilutions and, then, according to the properties of the virus—

(a) adding each to a separate tissue culture and looking for cytopathogenic effects;
(b) injecting each into a fertile egg and watching for death of the embryo;
(c) mixing each with a red blood cell suspension and examining for haemagglutination; or
(d) injecting each into an animal and watching for death (e.g. yellow fever) or some other effect (e.g. pustules from cowpox).

Another method of determining the number of infective units can be used if the virus grows in the chorioallantoic membrane or causes cell disintegration in agar-covered tissue cultures. It involves counting the lesions on the membrane, or the plaques in the culture, after a known volume of the suspension has been added and the test incubated (compare plate counting in bacteriology).

Interferon

When living cells are infected with live virus, or virus that has been inactivated by a non-drastic method such as low heat or ultra-violet light, they acquire resistance to infection by a second virus. This phenomenon is known as virus interference, and in 1957 Isaacs and Lindemann found that it was due to production by the host cells of a non-antigenic protein of low molecular weight which they named interferon.

Interferon can diffuse into and protect surrounding cells and is believed to act by blocking an early stage of virus synthesis. Its production seems to be a more or less general response of mammalian cells to viral infection and appears to play a major part in resistance to viral diseases. While antibodies are of prime importance in preventing reinfection (p. 378), interferon may function by assisting recovery from a first infection, i.e. at a time when antibody production is inadequate. An interesting piece of evidence, from several that support this theory, is the ability of cortisone both to increase susceptibility to infection and to inhibit the antiviral activity of interferon.

Because interferon is non-specific and free from toxicity, its suitability as an antiviral agent in animals and man is being investigated. Laboratory tests suggest that therapeutic applications will be very limited because, to be effective, it must be applied directly to infected cells or administered before or immediately after infection. Use in prophylaxis seems more promising, but so far the very large doses needed to protect animals have discouraged experiments in man.

Classification

There is no internationally recognised system of classification for viruses but suggestions have been made from time to time and recently a Provisional Committee for the Nomenclature of Viruses has proposed a scheme that has received considerable support. It is similar to the system used in biology and, therefore, involves subdivision of the phylum (viruses) into subphyla, classes, orders, families, genera, and species. The larger groupings are based on major differences such as the type of nucleic acid, the symmetry of the capsomeres and the presence or absence of an envelope. Division into families is related to geometrical factors, while antigenic properties and effects on living tissues are used to distinguish genera. The small abstract from the scheme given in Table 27.2 indicates its major features.

In the main, the families in the abstract have been limited to those that include species mentioned in the immunology section of this book.

The family Napoviridae includes the genus *Poliovirus* which contains the three strains of poliomyelitis virus.

Most of the species of the Myxoviridae and Paramyxoviridae have haemagglutinating properties. The two families differ sufficiently, e.g. in size, capacity to form filaments, and haemolytic ability, to justify the separate grouping. *Myxovirus influenza* (influenza virus) and *Paramyxovirus parotidis* (mumps) are familiar species from these families. *Pseudomyxovirus morbilli* (measles) belongs to a second genus within the Paramyxoviridae that is distinguished by the inability of its members to cause haemagglutination.

In the Herpesviridae is the virus of chicken pox (*Herpesvirus varicellae*) while the Poxviridae includes *Poxvirus variolae* (smallpox) and *P. vaccinae* (cowpox). An unusual feature of the Poxviridae is the insensitivity of the envelope to ether.

Table 27.2

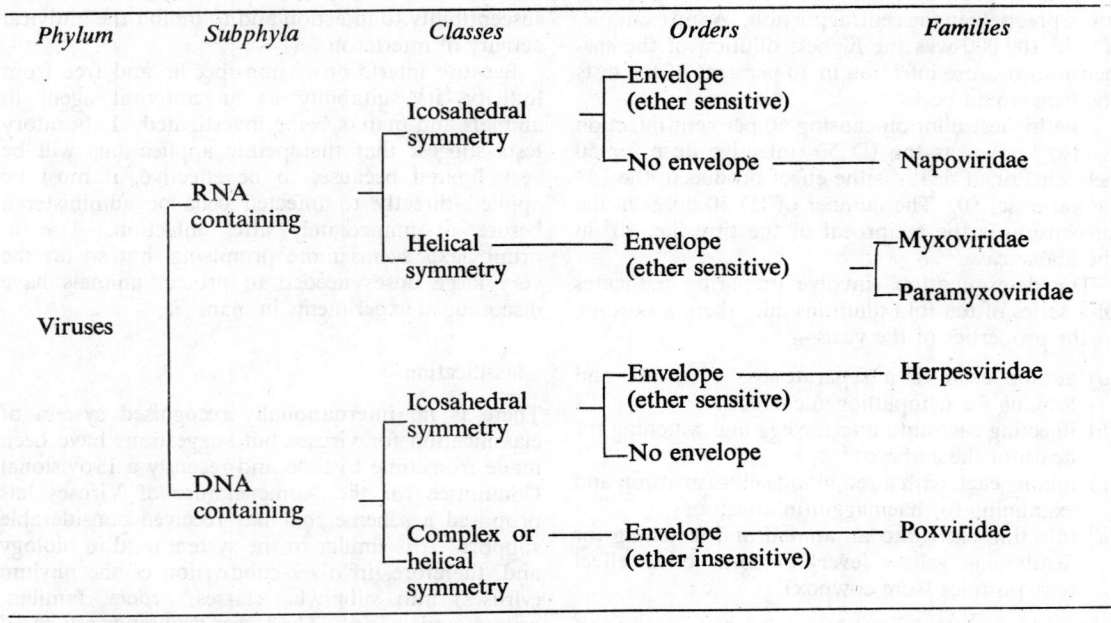

Phylum	Subphyla	Classes	Orders	Families
Viruses	RNA containing	Icosahedral symmetry	Envelope (ether sensitive)	
			No envelope	Napoviridae
		Helical symmetry	Envelope (ether sensitive)	Myxoviridae, Paramyxoviridae
	DNA containing	Icosahedral symmetry	Envelope (ether sensitive)	Herpesviridae
			No envelope	
		Complex or helical symmetry	Envelope (ether insensitive)	Poxviridae

D. Bacteriophages

Bacteriophages (more often called phages) are viruses that are parasitic on bacteria. They are highly specific and attack only a single bacterial species or even a particular strain of a species. Like viruses they are extremely small and cannot be seen under the light microscope. They are detected by two effects—

1. If material containing phages is added to a turbid culture of young and sensitive bacteria the latter are lysed and the culture becomes perfectly clear.
2. If a dilute suspension of phages is spread over a confluent growth of sensitive bacteria on an agar plate, clear areas of lysis are produced. Since each of these areas is caused by a single phage this technique can be used to count a phage suspension.

Under the electron microscope most phages resemble tadpoles in having well-defined head and tail portions. The head contains DNA and is surrounded by a protein coat made up of subunits like the capsid of a virus. In the T2 phage of *E. coli* the tail has a sheath, composed of protein subunits, a hollow core and a base plate that has projecting spikes and fibres (Fig. 27.14); the latter are wound round the end of the tail.

Mechanism of Infection

Contact between a phage and a bacterium is the result of random collisions and, if the two are complementary, adsorption occurs at specific receptor sites on the bacterial cell wall. In the T2

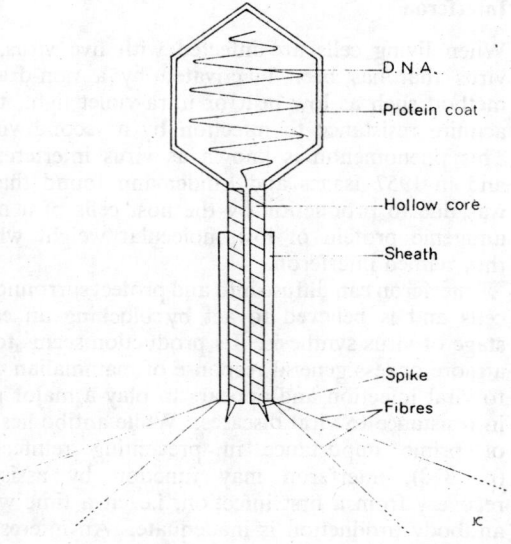

Fig. 27.14 Bacteriophage

phage attachment is through the tips of the fibres, which uncoil when contact takes place. Then the tail releases an enzyme that weakens the wall and allows the core of the tail to penetrate; sometimes this is assisted by contraction of the sheath. Finally, the DNA is injected into the cell leaving the rest of the phage attached to the surface.

The stages that follow resemble those of virus infection. The DNA directs the metabolic activities of the host to synthesis of phages and, after an eclipse phase of about 10 minutes, new phage particles start to appear. Production is complete in about 25 minutes from penetration and then, as a result of a gradual build-up of a lytic enzyme, the host cell bursts, freeing about 100 phages.

Phage infection is not always followed by lysis. Instead, the DNA becomes loosely attached to the chromosome of the bacterium and multiplies in step with the genes, thus becoming inherited by all the offspring. Phages that behave in this way are described as temperate, to distinguish them from virulent, or lytic, phages. The DNA component of the former is known as prophage.

Prophage-infected bacteria are resistant to lysis by the corresponding virulent phage. The prophage may become virulent again; although this is rare in nature it can be stimulated artificially by exposing the bacteria to mutagens such as ultra-violet light, ionising radiations, and nitrogen mustard. Because the bacteria have this potential for lysis they are known as lysogenic bacteria.

Sometimes the acquisition of a prophage confers a new property on the bacterium (lysogenic conversion). For example, the toxin-producing capacity of *Corynebacterium diphtheriae* is due to temperate phage infection.

In addition, it is possible for a genetic factor to be transferred from one bacterium to another (transduction) as a result of an error in phage synthesis which results in *host* DNA being incorporated in the new phages when the prophage becomes virulent again. Transfer of this DNA to the chromosome of another bacterium may confer a new characteristic; e.g. the ability to ferment a particular carbohydrate.

Applications, and a Danger

Bacteriophages, because of their specificity, are of considerable importance in the identification of bacteria (p. 323).

It was hoped that they would be useful in the treatment of diseases caused by the host bacteria but, although there is an oral preparation on the market containing phages specific for certain pathogens, products of this kind have given disappointing results; possibly because phage-resistant strains are present.

Their occurrence as contaminants in the production of antibiotics can be disastrous, and phage-resistant strains of certain antibiotic-producing organisms have had to be developed to overcome this problem.

BIBLIOGRAPHY

ADAMS, M. H. (1959) *Bacteriophages*. Interscience Publishers: New York and London.
BISSETT, K. A. (1955) *Cytology and Life History of Bacteria*. 2nd ed. Livingstone: Edinburgh.
BRAUN, W. (1965) *Bacterial Genetics*. 2nd ed. Saunders: London.
BURNET, F. M. (1960) *Principles of Animal Virology*. 2nd ed. Academic Press: New York and London.
CLOWES, R. (1967) *The Structure of Life*. Penguin Books: Harmondsworth.
COHEN, A. (1969) *Textbook of Medical Virology*. Blackwell: Oxford.
CRUICKSHANK, R. (1965) *Medical Microbiology*. Livingstone: Edinburgh.
DEAN, A. C. R. and HINSHELWOOD, C. (1961) *Growth Function and Regulation in Bacterial Cells*. Clarendon Press: Oxford.
DIFCO LABORATORIES (1953) *Manual of Dehydrated Culture Media and Reagents*. Difco Laboratories: Detroit.
GILLIES, R. R. and DODDS, T. C. (1968) *Bacteriology Illustrated*. Livingstone: Edinburgh.
GUNSALUS, I. C. and STANIER, R. Y. (Eds) (1960–62) *The Bacteria* (five volumes). Academic Press: New York.
GUNN, C. and CARTER, S. J. (1965) *Dispensing for Pharmaceutical Students* 11th ed. Pitman Medical: London.
HARRISON, K. (1965) *A Guide-book to Biochemistry*. 2nd ed. University Press: Cambridge.
HUGO, W. B. (1964) *An Introduction to Microbiology*. Heinemann: London.
OXOID LABORATORIES (1965) *Oxoid Manual of Culture Media*. 3rd ed. Oxoid Ltd.: London.
POSTGATE, J. (1969) *Microbes and Man*. Penguin Books: Harmondsworth.
ROSE, A. H. (1961) *Industrial Microbiology*. Butterworths: Oxford.
SOCIETY FOR GENERAL MICROBIOLOGY. Annual Symposia. University Press: Cambridge.
SOCIETY FOR GENERAL MICROBIOLOGY (1956) *Constituents of Bacteriological Culture Media*. University Press: Cambridge.
STANIER, R. Y., DOUDOROFF, M., and ADELBERG, E. A. (1963) *General Microbiology*. 2nd ed. Macmillan: New York.
STEPHENSON, M. (1949) *Bacterial Metabolism*. Longmans: London.

316 TUTORIAL PHARMACY

UMBREIT, W. W. (1962) *Modern Microbiology.* Freeman: London.

VINES, A. E. and REES, N. (1967) *The Microbes.* Pitman: London.

WILSON, G. S. and MILES, A. A. (1964) *Topley and Wilson's Principles of Bacteriology and Immunity.* 5th ed. Arnold: London.

ZDRODOVSKI, P. F. and GOLINEVICH, E. H. (1960) *The Rickettsial Diseases.* Pergamon: London.

REFERENCES

LEDERBERG, J. and TATUM, E. L. (1946) Gene recombination in Escherichia coli., *Nature, Lond.* **158**, 558.

MITCHELL, P. (1958) Strategy of chemotherapy:

membrane penetration and the therapeutic value of chemicals. *Symp. Soc. gen. Microbiol.,* **8**, 94–103.

MITCHELL, P. and MOYLE, J. (1956) Bacterial anatomy: Osmotic function and structure in bacteria. *Symp. Soc. gen. Microbiol.,* **6**, 150.

MITCHELL, P. and MOYLE, J. (1956) Permeation mechanisms in bacterial membranes. *Discuss. Faraday Soc.,* **21**, 258.

MONOD, J. (1949) The growth of bacterial cultures. *Ann. Rev. Microbiol.,* **3**, 371–394.

QUESNEL, L. B. (1960) Lag phase and population growth of bacteria. *J. appl. Bact.,* **23**, 99–105.

SOCIETY FOR APPLIED BACTERIOLOGY (1956) A symposium on anaerobic organisms. *J. appl. Bact.,* **19** (1), 112–180.

28

Bacteriological Methods

Cultural Techniques

MICRO-ORGANISMS may be grown in fluid or semi-solid media, or on solid media, and an account of the constituents and methods of preparation of culture media will be found in Gunn and Carter (1965). Semi-solid media are less widely used than the other two types but are valuable for isolating colonies of non-motile anaerobes. Fluid media (broths) for aerobic organisms are placed in tubes closed with cotton plugs or loose-fitting metal caps. Screw-capped bottles may also be used provided they are no more than one third full and the cap is left loose during incubation. Techniques for cultivating anaerobes are described on page 304.

Solid media are used in flat dishes (petri dishes) or in small wide-mouthed bottles. In dishes the organisms are mixed with the medium before it solidifies or are spread or dropped on to the surface after solidification. In bottles the medium may be allowed to set with the container vertical, when the organisms are inoculated with a straight wire (stab cultures), or with the container at an angle, to produce a slope, or slant, on which the bacteria can be spread. Large quantities of bacteria may be grown in special containers known as Carrell flasks or Roux bottles (Fig. 28.1).

A variety of special techniques are in use, as, for example, in the evaluation of disinfectants when it is necessary to take samples of bacteria from machinery or the skin. Commercially produced 'sausages' of solid media are available in a plastic skin; after exposing one end and applying it to the surface under test, the organisms that adhere are grown by removing a disc of the medium and incubating it in a petri dish to prevent drying-out.

TRANSFERENCES

The transfer of organisms from one container to another must be done aseptically, i.e. without introducing extraneous organisms (see Gunn and Carter, 1965). Suitable equipment includes—

Pipettes

Graduated pipettes or calibrated capillary dropping pipettes may be used. Three types of the latter are shown in Fig. 28.2.

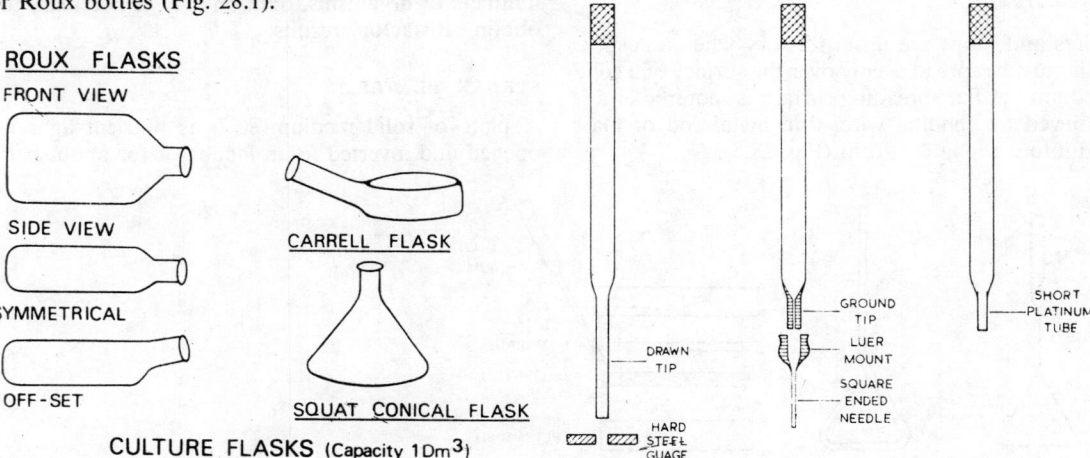

Fig. 28.1 Large volume culture flasks

Fig. 28.2 Capillary dropping pipettes

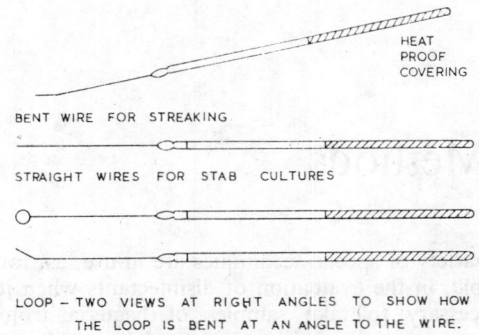

Fig. 28.3 Loops and wires

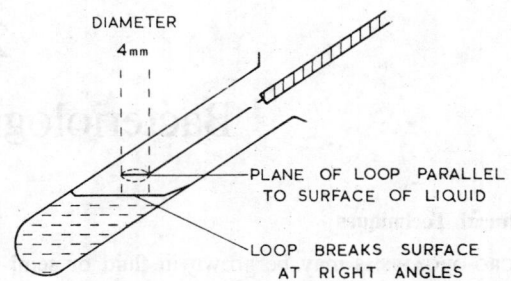

Fig. 28.4 Withdrawal of sample using loop

Wires and Loops

These are made from platinum or nichrome wire and are mounted in an insulated metal or glass handle (Fig. 28.3).

Wires are used straight (for making stab cultures) or slightly bent (for streaking a solid medium without damage to the surface). They are valuable for removing small amounts from a culture, particularly from colonies deep in a solid medium.

Loops are made by bending the end of a straight wire into a curve. For accurate work such as disinfectant testing, where the loop must pick up an accurate volume of liquid, the ring is formed around a rod of suitable diameter, and the end soldered. The loop is angled for ease of working and for precise work the plane of the loop should leave in a direction at right angles to the liquid surface (Fig. 28.4).

Spreaders

Wires and loops are unsatisfactory when a suspension must be spread evenly over the surface of a solid medium. A flat spreading surface is required and is achieved by bending wire, thin metal rod or glass rod into a triangular form (Fig. 28.5).

Membranes

If the concentration of organisms in a suspension is low, as in drinking water, the above methods are unsuitable. The organisms must be concentrated and this is best done by filtering a large volume of the liquid through a bacteria-proof membrane. Then the membrane is placed on a pad impregnated with a nutrient medium and incubated in a closed container (Fig. 28.5). Special units have been designed so that after filtration a culture medium can be introduced below the filter and the whole unit incubated.

Isolation of Pure Cultures

Before a bacterial species can be positively identified it must be obtained in pure culture (see Koch's work, p. 291). The following are some of the methods that can be used to isolate bacteria from a mixture. If the initial preparation contains large numbers of organisms, dilution may be necessary to obtain satisfactory results.

STREAK PLATES

A plate of solid medium such as nutrient agar is opened and inverted in an incubator for about half

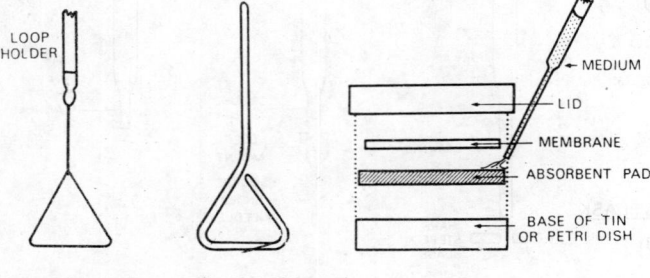

Fig. 28.5 Spreaders, and membrane incubation technique

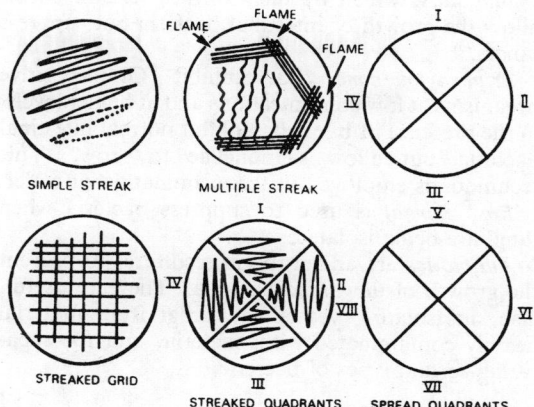

Fig. 28.6 Plate surface methods for obtaining isolated colonies

an hour, to dry the surface. Then, using a bent wire that has been flamed and allowed to cool between each set of streaks, lines are made in the manner shown in Fig. 28.6. Because each group of streaks obtains organisms only from the points at which the lines cross the previous set, there is progressive dilution of the organisms.

The plate is incubated in an inverted position and, provided the initial culture was dilute enough, isolated colonies will be found in the later sets of streaks. Material can be removed from these with a sterile wire and pure cultures set up. Inversion during incubation prevents condensate from the lid falling on to the surface of the medium and spreading the colonies. The preliminary drying also assists in this respect.

SPREAD PLATES

A more dilute suspension is necessary for this method. The base of a poured plate is marked into quadrants with a waxed pencil. A drop of culture is placed on the medium within one quadrant and spread over that area with a flamed spreader. Then the spreader is moved to the second quadrant and the organisms carried on it are spread over this area. The procedure is repeated for the third and fourth quadrants. After a few minutes to allow absorption of the liquid by the medium the plates are incubated inverted.

POUR PLATES

The initial suspension is diluted in 1 in 10 or 1 in 100 steps to a concentration of about 100 organisms/cm³. Volumes of 1 cm³ are pipetted into empty petri dishes and mixed with nutrient agar in the manner

illustrated in Fig. 28.7. The plate is gently moved five times in the directions shown, taking care not to splash medium between plate and lid. The temperature of the agar should not exceed about 47°C to avoid damaging the organisms. The oxygen tension varies at different levels of the medium and to avoid inhibition of aerobes near to the bottom of the dish the amount of agar should not exceed about 15 cm³ in a 75 mm petri dish. Because colonies in the agar are smaller than those on the surface and may also differ in shape, more experience is required for success with this technique. It has the advantage that quantitative estimates of the numbers of organisms in the original suspension can be made.

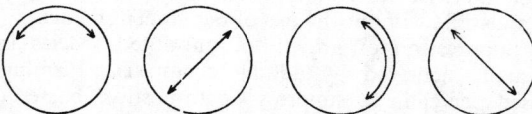

Fig. 28.7 The Milk Marketing Board method of mixing in plates

MICROMANIPULATION

Provided the species differ morphologically, a micromanipulator can be used to remove single organisms from a suspension on a microscope slide. A high degree of skill is needed.

HEAT DIFFERENTIATION

If a mixed culture is heated in a temperature-controlled water bath the number of heat-sensitive species in samples will decrease as time progresses. If temperatures above 70°C are used only spores will be isolated after about 10 minutes and further heating will separate the sporing species according to their heat tolerance.

Use can be made of optimum growth temperatures by incubating streak, spread or pour plates at a series of temperatures. Often different species will predominate at each temperature and, therefore, will be easier to isolate.

MOTILITY

If a mixed culture is inoculated at the bottom of a moist slope, which is then incubated upright, motile organisms can be recovered from the top of the slope which they have reached by swimming in the film of liquid on the surface.

MEMBRANE FILTRATION

If a dilute suspension is used, isolated colonies are obtained after incubation (*see* p. 318). Special stains can be applied to aid identification of the organisms.

ENRICHMENT (SELECTIVE) MEDIA

Even if some of the physical methods mentioned above do not achieve complete separation they make the culture much richer in one or more species. This can also be attained by chemical methods.

A medium is chosen that favours growth of the species of interest but depresses the growth of other organisms. Such methods are useful in the Public Health Service when the source of an epidemic is being traced; for example, sewage contains tremendous numbers of the normal bacteria of the human gut and to isolate a few typhoid organisms is virtually impossible without the use of enrichment media.

Suppression of growth of unwanted species is usually achieved by adding chemicals. Fleming used penicillin to suppress Gram-positive bacteria when he wished to isolate Gram-negative species. There are many other examples of which the following are a few—

Bile salts, which by their surface tension effects allow the growth of intestinal bacteria but suppress others.

Triphenylmethane dyes inhibit Gram-positive organisms at low concentrations and at higher levels, in the presence of bile salts, inhibit normal intestinal bacteria but allow salmonellae to grow. This technique is employed in the examination of water.

Rose Bengal is used to suppress bacteria when fungi are being isolated.

Antibiotics are added to virus cultures to prevent the growth of unwanted bacteria. They are useful, also, in isolating yeasts and fungi from material heavily contaminated with bacteria, and for separating certain types of bacteria.

SOIL ISOLATES

Most soil organisms can use very simple nutrients and will flourish in a medium containing mineral salts and an energy source, such as dextrose, whereas more exacting species will not grow.

IDENTIFICATION OF BACTERIA

Because bacteria are very small it is often difficult to differentiate between closely allied species. Usually a large number of tests are necessary to establish identity.

Sensory Characters

The shapes and colours of the colonies, their consistency and the odour of products of metabolism may help towards, at least, a partial conclusion. In evaluating the results of any test it should be remembered that the characteristics of an organism may change with age, the nature of the medium in which it is grown, the temperature of incubation, etc.

Microscopical Examination

Organisms may be examined in stained or unstained condition. Information may be obtained by the examination of unstained organisms suspended in a liquid, e.g. if a drop of a young fluid culture is suspended from a coverslip over a welled slide motility can be detected. The use of dark-ground or phase contrast illumination avoids the artefacts introduced by using stains. Very delicate bacteria, such as the syphilis spirochaete, are more easily seen under dark-ground illumination because the image is due to refraction of light but since a false impression of size is given, reliable measurements

cannot be made. Phase contrast is used to disclose detail in unstained specimens.

Simple staining with a single dye affords information about the morphology of the organism, but differential staining, which distinguishes different types, is more important.

Gram's Stain

The bacteria are first stained with a violet dye, e.g. crystal violet, and then treated with an iodine solution which fixes the stain to the cell. When washed with alcohol some organisms retain the stain (Gram-positive) while others lose it (Gram-negative). A counter stain, usually red, is then applied to stain the Gram-negative cells. This method, therefore, divides bacteria into two large groups.

Examples of Gram-positive genera are—

Micrococcus	*Corynebacterium*	*Bacillus*
Diplococcus	*Mycobacterium*	*Clostridium*
Streptococcus	*Staphylococcus*	

Examples of Gram negative genera are—

Vibrio	*Escherichia*	*Pseudomonas*
Proteus	*Salmonella*	*Pasteurella*
Neisseria	*Shigella*	*Bordetella*

ACID FASTNESS

Some organisms are not easily stained by the usual dyes, possibly because of a water-repellant outer layer or a high lipid content, but when stained they may retain the colour even when washed with acid. Such organisms are called acid-fast. Ziehl-Neelsen's method involves staining with hot concentrated carbol-fuchsin solution, washing with water and then treating with 25 per cent sulphuric acid followed by 98 per cent alcohol. Finally a counter stain is applied. The mycobacteria that cause leprosy and tuberculosis retain the red colour when treated with both acid and alcohol, i.e. are both acid and alcohol fast. Other members of the genus are acid fast only. Most bacteria are neither acid nor alcohol fast.

Special stains have been developed to show the presence of capsules, spores, flagella and cell inclusions.

Cultural Techniques

The appearance of the growth produced on or in suitable culture media is often very important in identification. Best results are obtained with fresh material and media that reproduce as closely as possible the natural environment of the organism; e.g. many pathogens grow better in media enriched with animal protein such as blood or serum.

GROWTH IN FLUID MEDIA

Useful features are colour, odour, evolution of a gas, presence of a surface pellicle or a deposit, and the nature of the turbidity. The turbidity may be flocculent, granular, stringy, irridescent, mucilaginous or merely a faint opalescence; its intensity at different depths may indicate the oxygen requirement of the organism.

GROWTH ON SOLID MEDIA

Plate Cultures

Identifying features include the size, shape, elevation, colour, degree of transparency and internal structure of the colonies. Some organisms produce a diffusible pigment that colours the medium if incubation takes place at the appropriate temperature (not necessarily the optimum temperature for growth of the organism).

Slope Cultures

These may show characteristic forms of growth, e.g. spreading, root-like and tree-like.

Stab Cultures

The growth radiating from the stab in a stab culture may be characteristic and its position may indicate if the organism is aerobic or anaerobic.

DIFFERENTIAL MEDIA

Differential media allow the growth of organisms other than those being identified but render the latter distinguishable. Blood agar is an example and by using it three classes of organisms may be distinguished—

(a) β-haemolytic, the colonies of which are surrounded by a clear zone of haemolysis. These include several important pathogens, e.g. *Streptococcus pyogenes*.

(b) α-haemolytic, where the haemolysis zone is much less distinct and the blood becomes green.

(c) Non-haemolytic, where there is no haemolysis. Some media are both differential and selective (p. 320), an example is McConkey's bile salt medium (Gunn and Carter, 1965).

OXYGEN REQUIREMENTS

Sometimes the position of the growth in a stab culture or in a tube of anaerobic broth, such as thioglycollate, gives an indication of the oxygen requirement or tolerance of an organism. For example, strict aerobes and strict anaerobes will grow at top and bottom respectively while facultative bacteria will grow throughout. Normal and damaged organisms may have different oxygen needs, e.g. aerobic bacilli harmed by heat treatment may grow in anaerobic but not in aerobic broths.

GROWTH TEMPERATURE

The optimum growth temperature and the temperature range over which growth takes place can be of diagnostic value. These are determined by inoculating the organisms into tubes of liquid media and incubating at a series of different temperatures. Water baths are used for this purpose because accurate temperature control is easier than with air incubators. A graph of temperature against quantity of growth (estimated from the opacity of the culture) is plotted and the optimum temperature read off.

OPTIMUM pH

The optimum pH and the range over which growth can take place may be determined by a method similar to the one described in the previous paragraph, taking care that the effect is due to pH alone.

Many organisms grow well in the range 5 to 8 but a few tolerate high and low pHs, e.g. *Vibrio cholerae*, pH 9 and lactobacilli, pH 3·5.

Chromatography and Electrophoresis of Cell Disintegrates

The organisms are grown in a defined medium, separated, washed and disintegrated. Chromatography or electrophoresis is carried out on the disintegrate and the constituents that are detected are compared with those from reference cultures. Electrophoresis is more widely used because better separations are obtained, particularly when enzymes are being investigated (*see* Norris, 1964).

Biochemical Reactions

Many biochemical reactions are helpful in the identification of a species.

CARBOHYDRATE FERMENTATION

Media containing fermentable carbohydrates (e.g. mono-, di-, tri- and polysaccharides, sugar alcohols and glycosides) are inoculated with the organism and incubated. Fermentation is indicated by the production of acid or gas or both. Acid is detected by including an indicator in the medium and gas is collected in a small inverted glass tube (a Durham tube) which must be full of the medium before the test begins. The spectrum of activity is often highly diagnostic and can be used to distinguish closely related bacteria.

PROTEIN BREAKDOWN

These tests depend on the ability of certain organisms to utilise proteins or their hydrolysis products. Signs of breakdown are—

(a) In cooked meat medium—blackening and digestion of the meat with foul odours.

(b) In gelatin, egg and serum media—liquefaction. If gelatin stabs are incubated at 25°C, a characteristic liquefaction pattern may be produced. When incubation at 37°C is essential, subsequent refrigeration will indicate if liquefaction has occurred.

(c) In peptone water—production of indole from the amino acid tryptophane, the indole being detected by its foul smell and a colour test.

NITRATE REDUCTION

This test is based on the ability of some organisms to use inorganic salts as sources of nitrogen. Some bacteria can reduce nitrate to nitrite (detected by the nitroso reaction) or nitrogen (collected in a Durham tube).

PRESENCE OF ENZYMES

Tests for the production of specific enzymes by bacteria have been extended in recent years (Norris, 1964). Examples of classical methods are tests to detect urease, by its ability to split urea into carbon dioxide and ammonia, and catalase, by the evolution of oxygen from hydrogen peroxide.

Serological Methods

If an animal is inoculated with a sub-lethal dose of an organism, antibodies are produced in its serum. Some of these antibodies (the agglutinins) are very useful in identification because they combine *in vitro* with the organism that stimulated their production, giving a precipitate. All that is necessary for rapid identification is a supply of agglutinin-containing sera prepared against standard organisms. An organism thought to be X should produce a precipitate with the anti-X serum. The test is usually carried out macroscopically, as follows—

Two separate drops of saline are placed on a clean slide (saline is used because the reaction will not take place if salts are absent). A trace of the unknown organism is added to both drops and anti-X serum is added to one. If the organism is X, flocculation occurs, i.e. small clumps of organisms become visible in a short time. The second drop is a control in case the organisms flocculate spontaneously in the saline.

COMPLEMENT FIXATION

If sheep red cells are injected into a rabbit, antibodies to the cells are produced in the rabbit's serum. This can be shown by adding sheep red cells to serum obtained from the rabbit, when the cells become lysed. However, if the serum is first heated at 56°C for half an hour no lysis occurs because the heating has destroyed a normal constituent of the serum, known as complement, that is essential for lysis to take place. Some antibacterial antibodies require the assistance of complement; these are known as complement-fixing antibodies. Sometimes there is no visible sign when an antibody 'attacks' a micro-organism but if the antibody requires the assistance of complement the take-up (fixation) of this from the surrounding serum indicates that the reaction has taken place. For example, organism Y is added to a serum containing anti-Y, complement-fixing antibody. The relatively large amount of complement in this serum is first destroyed by heating, as above, and then a very small amount of complement, all of which will be taken up if the reaction occurs, is added. After a suitable interval, red cells and red cell antibody are added when haemolysis or no haemolysis will indicate the presence or absence respectively of complement fixation.

FLUORESCENT ANTIBODIES

This is a very elegant method of detecting certain types of reaction between antibodies and bacteria. Antibodies labelled with a fluorescent dye, such as fluorescein isocyanate, are added to a film of the bacteria on a slide, left for about 15 minutes and then any uncombined material is washed off. If combination has taken place the organisms fluoresce brightly under the microscope when examined with ultra-violet light (*see* Walker and Batty, 1964).

RADIOACTIVE ANTIBODIES

Antibodies labelled with radioactive isotopes can be used in essentially the same way as fluorescent antibodies except that combination is detected by the blackening that takes place when a photographic film is exposed to the washed slide.

Use of Bacteriophages

Many bacteriophages (p. 314) are highly specific and will lyse only a particular species or variety. If an unknown organism is grown thickly on an agar plate and then touched with drops of a suspension of the bacteriophage specific for the organism it is suspected to be, the presence of clear regions in the culture after incubation will confirm the identification.

Spectrophotometry

Differences in the ultra-violet and infra-red spectra of the constituents separated from bacteria have been used in identification. The cultures and separative techniques must be standardised and a comprehensive set of reference curves is necessary.

Animal Inoculation

Some pathogens can be identified by infection of laboratory animals. The death of the animal confiims pathogenicity while a post-mortem may show features characteristic enough to confirm identity. If at the same time other animals are injected with the organism mixed with the specific antiserum, and these are unaffected, additional proof is provided.

The strictest criteria for the identification of an organism as the cause of a particular disease are still those laid down by Koch—

(*a*) It must be possible to isolate the organism from the tissues and body fluids of the diseased animal.

(*b*) It must be grown in artifical and pure culture for several generations.

(*c*) It must reproduce the disease in susceptible animals and be reisolated from them.

Generally, an organism can be identified without resorting to animal inoculation.

CLASSIFICATION OF BACTERIA

The earliest classifications of bacteria were based on morphological characters, but it soon became obvious that morphological similarity was often accompanied by marked physiological differences. Attempts to take staining reactions into account, especially the Gram and acid-fast techniques, produced a more useful system but it was not until many other factors such as cultural characters, biochemical and serological reactions and pathogenicity were included that the present useful systems were evolved.

The classification most widely used today is that of the American Society of Bacteriologists (*see* Bergey, 1957) although this has features that are not accepted by all authorities in this country.

Bacteria have similarities with the lower members of the fungi and algae of the plant kingdom and the protozoa of the animal kingdom. Since their differences from fungi are the least marked (e.g. unlike most bacteria the algae contain chlorophyll and the protozoa have a well-marked nucleus) they are put in the lowest class of the fungi, the *Schizomycetes*, so called because of the simple method of reproduction of its members—by splitting into two.

The class *Schizomycetes* is broken down into subdivisions of which the most important are Orders, Families, Genera, Species and Varieties. In accordance with the binomial system of the Swedish botanist Carl von Linné each organism is given two latin or latinised names. The first is the name of the genus and is given a capital letter, the second the name of the species which is not capitalised. If the species is divided into varieties this is indicated at the end of the name. To illustrate this we may take the causative organism of tuberculosis in man. It belongs to the order *Mycobacteriales*, the family,

Mycobacteriaceae, and the genus *Mycobacterium;* its specific name is *tuberculosis* and the human variety is termed *hominis*. Hence its full name is— *Mycobacterium tuberculosis*, var. *hominis*.

Since a detailed consideration of classification would be out of place in this book the following selection of orders, families and genera has been made to give prominence to organisms of importance in immunology and pharmacy and, at the same time, to indicate some of the more important factors used in classification.

The classification of higher plants is based largely on morphology and while, because of their small size and the consequent difficulty of distinguishing morphological features, physiological behaviour plays a considerable part in bacterial classification, it is on morphological characters that most of the main subdivisions of bacteria are based. The order *Eubacteriales* is distinguished from the *Actinomycetales* by the fact that the former have a very simple form while the latter usually show a branched hyphae-like structure. Several of the families are characterised by the shape of the cells (e.g. *Micrococcus* and *Enterobacteriaceae*), the position of the flagella (e.g. *Enterobacteriaceae* and *Pseudomonadaceae*), the presence or absence of spores (e.g. *Enterobacteriaceae* and *Bacillaceae*) etc. Genera are also separated by similar features, e.g. the cell shape (*Vibrio* and *Pseudomonas*), the grouping of cells (*Diplococcus, Staphylococcus* and *Streptococcus*) and whether or not the spore causes bulging of the cell wall (*Clostridium* and *Bacillus*).

The other factor that makes a large contribution to the division into major groups (orders and families particularly) is the Gram reaction. The genera *Neisseria* and *Diplococcus* both contain paired cocci but as the former are Gram-negative and the latter Gram-positive they are included in separate families. The rods of the families *Enterobacteriaceae* and *Bacillaceae* are distinguished similarly.

Other factors such as biochemical, serological and 'phage reactions, pathogenicity, cultural characters and other staining reactions find their chief applications in the differentiation of species.

Order: *Pseudomonadales*

Simple rigid cells.
Straight, curved or spiral rods.
Usually occur singly.
Usually motile by polar flagella.
Gram-negative.

FAMILY: *Pseudomonadaceae*

Straight rods.
Often produce water-soluble pigment.

Genus: *Pseudomonas*

Pseudomonas aeruginosa can infect wounds and burns. It produces a pigment that gives pus a characteristic bluish tint. It is hard to eradicate because it is very resistant to antibacterial agents; this is related to its ability to produce a wide range of enzymes that can utilise simple substrates.

FAMILY: *Spirillaceae*

Curved or spiral rods.

Genus: *Vibrio*

Comma shaped with a single polar flagellum. Includes *Vibrio cholerae* which causes cholera.

Order: *Eubacteriales*

Simple rigid cells.
Spherical or rod-shaped.
Occur singly or in pairs, clusters, chains or filaments.
Motile by peritrichous flagella or non-motile.
Only one family produces spores.
Gram-positive or Gram-negative.
Not acid fast.

FAMILY: *Enterobacteriaceae*

Motile or non-motile rods.
Gram-negative.
Ferment carbohydrates.

Genus: *Escherichia*

Ferment lactose.
Includes *Escherichia coli* which is commensal in the gut but pathogenic in the urinary tract; it can also cause gastro-enteritis. In the public health service it is used as an indicator of pollution with faeces.

Genus: *Serratia*

Very small pigmented rods.
Serratia marcescens produces a bright red pigment and, because of its small size, is used to test the efficiency of bacteria-proof filters.

Genus: *Proteus*

Highly motile rods.
Produce a characteristic seminal odour.
Ferment glucose but not lactose.
Proteus vulgaris is commensal in the bowel and can infect wounds. Like *Pseudomonas aeruginosa* is difficult to eradicate.

Genus: Salmonella

Rods that are usually motile.
Lactose is not fermented.
Antigenic structure is important in species differentiation.
Pathogenic, e.g. *Salmonella typhi*, which causes typhoid fever.

Genus: Shigella

Very similar to the salmonella but non-motile.
Responsible for bacillary dysentery.

FAMILY: *Brucellaceae*

Small ovoid or elongated rods.
Motile or non-motile.
Gram-negative.
Growth outside the animal body requires presence of body fluids in culture media.
Biochemical reactions poor.

Genus: Pasteurella

Non-motile.
Shows characteristic bi-polar staining.
Pasteurella pestis causes bubonic plague.

Genus: Bordetella

Ovoid rods.
Bordetella pertussis, which causes whooping cough, requires blood in the medium when first isolated.

FAMILY: *Micrococcaceae*

Spheres, occurring singly or in groups that may be characteristic.
Non-motile.
Usually Gram-positive.
May be pigmented.

Genus: Staphylococcus

On solid media the cells are arranged in grape-like clusters.
Pathogenic species ferment carbohydrates and liquefy gelatin.
Staphylococcus aureus causes boils, abscesses, styes, osteomyelitis and food poisoning. It produces an exotoxin (p. 376).

FAMILY: *Neisseriaceae*

Cocci, typically in pairs, with adjacent sides flattened.
Usually non-motile.
Gram-negative.

Genus: Neisseria

Several species are pathogenic, e.g. *Neisseria gonorrhoea* (the gonococcus) and *Neisseria meningitidis* (the meningococcus) which cause gonorrhoea and bacterial meningitis respectively.
Blood or serum is essential for growth (gonococcus) or enhances growth (meningococcus). Most strains grow better in an atmosphere enriched with carbon dioxide.

Genus: Lactobacillaceae

Cocci or rods, occurring singly, in pairs or in chains.
Generally non-motile.
Facultative or strict anaerobes.
Ferment carbohydrates with marked acid production.
Gram-positive.

Genus: Diplococcus

Cocci or ovoid rods.
Usually in pairs.
Some are capsulated.
Diplococcus pneumoniae causes a form of pneumonia.

Genus: Streptococcus

Cocci or ovoid rods.
Usually in chains.
Some are capsulated.
Some are highly pathogenic, e.g. *Streptococcus pyogenes* which causes scarlet fever and sore throat.

FAMILY: *Corynebacteriaceae*

Rods or club-shaped cells.
Mostly non-motile.
Gram-positive.

Genus: Corynebacterium

Slender or slightly curved rods often with clubbed ends.
Usually arranged in palisades.
Contain nitrogenous granules that stain characteristically.
Corynebacterium diphtheriae causes diphtheria; it produces a dangerous exotoxin.

FAMILY: *Bacillaceae*

Motile or non-motile rods.
Form endospores.
Gram-positive.

Genus: Bacillus

Aerobic.

Spores do not cause bulging of the cell wall.

A few species are pathogenic, e.g. *Bacillus anthracis* which causes anthrax. Several of the saprophytic species are of pharmaceutical interest, e.g. *Bacillus subtilis* and *pumilis*, used in antibiotic assays, *Bacillus megaterium*, used to produce penicillinase, and *Bacillus stearothermophilus* used to test steam sterilisers.

Genus: Clostridium

Anaerobic.

Spores cause bulging of the cell wall.

Many species are pathogenic, e.g. *Clostridium tetani*, which causes tetanus, *Clostridium botulinum*, responsible for a type of food poisoning, and *Clostridium oedematiens*, *septicum* and *welchii*, causal organisms of gas gangrene. All produce powerful exotoxins.

Order: *Actinomycetales*

Most resemble fungal hyphae and tend to branch.

FAMILY: *Mycobacteriaceae*

Cells rarely filamentous or branching.
Non-motile.
Gram-positive.

Genus: Mycobacterium

Straight or slightly curved rods.
Acid fast.
Often stain unevenly.
Some grow very slowly.
Some are pathogenic, e.g. *Mycobacterium tuberculosis*.

FAMILY: *Streptomycetaceae*

Cells filamentous and branching.
Very important commercially because some species of the genus Streptomyces produce antibiotics.

Order: *Spirochaetales*

Slender, non-rigid spiral forms.
Motile, but not by flagella.
Gram-negative.

FAMILY: *Treponemataceae*

Features essentially similar to those of the order.

Genus: Treponema

Many pathogens.
Treponema pallidum causes syphilis.

Genus: Leptospira

Leptospira icterohaemorrhagica causes Weil's disease (p. 404).

Order: *Mycoplasmatales*

Soft, fragile, pleomorphic cells without a distinguishable cell wall.
Do not appear to reproduce by binary fission but by spherical elementary bodies.
They are filterable and resemble viruses. Unlike viruses they can be grown on artificial culture media.
Non-motile.
Gram-negative.
Also known as the pleuropneumonia-like organisms (PPLO) because one species causes pulmonary disease. They have been found as contaminants of tissue cultures. The generic name is *Mycoplasma*.

COUNTING OF BACTERIA

The total number of organisms living and dead in a preparation is known as the total count, while the number of living organisms is called the viable count.

TOTAL COUNTS

Direct Methods

In these the number of cells is counted directly, usually by an optical method, but in one case, the Coulter Counter, by breaks in electrical conductivity caused as a cell passes through a tiny orifice.

BREEDS'S METHOD

A microscope slide marked with a square of known area, e.g. 2 cm², is used. A squared eyepiece micrometer is put into the eyepiece of a microscope and the size of one of the sides of a square is found with a stage micrometer. Hence the area of the square and the number of squares in the area marked on the slide is determined.

The suspension is diluted to give a countable number of organisms per eyepiece square and a known small volume, e.g. 0·1 cm³, is spread carefully and evenly over the square on the slide. This is allowed to dry and then fixed and stained. The number of organisms in about 40 squares, selected at random with a field finder, are counted. From the size of the squares in the eyepiece, the area of film on the slide, and the volume of suspension spread on to the slide, the number of organisms in the original suspension can be calculated, e.g.—

If the area of one eyepiece square is 0.0004 mm^2, the total number of squares in the total area of the film is $400/0.0004 = 10^6$.

If the mean number of organisms per eyepiece square is 10, the total number in the film will be 10^7.

Since this number was in 0.1 cm^3 the count of the original suspension is 10^8 per cm^3.

WRIGHT'S METHOD

Equal volumes of the suspension and blood are intimately mixed and a film is made on a slide. This is dried, fixed and stained and the number of bacteria and red cells in about 40 fields are counted. The number of red blood cells in the sample may be assumed to be 5×10^6 per cm^3 or, for more accurate work, can be counted in a haemocytometer. Alternatively, a commercial standardised blood sample can be used.

As the ratio of blood cells to bacteria on the slide is known, the number of bacteria per cm^3 in the suspension can be found by proportionality.

The sources of error in these methods are firstly, lack of homogeneity in the spread films (the Chisquared test can be used to detect this) and, secondly, the small volumes used, particularly in the Breed method. At least three replicates should be done.

COUNTING CHAMBER

This is a slide with a recessed area that is ruled in squares. A suitable dilution of the culture is made and a drop is placed on the recess and covered with a special plane cover-slip, taking care not to trap air bubbles. The bacteria are allowed to settle and then viewed by dark-ground or phase contrast illumination. Alternatively, they may be stained with crystal violet and examined by normal bright field illumination. Usually two slides are made and the numbers of organisms in 4 groups of 16 small squares are counted. If the mean number of organisms per square is assumed to be 10, the dilution of the original culture to get a suitable number per square is 100, the calculation is as follows (assuming a Thoma cell, Fig. 28.8, has been used)—

$$\text{Depth of recess} = \tfrac{1}{50} \text{ mm};$$
$$\text{Side of each square} = \tfrac{1}{20} \text{ mm}.$$

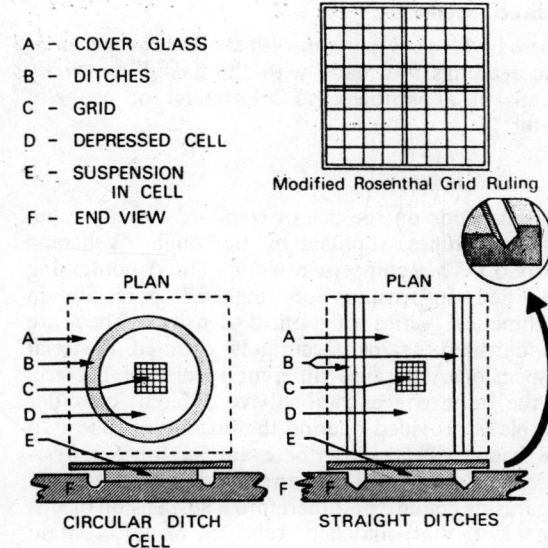

A – COVER GLASS
B – DITCHES
C – GRID
D – DEPRESSED CELL
E – SUSPENSION IN CELL
F – END VIEW

Modified Rosenthal Grid Ruling

PLAN   PLAN

CIRCULAR DITCH CELL   STRAIGHT DITCHES

Fig. 28.8   Haemocytometer cells

Therefore, volume above each square $= \tfrac{1}{20} \times \tfrac{1}{20} \times \tfrac{1}{50}$ mm^3 and this contains 10 organisms, i.e.—

$$\text{number of bacteria per mm}^3 = 20 \times 20 \times 50 \times 10 = 2 \times 10^5$$

Consequently, the original culture contained 2×10^7 bacteria per mm^3 or 2×10^{10} per cm^3.

COULTER COUNTER

The Coulter Counter, which is described on p. 181, can be adapted for counting bacterial suspensions.

MEMBRANE FILTRATION

Provided that the suspension is sufficiently dilute the membrane filtration technique (p. 318) can be employed for counting. The organisms retained on the filter are stained and then the membrane is dried and treated with immersion oil to make it transparent. The organisms in a suitable number of fields are counted under a microscope. The number of bacteria collected on the filter from a known volume of suspension can be calculated from a knowledge of the field area and the filtration area of the membrane. Membranes with a porosity of 0.45 μm are commonly used and the rate of filtration is controlled to produce an even distribution of bacteria over the membrane. The method is rather tedious but is particularly useful when the number of organisms in the preparation is very small, as in certain natural waters.

Indirect Methods

These involve comparison with standard suspensions and readings are made with the naked eye or by means of a photoelectric colorimeter or nephelometer.

VISUAL METHOD

This depends on the use of standard opacity tubes (Brown's tubes, supplied by Burroughs Wellcome and Co.) They comprise a set of 10 tubes containing solidified suspensions of unglazed porcelain in arithmetical series of optical density. They are standardised against accurately counted bacterial suspensions. Because different species of bacteria in the same concentration have different opacities a table is provided relating the opacity of tube 1 to the bacterial species. For example, for *Staphylococcus aureus* tube 1 corresponds to 600×10^6 organisms per cm³ and therefore a suspension of this organism that matched tube 6 would contain $6 \times 600 \times 10^6$ bacteria per cm³.

PHOTOMETRIC METHODS

Colorimetry

In this technique the amount of light absorbed by the suspension is measured and converted to numbers by reference to a calibration curve. The simplest instrument for this purpose is the colorimeter but a more

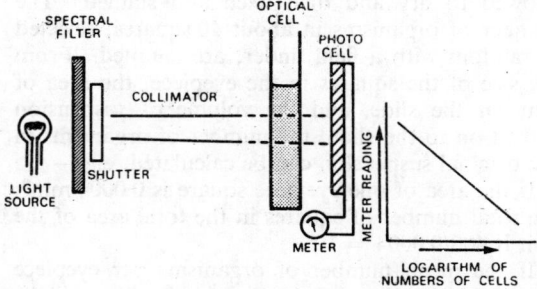

Fig. 28.9   Principles of the colorimeter and graph of response

sophisticated alternative is the spectrophotometer in which light of controlled wavelength is used. The method (Fig. 28.9) is relatively inefficient for low concentrations of bacteria because these do not materially affect the response of the light detector which in the absence of particles is receiving full light. At the other end of the scale the instrument becomes inaccurate when the suspension is so thick that organisms are obscured by others in the path of the light.

Nephelometry

The difference between this and the previous method is that the instrument measures light refracted by particles as the beam passes through the suspension. In the absence of bacteria no light reaches the detector. Nephelometers (Fig. 28.10) are more

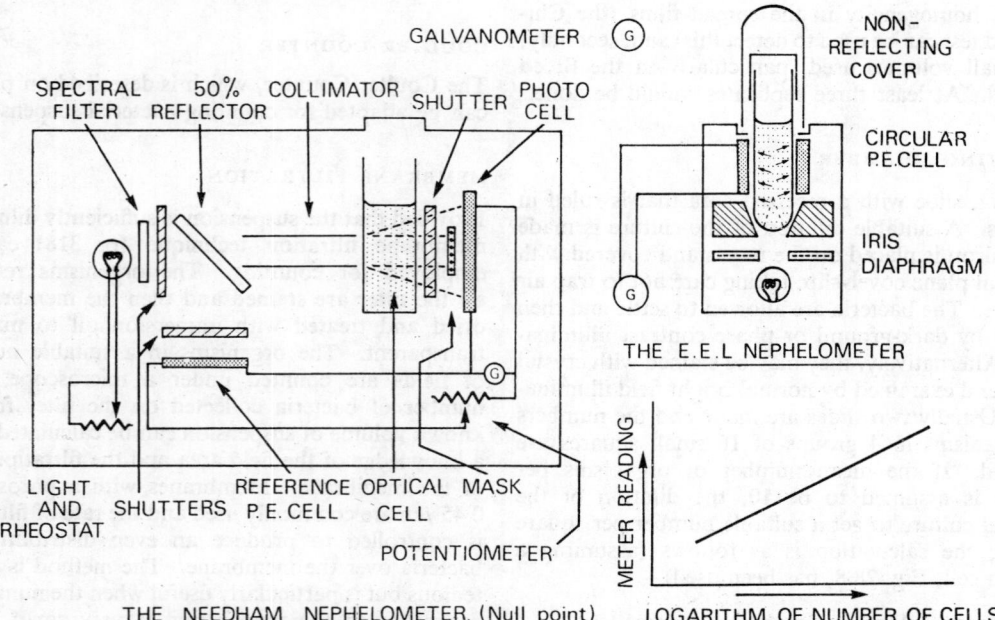

Fig. 28.10   Principles of nephelometers for estimating the numbers of bacterial cells

efficient than colorimeters for suspensions of low density but a point is soon reached where refracted rays are further refracted by other particles and the result is no longer quantitative.

PACKED CELL VOLUME

The suspension is centrifuged under defined conditions and the depth of the sediment is measured. The equivalent number of cells is obtained from a graph of cell numbers against packed cell volume. The method is not very accurate but is useful for thick suspensions.

DRY WEIGHT

The centrifuged cells from the previous method can be separated, washed free from culture medium by further centrifugations, and then dried in a desiccator at constant temperature. This weight can be related to numbers but for certain determinations (e.g. absorption or uptake studies) the dry weight itself is more useful.

VIABLE COUNTS

These are used to determine the number of living organisms in pharmaceutical products and in foods, and to find the number of bacteria surviving after exposure to a lethal agent.

Solid Media Techniques

These employ normal fluid media solidified with 1–2 per cent of agar. Confirmation that the agar does not interfere with the counting technique is necessary and this is particularly important when attempts are being made to grow organisms from unfavourable environments (Harris, 1963).

POUR PLATE METHOD

The suspension is diluted to contain about 200 organisms per cm³ and one cm³ quantities are plated as described on pages 317 and 319. When the plates have set they are incubated inverted for a suitable time and the colonies are counted.

SURFACE VIABLE METHOD

Plates from which the surface moisture has been removed (p. 318) are necessary.

Drop Technique (Miles and Misra, 1938)

The suspension is diluted to 20–80 organisms in 0·02 cm³ and usually three or four dilutions within this range are made. Using a dropping pipette set at a height of 10 mm from the agar surface, two drops of each dilution are dropped on to each plate at a rate of one drop a second, i.e. 6 to 8 drops per dish of normal size. After about 20 minutes the drops have been absorbed by the medium and then the plates are incubated inverted. Counts can be examined in a shorter time with this method, e.g. 8 hours, as against 24 hours with the pour plate method, for *E. coli*.

Spreading Technique

A suspension containing about 500 organisms per cm³ is desirable for this method. To each quadrant of a poured plate is added a 0·2 cm³ drop of the suspension. This is spread evenly over the quadrant with a spreader, taking care not to contaminate the other quadrants. After absorption of the liquid, the plate is incubated inverted and examined after the time recommended for the drop technique. A disadvantage of this method is the loss of organisms on the spreader; this can be allowed for by performing several replicates, using the same spreader for all the drops of one dilution, rejecting the count for the first drop and assuming that the carry-over is the same for each of the remainder.

Surface methods have a number of advantages—

(a) Counting is easier; colonies are approximately the same size, because they are on the surface of the medium and, therefore, in the same oxygen tension. In addition parallax errors, which confuse the counting of colonies in the depth of the agar, do not arise.

(b) Obligate aerobes, including fungi, that will not grow well below the surface of a solid medium, can be counted satisfactorily. For moulds a fungal medium is desirable.

(c) Colony characteristics on solid media are more pronounced when organisms are growing on the surface and, therefore, contaminants are more easily detected and differential counts on mixed cultures can be carried out more satisfactorily.

The main disadvantage of surface methods is the uncertainty that the small sample volumes represent the original populations in the suspensions.

ROLL TUBE METHOD

Originally roll tubes were prepared by adding the dilution of organisms to a small volume of nutrient agar in a test tube or boiling tube, shaking to mix the contents and rotating almost horizontally, under cold water or in a hollowed block of ice, until the medium had set in a thin film around the inside of

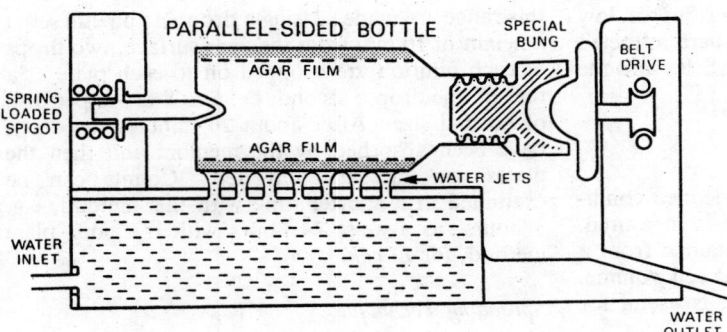

Fig. 28.11 Astell spinning bottle system

the tube. Nowadays, the Astell spinning bottle technique (Fig. 28.11) is preferred by most workers. After rolling, the bottles are incubated inverted for a time intermediate between those for pour and surface plates. A special illuminator, that facilitates counting, can be obtained. The ideal number of organisms is between 100 and 200 per bottle. The rubber stoppers should be loosened during incubation to prevent oxygen lack.

Membrane Filtration

This technique, which is outlined on p. 318, is useful when the number of organisms in the suspension is very low. Using a filter of 47 or 50 mm diameter, up to 200 colonies can be counted without difficulty. Care must be taken not to use too much medium for soaking the absorbent pad or liquid will creep round the edge of the filter and spread the colonies. By using a stereoscopic microscope and surface illumination counting can be done before the colonies run into one another. The method is widely applicable although there are a few organisms that are difficult to grow on membranes.

Fluid Media Techniques

A series of, usually 1 in 10, dilutions of the suspension are made in a suitable fluid medium. Dilution is continued to the point at which there is a low probability of an organism being present in the tube. The tubes are incubated and examined for signs of growth, usually turbidity. The result can be expressed as, for example, 'viable bacteria are present in a 1 in 10^4 but not in a 1 in 10^5 dilution' or it can be assumed that the last tube showing growth contains one organism and, by multiplying this by the degree of dilution a figure for the number of organisms per cm^3 obtained. Without replication this method is very inaccurate but with a satisfactory number of replicates and correct design, statistical methods can be used to provide a more reliable indication of the 'most probable number' of bacteria present.

Counting in fluid media is of value when organisms will not grow on solid media (e.g. coliforms in water). It is sometimes more convenient for anaerobes because, provided the medium is adequately reduced (p. 304), there is no need to incubate in an oxygen-free atmosphere, as with most solid media techniques.

Counting Anaerobes

The solid media methods of counting described above can be used for anaerobes provided that the containers are incubated under anaerobic conditions. Oxygen-free diluting fluids may be necessary, e.g. solutions containing reducing agents which have been boiled and cooled before use, or fluid anaerobic media.

Two special methods are—

(*a*) *The Miller-Prickett Tube.* In this the organism is mixed with nutrient agar in a tube that is flattened oval in section and has a longish narrow neck. The agar suspension fills the body of the tube and the neck is sealed with agar containing a reducing agent and an oxidation-reduction indicator. Colonies grow throughout the agar but can be seen for counting because the tube is so flat.

(*b*) *Ingram's Method.* This is essentially the same as the previous method except that normal tubes or bottles are used. After introducing the suspension in agar, a thick sterile black rod is placed down the centre of the container and the medium solidifies around this. Because the agar layer is relatively thin and the organisms are viewed against a black background, counting is facilitated.

For neither of these methods is incubation in an anaerobe jar essential.

Errors of Counting

SAMPLING ERRORS

These arise because bacteria are not evenly distributed in the material under examination. There should be very little variation between samples from mobile liquids provided these are shaken well immediately before the samples are removed. With solid, semi-solid or viscous preparations (e.g. surgical dressings and ointments) it is more difficult to ensure that the sample represents the whole and portions should be selected in a random manner and be adequate in number and size (*see* Sterility Testing, Gunn and Carter, 1965).

ERRORS OF DILUTING AND PIPETTING

Often considerable dilution is necessary to reduce the number of bacteria in a sample to a level at which counting is possible: At each stage error can occur. Some important precautions are—

1. The diluent must be chosen with care—

(*a*) It must not harm bacterial cells, e.g. it must have a satisfactory osmotic pressure and must be free from toxic heavy metals, such as copper ions from older types of metal stills.

(*b*) It must not encourage division of the cells. If a nutritive diluent, such as peptone water or broth, is used, it must be kept cool and the dilutions must be performed as rapidly as possible.

(*c*) It must not interfere with the measuring technique, e.g. a coloured diluent would affect the use of a colorimeter.

Common diluents are water (from an all-glass still), normal saline, $\frac{1}{4}$ strength Ringer's solutions and $\frac{1}{10}$ phosphate buffer of pH 7. Survival tests are carried out to show that the chosen diluent has no harmful effect on the organism.

2. The sterile diluent should be distributed aseptically into sterile containers. Sterilisation after packing can lead to changes in volume. Certain types of rubber liner can yield bactericidal impurities during autoclaving.

3. For critical work the temperature of the diluent should be kept constant throughout the dilution procedure.

4. Glassware must be scrupulously clean since traces of adsorbed detergent or disinfectant leached into the diluent could have disastrous effects on the count.

5. Dropping pipettes must be accurately calibrated. The size of the drop is influenced by the external diameter at the tip, by the temperature and surface tension of the liquid and by the rate of dropping. Calibration is by weighing numbers of drops and by checking statistically the variation within and between pipettes.

6. Before measurement, the suspension should be drawn up and down in the pipette several times to reduce loss of cells from deposition on the pipette wall.

7. Throughout, great care should be taken not to introduce contaminants.

ERRORS DUE TO THE CULTURE MEDIUM

The medium used for counting should be accurately reproducible and uniform throughout; it should give maximum and concordant counts from time to time and batch to batch. Statistical tests are necessary to confirm that these requirements are satisfied.

ERRORS OF COUNTING COLONIES

Small colonies may be missed if a lens is not used. If the number of colonies is large a hand tally or an electro-magnetic counter is helpful. The counting of large numbers is also facilitated by dividing the container into small areas with waxed pencil lines and counting each separately.

PERSONAL ERRORS

These are related to the carefulness and technical ability of the worker. They can often be reduced, e.g. by holding a dropping pipette in a stand instead of the hand, by timing the fall of drops with a metronome and by the use of aids for counting colonies. (For a comprehensive discussion of counting errors *see* Wilson, 1935).

A pharmaceutical microbiologist needs a working knowledge of statistics so that he can discuss with a trained statistician the design of his experiments and the interpretation of his results. A good design is of prime importance and when this has been devised the error of the technique should be estimated. The Chi-squared test (Index of Scatter) is used to confirm that experimental results do not differ significantly from those predicted by mathematical theory.

BIBLIOGRAPHY

AINSWORTH, G. C. and SNEATH, P. H. A. (1962) *Microbial Classification. 12th Symposium of the Society for General Microbiology.* Cambridge University Press.

BAILEY, N. T. J. (1959) *Statistical Methods in Biology.* English Universities Press, London.

BERGEY, D. H. (1957) *Manual of Determinative Bacteriology.* 7th ed. Williams and Wilkins Co. Baltimore.

COWAN, S. and STEEL, K. J. (1965) *Manual for the Identification of Medical Bacteria.* Cambridge University Press.

FISHER, R. A. and YATES, F. (1957) *Statistical Tables for Biological, Agricultural and Medical Research.* Oliver and Boyd, Edinburgh.

GIBBS, B. M. and SKINNER, F. A. (1966) *Identification Methods for Microbiologists Part A*. Academic Press, London.

GIBBS, B. M. and SHAPTON, D. A. (1968) *Identification Methods for Microbiologists Part B*. Academic Press, London.

GUNN, C. and CARTER, S. J. (1965) *Dispensing for Pharmaceutical Students*. 11th ed. Pitman Medical, London.

NORRIS, J. R. and RIBBONS, D. W. (1969) *Methods in Microbiology* (7 volumes.) Academic Press, London.

SALLE, A. J. (1961) *Fundamental Principles of Bacteriology*. 5th ed. McGraw-Hill, New York.

SHAPTON, D. A. and GOULD, G. W. (1969) *Isolation Methods for Microbiologists*. Academic Press, London.

SKERMAN, V. B. D. (1959) *A Guide to the Identification of the Genera of Bacteria*. Williams and Wilkins Co., Baltimore.

WILSON, G. S. (1935) *The Bacteriological Grading of Milk. Medical Research Council Special Report No. 206*. H.M.S.O., London.

REFERENCES

BAILLIE, A. and NORRIS, J. R. (1963) Studies of enzyme changes during sporulation in *Bacillus cereus* using starch-gel electrophoresis. *J. appl. Bact.*, **26**, 102–106.

HARRIS, N. D. (1963) The influence of recovery medium and incubation temperature on the survival of damaged bacteria. *J. appl. Bact.*, **26**, 387–397.

MCCRADY, M. H. (1918) Tables for the most probable numbers of coliform organisms in water samples. *Can. publ. Hlth. J.*, **9**, 201.

NORRIS, J. R. (1964) The classification of *Bacillus thuringiensis*. *J. appl. Bact.*, **27**, 439–447.

OUCHTERLONY, O. (1962) Diffusion in gel methods for immunological analysis. II. *Prog. Allergy*, **6**, 30–154.

PITTMAN, M. (1946) A study of fluid thioglycollate medium for the sterility test. *J. Bact.*, **51**, 19–32.

SOCIETY FOR APPLIED BACTERIOLOGY (1956) Symposium on anaerobic bacteria. *J. appl. Bact.*, **19**, 112–180.

TAYLOR, J. (1962) Estimation of bacterial numbers by a ten-fold dilution series. *J. appl. Bact.*, **25**, 54–61.

WALKER, P. D. and BATTY, I. (1964) Fluorescent studies in the genus Clostridium I. Location of antigens on the surface of *Clostridium sporogenes* during sporulation and germination. *J. appl. Bact.*, **27**, 137–139.

29

Dynamics of Antimicrobial Action

Action Rates of Antimicrobial Chemicals

QUANTITATIVE expressions for rates of disinfection date from the beginning of the twentieth century. Rideal and Walker (1903) and Chick (1908) carried out many determinations on the effect of chemicals on bacteria. Watson (1908) derived mathematical expressions from Chick's data and showed that the reaction rate could be expressed in the same form as a first order chemical reaction, the determinant being the number of cells in the culture. Interpretations of this kind that are based on theoretical mechanisms are called *mechanistic* theories. The resulting expression is—

$$K = \log(a/a - x) \times t^{-1}$$

where K is the rate constant;
   t is the time of contact before the sample is removed;
   a is the initial number of bacteria in the culture; and
   $a - x$ is the number of organisms in the same volume after exposure for time t.
For mathematical convenience, this equation is usually written in its log form and graphs are drawn of log number of survivors against log time of exposure in minutes. When killing occurs at a fast rate, the plot is a straight line; hence the term logarithmic order of death is often used to describe this type of death rate (Fig. 29.1).

Later workers, using lower concentrations of bactericides and, therefore, slower rates of kill, found that the plot was not straight but S-shaped (sigmoid), as in Fig. 29.2. Many suggestions were made and much experimental work was done in attempts to explain this type of curve. The same result is obtained in toxicity testing, when the number of animals killed by doses of a drug (in log units) are being investigated, and it has been shown that this response is obtained because the sensitivities of the animals to the toxic agent are not the same but follow a normal distribution. It therefore seemed possible that the resistance of a population of micro-organisms to a bactericide would also be distributed normally in relation to the log of the time of exposure, since the latter is a form of dosage. This assumption led to a mathematical treatment that took into account the variation in resistance in a population of organisms in a culture and produced a straight line graph. Because this

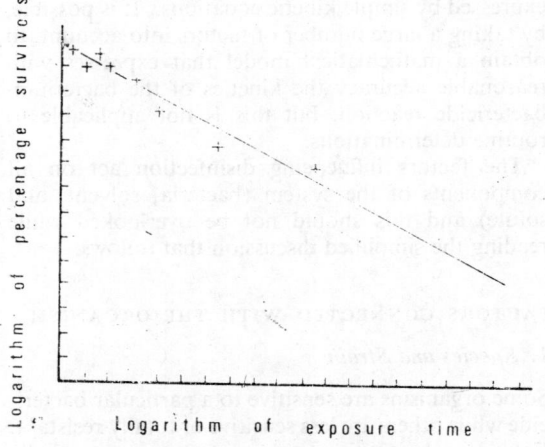

Fig. 29.1   The logarithmic order of bacterial death

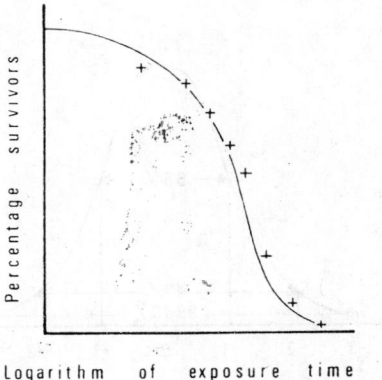

Fig. 29.2   A sigmoid time-survivor curve

interpretation allows for natural variation it is sometimes known as the *vitalistic* theory.

Figure 29.3 represents a normal distribution curve. The point 0 represents the mean resistance and −2 and +2 are spaced so that the distance of each from 0 along the log time axis represents two standard deviations (*see* a textbook on statistics). The part to the left of −2 represents 2·5 per cent, that between −2 and +2, 95 per cent and that to the right of +2, the remaining 2·5 per cent, of the area under the curve. This means that at the times corresponding to −2, 0, and +2, 2·5, 50, and 97·5 per cent respectively of the total population would be killed. Consequently, it is possible to express percentages of a population in terms of the standard error of the system. Gaddum (1933) used this technique in biological assays that involved the death of proportions of groups of animals and he called the numerical values derived from the normal distribution, normal equivalent deviates (NED). The 50 per cent value was designated zero and values to the left and right of this were given negative and positive values respectively. For the above example the following values would be allocated—

Per cent	NED
2·5	−2
50	0
97·5	+2

This interpretation produced a straight line with biological toxicity data, but in mathematical processing the negative sign was an encumbrance. Bliss (1934), working on population mortality statistics, suggested that it would be more convenient if 50 per cent were given the value of 5 instead of zero and 5 was added to all of Gaddum's NED values, so that a negative value would be rare. The new units so obtained were named

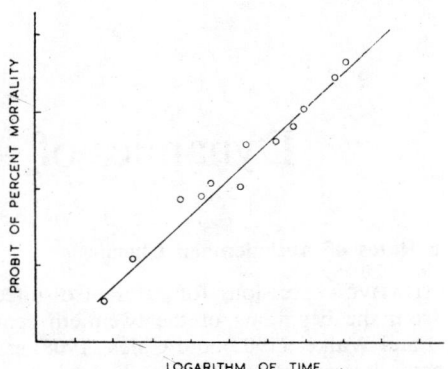

Fig. 29.4 Log time versus probit percent mortality

probability units, eventually shortened to *probits*, and, since about 1947, this system has been used in evaluating survivor data in studies of the action of bactericides. When probits are plotted against log time of exposure a straight line generally results (Fig. 29.4). Tables relating percentages to probits will be found in the statistical tables of Fisher and Yates (1957).

Although, in pharmacy and microbiology, the vitalistic theory has been widely applied to the destruction of bacteria by chemicals and by other lethal agents, it is not widely used outside these fields.

Factors Affecting Rate of Antimicrobial Action

The above discussion shows that the relationship between chemical and biological factors cannot be expressed by simple kinetic equations. It is possible, by taking a large number of factors into account, to obtain a mathematical model that expresses with reasonable accuracy the kinetics of the bacterium-bactericide reaction, but this is not applicable to routine determinations.

The factors influencing disinfection act on all components of the system (bacteria, solvent, and solute) and this should not be overlooked while reading the simplified discussion that follows.

FACTORS CONNECTED WITH THE ORGANISM

1. *Species and Strain*

Some organisms are sensitive to a particular bactericide while others are less sensitive or totally resistant. For example, Gram-positive bacteria are normally susceptible to penicillin whereas Gram-negative species are much less so. In addition, some bacteria

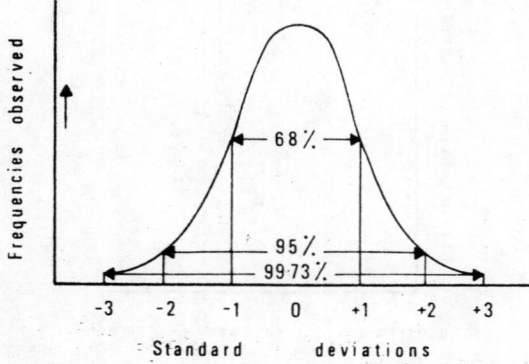

Fig. 29.3 Properties of the Normal (Gaussian) distribution curve

can develop resistance to a drug to which they were originally sensitive (*see* p. 308).

2. *Morphological State*

The spores of sporing organisms are more able than the vegetative forms to resist the action of chemicals. Higher resistance may also be found in bacteria with slime layers or capsules because these may prevent penetration of the bactericide into the cell. The water-repellant layer of the mycobacteria behaves similarly.

3. *Cultural State*

Ability to resist chemical action is usually low when an organism is in an active metabolic state, e.g. when the cells are actively dividing in the log phase of growth. This sensitivity may be due to even minor interference with the replication of nucleic acids and with protein synthesis having a profound effect on the continuation of high metabolic activity. This is well-illustrated by the action of antibiotics, such as tetracycline, which interfere with protein synthesis; small changes in protein synthesis and, therefore, enzyme production, result in marked changes in the sugar-utilising capacity of the cells. It is possible, also, that certain components of the cell are incompletely laid down and, if this happens in the wall, organisms will be more susceptible to chemicals at the point of division. Interference with cells in rapid division may cause activities to get out of phase; e.g. the genetic material may be synthesised at a rate different from that of other components and, therefore, the control mechanisms may break down.

4. *Previous History*

The nature of the culture medium influences the type of metabolite produced by the growing organism. Hugo and Stretton (1966) have shown that glycerol-containing media promote synthesis of lipids in certain organisms and that this results in increased resistance to penicillin. Another example is when bacteria are grown in medium rich in thiol groups; their protoplasm becomes rich in thiol-containing protein which can bind a higher concentration of metal ions such as Hg^{++} or As^{+++} before metabolism is blocked and inhibition of growth occurs.

FACTORS CONNECTED WITH THE REACTION MEDIUM

1. *Nature of the Medium*

Most bactericides are more active in aqueous solution than in an organic or oily solvent (*see*

Phenols). Secondly, if the determination is carried out in a nutrient medium the organisms may multiply making the reaction difficult to follow

2. *Inoculum Size*

If all of the organisms in the initial inoculum are alive, reaction rates may be accurately predicted as indicated in the section on Action Rates. This will not apply if the inoculum contains an appreciable number of dead cells. For example, if the bactericide is only slightly soluble its solution could become seriously depleted due to take-up of the chemical by the dead cells.

3. *Concentration of the Bactericide*

The effect of this is usually expressed by the equation—

$$K = C^n t$$

Where K is the rate constant; C is usually the concentration of the bactericide; n is the concentration exponent for the particular system; and t is the time required to produce a given result.

For a number of bactericides this equation holds true over a fairly wide range of concentrations but a better parameter to use for C would be the product of chemical activity (reactivity) and concentration, as used in more sophisticated calculations in chemical kinetics. Reactivity takes into account such phenomena as ionisation and intermolecular bonding when the chemical potential of a reactant in a system and, hence, its reaction rate is being determined. In very dilute solutions it bears a direct relationship to concentration but in more concentrated solutions departure from this is marked. (*See* a textbook of chemical thermodynamics for a more complete explanation.)

The simple equation presupposes that the chemical is inimical to the organism at all concentration levels. From studies of adsorption of chemicals at surfaces (*see* p. 42) and the kinetics of heterogenous catalysis in enzyme systems (*see* p. 96) it can be seen that the parameters are the same (Fig. 29.5). This means that in many cases there will be a minimal concentration below which no reaction will take place, because insufficient chemical reaches the enzyme receptors, and a maximal concentration above which the reaction rate does not increase, probably because the receptor sites have become saturated with the chemical or because steric interference prevents further adsorption.

The equation is useful—

(*a*) in deciding the type of bactericide to use in a particular situation;

(*b*) in choosing a method for recovering organisms

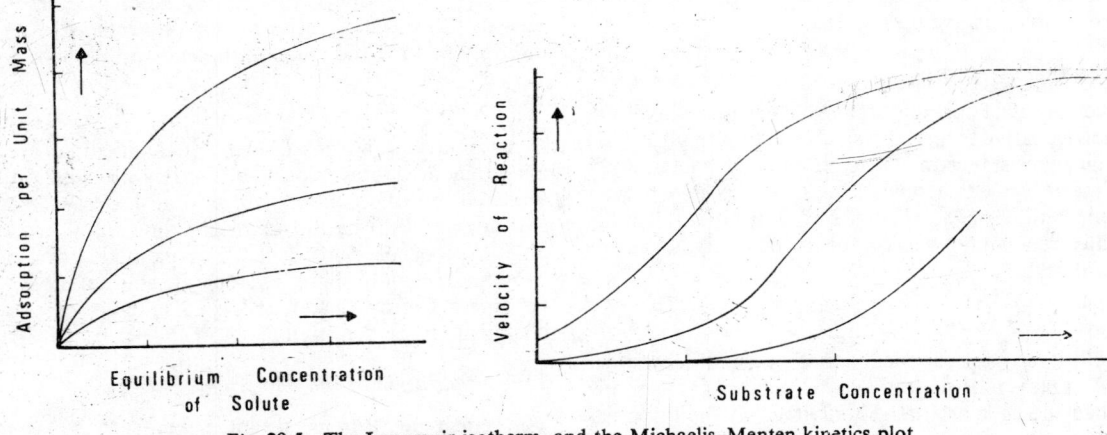

Fig. 29.5   The Langmuir isotherm, and the Michaelis–Menten kinetics plot

after contact with a bactericide in disinfectant tests;

(c) in choosing an inactivating agent for sterility tests.

The following example indicates how it can be used to solve a practical problem—

Example: A 1 per cent solution of a phenolic disinfectant, with a concentration exponent of 6, kills a culture in 10 minutes. In what time would a 0·5 per cent solution kill the culture, under the same conditions?

$K = C^n t$, ∴ for 1 per cent solution, $K = 1^6 \times 10$
$$= 10$$

K for 0·5 per cent solution

$= K$ for 1 per cent solution $= 10$

∴ for 0·5 per cent solution $10 = (0·5)^6 \times t$
$$= t/64$$
i.e. $t = 640$ min.

Examples illustrating the value of the equation in sterility testing are given by Gunn and Carter (1965). These show that the inhibitory effect of a bactericide in a disinfectant test or in sterility testing may be removed by dilution if the value of n is large; if the value is small, chemical neutralisation of the bactericide is preferable.

FACTORS CONNECTED WITH THE ORGANISM AND THE REACTION MEDIUM

1. *Temperature*

The effect of temperature on a chemical reaction may be predicted by the Arrhenius equation (*see* p. 97). When this is applied to antimicrobial reactions it is usually restricted to the range 15 to 45°C. This is because temperature has profound effects on the microbial cell; below 15°C enzyme activity is at a low level and above 45°C there is considerable inactivation of enzyme systems. Between 15 and 45°C the effect of temperature on the bactericide far outweighs any effect on the micro-organisms. The simplified form of the equation, as used in microbiology, is—

$$\frac{K_1}{K_2} = \theta^{(T_2 - T_1)}$$

where T_1 and T_2 are the lower and higher temperatures respectively and K_1 and K_2 are the corresponding reaction rates. The value θ is known as the temperature coefficient of the reaction. It is an exponential function, and for each 10°C change of temperature within the range mentioned above is closely allied to the value of n for the bactericide. It is of considerable value in deciding which bactericide to use in practice, particularly where a wide temperature range will be encountered or where temperatures of use are not accurately known.

In some sterilisation procedures used in the pharmaceutical and food industries the temperature must be kept low to avoid damaging the product; an antibacterial substance that is active at the temperature employed may be added at a non-toxic concentration to potentiate the heat treatment. In the production of the type of vaccine that contains dead organisms the sterilisation process must not damage the antigens (*see* p. 386) and, therefore, heat cannot be used in certain cases; one alternative is to kill the organisms by treatment, at room temperature, with a bactericide having a low temperature coefficient.

2. *pH*

The effects of the pH of the reaction mixture are complex and difficult to predict. Changes in pH can markedly affect the nature of the bactericide and its receptor sites in the bacterial cell. Sometimes, as with the triphenylmethane dyes, there is a profound change in the ionisation of the bactericide, resulting in dramatic changes in its activity. In one experiment the minimum inhibitory concentration (MIC) of crystal violet for *Staphylococcus aureus* in a peptone water medium at pH 7 was 1×10^{-7} molar, but when the pH was raised to 8 the MIC became 4×10^{-9} molar. Alterations in the pH or protein content of a medium may affect its buffering capacity because the buffering effects of different proteins at various pHs are not the same, due to differences in their iso-electric points. Consequently, statements of MIC values should be accompanied by a clear indication of the conditions under which they were obtained.

3. Oxidation-Reduction Potential

The oxidation-reduction potentials of reaction media are important where bactericides act by oxidation or reduction. Many antibacterial agents (e.g. the hypochlorites) oxidise bacterial proteins and the presence of reducing substances, in the form of protein or other organic matter, leads to considerable loss of activity and, sometimes, failure of the disinfection process. To prevent this, surfaces or equipment should be thoroughly cleaned before treatment with the disinfectant. When hypochlorite is used to treat water the *biological oxygen demand* (BOD) of the water is first estimated; then enough hypochlorite is added to neutralise this and leave an excess for killing the micro-organisms. In the dairy and food industries where hypochlorites are in regular use, great importance is attached to removing 'soil' before disinfection is attempted. Similar precautions should be taken when oxidising bactericides are being evaluated.

Potassium permanganate solutions are sometimes dispensed as mild antiseptics and care should be taken to avoid contact with bark corks because reducing substances in these can lower the potency of the solutions.

4. Reaction between Bactericides and Constituents of the Reaction Medium

(a) *Chemical.* A molecular species in the bactericide may combine with one in the reaction mixture, modifying the kinetics of the reaction. In some instances combination is incomplete and a reversible or equilibrium reaction takes place. An example is the inactivation of bactericides containing Hg^{++} ions by thiol-containing compounds such as proteins—

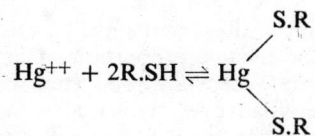

$$Hg^{++} + 2R.SH \rightleftharpoons Hg \begin{matrix} \nearrow S.R \\ \searrow S.R \end{matrix}$$

(b) *Physico-chemical.* If the reaction mixture is biphasic several major changes may occur—

Adsorption—When finely divided particles or droplets are present, molecules of the bactericide may be adsorbed and become unavailable for action on the bacteria unless a large excess is present in the solution. This problem arises in the preservation of suspensions.

Partition—When two liquid phases are present, as in a mixture of oil or water or in an emulsion, the important concentration is that in the aqueous phase in contact with the micro-organisms. If the bactericide is much more soluble in oil than in water its effects will be reduced in the presence of lipid materials. This is true of the highly substituted phenols that are used to preserve oil-in-water creams.

(c) *Biochemical.* Sometimes the bactericide acts on a specific metabolic pathway in the organism; this usually results in reversible blockage of the synthesis of an essential metabolite. Substances in the reaction mixture may remove such a blockage; a supply of the elaborated metabolite may be sufficient but often a high concentration of one of the precursors is more effective; in addition, if the metabolite or its intermediates can be produced from alternative starting materials sufficient of these may overcome the blockage.

5. Surface Effects

Surface active agents are often used in the formulation of pharmaceutical preparations that require preservation, and in the formulation of concentrated solutions of bactericides that are diluted before use. Hence their effects are very important and they vary with the bactericide and the surface active agent.

A. Bactericide with Marked Surface Activity

(a) Surfactant with same charge as bactericide

Because there is no ionic antagonism in this case, the bactericide is not inactivated by coacervation (*see* p. 60). There are three possibilities: firstly, the surfactant may not affect the bactericidal activity; secondly, the effects of bactericide and surfactant may be additive; and thirdly, there may be synergism, i.e. a more marked effect than would be expected from addition of the two actions.

(b) Surfactant with opposite charge to bactericide

This reduces the antibacterial effect to a degree that depends on the relative proportion of ions of the two substances. Where the proportion of bactericide is greater than one, compared with the surfactant, some antibacterial action will remain, but if the proportion is less than one the antibacterial activity will be lost through precipitation.

(c) Non-ionic surface-active agents (see below)

B. Bactericide without Marked Surface Activity

(a) Effects of ions of bactericide on ions of surfactant

The interactions will be as described in A, (a) and (b). They are of great importance in the formulation of creams as vehicles for ionic bactericidal agents such as the medicinal dyes, where incompatibilities between medicaments and surfactants can have serious effects on activity and appearance.

(b) Non-ionic surfactants

Often non-ionic surfactants are ethers, e.g. the polyethylene glycols and some sorbitan derivatives, and they may contain hydroxy groupings, e.g. all of the sorbitans. Hydrogen bonding takes place between these types of compound and —OH, —NH$_2$, and —COOH groups in bactericides. Because this bonding is reversible it does not completely inactivate the bactericide but the effects are hard to predict. Consequently, when a system containing such agents is being formulated, it is necessary to check the effectiveness of antimicrobial preservatives by inoculation with a suitable range of micro-organisms and storage under conditions similar to those that the product will encounter in practice. The storage life of the preparation is based on the results of these tests. Present knowledge of these systems does not allow transfer of information on stability from one formulation to another.

(c) Colloidal electrolytes

Many antimicrobial substances are only slightly soluble in water and must be solubilised by the use of colloidal electrolytes (see p. 61); alkali soaps of long chain fatty acids are often used, as in Lysol, B.P. Formulations of this type are issued as concentrates and diluted before use. The death time curves of these preparations are very complex, as was shown by Alexander and Trim (1946), Berry and Bean (1951) and Berry, Cook and Wills (1956) (see Fig. 29.6).

The shape of these curves is partly explained by postulating a biphasic system in the solution after

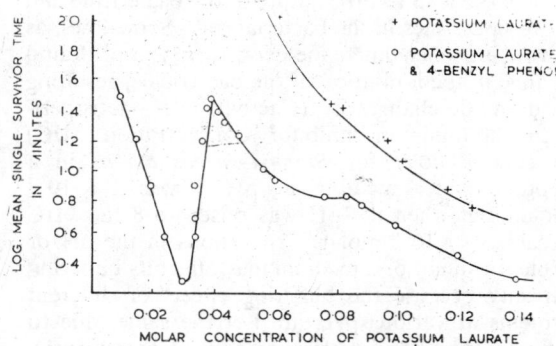

Fig. 29.6   The activities of benzylphenol-potassium laurate mixtures at 20°C

(*After Berry et al.*, 1956)

micelles have been formed, and a partition of the bactericide between the bulk phase (aqueous solution) and the micellar phase (equivalent to a non-aqueous phase) which results in loss of bactericidal activity (Evans and Dunbar, 1965). However, this theory does not account for the second increase in activity shown on Fig. 29.6. An alternative explanation can be suggested by considering the partition of soap between the bulk phase, the micellar phase and the surface of the micro-organisms. To assist this explanation the graph has been divided into three concentration zones; I, II, and III.

Zone I (below 0.03 mol/dm^3)

Here the soap occurs as single ions or small aggregates, such as doublets, tetrads, or more and these are adsorbed at the bacterial surface. This adsorption increases rapidly as the soap concentration increases and as a result the surface of the bacterium is altered leading to modifications of the cytoplasmic membrane and metabolic changes that facilitate penetration of the bactericide. Consequently, the killing time falls very rapidly as the soap concentration increases. Because there are no micelles present, the concentration of the bactericide in the bulk phase is constant and nearly at saturation point; therefore, bactericidal activity is high.

Zone II (0.03 to 0.045 mol/dm^3)

At the division between zones I and II (the critical concentration for the formation of micelles) the thermodynamic properties of the soap solution change. Most of the soap ions form into micelles, leaving less in the bulk phase; consequently, surface effects are reduced and this appears to continue throughout zone II. The micelle to bulk partition favours the concentration of many bactericides in the micellar phase and so the concentration in the bulk phase falls, lowering the activity of the system and increasing the death time, in spite of the fact that the soap concentration is increasing.

Zone III (above 0.045 mol/dm³)

In this zone the soap death-time curve and the soap-phenol death time curves are parallel and therefore the shape of this part of the curve appears to be determined by the soap concentration. It would seem that there is a second critical concentration value in the aqueous soap system where the number of free ions again increases proportionally to the increase in soap concentration. The result is probably similar to that in zone I. The phenol-soap curve is downwardly displaced in relation to the soap curve and as this displacement is approximately constant it suggests that the concentration of phenol in the bulk phase is fairly constant at the soap concentrations of zone III. This hypothesis cannot be confirmed at present because it is not possible to determine the concentrations of soap or phenol in the micelles.

This phenomenon is important in the dilution of concentrated solutions for use. A horizontal line in Fig. 29.6 represents the situation when a concentrated solution is being diluted; there is anomalous behaviour as the solution is diluted from right to left. First, there is an increase in death time, then a decrease and, finally, a sharp increase. Hence it is most economical to formulate for maximum activity at low concentration; that is, near to the critical concentration of soap for the formation of micelles (CMC). The preparation should also be formulated to give a broad curve of approximately equal activity about the CMC; this increases the chance of the preparation being active when diluted by an unskilled person.

BIBLIOGRAPHY

DEAN, A. C. R. and HINSHELWOOD, C. (1966) *Growth Function and Regulation in Bacterial Cells.* Clarendon Press, Oxford.

FISHER, R. E. and YATES, F. (1957) *Statistical Tables.* Oliver and Boyd, Edinburgh.

GADDUM, J. H. (1933) *Report on Biological Standards III. Methods of biological assay depending on a quantal response. Medical Research Council Special Report Series No. 183.* H.M.S.O., London.

RAHN, O. (1945) *The Injury and Death of Bacteria by Chemical Agents. Biodynamica No. 3.* Normandy, Missouri.

SOCIETY FOR CHEMICAL INDUSTRY (1965) *Surface Activity and the Bacterial Cell. S.C.I. Monograph No. 19.* Society for Chemical Industry, London.

REFERENCES

ALEXANDER, A. E. and TRIM, A. R. (1946) The biological activity of phenolic compounds. The effect of surface active substances upon the penetration of hexylresorcinol into *Ascaris lumbricoides var. suis. Proc. R. Soc.,* B133, 220–234.

BEAN, H. S. (1967) Types and characteristics of disinfectants. *J. appl. Bact.,* 30, 6–16.

BEAN, H. S. and BERRY, H. (1951) The bactericidal action of benzylchlorphenol in aqueous solutions of potassium laurate. *J. Pharm. Pharmac.,* 3, 639–655.

BERRY, H., COOK, A. M., and WILLS, B. A. (1956) The bactericidal activity of soap—phenol mixtures. *ibid,* 8, 425–441.

BERRY, H. and MICHAELS, I. (1950) The evaluation of the bactericidal activity of ethylene glycol and some of its monoalkyl ethers against *Bacterium coli. ibid,* 2, 27–38.

BLISS, C. I. (1934) The method of probits. *Science,* 78, 38.

CHICK, H. (1908) An investigation of the laws of disinfection. *J. Hyg., Camb.,* 8, 92–158.

CHICK, H. (1910) The process of disinfection by chemical agencies and hot water. *ibid.,* 10, 237.

EVANS, W. P. and DUNBAR, S. F. (1965) The effect of surfactants on germicides and preservatives. In *Surface Activity and the Microbial Cell. S.C.I. Monograph. No. 19.* See bibliography.

HUGO, W. B. and STRETTON, R. J. (1966) The role of cellular lipid in the resistance of Gram-positive organisms to penicillins. *J. gen. Microbiol.,* 42, 133–138.

JACOBS, S. E. and HARRIS, N. D. (1961) The effect of modifications in the counting medium on the viability and growth of bacteria damaged by phenols. *J. appl. Bact.,* 24, 172–181.

JACOBS, S. E. (1960) Some aspects of the dynamics of disinfection. *J. Pharm. Pharmac.,* 12, 9T–18T.

JENSEN, E. and JENSEN, V. (1938) Studies on the influence of various organic substances upon the phenol coefficient. *J. Hyg., Camb.,* 38, 141–149.

JORDAN, R. C. and JACOBS, S. E. (1944) Studies in the dynamics of disinfection. I. Distribution of resistance. *ibid.,* 43, 275–289. II. Calculation of the concentration exponent for phenol at 35°C. *ibid.,* 43, 363–369.

JORDAN, R. C. and JACOBS, S. E. (1945) III. The reaction between phenol and *Bact. coli.*: The effects of temperature and concentration with a detailed analysis of reaction velocity. *ibid,* 44, 210–220. V. The temperature coefficient of the reaction between phenol and *Bact. coli.* derived from data obtained by an improved technique. *ibid.*, **44**, 243–248. VI. Calculation of a new and constant temperature coefficient for the reaction between phenol and *Bact. coli. ibid.*, **44**, 249–255. VII. The reaction between phenol and *Bact. coli.* The effect of temperature on the usually accepted concentration exponent and the calculation of a more satisfactory exponent based on theoretical considerations. *ibid.*, **44**, 421–429.

RIDEAL, S. and WALKER, J. T. A. (1903) The standard-ization of disinfectants. *Jl R. sanit. Inst.*, **24**, 424–441.

WATSON, H. E. (1908) A note on the variation of the rate of disinfection with change in concentration of disinfectant. *J. Hyg., Camb.*, **8**, 536.

WITHELL, E. R. (1938) The evaluation of bactericidal action. *Q. Jl Pharm. Pharmac.*, **11**, 736–757.

WITHELL, E. R. (1942) The significance of the vari-ation in the shape of time-survivor curves. *J. Hyg., Camb.*, **42**, 124–183.

30

Evaluation Techniques in Microbiology

Definitions

BACTERICIDE (Germicide)

A CHEMICAL substance used to kill bacteria. The corresponding terms for viruses and fungi are virucide and fungicide respectively.

DISINFECTANT

A chemical used to destroy the biological agents that cause disease in man, animals, or plants. The term is commonly applied when destruction takes place in, or on, inanimate objects.

ANTISEPTIC

Strictly this is a chemical used to prevent sepsis (blood poisoning) but the term is normally used for a substance applied to the tissues of humans or animals to inhibit or destroy invading organisms.

INHIBITOR (Bacteriophrenic)

A substance that causes micro-organisms to grow at a slower rate than normal.

BACTERIOSTAT

A substance that holds the number of bacteria at a constant level (similarly, virustat and fungistat).

ANTAGONISER

A substance that prevents or reverses the action of an antimicrobial substance.

SANITISER

A chemical that reduces the number of organisms and destroys any that might cause disease in man or economically important animals. The term is generally applied to substances used to treat utensils and equipment in the food and drink industries.

ESSENTIAL METABOLITE

A nutritional substance essential for the growth and reproduction of a particular organism.

ANTIMETABOLITE

A substance that either opposes the action of a metabolite or prevents its assimilation by an organism.

In the evaluation of microbial chemicals some fundamentals must be decided—

1. What is Death of a Micro-organism?

Because so many methods have been used to evaluate bactericides, this apparently simple question does not have a simple answer. The criterion of death that is most often applied is inability of a sample of stated size, taken from a reaction mixture, to produce growth within a given time in a defined medium at a defined temperature. The signs of growth that are normally accepted are either turbidity in a liquid medium or colonies in, or on, a solid medium.

The factors that influence the capacity of a culture to demonstrate growth include—

(a) VIABILITY OF THE ORGANISM

Viability means ability to produce growth. If no growth is produced this does not mean that the organism is dead; nutrients necessary for the manifestation of life may be absent, e.g. if a key enzyme is missing, because of a mutation, the organism will not grow and will appear to be dead.

(b) PRESENCE OF INHIBITORS IN THE GROWTH MEDIUM

These may arise from two sources—
(i) *Constituents of the Medium.* Jacobs and Harris (1961) have shown that some agars inhibit the growth of organisms previously treated with bactericides.

(ii) *Transfer of Bactericide from the Reaction Mixture to the Recovery Medium.* If the resulting concentration is enough to inhibit the growth of surviving organisms the bactericide must be neutralised, or removed by filtering the organisms from the sample, washing and incubating the filter pad in a nutrient medium.

(c) NUMBER OF ORGANISMS IN THE SAMPLE TAKEN FROM THE REACTION MIXTURE

Near the point of extinction of a culture, prediction of the number of organisms likely to be removed in a sample of given size depends on the Poisson distribution. In deciding sample size and the number of replicates, knowledge of the probable number of survivors is necessary, as is illustrated by the following example—

In a disinfection experiment an inoculum of 5×10^6 organisms is added to 50 cm^3 of reaction mixture and it is expected that 0·1 per cent will survive. What size of sample must be taken to obtain growth in a tube of nutrient broth?

Original concentration of organisms in 1 cm^3 of reaction mixture $= 1 \times 10^5$.

If only 0·1 per cent survive, the final number in 1 cm^3 will be 1×10^2.

Therefore, the minimum size of sample that could be expected to contain an average of one organism is 1×10^{-2} cm^3, but, from the Poisson distribution it can be shown that survivors would be taken up in only three such samples out of every ten which means that the minimum sample size that will give growth in every tube is about 4×10^{-2} cm^3.

However, to be reasonably sure of obtaining survivors in each sample, the volume should be about 1×10^{-1} cm^3. Alternatively, if replicates of the minimum sample size are taken, about four would be necessary. At higher levels of kill the level of sampling must be raised accordingly.

(d) SENSITIVITY OF THE MEDIUM

Even if organisms survive bactericidal action they may be unable to grow in, or on, media that would support the growth of untreated organisms. Organisms from a hostile environment are often very exacting with respect to nutritional requirements.

(e) INCUBATION TEMPERATURE

Usually the recovery and growth of damaged organisms require a temperature different from the optimum for undamaged cells (Society for Applied Bacteriology, 1963). Generally a lower temperature is best during the early stage of incubation, because it slows down deleterious processes and allows repair to take place. Once recovery is well under way it is often beneficial to raise the temperature.

(f) INCUBATION TIME

After treatment by heat, irradiation or chemicals, repair precedes the reproduction of survivors. Onset of the normal growth curve for the organism is delayed and, therefore, an extended period of incubation is necessary.

Some methods of evaluation do not employ growth directly as a measure of survival; as with counting (*see* p. 326), other activities of micro-organisms can be used, and in such cases different criteria of growth and death must be established—

(a) *Respiration.* The effect of bactericidal action on the uptake of oxygen and evolution of carbon dioxide by an organism is determined in a Warburg respirometer or by using special electrodes. Since dead tissues take up some oxygen, this must be estimated and taken into account. In addition, the significance of different levels of oxygen utilisation must be established. An advantage of these techniques is that measurements can be made with a single substrate as the sole nutrient; this is useful in research into the effect of chemicals on specific enzymes.

(b) *Metabolite Determinations.* The uptake or release of a wide range of metabolites can be measured by radiochemical, colorimetric or spectrophotometric techniques but such methods are more suitable for research than routine work. It is often difficult to correlate the results with the survival of bacteria under stresses and to decide whether cessation of biochemical activity is the cause or consequence of death. Also, ability to produce certain metabolites does not always mean that an organism is capable of reproduction.

(c) *Optical Density.* Valuable information on the nature and kinetics of antibacterial activity may be obtained from optical density measurements using narrow wavebands of light.

Generally viable counts give reliable information provided culture media and incubation techniques are chosen carefully. When cells are aggregated in the natural state (e.g. streptococci) or as a result of chemical treatment, absolute results cannot be obtained; in these circumstances counts represent colony forming units, not individual cells. The validity of the results may be further reduced by breakdown of some of the aggregates during the shaking of dilutions prior to counting.

2. What is Bacteriostasis?

In the past emphasis has been placed on the determination of 'bacteriostatic values' for chemicals. The condition described in the definition of a bacteriostat (p. 341) is difficult to evaluate in practice because of the delicate balance in such a biological situation. A steady state in the number of bacterial cells may be—

(a) *static*, where the cells are in a condition of suspended animation. This is difficult to explain, especially if it is accepted that life is a dynamic state. A proportion of the cells would be expected to die from senescence.

(b) *dynamic*, where the number of dying cells is balanced by the number of new cells produced. This could not last for long because the chemical would cause selection of the most resistant mutants which would multiply and destroy the equilibrium. In addition, such a state depends on the medium being able to support growth, because division must occur; but many of the environments in which bacteriostasis takes place are non-nutritive.

Both states would contain a delicately poised and numerically stable population and would be easily upset. Marshal and Hrenoff (1937) and Berry and Parkinson (1955) found bacteriostasis difficult to define simply. In Fig. 30.1 the time axis (growth = 0) corresponds to the theoretical concept of bacteriostasis but, because its practical proof is difficult, the above workers suggested that the term be applied to any culture in which growth is occurring at a slower rate than normal. This is shown on the figure as 'zone of inhibition'.

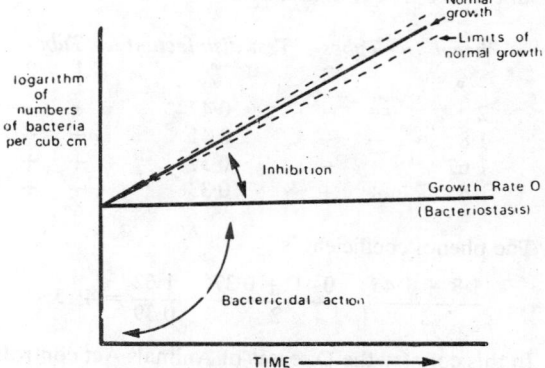

Fig. 30.1 The relationships between growth, death and inhibition in a bacterial culture

(After Marshall and Hrenoff)

Because of the difficulty of defining and proving bacteriostasis the term is less often used nowadays and bacteriostatic evaluations are called evaluations of minimum inhibitory concentrations.

Reasons for Microbiological Evaluations

1. *To Estimate Potency*

With some substances it is necessary to make an absolute declaration of potency (e.g. many antibiotics). Generally the necessary information can be obtained from a chemical determination, but in some cases this is not discriminating enough (e.g. liver products) and in others the difference between inactive and active forms shows only in a biological assay. Microbiological evaluation is used in these circumstances. As with all biological assays, the activity of the preparation is compared to the activity of a standard preparation.

2. *To Obtain a Phenol Coefficient*

In this type of determination the concentration of a disinfectant required to produce a particular result is compared with the concentration of pure phenol that gives the same result. Such tests are often used by manufacturers to confirm that variation between batches of a product is not excessive. Further, when an antibacterial preparation is being made to a fixed specification, a phenol coefficient may be part of the legal requirement. Phenol coefficients are reasonably valid for phenols and closely related substances, but much less so when the formulation contains soaps or when the mode of action of the test material differs markedly from that of phenol.

3. *To Confirm that Bactericides are Active at the Concentrations Recommended for Use*

These tests attempt to simulate conditions of use and, therefore, are called use-dilution tests, e.g. surface disinfectants are tested against films of micro-organisms dried on to suitable materials. An important application is in the food and dairy industries, where the performance of the test disinfectant is compared to that of hypochlorite. Attempts are being made to establish this type of test for antimicrobial substances used in hospitals.

4. *To Determine the Efficacy and Limitations of New Antimicrobial Substances*

So-called 'general disinfectants' have been common in the past; they were recommended for many purposes and carried impressive statements such as 'ten times as active as pure carbolic acid'. Generally these recommendations and comparisons were based on a single phenol coefficient test which gave very limited information (see p. 345) and did not justify the enthusiastic claims.

Nowadays, most manufacturers apply a series of proving tests to new antibacterial agents. These include determinations of—

(a) the phenol coefficient,
(b) the minimum inhibitory concentration for a range of organisms from the type of environment in which the agent will be used,
(c) the effect of organic matter, and
(d) acute and chronic toxicity.

METHODS OF EVALUATION

I. DISINFECTANTS

A. Phenol Coefficient Tests

In these determinations, the minimum concentration of pure phenol that produces viable sub-cultures at one time of sampling but non-viable sub-cultures at the next is compared to the minimum concentration of test disinfectant that produces a similar result. This comparison is expressed as a ratio and is called the phenol coefficient.

In these determinations the species or strain, cultural conditions and number of organisms, the temperature and time of exposure, the sample size, the nature of the recovery medium, and the time and temperature of incubation are fixed arbitrarily as part of the specification of the test.

1. SUSPENSION TESTS

The organism, as a suspension in an aqueous medium, is subjected to a standard concentration of phenol and to a range of concentrations of the disinfectant under test. The reaction takes place at a controlled temperature, samples of one loopful being removed to a standardised broth on several occasions during the reaction. The broth tubes are then incubated under controlled conditions and the results recorded as growth or no growth according to whether or not turbidity is produced. There are a number of variations—

(a) The Rideal Walker Test (BS 541:1934)

This uses a strain of *Salmonella typhi* that is prepared for the test in a specified way, using a standard broth. Serial dilutions of phenol and the disinfectant under test are inoculated with 0.2 cm^3 of the culture and standard loopfuls are removed into 5 cm^3 volumes of broth 2.5, 5, 7.5 and 10 minutes later and incubated at 37°C for 48 hours. The phenol coefficient is obtained by dividing the lowest concentration of disinfectant showing growth after 5 minutes but not after 7.5 minutes by the lowest concentration of phenol giving the same result. For example—

Concn. \ Time (min)		2·5	5	7·5	10
Phenol	1 in 95	+	+	−	−
Unknown	1 in 250	−	−	−	−
Unknown	1 in 300	+	−	−	−
Unknown	1 in 350	+	+	−	−
Unknown	1 in 400	+	+	−	−

The phenol coefficient is $\frac{400}{95} = 4.2$.

(b) The Chick Martin Test (BS 808:1938)

This test is more realistic because the reaction takes place in the presence of a controlled amount of organic matter in the form of a standardised suspension of yeast cells. Organic matter, which is often present under conditions of use, reduces the activity of many disinfectants.

The test organism and the incubation conditions are as for the Rideal Walker test but the reaction temperature is 20°C (instead of 17–18), the exposure time is 30 minutes, and duplicate samples are taken. The Chick Martin coefficient is the mean of the highest concentration of phenol showing growth (in both tubes) and the lowest concentration preventing growth, divided by the same mean for the disinfectant under test. For example—

Phenol %	Tubes 1	2	Test disinfectant %	Tubes 1	2
2	−	−	0·47	−	−
1·8	−	−	0·41	−	−
1·62	+	−	0·37	+	+
1·45	+	+	0·33	+	+

The phenol coefficient is

$$\frac{1.8 + 1.45}{2} \div \frac{0.41 + 0.37}{2} = \frac{1.62}{0.39} = 4.15.$$

In this country the Diseases of Animals Act controls the use of disinfectants in farming; the Chick Martin coefficient is the basis on which use dilutions are calculated (see p. 345).

(c) Other Tests

Further types of phenol coefficient test were developed in the United States of America. The Food and Drugs Administration (FDA) method of 1931 acknowledged the importance of information on activity against organisms other than *Salmonella typhi* and included a test for disinfectants used on the body, in which *Staphylococcus aureus* was the test organism and the reaction temperature was 37°C. Now the official method in America is that of the U.S. Association of Official Agricultural Chemists (AOAC); it is similar to the FDA method but more flexible. Three types of recovery media are permitted—

(i) Normal nutrient broth, for phenolic disinfectants the activity of which can be reduced to a non-inhibitory level by dilution in the recovery medium.

(ii) USP modified fluid thioglycollate medium, to neutralise the action of disinfectants containing mercurials, other heavy metals or bactericides that act by oxidation.

(iii) 'Letheen' medium, containing lecithin and the surface active agent, polysorbate 80, to neutralise quaternary ammonium compounds and chlorhexidine.

The medium giving the lowest phenol coefficient for the disinfectant under test is used. The test organisms are *Salmonella typhi* and *Staphylococcus aureus* of defined resistance to phenol. The British Standard test for black and white fluids (BS 2462:1961) is similar to the Rideal Walker test but the test organism is *Staphylococcus aureus*.

2. SURFACE FILM TESTS

Tests for disinfectants that are applied to surfaces are more realistic if they involve treatment of a film of bacteria dried on a suitable surface. Surfaces that have been used include cover slips (Jensen and Jensen, 1933), filter paper discs, and stainless steel plates or cylinders. The organisms are applied in a suspending agent containing organic matter such as protein. After an appropriate time the surface is incubated in a suitable medium. Occasionally this type of test is designed so that a phenol coefficient can be calculated but, more often, it is used in the determination of use dilutions.

Use Dilution Tests

It is important that a disinfectant should still be effective when diluted for use and the AOAC recommends that use dilutions of disinfectants should be at least as effective as 5 per cent phenol.

Generally, a dilution of twenty times the phenol coefficient is satisfactory. For example, for a disinfectant with a phenol coefficient of 4 this would be 1 in 4 × 20, i.e. 1 in 80. This method of calculation is unreliable where the concentration exponent of the disinfectant (*see* p. 335) differs from 5 and, if this is the case, the dilution can be calculated from the formula 2·5 [phenol coefficient × ($n-1$)], where n is the concentration exponent (calculated using *Salmonella typhi*). Use of this formula is complicated by lack of reliable values for n, apart from those published for phenols (Tilley, 1942).

The calculated dilution is checked by a surface film test, e.g. the AOAC test, used in the United States, and the Hoy Can test (1953), used for dairy disinfection in Great Britain.

CRITICISMS OF PHENOL COEFFICIENT TESTS

Choice of the Test Organism

In most tests only one organism is used. This is *Salmonella typhi* which is not very resistant to disinfectants and is not a very common pathogen nowadays. Results for this organism give only limited information on how the disinfectant will behave against other organisms. Coefficients for a range of organisms are desirable and this is acknowledged in some tests, e.g. the AOAC test, in which *Staphylococcus aureus* may also be used.

Absence of Organic Matter

Because of its adverse effect on the activity of many disinfectants, organic matter should be included in the tests. Of the suspension tests only the Chick Martin is satisfactory in this respect.

Long Intervals between Successive Samples

This leads to imprecision. For example, in theory, in the Rideal Walker test (in which samples are removed at intervals of 2·5 minutes) the phenol and comparable disinfectant dilutions could kill the organisms at just over 5 and just under 7·5 minutes respectively and still give the same end point.

Use of Death (Extinction) of the Inoculum as the End Point

The main argument in favour of extinction tests is that the function of a disinfectant is to destroy all organisms. In fact, absence of growth could simply mean that no organisms were present in the sample removed from the reaction mixture. The probability of this increases near to the end point, because only a few living organisms remain.

Tiny Sample Volumes

Generally, sampling is done with a platinum loop, to avoid carrying inhibitory concentrations of the bactericides into the recovery tubes; consequently, the sample volume is small. In addition, there can be considerable variation in the size of sample taken by the same and different workers (Sykes, 1965).

Lack of Replication

To reduce the significance of errors of the kind mentioned in the previous two paragraphs, replication is desirable.

Comparison of Dissimilar Substances

Since phenol coefficient tests are biological assays they should conform to the fundamental requirement of a biological assay, that like should be compared with like. For example, it is found that if the reaction time is varied quite different results are obtained if the bactericide under test is chemically dissimilar to phenol. This is a reflection of differences in concentration exponent.

Usually only One Reaction Temperature

In practice, disinfection takes place at a variety of temperatures and because bactericides have characteristic temperature coefficients their performance at the temperature of the test may fail to reflect their behaviour at other temperatures.

Absence of Information on Toxicity to Living Tissues

While data on toxicity are important for substances intended for personal hygiene and treatment of wounds, phenol coefficient tests are intended primarily for the control of substances used for the disinfection of inanimate materials. Consequently, this criticism is somewhat unfair.

ADVANTAGES OF PHENOL COEFFICIENT TESTS

1. They are inexpensive and can be performed quickly.
2. They give reproducible results in the hands of experienced workers.
3. They are valuable to—
   (a) eliminate useless products, and
   (b) supply standards for crude preparations, such as black and white fluids, for which chemical standards are difficult to set up.

B. Method of Berry and Bean (1954)

This is an extinction-time method in which, unlike the techniques described previously, the extinction-time is not fixed. Instead the time to kill the organisms at a fixed concentration of bactericide is determined. The end-point is assessed precisely by a multiple drop technique.

Using a Cook and Yousef (1953) type dropping pipette (see p. 317), a standardised suspension of *Escherichia coli* is inoculated into several dilutions of the bactericide and, immediately after mixing, a fixed number of drops from each dilution is transferred to a separate sterile tube. The tubes are returned to a water bath at 20°C, the temperature at which all the stages of medication are carried out. The reaction is allowed to continue for appropriate times after which broth is added to quench the reaction and the tubes are incubated and examined for growth. Replicates are performed and a mean death time is calculated.

Mather (1949) suggested that the method would be more valuable if the results were treated in the following way. The number of tubes showing no growth after a given reaction time is expressed as a probability of obtaining no growth; e.g. for three negatives out of ten the probability $(p) = 0.3$. From tables a value of y is obtained for each probability; $y = \log_e (-\log_e p)$. A graph is plotted of y against time of exposure, and the time at which $y = 0$ is the most probable time at which the number of surviving organisms in a sample taken from a reaction mixture has been reduced to an average of one. This value is called the Mean Single Survivor Time (MSST).

Advantages of this method include—

(a) Samples are taken from the reaction mixture before clumping occurs. Clumping is serious when certain species, e.g. *Pseudomonas aeruginosa*, are treated with solutions of phenols in soaps.

(b) Because sampling takes place immediately after inoculation with the organisms, the sample is removed while the population of organisms is large and, therefore, errors are smaller than when the reaction is sampled near to the point of extinction.

(c) The volumes of samples delivered by a dropping pipette are less variable than those withdrawn by a loop.

(d) Extensive replication.

(e) The quenching times are not chosen arbitrarily, as in other extinction methods, but are fixed small proportions of the expected MSST.

(f) Limits of error can be estimated from the results.

A disadvantage of dropping pipettes is that the volume delivered varies according to the surface tension of the liquid; this can be overcome by preliminary experiments to discover which of a range of needles delivers the correct volume of a particular dilution.

C. Nephelometric Method

Needham (1947) proposed a test in which a nephelometer (see p. 328) is used to estimate the survival of *Salmonella typhi* after exposure to a bactericide. A reference survivor curve is obtained from dilutions of the suspension containing 3,2 and 0·75 per cent of the original numbers in unit volume. Samples are removed from the reaction mixture into tubes of broth which are incubated at 37°C for 5 hours. At the same time tubes containing the three dilutions of untreated organisms are incubated under exactly the same conditions. After incubation the opacity of each tube is measured nephelometrically and from the results for the untreated organisms the reference curve is plotted and this is used to obtain the numbers of organisms in the 'treated' tubes.

An objection to this method is that damaged and untreated organisms may not reproduce at the same rate.

Although the short incubation time would have been an advantage in routine disinfectant testing, this technique is not used for this purpose because it is too sensitive.

D. Counting Methods

The difficulty of determining the end point precisely in phenol coefficient tests led several workers to suggest that a comparison of death rates, determined by viable counts, would give more accurate information, particularly if several disinfectant concentrations, bacterial species, and temperatures were used.

Because the presence of cells of exceptionally high resistance distorts the results of extinction methods, Withell (1942) recommended determination of the time to kill 50 per cent (LT50) of the organisms. Results are plotted as probits (see p. 334) against log time and the LT50 is read off from the graph. However—

(a) Viable counts are tedious at this end point, because of the large number of organisms present.

(b) Reduction of numbers to 50 per cent is of little practical significance.

(c) The relationship between log concentration and log time is not linear at the 50 per cent level. Consequently, other workers have suggested a 99 or 99·9 per cent mortality level as the end point.

Counting methods involve—

(a) Addition of the suspension to the disinfectant dilution.

(b) Sampling at suitable intervals into a liquid that neutralises the action of the bactericide.

(c) Dilution to a level suitable for counting the survivors. The dilutions are arranged so that, as far as possible, the counts are approximately the same, because this procedure gives the best value of Chi-squared.

(d) Inoculation into (pour plate or roll tube method) or on to (surface viable technique) suitable media.

(e) Counting of the colonies.

(f) Statistical evaluation of the result and its error.

E. Determination of Minimum Inhibitory Concentrations

Minimum inhibitory concentrations (MIC) are sometimes called bacteriostatic values, but for the reason given on page 343 the first term is preferable. The minimum inhibitory concentration of an antibacterial agent, for a particular organism, is the lowest concentration that just prevents growth of that organism.

(a) LIQUID DILUTION METHODS

Graded concentrations of inhibitor are prepared in broth and an accurate volume of a suspension of the organism is added to each. After shaking to mix, the dilutions are incubated, usually for 2–3 days at 37°C, and examined for growth.

The MIC lies between the lowest concentration inhibiting growth and the highest concentration allowing growth. The determination can be repeated, using a range of dilutions between these two values, if a more precise result is required.

Normally the dilutions are in geometric series (e.g. with a 1 in 10 or a 1 in 2 difference between successive tubes) but sometimes an arithmetic series is more suitable (Table 30.1). Tubes 6 and 7 are controls. Tube 6 contains no inhibitor and confirms that the culture is viable. Tube 7 contains the highest concentration of inhibitor but no organisms and is to detect precipitation caused by interaction of broth constituents and inhibitor; this could be confused with turbidity due to bacterial growth.

In expressing an MIC value the conditions under which it was obtained should be specified because the result is influenced by many factors including the strain, age and number of organisms, the nature and pH of the culture medium, and the temperature and time of incubation.

Table 30.1
Determination of the Minimum Inhibitory Concentration of Phenol for *Staphylococcus aureus* (arithmetic series)

The volumes are all in cm³

Tube	1	2	3	4	5	6	7
Double-strength broth	5	5	5	5	5	5	5
Phenol 1 per cent	4	3·5	3	2·5	2	0	4
Sterile water	0·8	1·3	1·8	2·3	2·8	5	1
Inoculum	0·2	0·2	0·2	0·2	0·2	0·2	0
Phenol concn. mg/cm³	4	3·5	3	2·5	2	0	4

When the antiseptic is to be applied to wounds, body fluids, e.g. blood and serum, may be added to the test medium to see if they affect the result.

(b) SOLID DILUTION METHOD

Cook (1954) described a method using nutrient agar. Dilutions of the bactericide are mixed with the molten medium and poured into petri dishes. After solidification, the surface of the agar is dried (*see* p. 318) so that it will rapidly absorb the drops of inoculum that are subsequently added to it. 15 cm³ of $\frac{4}{3}$ strength nutrient agar is convenient, the volume being made up to 20 cm³ with appropriate volumes of inhibitor and water. The advantages of this method are—

(i) Several different organisms can be tested on each plate.
(ii) Precipitation in the medium does not obscure the result.
(iii) Contamination is more easily detected, because colony features on solid media are more distinctive than turbidity differences in fluid media.

F. Proving Tests for New Disinfectants

In the United Kingdom very few tests are laid down by legislation. Nevertheless, manufacturers have to satisfy themselves that any product they wish to market is effective and safe. An official test that gives valuable guidance is the test for quaternary ammonium compounds described in BS 3286:1960. Its terms are very general but they include the

following features—

(*a*) Several test organisms; *Staphylococcus aureus*, *Pseudomonas aeruginosa* and *Escherichia coli* are recommended but other bacteria and, also, yeasts and moulds may be used.
(*b*) Several temperatures.
(*c*) A disinfection time of up to 30 minutes.
(*d*) Neutralisation of the antibacterial agent to avoid inhibition in the recovery tubes.
(*e*) Inclusion of organic matter.
(*f*) After reaction and neutralisation the samples are diluted to give 30 to 300 organisms in an agar plate. The data are presented as a graph of log concentration against log number of survivors at a fixed exposure time. From this the concentration representing a kill of something less than 100 per cent (e.g. 99·9) can be obtained. Replication is recommended and it is explicitly stated that the result should not be expressed as a coefficient. Limits of error should be stated.

This test cannot be used as a legal standard because it is written as a series of recommendations. It is not a full proving test but a sophisticated use dilution test for a variety of conditions of use.

In a full series of proving tests the following are recommended—

(a) A PHENOL COEFFICIENT TEST

This can be used to calculate a use dilution which should be checked experimentally.

(b) MINIMUM INHIBITORY CONCENTRATIONS

A range of organisms appropriate to the conditions of use should be tested. It is convenient to determine the effect of organic matter by this type of test.

(c) TOXICITY TESTS

Acute Toxicity. For antibacterial agents that are to be administered systemically, oral administration of large doses to small animals is a standard method of investigating toxicity. Tests are often performed on human leucocytes because they are delicate and must not be inactivated *in vivo* as they help to protect the body against bacterial invasion. Freedom from irritancy may be confirmed by instilling use dilutions into the eyes of rabbits.

Chronic Toxicity. Effects of application to the skin of animals over long periods are studied to detect contact dermatitis (such as is found after prolonged use of chloroxylenol solutions) and carcinogenicity.

G. In Vivo Tests

These are not of great value because of the extra variation introduced by the use of animals.

(a) INFECTIVITY TESTS

An example is the mouse-tail technique. The tip of the tail is infected, treated with bactericide, removed with sterile scissors, placed in a peritoneal pouch, and then the animal is watched for signs of infection. The animal replaces the incubator of *in vitro* tests and a recognisable syndrome replaces turbidity as the indicator of living organisms.

Among the uncertainties of this type of test are the influence of toxicity of the bactericide on the ability of the animal to survive infection, and the number of organisms required to initiate infection, which may not be the same for other animal species or for man.

(b) TESTS UNDER CONDITIONS OF USE

Examples are the hand washing tests that are sometimes used for skin disinfectants, particularly soaps. The resident flora of the skin is determined and the hand is disinfected; residual living bacteria are collected, e.g. by washing or by the sausage technique (*see* p. 317). After the washing technique the fluid is either plated directly or passed through a membrane filter which is then incubated in the usual way (*see* p. 318).

Results are seldom significant because of the variation in the skin flora from one individual to another. Application of a test culture to the skin is of little advantage because the contamination is superficial and is too easily reached by the disinfectant and removed after treatment.

The evaluation of aerial bactericides is discussed by Gunn and Carter (1965).

II. ANTIBIOTICS

1. Serial Dilution Methods

These are essentially the same as the dilution methods used to determine MICs. The dilution of the antibiotic under test that will inhibit the growth of a sensitive organism is compared with the dilution of a standard preparation that has the same effect. From knowledge of the potency of the standard the strength of the unknown can be calculated. Usually dilution in broth is most suitable but in some cases dilution in a nutrient agar is more satisfactory.

2. Diffusion Methods

Generally these are preferred to serial dilution methods because of the ease with which quantitative results can be obtained. They cannot be used when, because of adsorption by, or incompatibility with, the medium, the medicament does not diffuse freely.

A geometric series of dilutions is prepared for the antibiotic under test and for the standard preparation. Plates are seeded with the test organism and the medium is allowed to set on a perfectly horizontal surface so that the agar is constant in depth throughout the dish. The organism may be mixed with the agar before pouring or applied to the surface of the medium after it has set. The plates may be petri dishes or large flat dishes up to 0·5 m square.

The solutions are contained in—

(a) Cups cut in the medium using a sterile cork borer about 10 mm in diameter, the agar disc being removed by a vacuum device or a splayed-out steel pen nib.

(b) Cylinders of stainless steel, glazed porcelain, Pyrex glass or sterilisable plastic having an external diameter of about 8 mm and a height of about 10 mm. These are usually warmed so that they sink slightly, to a constant depth, when placed on the agar.

(c) Filter paper or cellulose discs, which absorb a fixed volume of solution.

(d) Standard ceramic insulation beads (fish spine beads) which attract a fixed volume when touched on the surface of the solution. The surface of the agar must be dry if this method is used.

The test and standard solutions are placed in the containers in random order, to prevent the bias that could be caused by a regular order of plating. The volume is critical for the cup method but is not significant when cylinders are used provided they are at least two-thirds full. Care is taken not to seal the tops of the cylinders with the lid of the plate.

The plates are left at room temperature for two hours to allow diffusion of the antibiotic to get ahead of growth of the organisms (*see* p. 351). Then they are incubated at the appropriate temperature, usually for about 16 hours.

After incubation, inhibition of growth can be seen as a clear zone around each container. The diameter of this is proportional to the log of the concentration of antibiotic. As soon as possible each diameter is measured and this is best done using an optical system that projects an image of the plate on to a large grid. Two diameters at right angles are used as a check on ellipticity of the zone.

The results can be processed in two ways—

. A graph is plotted of log concentration of standard against zone diameter and the results for the test preparation are plotted on the same graph. Provided the two lines are parallel, the relative potencies of the standard and test are represented by the horizontal distance between the two lines.

2. Parallelism between the two lines can be confirmed mathematically and the potency of the test obtained by calculation (*see*, for example, the B.P. assay of penicillin).

As with all bioassays the validity of the method should be confirmed and the error of the result indicated. Although it may be difficult, attempt should be made to use test and standard solutions of approximately equal strength, because the most accurate result is obtained under these circumstances.

The *Pharmacopoeia* includes a number of assays performed by microbiological techniques and other examples will be found in the Bibliography at the end of this chapter.

III. METABOLITES

Similar methods to those for antibiotics are used for certain metabolite assays except that enhancement, instead of inhibition, of growth is produced; hence these are sometimes called exhibition assays.

Features of the Assays of Antibiotics and Metabolites

Since these determinations are bioassays, the rules applying to such assays must be obeyed. The most important is that like must be compared with like and therefore a suitable standard preparation must be set up and a standardised technique followed. Many pharmaceutical preparations contain additives that aid formulation and if these interfere with the assay similar additions must be made to the standard. The main factors that affect the results of assays are—

Factors Associated with the Organism

An important consideration is whether a spore suspension or a suspension of vegetative cells will give the best result. Spores have been most satisfactory because spore suspensions retain their genetic characteristics for long periods in a refrigerator and, therefore, a large quantity can be stored ready for use and can be relied upon to be homogeneous in response. Spores are advantageous in diffusion assays for antibiotics. If the growth of the organism is delayed a little (as when spores have to change into vegetative forms before multiplication begins) the zones of inhibition are larger because outward diffusion of the antibiotic gets ahead of growth of the cells. In addition, the edges of the zones are more distinct when spores are used.

Genetic stability is especially important for assays in fluid media because a high mutation rate could cause changes in biochemical characteristics that might interfere with certain types of determination, such as vitamin assays. In antibiotic assays, contamination of the culture with the factor responsible for multiple antibiotic resistance can ruin the results.

The number of organisms in the inoculum determines the length of the lag phase of growth. This is important because the edge of the zone corresponds to a fixed concentration of the chemical and to the inhibition of a fixed number of organisms (the *critical number*) and represents a balance between the outward diffusion of the antibiotic and the inward growth of the cells.

In serial dilution techniques adsorption of the chemical on to living and dead cells may deplete the assay substance and, if the concentration in the liquid phase is low, may have a profound effect on the precision of the assay. For this reason, it is particularly important to control the number of dead as well as the number of living cells in the inoculum.

The medium must be standardised because its composition influences growth rates and the development of specific metabolic pathways. Changes in these pathways may be reflected in changes of activity of the chemical. Preparation of media from pure chemicals would seem the ideal solution, but synthetic media are expensive, difficult to prepare and some of their ingredients do not keep well. A satisfactory solution is to buy ready-made dehydrated media from specialist manufacturers and to request material from a single manufacturing batch. Heat sterilisation methods should not be varied. Sometimes special adjuncts are useful, e.g. non-ionic surfactants improve the zones of inhibition in some antibiotics assays.

For assays of metabolites the organism is prepared by cultivation on a medium containing a minimum, or no relevant metabolite, so that it responds well to graded doses of the test and standard during the assay. The medium must not become contaminated with the metabolite or its precursor(s) or the result will be invalidated. One possible cause of such contamination is the growth of organisms accidentally introduced to the medium during its preparation; consequently, strict aseptic technique is desirable.

Factors Associated with the Preparation of the Test and Standard Solutions

In diffusion assays maximum precision is obtained when the medium and assay solutions have the same pH. Buffers must be chosen carefully, to avoid incompatibilities with ions in the assay material; e.g. active material may be adsorbed on to the precipitate produced by reaction between calcium ions and phosphate buffer. Sometimes a chemical is active only near the limit of its solubility in water and this should be checked before dilutions are made. Solvents must have no bactericidal activity and should not exhibit synergism with the bactericide. Thorough mixing of the contents of tubes in serial dilution assays, before and after the addition of the inoculum, is essential to prevent false results due to local concentrations of medicament or organisms.

The precision of an assay depends on the accuracy with which test and standard solutions are prepared. As a check it is usual to duplicate the complete assay including the preparation of the solutions.

There is a straight line relationship between the log of the dose and the response and, therefore, dosage levels in the dilutions are usually arranged in geometric progression to give equal spacing of points on the log dose axis of the graph.

In the assay of metabolites, the material under test (e.g. a food) is often complex and a separation technique may be necessary before preparation of the test solutions. Care is needed to ensure that this is quantitative and reproducible.

Factors Associated with Diffusion

These are of importance only in the diffusion type assay because homogeneous solutions are used in tube dilution methods. The law representing radial diffusion of a solution from a reservoir through an agar gel (Eqn 30.1) is derived from Fick's law.

$$x^2 = 4Dt \ln (m_0/m) \qquad (30.1)$$

In this equation, x is the distance from the edge of the container to the edge of the zone of inhibition; D is the diffusion coefficient for the system; m_0 is the concentration of the solution in the reservoir; m is the concentration of solute at the edge of the zone, and t is the time of diffusion.

To obtain a straight line graph, log dose is plotted against x^2 while the relationship between time and diffusion is shown by plotting time (in hours) against x^2. In inhibition assays doses that produce zone diameters of between 12 and 30 mm overall are most satisfactory. One reason is that within this range it is permissible to simplify the processing of results by plotting zone diameter (instead of x^2) against log dose, or time. At first it is necessary to take five dose levels, but when it has been shown that there is a straight line response over a reasonable range of concentration only two levels of the test and two of the standard need be used, and this

makes statistical analysis easier. Such a design is known as a 2 by 2 assay (see the appendix on biological assays in the BP).

Because the growth of organisms is very rapid, zones of inhibition would be very small if plates were incubated immediately after addition of the assay solutions. Plates are left at room temperature for two hours before incubation to allow prior diffusion of the assay solutions. The resulting concentration gradients in the agar produce zones that are satisfactory in size and clarity of edge. If, after inoculation with the organisms, but before adding the solutions, the plate is dried by incubation for a short time, the zone diameters are reduced because growth of the organisms gets a good start before diffusion of the inhibitor begins. This decrease in the size of the zone becomes greater as the drying time is lengthened until a point is reached at which there is no zone. The minimum time required to produce this result is known as the *critical time*.

If the preparation under test contains sugars (as is the case with paediatric antibiotic syrups) the additional viscosity influences diffusion and its significance must be assessed (Kavanagh, 1963).

Factors Associated with Incubation Conditions and Reading of Results

The temperature of incubation should be high enough to give satisfactory growth and, therefore, distinct zones, without producing excessive temperature gradients or undue decomposition of the material under assay. There can be a large temperature gradient between the metal shelf of an incubator and the top plate of a stack of small petri dishes; this is prevented by restricting stacks to a maximum of four plates or by using bigger plates. For most antibiotic assays the time of incubation is critical; if too short, growth is insufficient to produce sharp edges to the zones; if too long, overgrowth of the organisms makes the edges less distinct. Zones should be measured immediately the plates are removed from the incubator, because overgrowth may occur even in a refrigerator.

Often, in tube assays, rapid cooling or addition of an inhibitor can be used to arrest growth of the organism and allow delayed reading of results. For measurements of optical density the temperature of all tubes must be the same because optical density changes with temperature. Cold containers may mist up in the warm instrument and produce false results. Unless the instrument is very stable (and, therefore, costly) drift of the calibration can lead to errors in later measurements; the effect of this is reduced by randomising the order in which readings are taken. When reading the results the operator should not know the test sequence, to avoid bias. Mechanical means of recording help to avoid inaccuracy due to fatigue.

BIBLIOGRAPHY

AMERICAN OFFICIAL AGRICULTURAL CHEMISTS (1960) *Official methods of analysis of the A.O.A.C.* 9th ed. A.O.A.C. Washington, D.C.

BARTON-WRIGHT, E. C. (1952) *Microbiological assay of the vitamin B complex and amino acids.* Pitman, New York and London.

BRITISH STANDARD 541:1934 *The technique for determining the Rideal Walker coefficient for disinfectants.* British Standards Institution, London.

BRITISH STANDARD 808:1938 *A modified technique for the Chick-Martin test for disinfectants.* British Standards Institution, London.

BRITISH STANDARD 2462:1961 *Specification for Black and White disinfectant fluids.* British Standards Institution, London.

BRITISH STANDARD 3286:1960 *Laboratory evaluation of the disinfectant activity of Quaternary Ammonium Compounds.* British Standards Institution, London.

GUNN, C. and CARTER, S. J. (1965) *Dispensing for Pharmaceutical Students.* 11th ed. Pitman Medical, London.

KAVANAGH, F. (Ed.) (1963) *Analytical Microbiology.* Academic Press, New York.

LAWRENCE, C. A. and BLOCK, S. S. (1968) *Disinfection, sterilization and preservation.* Henry Kimpton, London.

SOCIETY OF CHEMICAL INDUSTRY (1965) *Surface activity and the microbial cell.* S.C.I. Monograph No. 19. Society for Chemical Industry, London.

SYKES, G. (1965) *Disinfection and sterilization.* 2nd ed. Spon, London.

REFERENCES

BEAN, H. S. and BERRY, H. (1954) The estimation of bactericidal activity from extinction-time data. *J. Pharm. Pharmac.,* 6, 649–655.

BERRY, H. and PARKINSON, J. C. (1955) The effect of temperature on bacteriostasis. *J. Pharm. Pharmac.,* 7, 616–626.

COOK, A. M. (1954) The evaluation of antibacterial substances part I. *J. Pharm. Pharmac.,* 6, 629–637.

COOK, A. M. and YOUSEF, R. T. (1953) An improved pipette for bacterial suspensions. *J. Pharm. Pharmac.,* 5, 141.

CHURCHMAN, J. W. (1912) The selective bactericidal action of gentian violet. *J. exp. Med.,* 16, 221–247.

HOY, W. A. and CLEGG, L. F. L. (1953) Testing farm dairy detergent sterilizers using soiled ten gallon cans. *Proc. Soc. appl. Bact.,* 16, (i).

JACOBS, S. E. and HARRIS, N. D. (1961) The effect of modifications of counting medium on the viability and growth of bacteria damaged by phenols. *J. appl. Bact.,* 24, 172–181.

JENSEN, E. and JENSEN, V. (1933) Determination of the phenol coefficients of disinfectants by the coverslip method. *J. Hyg., Camb.,* 33, 485–494.

MARSHALL, M. S. and HRENOFF, A. K. (1937) Bacteriostasis. A review. *J. infect. Dis.,* 61, 42.

MATHER, R. L. (1949) Analysis of extinction-time data in bioassay. *Biometrics.,* 5, 127.

NEEDHAM, N. V. (1947) A photometric method for the comparative evaluation of disinfectants. *J. Hyg., Camb.,* 45, 1–11.

PRICE, P. B. (1950) The meaning of bacteriostasis, bactericidal effect and rate of disinfection. *Ann. N.Y. Acad. Sci.,* 53, 76–90.

SOCIETY FOR APPLIED BACTERIOLOGY (1963) Symposium on survival of bacteria. *J. appl. Bact.,* 26, 287–404.

SYKES, G. (1962) The philosophy of the evaluation of disinfectants. *J. appl. Bact.,* 25, 1–11.

TILLEY, F. W. (1942) An experimental study of the influence of temperature on the bactericidal action of phenols and alcohols. *J. Bact.,* 43, 521–525.

WITHELL, E. R. (1942) The evaluation of bactericides *J. Hyg., Camb.,* 42, 339.

31
Antiseptics, Disinfectants, and Preservatives

THIS chapter deals with chemicals used to prevent and treat disease. The order is arbitrary and does not indicate efficacy or usefulness. Brief dis-cussions of structure—activity relationships are included but, in a general textbook, are necessarily brief.

ANTISEPTICS AND DISINFECTANTS

Acids and Alkalis
STRONG ACIDS

These dissociate completely in dilute solution, producing hydrogen ions that have a very strong affinity for water. Their antibacterial activity is due to irreversible denaturation of proteins (at a pH of about 1, the pH of strong mineral acids) or to withdrawal of water from the bacteria. Concentrated acids kill all bacteria in a very short time; weak solutions destroy most vegetative forms, an important exception being *Mycobacterium tuberculosis* which, because of its water-repellant outer layer, resists penetration by quite concentrated acids (*see* Acid-fast staining). In spite of their efficiency, strong acids are not widely used as bactericides because of the difficulty of handling them safely.

WEAK ACIDS

These dissociate to a limited or negligible extent in aqueous solutions and as few hydrogen ions are produced they act differently from strong acids. Little is known of the mechanism(s) by which undissociated acids attack bacteria.

Weak acids are widely used in preservation (e.g. benzoic, acetic, sorbic, and propionic) and in the treatment of skin conditions (e.g. undecanoic and boric). Boric acid has been widely used in dusting powders and ointments but its use is no longer recommended because enough can be absorbed to cause toxic effects, particularly in infants. Preparations containing weak acids and surface active agents are used to treat stainless steel equipment in the catering and dairy industries. Above pH 3 there is a rapid decrease in activity.

STRONG ALKALIS

These are completely dissociated, particularly in dilute solutions, and hydroxonium ions, which like hydrogen ions have a strong affinity for water, are formed. Their mode of action resembles that of strong acids but alkali metal hydroxides are good detergents and penetrate well, even into mycobacteria. Strongly alkaline solutions are of considerable value in disinfection processes. Lye, a natural liquor from the alkali industry, is used in one system of dairy hygiene. Solutions with a high percentage of sodium hydroxide are useful for clearing and disinfecting drains blocked with organic debris, provided the glaze on the pipes is not of the boric acid type. Stainless steel surfaces may be cleaned and disinfected with trisodium phosphate. Because alkalis are non-toxic, when adequately diluted, and leave no residual odour, they are suitable for treating floors etc. in food factories where layers of fatty material may accumulate. Like strong acids they are corrosive and must be handled with care.

WEAK ALKALIS

Most, like the weak acids, are only slightly dissociated; some (e.g. sodium bicarbonate) are salts of a strong alkali and a weak acid. Quicklime is used as an anti-infective agent in agriculture and borax (sodium borate) is recommended for the control of foot and mouth disease.

Halogens and Derivatives
CHLORINE

Chlorine gas, liquified under pressure, is one of the most frequently used bactericides. It combines readily with water to form hypochlorous acid, which in the undissociated form is thought to be the active agent in disinfection with chlorine. Because of its powerful oxidising properties it can replace natural hydrogen acceptors and cause denaturation of proteins, particularly in the cell membrane; this interferes with transport across the membrane and reduces or halts metabolism. For many applications the gas is too dangerous and compounds that release hypochlorous acid are used instead.

Hypochlorites

The use of hypochlorites in the control of disease is older than the germ theory. A crude material containing calcium hypochlorite (bleaching powder) was used but this material, which when fresh contains 30–40 per cent available chlorine, is strongly hygroscopic and quickly loses much of its activity; in addition, it attacks card or metal drums. Nowadays this has largely been replaced by hypochlorite solutions prepared by electrolysis of brine. There are two types of solution on the market. The first is concentrated and has a chlorine content of about 20 per cent; a stabiliser is included. It is intended to be diluted with water before use and is widely used in the food and dairy industries. Its pH is about 9 but this is reduced by dilution, with consequent increase in activity. The second type consists of more dilute solutions prepared for personal use and sterilisation in the home, e.g. feeding bottles. Usually the pH is buffered near to neutrality and consequently these solutions are less stable than the concentrates and have to be stored carefully, particularly after the bottle has been opened.

Chloramines

The inorganic chloramines are made from chlorine and ammonia. For swimming pools, liquid ammonia and liquid chlorine are used, the ammonia being dissolved first, followed by the chlorine. Because the monochloramine is not very active the proportions are adjusted to produce the dichloro derivative which is more effective.

$$NH_4^+ + HOCl = NH_2Cl + H_2O + H^+$$
$$NH_2Cl + HOCl = NHCl_2 + H_2O$$

Because these reactions are reversible the chloramines form reservoirs of chlorine. They are less active than hypochlorous acid especially against viruses but this can be overcome by superchlorination, a process in which an excess of chlorine (up to 50 ppm) is fed into the system. This technique is applied to the emergency sterilisation of water supplies, particularly in war or after natural disasters, and is very effective, even killing spores of bacilli in a few minutes. After treatment, a dechlorinating agent, such as sodium thiosulphate, is added to make the water palatable.

Organically-combined Chlorine

Chlorine combines with certain nitrogen-containing chemicals to produce compounds that provide a depot of chlorine for sustained antibacterial activity; unlike the inorganic chloramines they are stable in the dry state. The two best known are—

Chloramine T CH_3—⟨⟩—$SO_2.Na:NCl.3H_2O$

Dichloramine T CH_3—⟨⟩—$SO_2.NCl_2$

These can be prepared in tablet form and are much more convenient than simple chloramines for emergency water sterilisation. Halazone is an analogue of dichloramine T in which the toluene moiety is replaced by benzoic acid. Chlorine derivatives of azodicarbonamidine, isocyanuric acid and hydantoin are also used and have high stability to pH change.

Factors Affecting the Action of Chlorine Compounds

Concentration. The action is stoichiometric for much of the concentration range and the value of n is approximately 1.

pH. Often the effect of pH on chlorine activity is so marked (Fig. 31.1) that the concentration

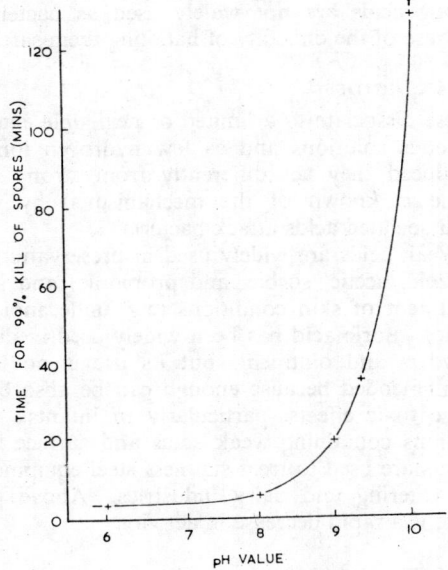

Fig. 31.1   The influence of pH on bactericidal efficiency of hypochlorite solutions on *B. metiens* spores
(*Rudolph and Levine*, 1941)

effect is of secondary importance. The more complex organic derivatives are more tolerant of pH change.

Temperature. The temperature coefficient is about 2 per 10°C rise over the range 20–50°C and the chemical stability of chlorine solutions is good within this range.

Advantages of Chlorine Compounds

1. At effective concentrations they are almost odourless and tasteless and this is of value in the sterilisation of water and in the food industry.

2. They are sporicidal at concentrations as low as 0·05 ppm and will destroy viruses under favourable conditions.

3. Certain organic forms provide a depot effect and are non-irritant to tissues.

4. The toxicity of dilute solutions is very low and, therefore, they can be used safely for dairy and food utensils and feeding bottles.

5. The stability of hypochlorite solutions (at pH 9) and organic chlorine derivatives is good. Both products are convenient to use.

6. They have cleaning and deodorising properties that are useful in wound treatment, particularly if putrefaction has taken place.

7. They are cheap to use because very low concentrations are active.

Disadvantages of Chlorine Compounds

1. They are said not to penetrate organic matter or bacterial cells, particularly those of fatty species such as mycobacteria.

2. Solutions are corrosive to metals (even stainless steel), textiles and biological tissues. Unnecessarily concentrated solutions should be avoided and susceptible materials, such as rubber in dairy equipment, should be checked regularly.

3. Chlorine combines with organic matter and, except when N-chlorine compounds are formed, this results in loss of activity.

4. Chlorine can be tasted at very low concentrations; e.g. tea made with water containing only 4 ppm is unpalatable. Combination with types of phenol-containing organic matter in water gives an unpleasant appearance although the water may be perfectly safe to use.

IODINE

Iodine has been used as an antibacterial agent for many years and is still one of the best bactericides for the skin. Free iodine is the most active constituent of iodine preparations. The element is almost insoluble in water, but aqueous solutions may be prepared by dissolving it in a concentrated solution of potassium iodide and diluting to the required strength. In solutions of this type part of the iodine is in the form of the relatively inactive complex ion, I_3^-; hence it is advisable to keep the amount of iodide as low as is compatible with stability. Most individuals tolerate iodine well, but a minority show sensitivity and in a few, respiratory failure may occur. This toxicity led to virtual abandonment of aqueous solutions but recently there has been a revival of interest in iodine, due to the development of the iodophores.

Iodophores

These contain iodine combined with complex organic chemicals. In the early forms, non-ionic surface active agents (e.g. polyoxyethylene derivatives) were used to 'carry' the iodine. Later, a combination of iodine and polyvinylpyrrolidone (PVP) proved more successful. Activity at least equivalent to iodine-potassium iodide solutions of the same iodine content has been reported. The number and severity of toxic reactions has been greatly reduced. The activity of this type of formulation is highest on the acid side of neutral and the inclusion of phosphoric acid has been advantageous in preparations for dairy use. The principal advantages of iodophores are—

1. Their toxicity is relatively low.

2. Preparations for skin disinfection leave enough stain on the skin to show the surgeon that the surface has been treated but this, unlike the stain left by many other skin preparations, can be removed with soap and water.

3. Preparations with an iodine content of 1 per cent are sporicidal in 2·5 hours (Gershenfeld, 1962).

4. They are compatible with soaps.

Iodine preparations are the most useful skin disinfectants, most organisms resident in the skin being killed by treatment with a 1 per cent aqueous solution for 30 seconds (Story, 1952).

Phenols

Phenol (carbolic acid) has been extensively used in chemical disinfection since the time of Lister. Now it has largely given way to mixtures of phenols distilled from coal, which are cheap, or to substituted phenolic substances of lower toxicity but greater antimicrobial activity. Phenol remains the standard with which other bactericides are compared in several official tests (*see* Chapter 30). It is non-selective against vegetative cells but has poor activity against spores. It is soluble up to 6 per cent

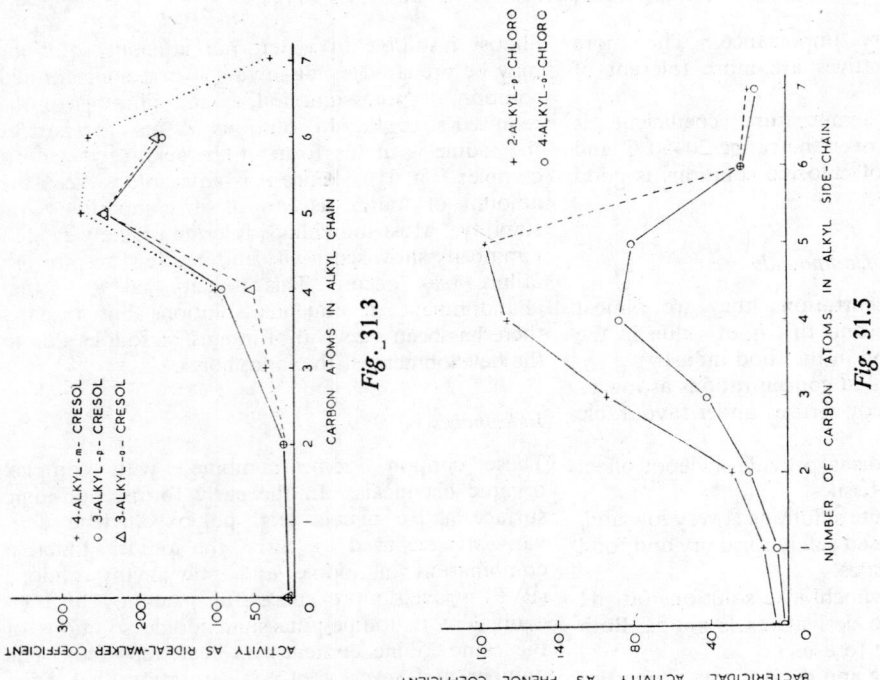

Fig. 31.3

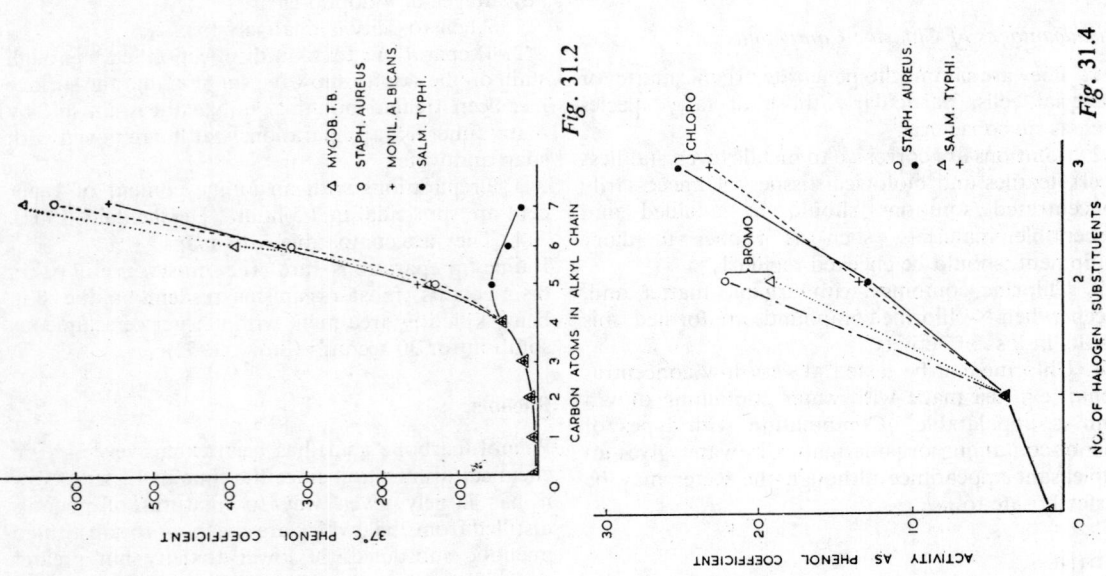

Fig. 31.5

Fig. 31.2

Fig. 31.4

Fig. 31.2   Bactericidal activities of N-alkyl phenols
Fig. 31.3   Bactericidal activities of alkyl cresols
           (*Data from Coulthard et al., 1930*)
Fig. 31.4   Bactericidal activities of halogenated phenols
Fig. 31.5   Bactericidal activities of chlorinated alkyl phenols

in water; a 20 per cent solution by weight of water in phenol (liquefied phenol) has been used as a concentrate. Phenol causes necrosis of tissues and care should be exercised when preparing solutions from it.

The simplest homologues of phenol are ortho-, meta-, and para-cresol and there is little difference between their antibacterial activities. Cresol BP is a natural mixture of the three obtained by fractional distillation of coal tar; for use this is solubilised with soap (see Lysol BP). The next in order of complexity are the xylenols (dimethyl phenols) and their chloro substitution products such as para-chlorometaxylenol BPC.

Figures 31.2 to 31.5 indicate some of the relationships between structure and activity in the phenols—

1. Activity increases with the number of carbon atoms in the alkyl chain.

2. A branched side chain with the same number of carbon atoms as an unbranched chain has lower activity.

3. For *Salmonella typhi*, the highest phenol coefficient is at a chain length of 5 carbon atoms (e.g. n-amyl). Because the chain length for peak activity is not the same for different organisms, Klarmann et al (1934) named this phenomenon 'quasi-specificity'. Originally, on the basis of the RW test, chloroxylenol disinfectants were credited with very high activity. Later it was found that the coefficients were too high because of an unsuspected reaction between the bactericides and the broth. This was most marked when staphylococci were used as the test organisms and closer scrutiny showed that the activity of chloroxylenol against these organisms was lower than had previously been assumed. As a result, this type of disinfectant lost the important place it had gained in midwifery and obstetrics.

The following additional points emerge from the graphs for halogen-substituted phenols (Figs. 31.4 and 31.5)—

1. Chlorination and bromination of phenol produce approximately the same increase in activity.

2. Ortho and para halogenation produce about the same increase in activity but meta compounds are less active.

3. The activity of a particular nucleus increases in proportion to the number of halogen atoms in that nucleus.

By selecting an appropriate range of tar acids, formulations can be prepared with RW values tailored to specification. However, Sykes (1965) warns against taking this process too far, since the production of a bactericide with a high coefficient for *Salmonella typhi* does not always mean that the activity will be as high against other more common

pathogens (e.g. streptococci and staphylococci); this quasi-specificity increases with the phenol coefficient.

At pH 10 and above phenols usually dissociate to form phenate ions that are almost inactive. The practice of using sodium hydroxide solution to solubilise phenol for gargles etc. results in decreased activity and at a 1:1 molecular ratio the solution has no antimicrobial activity, although it remains a good local anaesthetic. Minimal quantities of alkalis should be used for solubilisation.

The action of phenols on micro-organisms appears to be non-specific and is believed to be due to protein denaturation. It is uncertain how this denaturation takes place; possibly the phenol enters the cytoplasmic membrane, disrupting its structure and functions. The hydroxy group of a phenol could form a hydrogen bond with a suitable receptor in a protein of an enzyme system, the rest of the phenol molecule then constituting a physical barrier to attachment of the normal substrate. Additionally, the attachment of many phenol molecules to a protein might force open the folds in its structure and cause dysfunction. Both these effects would be potentiated by increase in length of a side chain. No satisfactory explanation of quasi-specificity follows from these theories.

BISPHENOLS AND DIPHENYLS

Representatives of these groups of phenolic compounds have recently found uses as bactericides. The diphenyls are derived from—

and the bisphenols from—

Important facts about the derivatives of these compounds are—

1. Derivatives with a hydroxyl group in both rings are more active than derivatives with a hydroxyl in one ring, but inclusion of further hydroxyl groups gives no additional increase in activity.

2. Usually, the 2:2' hydroxy compounds are more active than any other combination of two hydroxyl groups, except in the stilbene derivative where the 4:4' derivative is the best.

3. Increase of chain length up to the equivalent of C_4 in the bridging group R of the bisphenols enhances activity.

4. Halogenation increases activity, particularly against fungi. Dichloro-derivatives are most active against Gram-negative cells and fungi while hexa-chloro-derivatives are more active against Gram-positive organisms.

5. The sodium salts are only slightly less active than the parent phenol and so alkalis may be used for solubilisation.

Solubility problems limit the use of diphenyls in disinfection but *o*-phenyl phenol has been used successfully. Several bisphenol preparations are on the market, the 2:2′ dihydroxychloro-derivatives being most popular. The dichloro-, tetrachloro-, and hexachloro-derivatives have also been used, because of their relatively low toxicity and also because of the residual antimicrobial activity left on the skin and on textiles, which is useful in reducing cross-infection from the hands and hospital bedding.

Compounds of a similar nature, e.g. bithionol, have been used as aerosols to reduce the microbial flora in the atmosphere of theatres and burns units.

FORMULATIONS CONTAINING PHENOLS

Although many phenols are fully active in saturated aqueous solutions, they are not very useful in this form because heavy inocula or large amounts of organic matter deplete such solutions causing loss of activity. In most commercial preparations the phenols are solubilised with soaps and the physical and biological problems associated with such formulations have been discussed by Bean and Berry (1951) and Berry and Stenlake (1942). Despite the difficulty of explaining their mode of action these products are widely used, particularly as household disinfectants.

Solution of Cresol with Soap (Lysol BP)

This contains 50 per cent of cresol solubilised with the sodium or potassium salt of one or more fatty acids. A soap made with linseed oil is used in the specimen formula in the BP because this oil is cheap and relatively efficient. Berry and Stenlake (1942) investigated the suitability of various natural oils and found that coconut oil gave the highest RW coefficients; however, cost prevents its use. The RW coefficients of lysol generally range from 3 to 4, depending on the oil used to make the soap.

Lysol is very effective against vegetative organisms because it has bactericidal and detergent properties. Its chief disadvantage is that strong solutions are necrotic to animal tissues; even 5 to 10 per cent aqueous solutions irritate the skin of many people.

Products without this disadvantage are now available (e.g. Sudol) but because these contain phenols of higher molecular weight they show a degree of quasi-specificity.

Black Fluids

These contain the higher boiling fractions of the tar acids and sometimes chlorinated derivatives from tar acids or petroleum distillation are added to adjust the RW coefficient. Details of the criteria used in selecting these distillates are discussed by Sykes (1965) and Finch (1958). Usually the phenolic constituents are solubilised by soaps of crude fatty or resin acids and sulphonated crude castor oil (turkey red oil) is added to minimise precipitation when the fluids are diluted with hard water. Normally, the phenol content is between 15 and 35 per cent.

Black fluids form good emulsions when diluted with soft water but with hard water produce an unpleasant black scum which, however, can be a reservoir of activity in certain circumstances. They are non-selective, relatively non-toxic when diluted, but they have strong odours and they stain linen. They are used as general household disinfectants in situations where the powerful odour is not important, e.g. for drains, and as soil disinfectants and winter sprays in horticulture.

White Fluids

These are emulsions prepared from slightly more refined tar acids than are used in black fluids; crude protein material is used as the emulsifying agent and turkey red oil is added as a stabiliser (see above). Dilution produces a weaker emulsion that is less susceptible to the action of hard water than the emulsion produced by diluting a black fluid. Because they do not stain they can be used to disinfect linen. Other applications include wound treatment in animals and sheep dips.

The turkey red oil dissolves some of the phenols and on dilution forms emulsified droplets or small globules that act as a reservoir of phenol from which the aqueous solution is replenished as it becomes depleted.

PREPARATIONS OF CHLORINATED PHENOLS

A number of these were introduced in the 'thirties. Most were formulations of chloroxylenol in a castor oil soap and contained terpineol as a carrier of the phenol on dilution and to give odour. Because of their low toxicity and pleasant odour they were widely used as disinfectants in the home and, for the same reasons and because of reported persistence of activity, in obstetrics and gynaecology. Later a small amount of dichloroxylenol was included to increase activity against staphylococci and it was found necessary to choose the soap carefully to obtain a product effective against *Pseudomonas aeruginosa*. Due to these deficiencies and the quasi-specific effect mentioned on p. 357, these preparations are now less widely used, particularly in obstetrics and gynaecology.

SOAPS CONTAINING PHENOLIC COMPOUNDS

A number of phenols have been formulated in soaps but most have very little activity in this form. Formulations containing chlorinated diphenyls or bisphenols are more effective, particularly because traces are left on the skin where they exert a prolonged action. They reduce but do not eliminate the skin flora and they have caused dermatitis in some individuals.

Alcohols

Ferguson and Pirrie (1948) have compiled tables of the bactericidal concentrations of a homologous series of alcohols and information from these is plotted in graphical form in Fig. 31.6. This shows that activity increases with length of carbon chain, but it is not always possible to take advantage of this because solubility decreases with chain length.

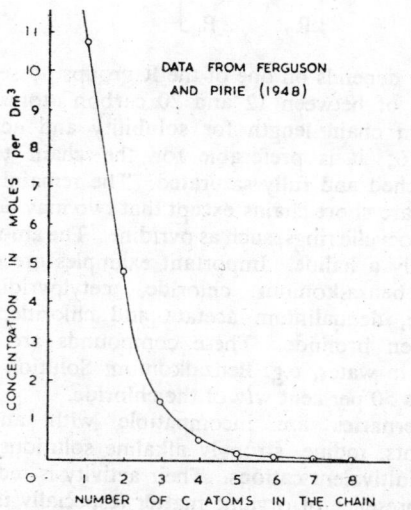

Fig. 31.6 Bactericidal activity of a homologous series of alcohols against *Salmonella typhi*

The probable mode of action of alcohols is denaturation of protein and effects and mechanisms similar to those for phenols would be expected. Structure-activity relationships are also similar except that alcohols do not produce compounds equivalent to the phenates.

Problems of toxicity and solubility result in only two monohydric acyl alcohols (ethyl and isopropyl) finding use as bactericides or preservatives. The concentration of ethyl alcohol that kills most rapidly is 70 per cent (Morton, 1950) and the minimum lethal concentration for some organisms is as low as 7·5 per cent. Sykes (1965) states that the action is bactericidal, i.e. irreversible. Alcohols show very little activity against spores. Isopropyl alcohol is about as effective as ethyl alcohol at the same concentrations.

The effect of a chlorine atom in the structure of an alcohol is shown by chlorbutol (chlorbutanol) which is active at about 0·5 per cent. Formerly, it was recommended as a preservative in eye drops and injections but now it is rarely used for these purposes because—

1. It has a fairly strong camphor-like odour.
2. It is hydrolysed in solution, particularly during heat sterilisation and if the pH is below 4.
3. Its solubility in water at 20°C is only about 0·5 per cent and so there is little margin for error because the effective strength is approximately the same.
4. It is volatile in steam.

PHENYL AND ARYL SUBSTITUTED ALCOHOLS

Phenylethyl alcohol, 0·5 per cent, is sometimes used as a preservative for eye drops. Benzyl alcohol, in a concentration of 0·9 per cent, is a suitable preservative for injections, particularly when a weak local anaesthetic effect is useful. Chlorine derivatives of benzyl alcohol have been studied by Carter *et al.* (1958); trichlorobenzyl alcohol was the most effective but 2:4 dichlorobenzyl alcohol was the least toxic and has been used in mouthwashes and gargles.

GLYCOLS

Triethylene and propylene glycols were originally used as solvents in the formulation of bactericidal aerosols. Later they were found to be only slightly less active than the complete aerosols. The triethylene compound is about 40 times as active as the propylene compound as an aerial bactericide but is more toxic and cannot be used in rooms occupied by people or animals. (*See also* Gunn and Carter, 1965.)

GLYCEROL

At high concentrations (50 per cent or more) glycerol is an effective antibacterial agent but at lower concentrations some organisms can use it as an energy source.

Formaldehyde

This compound, usually in the form of Formalin, B.P. (about 40 per cent of formaldehyde gas in water) has been widely used as a fumigant, for disinfecting rooms, and as a preservative of pathological specimens. Formalin lozenges were once popular for treating mouth and throat infections.

It is a powerful reducing agent, exerting most of its action on protein and protein-like materials; for this reason its use on mucous membranes has been discouraged. Its use for sterilisation has been discussed by Gunn and Carter (1965).

Hydroxy-acids and their Esters

Lactic acid is widely used to preserve foods; often (e.g. in yoghourt and sauerkraut) it is generated *in situ* by fermentation with a suitable strain of lactic acid organisms.

In pharmacy the methyl, ethyl, propyl and butyl esters of parahydroxybenzoic acid are used as antifungal preservatives. In all cases the effective concentration is near to the saturation concentration in water; to overcome this, mixtures of the esters may be used; the methyl and propyl esters are said to exhibit synergism. Because some species of *Pseudomonas* can utilise parahydroxybenzoates, these esters are unsuitable for preserving eye drops. They are also unsatisfactory as preservatives of oil-in-water creams made with emulsifying agents of the polyethylene glycol type, because preservative is lost through hydrogen bonding to the emulgent.

Surface Active Agents

Synthetic detergents were first developed in the First World War when, because fats were short, it became necessary to find alternatives to soap. There are three major classes (*see* p. 41) but only the cationic type is of significant value in disinfection.

ANIONIC AGENTS

These are excellent detergents but, although they mechanically remove dirt, including bacteria, their bactericidal activity is poor. Some, for example the crude fatty acid soaps, have a pH of about 10 which is bactericidal, but toilet soaps have very little antibacterial activity. Some long chain fatty acid soaps have slight activity, those from saturated and unsaturated acids being more active against Gram-positive and Gram-negative organisms respectively. Synthetic compounds such as sodium cetyl sulphate have virtually no antimicrobial properties.

NON-IONIC AGENTS

Although valuable as detergents and emulsifying agents, these have no value as antibacterials. They are useful, however, in the formulation of bactericides that are not very soluble in water (e.g. iodophores). Their detergent activity may break up aggregates of certain organisms and render them more susceptible to attack by other chemicals.

CATIONIC AGENTS

This is a very important group of bactericides. They are not very good detergents, particularly at the low concentrations that are effective in killing bacteria. Additions (such as polyphosphate salts) may be made to improve their detergency, particularly when hard water is used for dilution; these preparations are known as detergent sanitisers.

The most satisfactory bactericides are the quaternary ammonium compounds which have the general formula—

$$\left[\begin{array}{cc} R_1 & R_2 \\ & N \\ R_3 & R_4 \end{array} \right]^{+} \quad X^{-}$$

Activity depends on one of the R groups possessing a chain of between 12 and 20 carbon atoms, the optimum chain length for solubility and activity being 16; it is preferable for the chain to be unbranched and fully saturated. The remaining R groups are short chains except that two may belong to heterocyclic rings, such as pyridine. The anion X^{-} is usually a halide. Important examples are cetrimide, benzalkonium chloride, cetylpyridinium chloride, dequalinium acetate and chloride, and domiphen bromide. These compounds are very soluble in water, e.g. Benzalkonium Solution BPC contains 50 per cent w/v of the chloride.

Quaternaries are incompatible with anionic detergents, iodine, strongly alkaline solutions and some multivalent cations. Their activity is reduced in the presence of organic matter (especially if this contains phospholipids, as is the case with milk, blood, serum, sebaceous secretions and egg yolk) and some non-ionic detergents (particularly poly-sorbate 80 and Lubrol W). They are most active against Gram-positive organisms and have very little activity against spores. *Proteus vulgaris* and *Pseudomonas aeruginosa* are very resistant; the last-named can survive in a concentration of 1 in 100 while Gram-positive cells are destroyed by 1 in 30 000. High resistance is also shown by *Mycobacterium tuberculosis* and viruses, but many fungi are sensitive.

Because low concentrations are effective, these agents are not very toxic, even on ingestion; however, they should not be used as wet dressings because of the risk of sensitisation.

They are widely used as disinfectants in the dairy, food and brewing industries because they are almost odourless and tasteless. They find many applications in pharmacy. A 0·01 per cent solution of benzalkonium chloride is recommended as a preservative for certain eye drops; silicone rubber must be used for the teats of the dropper bottles because quaternaries attack most rubbers. They are unsuitable as preservatives for injections because even low concentrations are haemolytic.

Bacteria may develop resistance to quaternary ammonium compounds, and strains that can resist about 40 times the normal bactericidal concentration have been isolated from weak solutions.

Because these agents are strongly adsorbed on to surfaces, materials such as glassware, plastics and fabrics may remain bactericidal even after several washings. Residual activity on hospital blankets is helpful in the control of cross-infection, particularly as pyogenic cocci are very sensitive to quaternaries. On the other hand, this adsorption has led to the allocation of excessively high antibacterial activities to quaternary ammonium compounds, because molecules adsorbed on to bacteria continue to act after the organisms have been transferred to recovery media. To overcome this problem, British Standard 3286:1960 suggests the use of lecithin (a phospholipid) and polysorbate (Tween) 80 or Lubrol W (non-ionic surface active agents) as inactivators.

Dyes

The dyes that were developed as a result of the work of Ehrlich include derivatives of acridine, pararosaniline and quinoline. Their importance has waned since the advent of antibiotics but some are still in use and are of particular interest because of structure-activity relationships and because of their importance in investigational microbiology (*see* p. 320).

ACRIDINES

The parent molecule (acridine) is a tricyclic nitrogen-containing ring system. In the active form of this

compound the nitrogen forms a quaternary type of cation which is associated with a suitable anion such as chloride (e.g. Aminacrine hydrochloride BP) or hemisulphate (e.g. Proflavine hemisulphate BP). Substituents that promote ionisation increase potency. In addition, the molecule must lie in a flat plane with no groups projecting above or below it; this is because the action of the acridine molecule is to fit between base groups in the DNA molecule of the genetic apparatus of the organism. This penetration, known as intercalation, disrupts the genetic code and interferes with protein formation and DNA replication, thus upsetting the control of the cell.

Amino groups are best for promoting ionisation of the N group without undue increase in toxicity, and the most effective position is 9, followed closely by 3 and 6. 9-Aminoacridine (aminacrine) is 100 per cent ionised at pH 7·3 and does not stain badly; it is used in obstetrics and gynaecology. Acridines are effective against pyogenic cocci and the gas-gangrene clostridia at concentrations as low as 1 in 100 000; they have also been employed in the treatment of trypanosomal diseases. They were widely used as powders (sometimes in association with sulphonamides) or as dressings (in the form of oily emulsions); this continued into the early years of the Second World War, but later they were superseded by systemic treatment with penicillin. Two disadvantages that were not discovered for some time and which made them unsuitable for large wounds, are toxicity to leucocytes and retardation of the granulation (healing) process.

PARAROSANILINE (TRIPHENYLMETHANE) DYES

In these compounds, the basic molecule (triphenyl-methane) has varying numbers of amino groups, with both hydrogen atoms substituted, on two or more of the phenyl rings; X may be Cl or HSO_4. R is CH_3 in malachite green and C_2H_5 in brilliant green.

Antibacterial activity is due to the cation and the associated quinonoid ring. The mode of action is uncertain but it appears that these dyes can poise the oxidation-reduction potential at a point unfavourable to growth of organisms. This poising is eventually overcome by the metabolic activity of the cells and when it has been completely nullified the culture can grow again. At high pH values a leuco base is formed which is inactive, but between neutrality and pH 9 there is a marked increase in activity against most bacterial species (Adams, 1967a) although it has been shown that there is no appreciable change in the sorption of dye on the cells within this range (Adams, 1967b).

These dyes are active against bacteria and fungi and are taken up and retained more readily by Gram-positive than by Gram-negative cells; the ratio of concentrations required to inhibit Gram-positive and Gram-negative cells is about 1:100. The action is said to be entirely inhibitory, the cells being held in a state of suspended animation (*see* p. 343)

They still find limited uses in medicine, particularly as paints for application to fungal infections such as ringworm.

Metals, their Salts and Organic Derivatives

Certain metals, particularly gold, silver and copper, in a pure, clean state, yield minute quantities of ions to aqueous solutions and these exert an antimicrobial (oligodynamic) effect. Water contaminated with about 20 000 organisms per cm^3 and stored in copper vessels for about six hours, fails to produce colonies on agar, and water prepared in copper stills may cause false results in bacterial counts. It is reported that King Darius of ancient Persia had his drinking water carried to battle in silver vessels; hence it is possible that the oligodynamic effect was known long ago.

Silvered gravel beds were used in army water tankers during the last war, as the last stage of purification of drinking water. Colloidal silver preparations have been used in eye drops and for bladder irrigations, but damage can be caused by the action of silver on proteins, particularly in the eyes.

MERCURY

From the bacteriological point of view this is the most important of the heavy metals. The oligodynamic effect, although evident, is not widely used because of the high toxicity of mercury. Most mercury compounds depend on a very slight degree of ionisation to yield the toxic mercuric ion. This ion may combine reversibly with sulphydryl groups of proteins and polypeptides in the substrate and so prevent their utilisation by the organism. Alternatively (Richards and el Khouly, 1967) they may combine with sulphydryl-containing receptor sites on enzymes and block take-up of the substrate.

The action of mercurials was thought to be bactericidal until Brewer (1939) demonstrated that recovery of cells was much improved if thioglycollate medium was used instead of the conventional nutrient broths. Cook and Steel (1959) showed that even better recoveries could be obtained if the thioglycollate broth was made under carefully controlled conditions and they concluded that the action of mercury was largely reversible, i.e. was inhibitory or bacteriostatic. Because inorganic mercury salts, such as the chloride and oxycyanide, are very toxic, their use is strictly limited, but organic derivatives of mercury are used as preservatives in injections, eye drops, and creams and as antiseptics in topical applications. The organic compounds in common use are phenylmercuric salts (nitrate, acetate, or borate) and thiomersal. They are used at low concentrations, 0·001 to 0·002 per cent for phenylmercuric salts and 0·01 to 0·02 per cent for thiomersal. At these concentrations toxicity to tissues is low although prolonged use of eye drops preserved with mercurials can lead to slight deposition of metallic mercury on the cornea. Thiomersal has been used, in alcoholic solution, as a paint for the treatment of fungal infections of the skin; it is a popular preservative for vaccines because it does not greatly impair their antigenicity.

Salts of zinc, copper, and aluminium are astringents, i.e. they precipitate proteins, and, therefore, are mild antiseptics. Lotions containing them are sometimes used to promote the healing of varicose ulcers.

Chlorhexidine

This bactericide was discovered during research into the biological properties of guanidine compounds following the introduction of Paludrine as an antimalarial. It is a very strong base and, to obtain solubility in water, is used as its salts. The acetate and hydrochloride are official together with a 20 per cent solution of the gluconate. The salts are not very soluble in water—acetate, 1 in 55; hydrochloride, 1 in 1700; both at 20°C. Slightly better solubility is obtained by using ethyl alcohol as solvent and in some preparations the hydrochloride is dissolved in propylene glycol.

Chlorhexidine is relatively non-toxic and has a good spectrum of activity against bacteria; the

MIC in blood media is about 1 in 200 000 for Gram-positive organisms and about 1 in 40 000 for Gram-negative bacteria, including many strains of *Pseudomonas aeruginosa*. At 1 in 10 000 and higher concentrations it is bactericidal in 10 minutes but alcoholic solutions are necessary to obtain the same result with *Mycobacterium tuberculosis*. It is not a good sporicide or virucide but will inhibit pathogenic fungi at about 1 in 1000. Maximum activity is shown at pH 8.

It is widely used in hospitals for skin preparation before surgery, for cleaning wounds and in lubricants for obstetrics and gynaecology. The acetate is used at a concentration of 0·01 per cent as a preservative for eye drops. A number of strains of *Pseudomonas* have developed resistance but the incidence is small. Dilute solutions demonstrate the unusual phenomenon of a fairly rapid kill at first, followed by prolonged survival of the remaining cells.

Because chlorhexidine is incompatible with anionic surface active agents, creams containing it should be formulated with cationic emulsifiers or a methylcellulose gel or, if the choice is made carefully, a non-ionic agent. (Some non-ionic agents are used to neutralise the activity of chlorhexidine in tests for sterility and bactericidal activity.)

ANTIMICROBIAL PRESERVATIVES

The use of preservatives in sterile products is discussed by Gunn and Carter (1965) and individual compounds have been mentioned in earlier parts of this chapter. The function of an antimicrobial preservative is to prevent the growth of unwanted micro-organisms in pharmaceutical preparations without introducing untoward effects. In choosing a satisfactory chemical consideration should be given to the following—

The Type(s) of Micro-organism likely to be Present and the Effects they may have on the Product

For example, products from animal sources may contain pathogens. A mild epidemic of typhoid fever in Sweden was traced to thyroid tablets contaminated with *Salmonella typhi*. Spores of tetanus and gas gangrene have been isolated from gelatin. Plant products, such as starches, may contain organisms from the soil; a few of these are pathogenic. e.g. clostridia and *Bacillus anthracis* but many more can cause spoilage of pharmaceutical products. Soil organisms are common in dust which may gain access to a preparation during processing or packaging. Containers or closures may cause contamination; spores can exist between the wad and liner of a screw-capped container and cork is a common source of mould spores. The product may also be contaminated by the user. The preservative must prevent accidental contamination from causing serious or even dangerous decomposition of the product throughout its accepted storage life.

The Nature of the Medicament

The preservative must not affect the chemical, physical, or pharmacological properties of the medicament.

The Nature of Adjuncts

In colloidal systems adsorption of the preservative may take place; in biphasic systems partition may occur; and in any system there may be combination between adjunct and preservative that renders the latter ineffective.

The Properties of the Preservative

The distribution of the preservative must be homogenous and where there is a multi-phase system, satisfactory solubility in the bulk phase is preferable. A sparingly soluble preservative, although active in saturated solution in the bulk phase, may become depleted by chemical or physical mechanisms to a point where its antimicrobial activity is lost. The relevant mechanisms are adsorption on to particulate matter, solution in plastic materials or outward diffusion through rubbers or plastics. Some chemicals such as chlorbutol may hydrolyse on storage, particularly if the pH is unfavourable. Preservatives may react with substances leached from the container; common sources of extractives are cork, plastics (from which plasticisers may be leached) and glass (which may yield alkali).

The Nature of the Container

Ideally the container should be impervious to micro-organisms and preservatives but some leakage takes place from most containers except those sealed by fusion of glass. The problem is most acute in dispensing when bottles, vials and jars, and, particularly, screw caps are re-used. When loss is unavoidable, enough excess preservative should be included to ensure a reasonable storage life and the product should carry an appropriate expiry date.

The Climate and Microbial Flora of the Country to which the Product is being Exported

Products for export to countries with climates and microbial flora different from the country of origin must be tested in those countries or, if this is not practicable, by carefully simulated conditions in the laboratory.

Preservatives Used in Official Preparations

ACIDS, SALTS AND ESTERS

	Percentage
Benzoic acid	0·1
Benzoic acid solution BPC	2·0
Salicylic acid	4·0
Sorbic acid	0·2
Sodium benzoate	0·1
Butylhydroxybenzoate	0·01 (in water) 0·15 (in oils and creams)
Ethylhydroxybenzoate	0·05 (in water) 0·15 (in oils and creams)
Methyl and propyl hydroxybenzoates	0·1 (in water) 0·2 (in oils and creams)
2:1 mixture of methyl and propyl hydroxybenzoates	0·06 and 0 03 respectively

ALCOHOLS

Benzyl alcohol	0·9
Chlorbutol	0·5
Ethyl alcohol	15·0
Glycerol	50·0
Phenylethyl alcohol	0·5
Propylene glycol	30·0

PHENOLS

Chlorocresol	0·1
Cresol	0·3
Phenol	0·5

MERCURIALS

Phenylmercuric acetate, borate, or nitrate	0·002
Thiomersal	0·02

OTHER AGENTS

Benzalkonium chloride	0·01
Cetrimide	0·001
Chlorhexidine	0·01
Chloroform	0·02
Formaldehyde	Equivalent of 4·0
Sucrose	66·7
Sulphur dioxide	420 ppm

BIBLIOGRAPHY

ALBERT, A. (1968) *Selective Toxicity*. 4th ed. Methuen, London.

FINCH, W. E. (1958) *Disinfectants, their Values and Uses.* Chapman and Hall, London.

GENERAL MEDICAL COUNCIL OF GREAT BRITAIN (1968) *The British Pharmacopoeia*. Pharmaceutical Press, London.

GUNN, C. and CARTER, S. J. (1965) *Dispensing for Pharmaceutical Students*. 11th ed. Pitman Medical, London.

LAWRENCE, C. A. and BLOCK, S. S. (1968) *Disinfection, Sterilization and Preservation*. Henry Kimpton, London.

MARTINDALE (Ed. R. G. TODD) (1967) *Extra Pharmacopoeia*. 25th ed. Pharmaceutical Press, London.

THE PHARMACEUTICAL SOCIETY (1968) *The British Pharmaceutical Codex*. Pharmaceutical Press, London.

SCHNITZER, R. J. and HAWKING, F. (1964) *Experimental Chemotherapy Vols. I, II, and III*. Academic Press, New York.

SEXTON, W. A. (1963) *Chemical Constitution and Biological Activity*. Spon, London.

SOCIETY OF CHEMICAL INDUSTRY (1965) *Surface Activity and the Microbial Cell. S.C.I. Monograph No. 19*. Society of Chemical Industry, London.

SYKES, G. (1965) *Disinfection and Sterilizatioh..* 2nd ed. Spon, London.

REFERENCES

ADAMS, E. (1967a) The antibacterial action of crystal violet. *J. Pharm. Pharmac.*, **19**, 821–826.

ADAMS, E. (1967b) The effect of pH on the bactericidal activity of crystal violet. *ibid.*, **19**, 203S–208S.

ADAMS, E. (1968) The binding of crystal violet by the nucleic acids of *Escherichia coli*. *ibid.*, **20**, 18S–22S.

BEAN, H. S. and BERRY, H. (1951) The bactericidal activitv of phenols in aqueous solutions of soaps

II. The bactericidal activity of benzylchlorphenol in aqueous solutions of potassium laurate. *ibid.*, **5**, 632–639.

BERRY, H. (1944) The antibacterial value of phenoxetol. *Lancet*, **247**, 175.

BERRY, H. and STENLAKE, J. B. (1942) Variations in the bactericidal values of Lysol B.P. *Pharm. J.*, **148**, 112.

BREWER, J. H. (1939) The antibacterial effects of the organic mercurial compounds. *J. Am. med. Ass.*, **112**, 2009.

CARTER, D. V., CHARLTON, P. T., FENTON, A. H., HOUSLEY, J. R., and LESSEL, B. (1958) The preparation and the antibacterial and antifungal properties of some substituted benzyl alcohols. *J. Pharm. Pharmac.*, **10**, 149T–157T.

COOK, A. M. and STEEL, K. J. (1959) Antagonism of the antibacterial action of mercury compounds. IV. Qualitative aspects. *ibid.*, **11**, 162T–168T.

COOK, A. M. and STEEL, K. J. (1960) V. Quantitative aspects. *ibid.*, **12**, 219–226.

COULTHARD, C. E., MARSHALL, J. and PYMAN, F. L. (1930) The variation of phenol coefficients in a homologous series of phenols. *J. chem. Soc.*, 280–291.

DAVIS, J. G. (1960) Chemical Disinfection. *J. Pharm. Pharmac.*, **12**, 29T–40T.

FERGUSON, J. and PIRIE, H. (1948) The toxicity of vapours to the grain weevil. *Ann. appl. Biol.*, **35**, 532–550.

FILDES, P. (1940) The mechanism of the antibacterial action of mercury. *Br. J. exp. Path.*, **21**, 67–73.

GERSHENFELD, L. (1962) Povidone iodine as a sporicide. *Am. J. Pharm.*, **134**, 78–81.

KLARRMAN, E. G., SHTERNOV, V. A., and GATES, L. W.

(1934) The bactericidal and fungicidal action of homologous halogen phenol derivatives and its 'quasi-specific' character. *J. Lab. clin. Med.*, **19**, 835–851. *ibid.*, **20**, 40–47.

MORTON, H. E. (1950) The relationship of concentration and germicidal efficiency of ethyl alcohol. *Ann. N.Y. Acad Sci.*, **53**, 191–196.

PITTMAN, M. (1946) A study of fluid thioglycollate medium for the sterility test. *J. Bact.*, **51**, 19–32.

RICHARDS, J. P. and EL KHOULY, A. E. E. (1967) Recovery of phenylmercuric nitrate treated bacteria. *J. Pharm. Pharmac.*, **19**, 209S–215S.

RUEHLE, G. C. A. and BREWER, C. M. (1931) *U.S. Food and Drug Administration Methods of Testing Antiseptics and Disinfectants. Circular No. 198.* U.S. Dept. of Agriculture, Washington, D.C.

RUSSELL, A. D. (1967) Preservatives in pharmacy. *J. Hosp. Pharm.*, **24**, 262–265.

RUSSELL, A. D., JENKINS, J. and HARRISON, I. H. (1967) The inclusion of antimicrobial agents in pharmaceutical products. *Adv. appl. Microbiol.*, **9**, 1–38.

STORY, P. (1952) Testing skin disinfectants. *Br. med. J.*, **2**, 1128–30.

THOMAS, G. W. and COOK, E. S. (1947) The action of phenylmercuric nitrate IV. The ability of sulphydryl compounds to protect against the germicidal action. *J. Bact.*, **54**, 527–534.

VARIOUS AUTHORS (1968) Biocides and sterilization. *Process Biochem.*, **3**, 23–37.

WEDDERBERN, D. L. (1964) Preservation of emulsions against microbial attack. *Adv. Pharm. Sci.*, **1**, 195–264.

WILSON, G. S. (Chairman) (1958) Report of committee. Disinfection of fabrics with gaseous formaldehyde. *J. Hyg.*, *Camb.*, **56**, 488–515.

32

Antibiotics

THIS major group of chemotherapeutic agents was introduced in Chapter 26.

Manufacture

Antibiotics may be manufactured by a fermentation process (most antibiotics), by fermentation followed by chemical synthesis (certain penicillins), or by synthesis (chloramphenicol).

The fermentation process involves growing the organism in a nutrient broth under optimum conditions, followed by extraction of the antibiotic or its precursor from the growth medium and/or the mycelium. The general principles can be illustrated by reference to the production of penicillin.

Originally the mould was cultivated on the surface of a liquid medium in numerous small flasks (each of about 500 cm³ capacity) shaped to facilitate stacking and having a special neck through which inoculation could take place aseptically. Thousands of flasks were necessary to obtain adequate amounts of antibiotic and the handling problems during washing, sterilisation, filling, inoculation and bulking made the process tedious and uneconomic. Today antibiotics are made by deep (submerged) culture in which the mould is encouraged to grow deeply submerged in a large tank of medium.

CHOICE OF ORGANISM

The organism should give high yields of antibiotic from economic sources of nutrients and should not produce excessive amounts of substances chemically related to the antibiotic because separation may be difficult.

The original Fleming strain of *Penicillium notatum* is probably not used nowadays. Strains of *Penicillium chrysogenum* have been successful in deep culture. High-yielding natural strains are often genetically unstable and are also unable to resist attack by biological agents such as bacteriophages. More reliable strains are obtained by subjecting cultures to physical or chemical mutagens such as X-rays, ultra-violet light or nitrogen mustard. Variation of the new strains must be prevented,

usually by freeze-drying the spores followed by storage in the dark.

CHOICE OF MEDIUM

The basis of most fermentation media is corn steep liquor, the fluid obtained from the steeping of maize prior to starch extraction. It provides a variety of nutrients and has good buffering capacity. For most fermentations, particularly those involving fungi, additional sugar (normally lactose or glucose) is needed as a source of energy for mycelium production. Occasionally, when the nitrogen demand is high, soya bean, or peanut, meal may be added. Buffering salts may be required when the antibiotic is pH sensitive.

To improve the yield of a particular penicillin a precursor (a preformed part of the molecule) may be added, e.g. phenylacetic acid for benzylpenicillin and phenoxyacetic acid for phenoxymethylpenicillin.

CULTIVATION OF THE ORGANISM

A slope is inoculated with spores from the master (e.g. freeze-dried) culture. After incubation, the growth is checked for freedom from contamination and variation. A spore suspension made from the slope is transferred to culture flasks, several litres in capacity, which are incubated to obtain a large crop of spores. The flasks are shaken during incubation to ensure that enough air is available to the aerobic mould.

The suspension in the flasks is used to inoculate a 2000 dm³ tank, known as the seed vessel; this is a small version of the fermenter. After further incubation, sterile compressed air is used to blow the contents through sterile pipes into huge fermentation tanks (fermenters) with a capacity of 50 000 dm³ or more. The growth of the mould is allowed to continue until a satisfactory level of antibiotic has been reached.

AERATION

Because the moulds (usually species of *Penicillium* and *Streptomyces*) used in antibiotic production are aerobic they will not grow well deep in a tank of medium unless they are supplied with plenty of oxygen. This is achieved by pumping in large volumes of air through an inlet (sparger) at the bottom of the fermenter. The sparger introduces the air as streams of bubbles that are further broken down and distributed by a high-powered stirrer (agitator). The resulting tiny bubbles dissolve readily to replace the oxygen absorbed from the liquid by the mould. Because of their protein content, culture media froth readily, particularly when aerated, and this is reduced by antifoaming agents such as silicone fluids, vegetable oils or octadecanol.

STERILISATION

The culture medium, vessels, pipe-lines and air must be sterile to prevent contamination by extraneous organisms that might reduce yields and produce unwanted metabolites. In the case of penicillin, penicillinase-producing organisms would rapidly destroy the antibiotic.

The fermenter, seed vessel and pipe-lines are usually sterilised by steam under pressure. Sterilisation of the medium may be carried out in the fermenter or in a separate vessel. In the fermenter, high pressure steam is passed into a heating jacket or through heating coils inside the tank. External sterilisation may be by a high-temperature, short-time method (*see* Gunn and Carter, 1965). Afterwards the hot medium is reduced to fermentation temperature, usually by passing cooling water through the internal coils.

Contamination during the process is prevented by careful design. For example, the point at which the stirrer enters the tank is surrounded by a jacket containing high pressure steam. Ports that must be opened for sampling during fermentation have two valves with the intervening pipe kept under steam. The valves act as a contamination barrier like the double doors at the entrance to an asepsis laboratory (*see* Gunn and Carter, 1965).

Because the demand for oxygen is high, a continuous method of air sterilisation is appropriate. A compressor of high capacity and capable of high compression is often used because the pressure necessary to provide the sterilisation temperature is also adequate to force the air through the medium against the head of pressure in the fermentation tank. As an added precaution, the air is passed through a sterilising filter (Gunn and Carter, 1965) immediately before entry to the tank.

TEMPERATURE CONTROL

Part of the energy produced by carbohydrate breakdown during the metabolism of the mould is liberated as heat. This must be controlled because high temperatures inhibit the mould and destroy the antibiotic. An optimum temperature (about 24°C for penicillin) is maintained by passing cooling water through coils or a jacket, or simply by running cold water over the surface of the fermenter.

ISOLATION OF THE PRODUCT

After fermentation the mycelium is removed by a rotary filter (Figs. 20.8 and 20.9). The antibiotic is obtained from the filtrate by adjustment to a pH at which the acid or base (depending on the nature of the antibiotic) is liberated, followed by removal of unwanted substances and extraction of the active material with a solvent system in, for example, a Podbielniak counter current machine (*see* p. 251). In some cases, where the free acid or base is unstable, impurities are separated from the salt by chromatographic or ion exchange techniques; the extraction of streptomycin is an illustration of this.

The crude product of extraction is purified in a variety of ways. Sometimes a complex salt is formed, e.g. the N-ethylpiperidine salt of penicillin, and from this a simple salt of the antibiotic is obtained by double decomposition, the last recrystallisation being done under aseptic conditions. The final drying is under vacuum and may involve freeze-drying. For freeze-drying the liquid may be packed in its final containers previously, but often drying is carried out in bulk and afterwards the powder is aseptically filled into vials.

Penicillins

These are the potassium, sodium or, occasionally, other metallic salts of derivatives of 6-aminopenicillanic acid (6-apa)—

$(CH_3)_2.C$———$CH.COOH$

$\longleftarrow$ ············· thiazolidine ring

S   N *

CH   CO $\longleftarrow$ ············· β-lactam ring

CH

NH$_2$

* point of hydrolysis by penicillinase (β-lactamase).

The penicillins are amides with various acyl groupings replacing one of the hydrogen atoms of the 6-amino group (*see* Table 32.1). They are produced by fermentation followed by chemical synthesis or by fermentation alone.

1. FERMENTATION AND SYNTHESIS

6-apa is obtained by one of the following methods and the required penicillin is synthesised from it by acylation of the 6-amino group.

(a) Direct Method

A special strain of *Penicillium chrysogenum* that gives good yields of 6-apa is grown in deep culture. Maximum production is obtained when the culture is aerated at 60 per cent of the normal rate for a penicillin fermentation (Batchelor *et al.*, 1959 and Cole, 1967, 1968).

(b) Indirect Method

Phenylacetic acid (precursor for benzylpenicillin) is added at intervals to a *Penicillium chrysogenum* fermentation. Later, *Escherichia coli*, which produces an acylase enzyme that breaks down benzylpenicillin to 6-apa is added. This method gives better yields than the direct method.

2. FERMENTATION ALONE

The procedure is similar to the indirect method above but *Escherichia coli* is not added and a precursor, corresponding to the type of penicillin required, is used.

Table 32.1 shows that the penicillins differ with regard to three important properties—

1. Stability in Acid pHs

If, as with benzylpenicillin, the molecule is hydrolysed by acid, the antibiotic will be destroyed by the gastric juice. If oral administration is essential the preparation must be buffered.

2. Resistance to Penicillinase

Many organisms develop resistance to penicillin by acquiring the ability to synthesise penicillinase which breaks the β-lactam ring in the molecule. For some other organisms (including several common airborne bacteria) penicillinase is one of their normal complement of enzymes. Some penicillins are resistant to penicillinase and those that are not must be protected by aseptic handling and, where appropriate, by the inclusion of bactericides in their preparations.

3. Antibacterial Spectrum

Earlier penicillins, such as benzyl- and phenoxymethyl-penicillins have a narrow spectrum of anti-bacterial activity which is largely confined to Gram-positive species. Ampicillin, one of the newer penicillins, is active against a much wider spectrum of micro-organisms.

TOXICITY

Compared with most other antibiotics, the toxicity of penicillins is very low but a few patients have died from anaphylactic shock (p. 402) due to extreme sensitivity. A significant number of people show milder allergic reactions, most often an irritating rash; this is not confined to patients but also occurs in pharmaceutical or medical staff who have to handle these antibiotics in their work.

MODE OF ACTION

Penicillin interferes with the formation of cell walls in dividing cells (Park and Wise, 1965; Park, 1966). The last stage in cell-wall formation is the cross-linking of units of a linear molecule, N-acetyl muramic acid. This cross-linkage gives the wall its strength and in its absence the organism cannot form cross walls and new cells are not produced. Long filamentous forms result and the existing walls stretch until they split, liberating the contents (a naked mass of protoplasm known as a protoplast) which, unless the surrounding medium is hypertonic, bursts causing death of the organism. It is possible that wide spectrum penicillins destroy bacteria by another mechanism.

DEVELOPMENT OF RESISTANCE

Resistance to antibacterial agents can develop in several ways (*see* p. 308). It is avoided by adequate dosage and discriminate use of the antibiotic. Because organisms exposed to inadequate concentrations may become resistant and because it is difficult to control the dose of topical preparations, topical use of penicillin is considered unwise and ointments, creams, eye ointments and lozenges are no longer official.

Procaine benzylpenicillin and ampicillin are permitted as additives to animal foodstuffs because they hasten fattening. It is debatable that antibiotics used to treat diseases should be employed in this way, because of the danger of inducing resistance in pathogenic organisms.

The number of penicillin-resistant staphylococci is increasing and is a source of anxiety to the medical profession.

The formulation of penicillin preparations, including depot forms of penicillin, is discussed by Gunn and Carter (1965).

Table 32.1
Penicillins

Name	Chemical nature	Solubility in water	Hydrolysed by:		Active against:	Remarks
			Acid	Penicillinase		
Ampicillin	6-[D(—)-α-aminobenzyl]-penicillanic acid or its sodium salt	Acid + + (soluble) Salt + + + (very soluble)	—	+	Gram + and — organisms but not Pseudomonas sp.	Given orally (acid) or by injection (salt)
Benethamine penicillin	N-benzylphenethylamine salt of benzylpenicillin	—	—	+	Gram + organisms	Depot effect lasting 3–4 days. Given as intramuscular suspension
Benzathine penicillin	NN'-dibenzylethylenediamine salt of benzylpenicillin	—	—	+	Gram + organisms	Depot effect lasting 7 days or more. Given orally or as intramuscular suspension
Benzylpenicillin (Penicillin G)	Sodium or potassium salt of 6-[benzyl]penicillanic acid	+ + +	+	+	Gram + organisms	Most reliable form by injection
Carbenicillin	Disodium salt of 6-(α-carboxy-phenyl-acetamido) penicillanic acid	+ + +	+	+	Gram + and — organisms including Pseudomonas sp.	Given by intravenous or intramuscular injection
Cloxacillin sodium	Monohydrate of the sodium salt of 6-[3-(2-chloro-phenyl)-5-methylisoxazole-4-carboxyamido] penicillanic acid	+ + +	—	—	Gram + organisms	Used against penicillinase-producing staphylococci. Given orally in capsules or by intramuscular injection
Methicillin sodium	Monohydrate of the sodium salt of 6-(2,6-dimethoxy-benzamido) penicillanic acid	+ + +	+	—	Gram + organisms	Given by intramuscular injection
Phenethicillin potassium	Mixture of potassium salts of 6-[L(—) and D(+)-α-phenoxy-propionamido]penicillanic acid	+ + +	—	+	Gram + organisms	Given orally
Phenoxymethyl penicillin (Penicillin V)	6-Phenoxyacetamido penicillanic acid and its potassium and calcium salts	Acid — Salts + + +	—	+	Gram + organisms	Widely used orally
Procaine benzylpenicillin	Procaine salt of benzyl-penicillin	—	+ (slow)	+	Gram + organisms	Depot effect lasting 1–2 days. Gives as intramuscular suspension

Streptomycin

This complex organic base is produced by growing *Streptomyces griseus* in deep culture. The official salt is the sulphate and its formula will be found in the BP.

The base is very unstable and, to prevent its liberation during extraction from the fermentation liquor, ion exchange techniques are used for its purification. Dry salts are stable for at least two years at below 30°C. Injections should be buffered between pH 3 and 7 and sterilised by filtration or prepared aseptically; stored in the dark at not more than 20°C they retain their potency for 18 months. Solutions become yellowish on exposure to light.

Absorption from the gut is insignificant and the drug must be given parenterally by intramuscular or intrathecal injection. It is a narrow spectrum antibiotic acting chiefly against Gram-negative bacteria, but it is also effective against *Mycobacterium tuberculosis* (Gram-positive). Streptomycin is most important in the treatment of tuberculosis but is sometimes used for urinary infections caused by Gram-negative organisms, and for gonorrhoea where, because (unlike penicillin, which is also active against the gonococcus) it has no action against *Treponema pallidum*, it does not obscure concurrent infection with syphilis.

Resistant strains develop quickly and some organisms become dependent on the drug. The simultaneous administration of the antitubercular drugs, calcium or sodium aminosalicylate (PAS), in cachets, and/or isoniazid (INH), in tablets, helps to prevent these changes. If treatment is prolonged streptomycin damages the eighth cranial nerve, causing deafness, difficulty in balancing and severe headaches. Simultaneous use of several antitubercular drugs reduces the risk of these effects by permitting the dose of streptomycin to be lowered.

Tetracyclines

Tetracycline, the parent antibiotic of this group, has an unusual chemical structure based on four benzenoid rings (*see* the BP). Also official are oxytetracycline (the 5-hydroxy derivative), chlortetracycline (the 7-chloro derivative) and demethylchlortetracycline (chlortetracycline without the 6-methyl group). Originally oxytetracycline and chlortetracycline were known as terramycin and aureomycin respectively. The tetracyclines are produced by submerged culture of *Streptomyces viridifaciens* (tetracycline), *Streptomyces aureofaciens* (the two chloro derivatives) and *Streptomyces rimosus* (oxytetracycline). Demethylchlortetracycline is the most stable, gives the highest blood levels and is the most active against *Pseudomonas aeruginosa* and *Proteus vulgaris*.

The tetracyclines are broad spectrum antibiotics, acting on a wide range of organisms including Gram-negative bacteria, mycoplasmata, spirochaetes, rickettsia and some larger viruses. Their activity against yeasts and fungi is low. They are usually given orally but in emergencies may be administered by slow intravenous infusion or by intramuscular injection. Because intramuscular injections are painful, procaine is usually added as an anaesthetic. The oral preparations are capsules of each of the four forms (as hydrochlorides), tablets of tetracycline (hydrochloride) and oxytetracycline (dihydrate), a mixture of tetracycline, and liquid forms of demethylchlortetracycline. The parenteral products are injections of tetracycline hydrochloride (with and without procaine hydrochloride) and an injection of oxytetracycline hydrochloride; these

are prepared aseptically shortly before use because solutions are very unstable even at refrigerator temperatures. The main topical preparations are chlortetracycline ointment and eye ointment, which are made with non-aqueous bases.

A side effect of prolonged treatment with tetracyclines is overgrowth of yeasts and moulds in the alimentary tract. Because the natural bacterial flora of the gut is depressed by the antibiotic the fungi find conditions more favourable for their growth. They proliferate in the mouth and lower gut causing discomfort, irritation and diarrhoea. Tetracyclines also interfere with the growth of teeth and should not be given to pregnant women or children under 12, unless no other drug will control the infection.

Their main mode of action is chelation of light divalent ions such as magnesium. Ribosomes are the primary sites of inhibition because they contain high concentrations of magnesium ions. Since ribosomes are concerned with protein synthesis, this is interrupted by the tetracyclines, leading to enzyme deficiencies and disruption of metabolism. Resistance develops relatively slowly but when it occurs organisms resistant to one member of the group are also resistant to the others; this is known as cross resistance.

Chloramphenicol

Compared with most other antibiotics, chloramphenicol has a simple chemical structure (*see* the BP) and, therefore, was the first antibiotic to be synthesised. Formerly it was obtained from *Streptomyces venezuelae* but now all the chloramphenicol used in this country is synthetic.

Because it is effective orally, is only slightly soluble in water and has an extremely bitter taste, it is usually administered in capsules. For children too young to take capsules, the palmitate or cinnamate is formulated in an aqueous suspension; because these derivatives are extremely insoluble they are virtually tasteless. In the treatment of certain acute conditions such as meningitis, septicaemia or severe whooping cough, intravenous infusion or deep intramuscular injection may be used; for these purposes the soluble sodium succinate derivative is used.

Although chloramphenicol is a broad spectrum antibiotic its use is severely restricted because it damages the haemopoietic system causing agranulocytosis and sometimes fatal aplastic anaemia. Systemic administration is virtually limited to the treatment of typhoid and paratyphoid fevers for which it is the most effective drug available. It should not be used for carriers of typhoid, because long treatment may be required.

Ear drops, with propylene glycol as the solvent, aqueous eye drops, containing a borax-boric acid buffer, and an eye ointment, in a non-aqueous base, are available. Aqueous solutions are stable if protected from light.

Chloramphenicol acts by interfering with protein synthesis.

Erythromycin

This is manufactured by growing *Streptomyces erythreus* in deep culture. It is only slightly soluble in water and the three derivatives that are also used in pharmacy (the estolate, stearate and ethyl carbonate) are almost insoluble.

The base and the stearate are administered in tablets, the estolate is given in capsules, and the stearate and ethyl carbonate (which are less bitter than the base) are used as a flavoured suspension, prepared shortly before use by adding water to dry granules.

It is a narrow spectrum antibiotic with activity similar to penicillin and its main use is for treating patients who have penicillin-resistant infections or who are allergic to penicillin.

Erythromycin belongs to a group of antibiotics known as the macrolides which also includes carbomycin, spiramycin and oleandomycin. All of these act by blocking protein synthesis. Resistance is not a great problem with erythromycin, because of its limited applications. Cross resistance occurs with the macrolides.

Cycloserine

Cycloserine is obtained by growing either *Streptomyces orchidaceous* or *Streptomyces garyphalous* in submerged culture or, because it has a relatively simple structure, by synthesis.

It is water soluble and has a broad spectrum of activity. Its main use is for treating pulmonary tuberculosis caused by strains resistant to streptomycin. It is administered orally in tablets or capsules and is combined with PAS or INH to prevent the emergence of resistant strains and reduce toxic effects. It damages the central nervous system leading to headaches, giddiness and epileptic convulsions, but generally these effects subside when the drug is withdrawn. It acts by interfering with the synthesis of bacterial cell walls.

Neomycin Sulphate

This is a mixture of the sulphates of antibiotics obtained by growing *Streptomyces fradiae* in deep culture. It is hygroscopic and soluble in water. The powder, tablets and aqueous solutions should be protected from light and stored below 30°C.

It has a broad spectrum of activity and although it has not been completely purified it is known to be chemically similar to streptomycin. It is poorly absorbed when taken by mouth but is useful for pre-operative sterilisation of the gut and for the treatment of gastro-intestinal infections. Alone, or with anti-inflammatory steroids, it is widely used topically in ointments, creams, ear drops and eye drops. Exceptionally, intramuscular injections are given to treat infections resistant to other antibiotics. Systemic use is avoided if possible because neomycin damages the kidney and the eighth cranial nerve. The nerve damage is usually irreversible. Prolonged oral administration may lead to fungal overgrowth in the gut. Reports of development of resistance are few and, surprisingly, there is no evidence of cross resistance with streptomycin.

Viomycin

This antibiotic is used in the form of the sulphate and is produced by certain strains of *Streptomyces griseus var. purpurea*. The sulphate is very stable, slightly hygroscopic and very soluble in water. Aqueous solutions have a storage life of one week at room temperature and one month between 2 and 10°C.

It is used by intramuscular injection to treat tuberculosis caused by strains resistant to streptomycin. As with streptomycin, it is given with PAS or INH. Toxic symptoms are uncommon but the drug is contraindicated in patients with kidney malfunction.

Novobiocin

This is an acidic substance produced by certain strains of *Streptomyces niveus*. The sodium and calcium salts are used in medicine; the former is very soluble in water (1 in 5) while the solubility of the latter is only 1 in 300.

It has a narrow spectrum of activity but is particularly effective against *Staphylococcus aureus*. Its main uses are the treatment of staphylococcal infections resistant to penicillin, and the treatment of patients sensitive to other antibiotics. It is administered as tablets or as a fine suspension of the calcium salt. Toxic symptoms, such as skin rashes, are common and novobiocin should not be given to infants under six months because it interferes with the conjugation of bilirubin. Bacteria rapidly develop resistance to it.

Table 32.2
Other Official Antibiotics

Name	Water solubility	Dose forms	Activity spectrum	Toxicity	Development of resistance	Remarks
Bacitracin	+++ (very)	Topical preparations	Wide	Nephrotoxic if given systemically	Slow	Very occasionally given by mouth for intestinal disinfection. In extreme emergency injected intramuscularly
Cephaloridine	+++	Intramuscular injection	Wide, including penicillinase-producing staphylococci	Rashes, as for penicillin	In Gram + organisms (slowly). Cross resistance to ampicillin	Used for penicillin-sensitive patients and penicillin-resistant infections
Colistin sulphate and Colistin sulphomethate sodium	+++	Tablets (sulphate) Injection (sulphomethate)	Gram – organisms, particularly *Ps. aeruginosa*	As for polymixin	Rare	Poorly absorbed in the gut
Framycetin	+++	Eye drops and ointment; paraffin gauze dressing	Mainly staphylococci	As for neomycin	Frequent. Cross resistance to neomycin	
Sodium fusidate	+++	Capsules	Gram + organisms and Gram – cocci	Slight gastric irritation	Frequent	Used for staphylococcal infections resistant to penicillin
Gentamycin	++	Intramuscular injection Ointment	Gram – organisms	—	Slow	
Kanamycin sulphate	+++	Capsules Intramuscular injection	Mainly Gram – organisms	High; rashes, vomiting, kidney damage and irreversible deafness	Serious with *Mycobacterium tuberculosis*	Mainly restricted to infections resistant to safer antibiotics
Paromomycin sulphate	+++	Capsules	Wide	Diarrhoea, deafness, intestinal overgrowth of insensitive organisms	No reports	
Polymixin B sulphate	+++	Intramuscular injection	Gram – organisms	Nephrotoxic Mildly neurotoxic	No reports	
Sulphomyxin sodium	+++	Intramuscular injection	Gram – organisms	Nephrotoxic and mildly neurotoxic, but less marked	No reports	
Triacetyloleandomycin	–	Capsules Tablets	Gram – organisms	Hypersensitivity, gastro-intestinal irritation, liver damage	Cross resistance to erythromycin	
Vancomycin hydrochloride	+ (slightly)	Intravenous injection	Gram + organisms, especially staphylococci	Impaired hearing, Contraindicated in kidney conditions and in thrombophlebitis	Slow	Incompatible with penicillin

Griseofulvin

This is an antifungal antibiotic produced by certain strains of *Penicillium griseofulvus*. Because its solubility is low it is usually administered as tablets made from very fine particles of the drug (*see* p. 113).

Its activity is restricted to fungi with chitinous cell walls, e.g. dermatophytes of the genera *Trichophyton*, *Dermatophyton* and *Microsporum*. It accumulates in the keratinous layers of the dermis on which the fungi live, and exerts a fungistatic action; consequently the fungi do not grow and are sloughed off with the outer layers of the skin. As the latter process takes about three weeks, treatment should be continued for this time.

There is little evidence of acute toxicity but as griseofulvin appears to influence mitosis it should not be used for prolonged treatment.

Nystatin

This is produced by certain strains of *Streptomyces noursei* and it belongs to a class of chemicals known as polyenes. It acts against yeasts and certain filamentous fungi. It is almost insoluble in water and very little is absorbed following oral administration. Tablets or suspensions, lozenges, soluble tablets or compressed pessaries, and ointments are used for the treatment of gut, oral, vaginal, and skin infections respectively.

Development of resistance is uncommon and usually of short duration. Nystatin appears to act by forming an irreversible complex with sterols in the cell membranes of susceptible fungi.

Other Antibiotics

Table 32.2 lists some of the interesting features of other official antibiotics. Apart from cephaloridine and sulphomyxin, which are semi-synthetic, they are all prepared by fermentation using a suitable organism.

BIBLIOGRAPHY

ALBERT, A. (1968) *Selective Toxicity*. 4th ed. Methuen, London.

CASIDA, L. E. JNR (1968) *Industrial Microbiology*. Wiley, New York.

GENERAL MEDICAL COUNCIL (1968) *The British Pharmacopoeia*. Pharmaceutical Press, London.

GOLDBERG, H. S. (Ed.) (1959) *Antibiotics, their Chemistry and Non-medical Uses*. Van Nostrand, Princeton.

GOTTLIEB, D. and SHAW, P. D. (1967) *Antibiotics: 1, mechanism of action*. Springer-Verlag, Berlin.

GUNN, C. and CARTER, S. J. (1965) *Dispensing for Pharmaceutical Students*. 11th ed. Pitman Medical, London.

HEROLD, M. and GABRIEL, Z. (1966) *Antibiotics—Advances in research, production and clinical use*. Butterworths, London.

MARTINDALE (Ed. R. G. TODD) (1967) *Extra Pharmacopoeia*. 25th ed. Pharmaceutical Press, London.

NEWTON, B. A. and REYNOLDS, P. E. (1966) *Biochemical Studies of Antimicrobial Drugs. 16th Symposium of the Society for General Microbiology*. University Press, Cambridge.

PHARMACEUTICAL SOCIETY OF GREAT BRITAIN (1968) *The British Pharmaceutical Codex*. Pharmaceutical Press, London.

RAINBOW, C. and ROSE, A. H. (Eds) (1963) *Biochemistry of Industrial Micro-organisms*. Academic Press, London.

SCHNITZER, R. J. and HAWKING, F. (1964) *Experimental Chemotherapy. Vols. I, II, and III*. Academic Press, New York.

WAKSMAN, S. A. (Ed.) (1958) *Neomycin, its nature and practical application*. Williams and Wilkins, Baltimore.

WAKSMAN, S. A. and LECHEVALIER, H. A. (1962) *The Actinomycetes. Volume III. Antibiotics of Actinomycetes*. Williams and Wilkins, Baltimore.

REFERENCES

BATCHELOR, F. R., DOYLE, F. P., NAYLER, J. H. C., and ROLINSON, G. N. (1959) Synthesis of penicillin: 6-amino-penicillanic acid in penicillin fermentations. *Nature, Lond.*, **183**, 257.

CALAM, C. T. (1967) Media for industrial fermentations. *Process Biochem.*, **2**, 19–22 & 46.

COLE, M. (1967) Microbial synthesis of penicillins and 6-amino-penicillanic acid, Part I. *Process Biochem.*, **1**, 334–338; Part II. *ibid.*, **1**, 373–377; Part III. *ibid.*, (1968) **2** (4), 35–41 & 46.

FRANKLIN, T. J. Mode of action of the Tetracyclines in *Biochemical studies of antimicrobial drugs* by Newton, B. A. and Reynolds, P. E. University Press, Cambridge, 192–212.

GOLL, P. H. (1966) Microbiological processing of steroids. *Process Biochem.*, **1**, 201–205.

LONG, L. M. and TROUTMAN, H. D. (1949) Chloramphenicol VI. A synthetic approach. *J. Amer. chem. Soc.*, **71**, 2469.

PARK, J. T. (1966) Some observations on murein synthesis and the action of penicillin, in *Biochemical Studies on Antimicrobial drugs* by Newton, B. A. and Reynolds, P. E. University Press, Cambridge.

PARK, J. T. and WISE, E. M. (1965) Penicillin: its

basic site of action as an inhibitor of a peptide cross-linking reaction in mucopeptide synthesis. *Proc. natn. Acad. Sci. USA.*, **54**, 75–81.

PERLMAN D. (1967) Microbial production of therapeutic compounds. Chap. 11 in *Microbial Technology*. Ed. by Peppler, H. J. Rheinhold, New York.

SMRT, J., BERANEK, J., SICHER, J., SKODA, J., HESS, V. F. and SORM, F. (1957) Synthesis of L-4-amino-3-isoxazolidinone, the unnatural isomer of cyclo-serine, and its antibiotic activity. *Experientia*, **13**, 291.

SYKES, G. (1966) Sterilization processes and problems. *Process Biochem.*, **1**, 268–272.

WOODS, D. D. (1940) The relation of p-amino-benzoic acid to the mechanism of action of sulphanilamide. *Br. J. exp. Path.*, **21**, 74.

WOODS, D. D. (1962) The biochemical mode of action of the sulphonamide drugs. *J. gen. Microbiol.*, **29**, 687–702.

33

Immunology

IMMUNOLOGY is the study of immunity. Immunity, in its microbiological sense, is the capacity of the body to resist infection.

INFECTION

When micro-organisms successfully invade the body and cause damage to the tissues, infection is said to have occurred. Consequently, diseases produced by micro-organisms are called infectious diseases.

Infection may take place by—

1. *Physical Contact with a Diseased Person or Animal*

As the causal organisms have only a brief existence outside the human body, venereal diseases are almost always contracted in this way. Rabies is transferred to man through the bite of an infected dog.

Strict precautions are essential for the protection of hospital medical staff, who are at particular risk when treating patients with infectious diseases.

2. *Droplet Infection*

Coughing, sneezing and even quiet talking cause expulsion from the respiratory tract of fine droplets containing micro-organisms which may be inhaled by individuals nearby. It is by this mechanism that respiratory diseases are often transmitted.

3. *Dust-borne Infection*

Some disease-producing bacteria, e.g. *Mycobacterium tuberculosis*, remain alive for long periods in the dried condition, and contaminated dust stirred up by cleaning processes may infect wounds or be inhaled.

4. *Contact with Contaminated Articles*

Clothes, bedding, handkerchiefs, towels, toys and other items recently contaminated by a diseased person are sources of infection, either through contact or via the microbe-laden particles discharged from them, into the air, by movement.

5. *Hand Infection*

The hands are a major potential means by which micro-organisms from saliva, nasal mucus, skin infections, and even faeces are transferred to other individuals and to food.

6. *Arthropod Vectors*

Some disease-producing organisms are transmitted by insects (e.g. flies and mosquitoes) and other arthropods (e.g. fleas and ticks).

In certain cases the vectors simply act as accidental carriers of the organisms from filth to food or to the human host. In this way, plague and typhoid fever are transferred by fleas and house-flies respectively.

In other cases, the micro-organisms are transmitted by blood-sucking arthropods and spend part of their life cycle in the vector. Examples are the transmission of malaria by the *Anopheles* mosquito, yellow fever by the *Aëdes* mosquito, sleeping sickness by the tsetse fly, and murine typhus by the rat flea.

Factors Influencing Infection

The ability of a pathogenic organism to cause infection depends on a number of factors—

A. VIRULENCE

This may be described as the capacity of a micro-organism to invade the body, establish itself in the tissues, and harm the host

Harm to the host may be caused in two ways. Firstly, multiplication of micro-organisms in the tissues may cause mechanical destruction of cells or, through interference with normal metabolism, lead to inflammation and other harmful effects. Secondly, the organism may produce poisons (toxins) that directly damage the host.

Ability to invade is called invasiveness or aggressiveness, while capacity to produce toxins is known as toxigenicity. Organisms possess these qualities to varying degrees; for example, *Clostridium tetani* can enter the body only through an injury and, therefore, its invasiveness is low; but when established it has high toxigenicity because it produces a very powerful toxin. On the other hand, pneumococci enter the body easily and multiply readily but have very limited capacity for toxin production.

The reasons for differences in invasiveness are not well understood. One factor that is clearly important in assisting the establishment of certain micro-organisms, e.g. the meningococci and pneumococci, is the possession of a capsule which appears to interfere with certain defence mechanisms of the host, particularly phagocytosis (q.v.).

Bacterial Toxins

There are two kinds of bacterial toxin—

(a) Exotoxins—so-called because they diffuse freely through the bacterial cell wall into the medium in which the organisms are growing.
(b) Endotoxins—so-called because they are retained within the bacteria and are freed only when the cells die and start to disintegrate.

EXOTOXINS

These have the following characteristics—

(i) They are the products of the metabolism of actively growing bacteria.
(ii) They are produced mainly by Gram-positive bacteria.
(iii) They are water-soluble and can pass into the surrounding medium. This provides a means of separating the toxin from the cells, since the latter can be removed on a bacteria-proof filter through which the toxin-containing medium will pass.
(iv) Chemically, they are high molecular weight proteins, and some are enzymes. Like many proteins and enzymes, they are relatively thermolabile and lose activity at about 60°C.
(v) Usually they are extremely toxic to the body. Botulinus toxin, produced by *Clostridium botulinum*, an organism responsible for a particularly dangerous type of food poisoning, is the most toxic substance known. It has been estimated that 1 mg is enough to kill about 20 million mice.

When exotoxin-producing bacteria grow in the body, the toxins are carried in the blood stream to all parts, and often the most serious consequences of infection are due to the effects of the toxins rather than the damage to the tissues invaded by the bacteria. In diphtheria, for example, the causative organism grows in the throat producing a membrane that may cause asphyxiation, but the general toxaemia caused by the circulating exotoxin is normally more serious.

The general effects of exotoxins are often most pronounced on the nervous system and the heart. For example, tetanus exotoxin is neurotoxic and causes severe muscular spasms. Other toxins cause death of the tissues (necrotoxins), intestinal damage (enterotoxins), haemolysis (haemolysins) and destruction of white blood cells (leucocidins). A few have more specific effects, like the erythrotoxin of scarlet fever that causes the scarlet rash characteristic of the disease.

Exotoxin-producing bacteria that are of particular importance in immunology include *Clostridium botulinum*, *Clostridium tetani* (tetanus), *Clostridium perfringens*, *septicum* and *welchii* (gas gangrene) and *Corynebacterium diphtheriae* (diphtheria).

ENDOTOXINS

These differ from exotoxins in several important respects—

(i) They are structural elements of bacteria.
(ii) They are contained in most bacterial cells but the greatest amounts are found in Gram-negative bacteria.
(iii) They are not excreted into the surrounding medium and are liberated only when the cells die or disintegrate.
(iv) Chemically they are complexes of phospholipid, polysaccharide and protein, most of which are thermostable.
(v) They are much less toxic.

Endotoxin-producing bacteria of interest in immunology include *Vibrio cholerae* (cholera), *Pasteurella pestis* (plague), *Salmonella typhi* (typhoid), *Salmonella paratyphi* (paratyphoid) and *Bordetella pertussis* (whooping cough).

Enzymes Associated with Virulence

Some bacterial toxins possess an activity that potentiates their virulence. For example, *Clostridium welchii* alpha toxin has lecithinase activity (*see* below). Alternatively, bacteria may liberate one or more enzymes or similar substances that facilitate invasion by the organism or increase the damage caused by the toxin.

Hyaluronidase

This enzyme, which is also known as the spreading factor, reversibly catalyses the breakdown of hyaluronic acid, a major component of the cement between tissue cells. As a result the viscous cement becomes fluid and bacteria and their toxins can more easily spread throughout the body.

Collagenase

Collagenase disintegrates collagen, a constituent of muscle, cartilage and bone.

Lecithinase

An important constituent of cell membranes is lecithin. Lecithinase activity results in the haemolysis of erythrocytes and the necrosis of other cells.

Coagulase

Certain highly pathogenic strains of *Staphylococcus aureus* produce this enzyme which clots plasma and surrounds the bacteria with a barrier of fibrin that protects them against phagocytosis.

Haemolysins

Many bacteria, e.g. streptococci and clostridia, produce enzymes or other substances that destroy red blood cells.

Leucocidins

Leucocytes (white blood cells) have important roles in the body's defences against bacteria. Leucocidins inactivate or destroy them and so aid bacterial invasion.

Changes in Virulence

Since natural differences in virulence are found in different strains of bacteria it is essential to use strains of the correct virulence for the manufacture of immunological products.

Virulence may be artificially altered thus:

1. Increased (exalted)—by successive fairly rapid transfers from one susceptible host to another.

2. Decreased (attenuated)—

(a) By growing the organism under artificial conditions in laboratory culture media. Usually an organism is most virulent when first isolated from its host, and unless it is grown on a medium that closely simulates its natural environment (e.g. a medium well enriched with sources of animal protein) it will often lose virulence (see BCG vaccine).

(b) By growing the organism at an unfavourable temperature. (See Pasteur's work on anthrax vaccine.)

(c) By growing the organism in an unnatural host (see Yellow fever vaccine). Virulence for man may be lost after repeated passages through laboratory animals.

(d) By drying (see Rabies vaccine).

B. THE NUMBER OF ORGANISMS

The number of organisms required to produce disease varies with the species and resistance of the host and the species, or strain, and virulence of the infecting micro-organism; but, in general, the larger the number of organisms the greater the chance of infection being established.

The number of organisms required to cause death or a characteristic sign of infection is sometimes used as an indication of the virulence of the bacteria, rickettsia or viruses used in immunological preparations. (See Testing of immunological products.)

C. ROUTE OF ENTRY

In many diseases infection will not occur unless the organism enters the body by a particular route, e.g. typhoid (alimentary tract), gonorrhoea (genitourinary tract) and diphtheria (respiratory tract).

D. THE RESISTANCE OF THE HOST

The body has a number of lines of defence against infection—

1. Prevention of Entry

This is achieved by the design of body structures (e.g. the nasal passages which effectively trap organisms); by the impermeability to microorganisms of the intact and healthy skin and mucosae; by competition from the natural microbial flora of the host; and by the antimicrobial activities of the secretions bathing the surfaces of the body. The mucus covering of mucous membranes collects and retains micro-organisms and, then, action of cilia in the respiratory tract, aided by coughing and sneezing, or peristaltic activity in the gut, removes them from the body. The fatty acids in the skin, the pH of the gastric juice, and the enzyme lysozyme in tears and sweat, all inhibit or destroy microorganisms.

2. Phagocytosis

Organisms that manage to invade the tissues are attacked by cells known as phagocytes which have the ability to engulf inert or living material, a process known as phagocytosis. There are two types of phagocyte—

(a) Fixed

These belong to the reticulo-endothelial system of cells that line blood spaces in various parts of the body, including the spleen and liver. They are known as macrophages and, amoeba-wise, they ingest micro-organisms from the blood as it passes.

(b) Wandering

The most important of these is the neutrophil type of polymorphonuclear leucocyte which moves about in the blood and, in response to inflammatory changes caused by the presence of micro-organisms in the tissues, mobilises at the site of infection, passes out of the capillary wall, and attacks the invaders. The leucocytes, like the fixed macrophages, engulf the organisms and render them harmless. Together with large numbers of fellow leucocytes that are destroyed in the attack they contribute to the formation of pus.

In some cases, e.g. with capsulated and other pathogens of high virulence, the phagocytes may be chemotactically repelled, leaving the organisms free to cause disease.

An essential feature of phagocytosis, distinguishing it from the defence mechanism to be discussed next, is that it is non-specific; i.e. it is directed against all micro-organisms.

3. Antibody Production

The body does not rely on phagocytosis alone for the destruction of pathogens that have successfully invaded the tissues. It produces substances known as antibodies that are antagonistic to pathogenic micro-organisms and their toxins. Antibodies may be defined as substances formed in the body in response to the presence of foreign proteins and certain other materials in the tissues. Unlike phagocytes, antibodies are highly specific and attack only the specific substances (i.e. micro-organism or toxin) that stimulated their production. Materials that when introduced into the body lead to antibody production are called antigens.

Chemically, antibodies belong to a class of proteins known as globulins, of which three types are known: alpha, beta, and gamma. Most antibodies are gamma globulins but some are beta. They are produced, particularly in the lymph nodes, by cells of the reticulo-endothelial system.

The way in which antibodies are formed is imperfectly understood. The most popular explanation is the template theory. According to this the antigen molecule acts as a pattern (template) for the synthesis of antibody globulin, the surface groups of the latter being shaped to key into complementary groups of the antigen. After formation, the antibody globulin is released to free the template for further antibody production.

Another theory has been proposed by Burnet. He believes that the information required to produce a new protein could not be provided via an external source but must be part of the host's genetic make-up. He suggests that groups of cells capable of producing an individual antibody already exist in the body and that the action of the antigen is to activate the appropriate group.

ANTIGEN-ANTIBODY REACTIONS

The reactions between antigens and antibodies fall into a number of classes, some of which are summarised in Table 33.1. It will be noticed that in most cases the antibodies are named according to the nature of the reaction.

The lysis of bacterial cells by bacteriolysins is different from the other three reactions in requiring the presence of a substance, normally found in blood and body fluids, known as complement. This constituent, which is a complex of several components, is non-specific and is responsible for the lysis. However, it cannot act until the organisms have combined with their specific bacteriolysins; i.e. the effect is complementary, hence its name.

Table 33.1

Antigen	Antibody	Nature of reaction
Exotoxin	Antitoxin	Neutralisation of the toxin. Exhibited, if the toxin and antitoxin are present in the correct proportions, by the appearance of a flocculent precipitate (floccules).
Bacterial cells	Agglutinin	Clumping (agglutination) of the cells.
Endotoxin	Precipitin	Precipitation of the toxin.
Bacterial cells	Bacteriolysin	Lysis of the cells.

Summarising—

Bacteria + specific bacteriolysin → No lysis
Bacteria + complement → No lysis
Bacteria + specific bacteriolysin
+ complement → Lysis of the
bacteria.

A further antibody of special interest is known as opsonin. Opsonins make pathogens more susceptible to phagocytosis but, unlike phagocytes, they are highly specific.

Originally it was believed that a particular antigen could give rise to several antibodies each capable of taking part in a different antigen-antibody reaction. It is now clear that in most cases a single antigen produces only one type of antibody which is able, under appropriate conditions, to carry out all the various reactions except where, as sometimes happens, it is deficient in the capacity to take part in one or more.

To provide adequate protection against pathogenic bacteria the body needs to produce antibodies that can—

(i) Neutralise exotoxins.
(ii) Prevent or inhibit the disintegration of endotoxin-producing bacteria.
(iii) Inactivate any liberated endotoxin.
(iv) Destroy the bacteria.

Reference to Table 33.1 shows that the range of available antibodies adequately covers this need. Exotoxins are rendered harmless through neutralisation by antitoxins. Agglutination delays disintegration, and also facilitates phagocytosis by decreasing the mobility of the cells. Endotoxin, liberated by disintegration, may be precipitated by precipitins and thereby inactivated. Destruction of bacterial cells is accomplished by the combined actions of bacteriolysin and complement, while the activity of specific opsonins assists phagocytosis.

Antibodies antagonistic to viruses and rickettsiae, but often with modes of action different from antibacterial antibodies, can also be produced by the body.

IMMUNITY

Natural (Constitutional) Immunity

This is resistance to disease possessed as part of an individual's constitutional make-up. It results in differences between species, races and individuals.

1. Species

Man is susceptible to plague but fowls are not. Dog distemper does not infect man. Typhoid fever is a serious disease in humans but mice are not affected.

2. Race

Negroes have a high resistance to yellow fever but white men are very susceptible. The Caucasian race is more resistant to tuberculosis than negroes or American Indians.

3. Individuals

It is well known that some people are more resistant than others to colds and skin infections.

The reasons for differences in natural immunity are not well understood.

Acquired Immunity

Natural immunity is inadequate for protection against many microbial diseases and during lifetime additional immunity is acquired either actively, due to stimulation of the individual's antibody-producing cells (active immunity), or passively, as a result of the introduction of antibodies from another person or animal (passive immunity).

ACTIVE IMMUNITY

This can be naturally acquired or artificially *stimulated*—

1. Naturally Acquired Active Immunity

This results from natural infection by pathogens which may or may not result in clinically recognisable disease.

(a) Following Clinical Infection

When a patient recovers from certain diseases he is left with a high degree of immunity. In the cases of diphtheria, smallpox, and poliomyelitis, for example, this persists for life. For a number of diseases, however, the immunity is of short duration, e.g. after influenza, pneumonia, and gonorrhoea.

(b) After Sub-clinical Infection

Sometimes invading organisms, possibly because the number is small, cause no clearly distinguishable signs of the disease. Nevertheless, the individual becomes immune, presumably because the antibody-producing cells have received an adequate stimulus.

Table 33.2

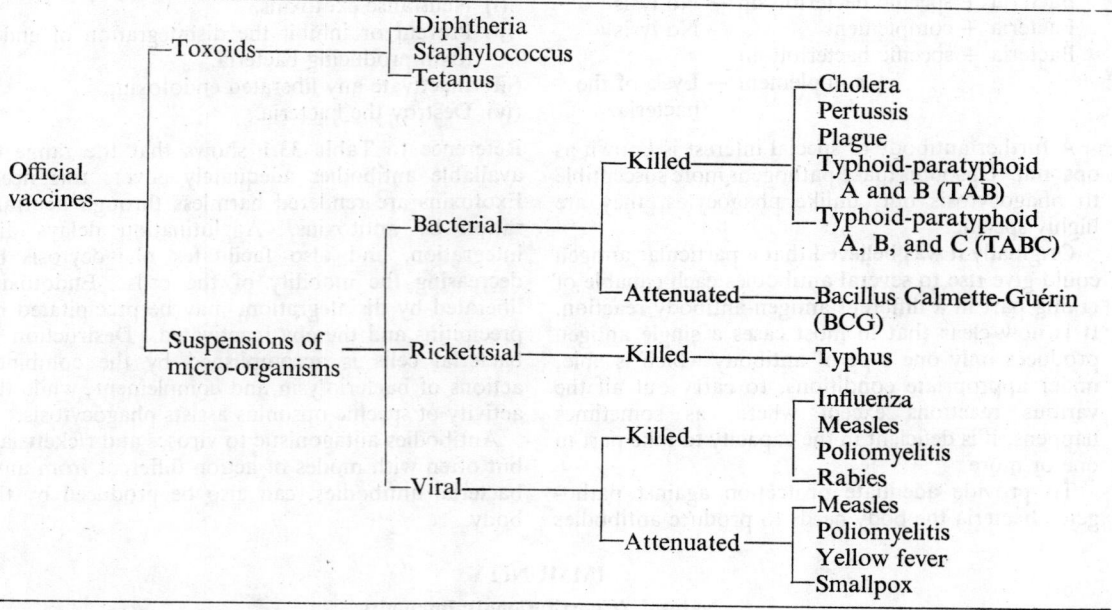

Children in slum areas, because of more frequent exposure to sub-infection, often develop immunity to a variety of diseases more quickly than children in more affluent areas.

2. Artificially Stimulated Active Immunity

The aim of artificial active immunisation is the stimulation of antibody production by safe means. This is achieved by the administration, usually by injection, of antigens. The antigens used are micro-organisms or their products and the preparations containing them are known as vaccines.

Vaccines are of two types—

(*a*) *Toxoids*. These are bacterial exotoxins modified so that their toxicity is destroyed or reduced to a safe level.

(*b*) *Suspensions of Micro-organisms*. These consist of micro-organisms that have either been killed or, if this treatment affects their antigenicity (i.e. capacity to stimulate antibody production), attenuated.

A summary of the official vaccines is given in Table 33.2. For simplicity this includes only two (TAB and TABC) of the official mixed vaccines. These are made by mixing more than one vaccine and are used to induce immunity to several diseases at the same time.

PASSIVE IMMUNITY

Like active immunity this can be naturally acquired. It can also be artificially *produced*.

1. Naturally Acquired Passive Immunity

Antibodies for diseases to which the mother is immune may be transmitted to the foetus via the placental blood and give immunity to the infant for several months. For example, babies show high resistance to chickenpox, diphtheria, measles, and scarlet fever but usually this is lost by the time the child is about six months old.

2. Artificially Produced Passive Immunity

This is effected by injection of antibodies produced in an animal, usually the horse. Occasionally, a human source is used, e.g. human normal immuno-globulin injection, which contains the rubella (german measles), measles and certain other antibodies from human plasma.

Antibody-containing preparations are known as antisera, sera or immune sera and the official products include preparations containing—

(*a*) Antitoxic antibodies, i.e. antibodies that neutralise exotoxins. Products containing these are generally called antitoxins; e.g.

Botulinum antitoxin
Diphtheria antitoxin
Gas-gangrene antitoxin (oedematiens)
Gas-gangrene antitoxin (septicum)
Gas-gangrene antitoxin (welchii)
Mixed gas-gangrene antitoxin
Staphylococcus antitoxin
Tetanus antitoxin

(*b*) Antibacterial antibodies, i.e. antibodies that combat endotoxin producing bacteria; e.g. Leptospira antiserum.

(*c*) Antiviral antibodies, i.e. antibodies that combat viruses; e.g. Rabies antiserum.

Human normal immunoglobulin injection B.P. contains the purified antibodies from human plasma.

COMPARISON OF ACTIVE AND PASSIVE IMMUNITY

Active immunity develops slowly and, normally, it is not fully effective for several weeks. This is because training the antibody-producing cells takes a considerable time. Nevertheless, once developed, this type of immunity is long-lasting and often gives protection for many years. Even when it begins to fade, a booster dose of antigen quickly restores an effective antibody level.

Passive immunity, on the other hand, can be established relatively quickly. The time depends on the route and ranges from immediately, by intravenous injection, to perhaps 48 hours if given subcutaneously. However, passive immunity is very short-lived because the body recognises the antibodies as foreign and gradually eliminates them. In consequence, protection is lost within two to three weeks. An exception is when human antibodies are used (e.g. human immunoglobulin), then the rate of elimination is much slower. Because of these differences active and passive immunisation have different applications.

Active immunisation is mainly used for the prevention of disease, by inducing a lasting immunity before the person is exposed to infection. There are some exceptions; e.g. when smallpox is suspected, early administration of the vaccine reduces the severity of the disease if contracted, possibly by potentiating the antigenic effect of the infecting viruses and thereby promoting more rapid formation of antibodies.

The value of preventative immunisation is beyond dispute. At one time almost every child in Europe contracted smallpox and it claimed one death in every thirteen; those who survived were disfigured or blind. Today the disease is almost unknown in countries where vaccination is compulsory. The horrible and dangerous disease diphtheria has been virtually eliminated from England by the strongly encouraged, voluntary immunisation of infants. The control of whooping cough, poliomyelitis, and tuberculosis has been greatly improved by immunisation procedures. Lastly, many servicemen, exposed to insanitary conditions in war, owe their lives to the protection given by typhoid, cholera, and plague vaccines.

While the main application of active immunisation is in prophylaxis, passive immunisation is used both prophylactically and therapeutically.

1. *Prophylactically*—to give immediate, but temporary, protection to individuals exposed to infection. A good example is the administration of human immunoglobulin to pregnant women who are exposed to rubella infection during the early months of pregnancy. An attack of the disease at this time can seriously damage the foetus.

Other slightly different examples are—

(*a*) The use of tetanus and gas-gangrene antitoxins to prevent the corresponding diseases after road accidents or sports-field injuries. The spores of the clostridia that cause these infections are found in the soil and if they gain access to deep wounds, such as compound fractures, in which there has been extensive tissue damage and, therefore, necrosis, they find suitable anaerobic conditions for growth.

(*b*) The use of rabies antiserum to protect a person bitten by a dog when there is any suspicion that the animal might have rabies.

2. *Therapeutically*—to treat an acute disease. A susceptible individual when attacked by a virulent pathogen is unable to respond quickly enough to the antigenic stimulus provided by the organism. As a result his production of antibodies cannot keep pace with the infection, and he may die. Passive immunisation, by immediately providing a high concentration of the appropriate antibodies, significantly increases the chance of recovery. Botulinum and diphtheria antitoxins and leptospira antiserum are examples of products that are used in this way.

In the succeeding sections antigen-containing and antibody-containing preparations will be discussed in more detail and some attention will be paid to a group of preparations used for diagnostic purposes in immunology, e.g. to decide if someone is immune to a particular disease.

SUMMARIES

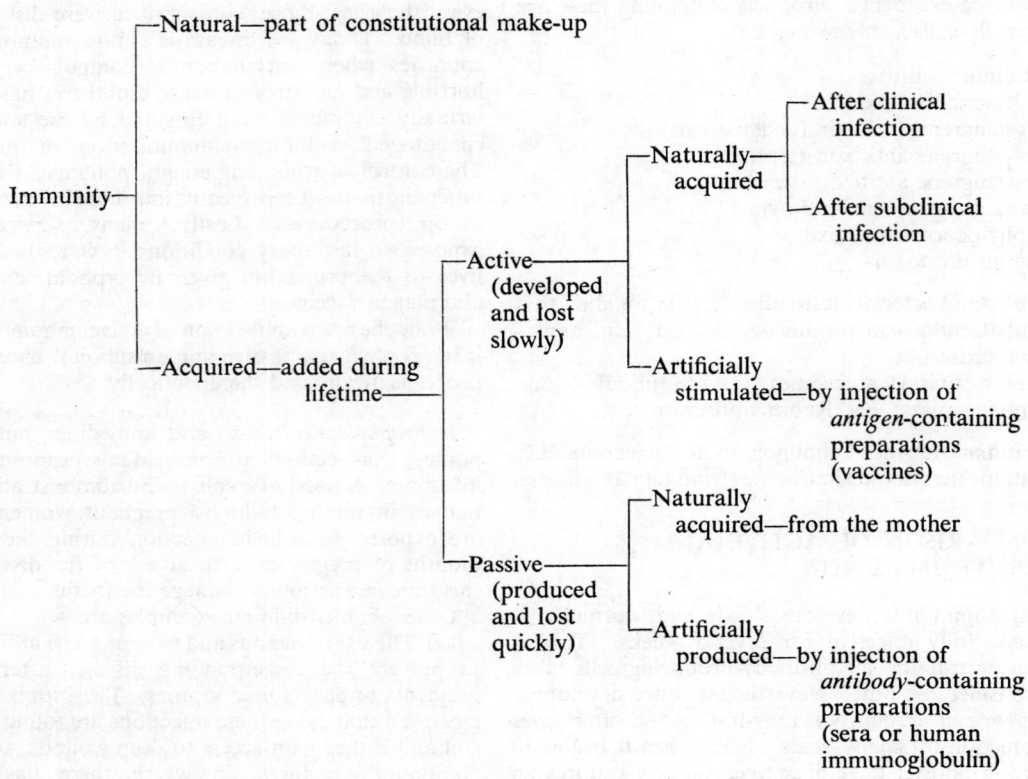

Antigen-containing preparations	Antibody-containing preparations
Stimulate active immunity	Give passive immunity
Patient produces antibodies	Patient receives antibodies
Immunity develops slowly	Immunity produced quickly
Lasting effect	Temporary effect
Used for long-term prophylaxis	Used for short-term prophylaxis and therapeutically

ANTIGEN-CONTAINING PREPARATIONS (VACCINES)

Only rarely can unmodified toxins or normal pathogenic strains of organisms be used safely as immunising agents.

Until fairly recently there was an official vaccine for scarlet fever, a disease caused by the exotoxin-producing organism, *Streptococcus pyogenes*. Attempts to convert this toxin into a toxoid with satisfactory antigenicity were unsuccessful and so the preparation consisted of unmodified toxin. The course had to be started with a tiny dose, to avoid severe reactions, and to build this up gradually to a satisfactory level necessitated more injections than are required with other prophylactics. This preparation is seldom used now because the disease can be controlled satisfactorily by chemotherapy.

Normally, the toxin or micro-organism is modified in some way to destroy its toxicity, or reduce this to a safe level, without at the same time decreasing its antigenicity.

Toxoids

The toxoids used as vaccines are toxins that have been incubated with formalin. This treatment completely destroys their toxic properties without causing significant loss of antigenic qualities. It appears that the formalin acts directly on the toxic groups (possibly, but not certainly, due to combination with free amino groups) without affecting the antigenically-active sites.

An interesting way of appreciating the general problems that have to be faced in the commercial production of toxoids is to examine in some detail the preparation of one of the official products. As the control of diphtheria in this country is one of the outstanding achievements of preventative immunisation it is logical to choose diphtheria vaccine.

DIPHTHERIA VACCINE (DIPHTHERIA PROPHYLACTIC)

Preparation of the Toxin

A suitable strain of *Corynebacterium diphtheriae* is grown on a liquid medium which must *not* be made with broth prepared from horse muscle. This is because the presence of horse protein in the toxin, and hence in the toxoid preparations made from it, might sensitise the recipient to horse serum and so make dangerous the subsequent injection of sera, which are made in horses (p. 402).

After incubation under optimal conditions until toxin production has reached a satisfactory level, the bulk of the organisms are removed on paper pulp (to prevent rapid clogging of the bacteria-proof filter used in the next stage) and the filtrate is sterilised, using, for example, fibrous pads or ceramic candles.

Conversion to Toxoid

Formaldehyde solution (formalin) is added and the mixture incubated at 37°C until the toxicity has been removed; this takes two to three weeks. The resulting material is known as Formol Toxoid (FT). For many years this product was used in unpurified form (also called Anatoxin); it was an excellent antigen but it often caused severe reactions, particularly in adults. More recently a number of purification techniques have been developed and the products are relatively free from side effects but are weaker prophylactics and less stable. Nevertheless, they are widely used in certain other forms of diphtheria vaccine and in mixed vaccines. In future references they will be called purified formol toxoids.

Preparation of Other Forms of Toxoid

TOXOID-ANTITOXIN FLOCCULES (TAF)

The reactions caused by crude formol toxoid are due partly to broth constituents and partly to metabolic products of the organism. If suitable amounts of toxoid and antitoxin are mixed, floccules are obtained that contain almost all of the antigenic activity and when separated and washed are free from contamination with broth and metabolites.

This product is known as toxoid-antitoxin floccules and is the least likely of all the forms of diphtheria vaccine to cause reactions. It is especially valuable for adults, who are much more sensitive than young children to the reaction-causing constituents of immunological preparations, but it is a weaker antigen than some of the alternative forms and, therefore, three, instead of two, doses must be given. Because it contains diphtheria antitoxin, which is made from horse serum, there is a slight risk of sensitisation.

It may seem strange that a neutralised product has any significant activity. This is because neither toxoid nor antitoxin is damaged when they combine. Therefore, the combination can dissociate under suitable conditions, e.g. after the floccules have been injected into the body, leaving the toxoid free to stimulate antibody production.

The following method of preparation is used: 80 units of antitoxin are added to 100 units of toxoid, i.e. the toxoid is slightly under-neutralised. After leaving for about three weeks to allow the floccules to form and settle, the supernatant liquid is decanted. Filtration would be difficult because of the protein nature of the precipitate. The floccules are then washed with saline, by decantation, until the washings are colourless, and resuspended in saline containing a bactericide.

ALUM PRECIPITATED TOXOID (APT)

This preparation resulted from the discovery that slow absorption of precipitated toxoids from the site of injection and slow excretion from the body led to increased antigenic activity. Its development was also associated with attempts to make purer toxoids.

High quality formol toxoid is treated with charcoal to remove (a) colouring matter, and (b) some of the non-specific (i.e. non-toxoid) impurities that might cause reactions. After filtration, to separate the charcoal, a suitable concentration of alum is added. This reacts with bicabronate, phosphate and protein impurities in the toxoid to produce a precipitate containing aluminium hydroxide and phosphate. The toxoid is adsorbed on to this mineral carrier.

The precipitate, which is washed and suspended in saline containing a bactericide, provides, because of its insolubility, a depot in the tissues from which the antigen is slowly released to give a prolonged stimulus.

Substances that, like alum, potentiate the effect of antigens are called adjuvants.

APT produces much higher antibody levels than FT or TAF and, therefore, two doses are sufficient. It is free from sensitising horse protein and contains toxoid of improved purity. Adults and older children may show local reactions to the carrier and there is a slight risk of provoking paralytic polio-myelitis in the limb in which the injection is given if the child is immunised during a poliomyelitis epidemic. In spite of its high efficiency it has been largely replaced by combined prophylactics because these are more convenient.

PURIFIED TOXOID ALUMINIUM PHOSPHATE (PTAP)

The main difference between this preparation and APT is that it contains a much purer form of toxoid. This is obtained—

(a) by using a semi-synthetic medium in the preparation of the toxin, to exclude as much non-specific material as possible;

(b) by a complicated purification of the toxoid involving the use of magnesium hydroxide, to precipitate colour, phosphate, and some protein, and ammonium sulphate and cadmium chloride as protein precipitants.

The separation of much of the unwanted protein reduces the likelihood of reactions but also removes the impurities that give a precipitate with alum; therefore, it is necessary to use a preformed carrier, pure hydrated aluminium phosphate.

Like APT, PTAP is an excellent antigen due to its depot effect; however, it also carries the small risk of provocative poliomyelitis and has suffered from the advent of combined prophylactics.

Because the toxoid is very pure and can be freeze-dried, a form in which it is very stable, the production of batches of uniform potency is greatly facilitated.

Purified toxoid aluminium hydroxide (PTAH) is an essentially similar preparation in which the aluminium phosphate has been replaced by aluminium hydroxide gel.

PURIFIED DIPHTHERIA FORMOL TOXOID IN COMBINED PROPHYLACTICS

The Ministry of Health recommends that children should be immunised against four infectious diseases (diphtheria, tetanus, pertussis, and poliomyelitis) during the first year of life. If each prophylactic is given separately, the large number of injections and attendances involved become a burden on children, parents, doctors, and record-keepers and, therefore, it is customary to use a combined vaccine containing either diphtheria, tetanus and pertussis antigens (triple antigen) or these three plus poliomyelitis antigens (quadruple antigen).

Purified diphtheria formol toxoid (FT) can be used successfully in these preparations because although it is less active alone than any of the three adsorbed forms its effect is potentiated by the presence of the dead pertussis bacteria which appear to act, like alum salts, as an adjuvant and, therefore, a good antibody response is obtained.

SUMMARY

The aims in the production of a satisfactory toxoid can be summarised as follows—

1. To produce a preparation free from specific toxicity (by conversion to toxoid).

2. To eliminate impurities responsible for non-specific reactions (by improving the culture medium used for growing the organisms and by applying modern techniques in purifying the toxoid protein).

3. To maintain antigenicity at a high level and, if possible, to improve it by using adjuvants.

4. To keep constant watch for adverse side effects from new developments (e.g. provocative poliomyelitis and tissue reactions from mineral carriers).

OTHER OFFICIAL TOXOIDS

Tetanus Vaccine

This is prepared from the exotoxin of the anaerobe *Clostridium tetani* and is available in all the forms described under diphtheria vaccine except TAF.

The activity of purified tetanus vaccine FT, like that of its diphtheria counterpart, is increased by administration with killed organisms and, therefore, this form is used in combined prophylactics containing microbial suspensions. In addition to the pertussis preparations (*see* Diphtheria vaccine) there is also, in this case, a mixed vaccine, containing the organisms responsible for typhoid and paratyphoid fevers, which is used to protect servicemen against these diseases and tetanus.

An interesting feature of the history of this preparation, that underlines the importance of control of media composition in toxoid production, was the discovery that a protein constituent (Witte's peptone) of the broth was the cause of serious sensitisation to protein, leading to anaphylactic shock. Replacement of this ingredient eliminated the problem.

There is an official requirement for the simple vaccine that when no particular form is prescribed, PTAP or PTAH must be supplied—a reflection of the superior qualities of these preparations.

Staphylococcus Toxoid

This is made from the exotoxin (alpha-toxin) of *Staphylococcus aureus* and it is occasionally given to susceptible individuals to prevent boils and other recurring local staphylococcal infections. It has largely been replaced by antibiotic therapy.

There is only one form, a formol toxoid. Unlike the corresponding diphtheria and tetanus preparations, it is not obligatory to remove completely the specific toxicity of the toxin during toxoiding but it must be reduced to a low level at which certain dangerous properties of the alpha-toxin have been destroyed, i.e. its ability to cause in the rabbit, haemolysis of red blood cells, necrosis of the skin, and death after intravenous injection.

The word vaccine is not used in the official name of this preparation because suspensions of killed *Staphylococcus aureus* cells are available and known as vaccines. Although these are not official or widely used it is necessary to avoid confusion between the two preparations.

Occasionally, autogenous vaccines are made from *Staphylococcus aureus*. This type of preparation contains organisms freshly isolated from the patient who is to receive the product.

Suspensions of Micro-organisms

This form of vaccine may be prepared from bacteria, rickettsia, or viruses. In some cases the organisms are living, in others they are dead. Like toxoids they may be—

Simple—prepared from one species or variety; e.g. plague vaccine, made from one species, *Pasteurella pestis*.

Mixed—mixtures of two or more simple vaccines; e.g. typhoid-paratyphoid A and B vaccine, made by mixing three simple vaccines, one from *Salmonella typhi* and two from *Salmonella paratyphi*.

Sometimes a further distinction is made—

Univalent—prepared from one strain (e.g. an immunological type) of one species; e.g. yellow fever vaccine is made from the 17D strain of yellow fever virus.

Polyvalent—prepared from more than one strain (usually of one species); for example:

(*a*) Cholera vaccine is made from the two main serological types of *Vibrio cholerae*, Inaba and Ogawa.

(*b*) Poliomyelitis vaccine is made from types I, II, and III of poliomyelitis virus.

(*c*) TAB vaccine, which is both mixed (*see* above) and polyvalent (because it contains the A and B strains of *Salmonella paratyphi*).

VARIATION IN MICRO-ORGANISMS

Chapter 27 explains that bacterial variation is often accompanied by loss of antigens from the cells. Non-capsulated variants of capsulated strains and organisms that have undergone the S to R, H to O and other variations have all lost important antigens. As a result, the non-capsulated, R and O forms of bacteria are often much less virulent than the capsulated, S and H forms. Therefore, it is essential not to use these variants in the manufacture of immunological products. Because of the deficiency in antigens they are unable to stimulate the production of antibodies effective against the virulent strains and, if used for immunisation, will produce little or no immunity. The same problem arises if non-virulent strains of viruses or rickettsia are used.

To guard against the use of variants in immunological preparations the Pharmacopoeia makes very careful specifications which include—

1. The exact strain or strains to be used; for example—

Cholera vaccine—smooth strains of the two main serological types.
TAB vaccine—strains of *S. typhi, S. paratyphi A* and *S. paratyphi B* that are smooth.
Plague vaccine—capsulated form of *Pasteurella pestis.*
Typhus vaccine—virulent rickettsiae.
Influenza vaccine—strains that are non-infective but retain their antigenic properties.
Yellow fever vaccine—the strain of yellow fever virus known as 17D which is virulent for mice.

2. The antigens that must be present—

Cholera vaccine—all strains must contain, in addition to their type O antigens, the heat-stable antigen common to Inaba and Ogawa.
TABC vaccine—strains that have their full complement of O and H antigens and, in the case of *S. typhi* and *S. paratyphi C* contain also the Vi antigen.

3. The time of harvesting—

BCG vaccine—after not more than 14 days.
Plague vaccine—when capsule production appears to be at maximum.
Measles vaccine (inactivated)—the final vaccine represents not more than 10 passages from seed.

There is another extremely important aspect of variation. In several vaccines that contain suspensions of organisms the cells are not dead but are attenuated. If variation towards greater virulence occurred in these strains the results could be disastrous. Thorough checks are maintained on stock cultures and on the vaccines during manufacture to ensure that such a dangerous change does not remain undetected.

Freeze-drying is the best way to prevent variation in micro-organisms required for vaccine production. In this condition the antigenic and other properties of the cells remain unchanged indefinitely.

KILLED BACTERIAL SUSPENSIONS

The methods used for preparing the killed bacterial vaccines are essentially the same. Each strain is carefully checked for freedom from variation and absence of contaminating organisms; then it is inoculated on to a solid or into a liquid medium and incubated under optimum conditions for one to three days.

At the end of this time the cells are either—

(*a*) washed from the solid medium with sterile saline and centrifuged to remove pieces of agar detached during the washing off, or
(*b*) deposited from the liquid medium by centrifugation and, after removal of the supernatant fluid, washed free from broth constituents, which might cause reactions on injection, and resuspended in saline.

Sterilisation of the Suspension

The bacteria may be killed in one of two ways—

1. BY HEAT

Low temperatures are essential to avoid damage to the antigens. The usual treatment is 56°C for one hour. As this exposure cannot be relied upon to kill all contaminating organisms, particularly spores, strict asepsis is necessary throughout manufacture.

2. BY CHEMICAL BACTERICIDES

The organisms are killed chemically when heat treatment affects antigenicity (e.g. plague vaccine). Chemical methods are also allowed, as an alternative to killing by heat, where the accumulated evidence fails to confirm that one method is better than the other (e.g. pertussis, cholera, TAB and TABC vaccines). Formalin, approximately 0·5 per cent, is most often used (e.g. for plague and pertussis) but in some cases other bactericides are more suitable (e.g. phenol (cholera), thiomersal (alternative for pertussis) and 75 per cent alcohol (TAB and TABC)).

STANDARDISATION OF THE SUSPENSION

The total number of organisms per ml is determined either directly, using a Helber cell, or indirectly, by an opacity method such as Brown's tubes or a photoelectric nephelometer (*see* Chapter 28). The preparation is then diluted appropriately, using a diluent that minimises loss of antigenicity and contains a suitable preservative bactericide.

Official Killed Bacterial Vaccines

CHOLERA

Cholera is a very serious intestinal infection caused by the spirillum *Vibrio cholerae* and characterised by profuse diarrhoea. The vaccine is used for travellers to certain tropical countries, particularly India, where the disease is endemic. Protection is short-lived—only about six months.

In production of the vaccine, good antigenicity depends on selection of suitable strains; hence the detail given in the *Pharmacopoeia* in this connection.

A less severe form of cholera has become widespread in the far east. This is caused by the so-called *eltor* variants, and the *Pharmacopoeia* also includes a vaccine (Eltor vaccine) prepared from these, and a mixed preparation containing Cholera and Eltor vaccines.

Sometimes a mixture of cholera and TAB vaccines is used in the armed services.

PERTUSSIS

Whooping cough, caused by *Bordetella pertussis* is a common disease of childhood that, because babies receive virtually no pertussis antibodies from their mothers, is particularly dangerous in infancy. Production of a satisfactory vaccine has been difficult, but present-day products give a high degree of immunity. However, they are not as reliable as the diphtheria, tetanus and poliomyelitis prophylactics.

The disease can be caused by several antigenically-different strains of the organism and for high grade protection it is advisable to include all of these in the vaccine. S to R variation must be prevented.

To obtain a satisfactory product it is also necessary to avoid over-long incubation, unsuitable methods of harvesting, and harmful sterilising agents (e.g. phenol) or preservatives. Even washing the cells free from broth may remove important antigenic substances. After preparation the vaccine may show abnormal toxicity in animal tests, and this is removed by cold storage for up to three months.

It is used most often in the form of triple or quadruple antigen in which it has an adjuvant effect.

PLAGUE

Plague (the Black Death) is caused by *Pasteurella pestis* which is transmitted to man by the rat flea. It is unlikely to become a serious hazard again because of improved hygiene, rat-proof buildings, and the availability of powerful rodenticides and insecticides.

In the U.K. the vaccine is used for protecting service personnel posted to areas where plague is endemic and for special groups of workers such as those engaged in research on biological warfare. Immunity is short-lived and re-immunisation is desirable at about six-monthly intervals.

The most notable feature of the preparation of this vaccine is the care taken to obtain the maximum amount of capsular antigen.

TAB AND TABC

These mixed polyvalent vaccines are used in the prophylaxis of enteric infections. TAB is made by mixing simple vaccines of *Salmonella typhi*, *S. paratyphi A* and *S. paratyphi B*. TABC contains *S. paratyphi C* in addition.

S. typhi and *S. paratyphi C* have a special surface antigen, the Vi antigen, that increases the virulence of the cells. They are, for example, more resistant to phagocytosis.

There are two variations in the method of preparing these vaccines. In the first, the bacteria are destroyed by heat, and phenol is used as the preservative in the final preparation. In the other, the organisms are killed by exposure to 75 per cent alcohol and the preparation is preserved with 25 per cent alcohol. The Vi antigen is better conserved in alcohol-treated vaccines. In practice, however, it appears that while alcohol-treated vaccines give better protection to mice, heat-killed, phenolised vaccines are superior in man.

Lately, the value of the paratyphoid components has been questioned because the paratyphoid fevers are often much milder than typhoid fever.

These vaccines reduce the risk of typhoid fever by about 75 per cent. Immunity is most likely to break down when the body is exposed to heavy infection, e.g. from contaminated food, which will support multiplication of the organisms. Protection is relatively short-lived, and re-immunisation after six months to a year is advisable. They are used in the services and for travellers to insanitary areas in the tropics and sub-tropics.

TAB is also used mixed with tetanus vaccine (TABT vaccine) and with cholera vaccine (TAB and Cholera vaccine). The name of the latter must not be abbreviated to TABC to avoid confusion with the typhoid-paratyphoid vaccine containing *S. paratyphi C*. In the mixture containing tetanus vaccine the bacterial cells potentiate the antigenic activity of the toxoid.

LIVING BACTERIAL SUSPENSIONS

Manufacture of a satisfactory dead vaccine is not always feasible. In some cases the sterilisation method damages the antigens while in others it is possible that immunity-stimulating antigens are produced only when the organism is multiplying in the body.

One alternative might be to use a fully virulent strain of the organism, e.g. by an unusual and, therefore, safer route of infection (*see* Smallpox Vaccine), but this is impracticable because of the risk of serious disease. A more acceptable method is to weaken (attenuate) the organism so that it is safe to administer to man but is still able to stimulate antibody production.

The problem of producing strains that are safe, possess good immunising potency, and have no tendency to revert to the highly virulent forms are considerable and, in some cases insoluble, but attenuated strains have been used successfully in one bacterial and several viral vaccines. The bacterial vaccine is BCG.

BACILLUS CALMETTE-GUÉRIN (BCG) VACCINE

This is a suspension of living cells of a strain of *Mycobacterium tuberculosis* known as the bacillus of Calmette and Guérin. Calmette and Guérin were French bacteriologists; they investigated attenuated rather than dead vaccines because Calmette had worked under Pasteur who had been very successful with this type of preparation in anthrax and rabies. A bovine (cattle) strain was selected in the hope that it would be safer for man than the human variety. It was grown on a medium containing ox bile as this had been found to reduce the virulence of organisms in cultures in which it had been used to break up clumps of cells. It was subcultured on this medium for thirteen years, by which time it had become safe to administer to humans and was stable.

Originally it was given orally but, due to unreliable absorption from the gut, the intracutaneous route is now used. The living nature of the cells is demonstrated by the production of a characteristic lesion at the site of injection, but this remains localised, unlike infections by the virulent strains.

Preparation

A factor that makes a great impact on the preparation and testing of attenuated vaccines is the importance of preventing and detecting contamination of the product with virulent strains. Once in the history of BCG vaccine a virulent culture of the human variety was used by mistake, and of approximately 250 inoculated children over 25 per cent died (the Lübeck disaster). In consequence, particularly strict regulations are laid down for the manufacture of this type of preparation. These include use of a completely self-contained laboratory suite in which no living organisms except the BCG strain are allowed, superlative air-conditioning, and regular X-ray examinations of staff to prevent contamination with virulent human tubercle bacilli.

The methods used to prepare dead and living bacterial vaccines are essentially the same except

that for living preparations—

(i) there is no sterilisation stage,
(ii) the viability of the cells must be maintained,
(iii) standardisation is on the basis of a viable count.

Before use, the strain is rigorously checked for antigenicity and freedom from pathogenicity. It is then grown on a liquid medium for not more than 14 days, older cultures being less efficient antigens. Then the organisms are separated by centrifugation, washed, and suspended in a vehicle that preserves antigenicity and viability for as long as possible. The resulting liquid vaccine has been replaced by a freeze-dried form because the former has serious disadvantages—

1. Even when stored under ideal conditions (2 to 10°C and protected from light) it rapidly deteriorates, due to loss of viability, and is unfit for use after 14 days from harvesting.
2. Because of its short life, control tests, including the vital test for virulence (which takes six weeks to complete) cannot be finished until after the vaccine has been issued for use. The compromise adopted to deal with this unsatisfactory situation was to attempt to stop further use of the batch as soon as failure of any test became known and to investigate thoroughly the method of manufacture before any further batches were made.

The freeze-dried preparation, when stored under the same conditions as the liquid form, retains its potency for at least a year and, therefore, all the tests can and must be completed before issue.

The application of freeze-drying to vaccines presents a number of difficulties—

(a) The product may be so unsightly that it is pharmaceutically unacceptable.
(b) The material may be so fluffy that part of the contents is lost when the vacuum is released in the drying chamber.
(c) It may be very difficult to obtain a clump-free homogenous suspension when the vaccine is reconstituted with sterile saline or water.

BCG tends to clump badly when grown in conventional liquid media, and for a number of years the preparation of a homogeneous suspension depended on grinding these clumps with steel balls in a small sterile mill. To overcome this problem a non-ionic surfactant (a polyoxyethylene ether) was included in the growth medium. This caused the organisms to grow throughout the medium instead of as a tough surface pellicle and it largely eliminated clumping problems at all stages, including reconstitution of the freeze-dried material. It also improved the appearance of the product. Fluffiness was reduced, and reconstitution assisted by the inclusion of dextran in the suspending medium that was used for drying the cells. This medium also contained glucose which prevents excessive drying and, in the correct concentration, allows retention of the optimum amount of moisture.

Nowadays, a new needleless technique of inoculation, involving penetration of the skin by a high pressure jet of the preparation, is often used for mass vaccinations. Percutaneous BCG vaccine is used in this method.

The use of the BCG vaccines will be discussed in connection with the tuberculins—agents used to diagnose susceptibility to tuberculosis.

VIRAL SUSPENSIONS

Virus Immunity

A striking feature of the immunity following recovery from virus diseases is that very often it is lifelong, e.g. after measles, mumps, smallpox, and yellow fever. This may be due in large part to the way in which many viruses infect the body. They enter through mucous membranes, often of the respiratory tract, and are transported to all parts of the reticulo-endothelial system by wandering phagocytes which, although they ingest the viruses, can destroy only those of low virulence. The long incubation period (commonly two to three weeks) that is characteristic of viral diseases follows and during this time the viruses are providing a continuous and strong antigenic stimulus in the system that actually produces antibodies. This could explain the long-lasting immunity. Eventually, the viruses are freed into the blood stream and carried to the sites in which the disease becomes manifest.

The immunity is further strengthened because the antibodies circulating in the blood are excellently situated to inactivate viruses as they travel through the blood stream on their way to or from the reticulo-endothelial system. In many bacterial infections the organisms remain outside the bloodstream where they are less vulnerable to antibody attack.

It has been suggested that the solidity of viral immunity might be the result of persistence in the tissues of viruses in non-infective form, after the host has recovered from the disease.

For a number of viral diseases, however, immunity is very short-lived. The common cold and influenza are well-known examples. In these infections the viruses are usually confined to the epithelial cells of the respiratory tract and are carried from one cell to another by mucus. As a result, the antigenic stimulus is less direct and much weaker. After

development of immunity the presence of antibodies in the blood stream is relatively unimportant (although they may prevent penetration of viruses into deeper tissues); they must pass out into the mucus to be effective. As the appropriate host cells can be reached easily by the invading viruses the incubation period and, therefore, the duration of the antigenic stimulus is usually short.

However, it is possible that inadequate production or non-persistence of antibodies is less responsible for the short immunity in respiratory infections than the ability of the viruses to change into antigenically different variants. While the viruses of diseases that are followed by long immunity are antigenically stable, respiratory viruses frequently give rise to new antigenic types against which the antibodies of other types are ineffective. This is reflected in the preparation of viral vaccines. Only one strain need be used if the disease is caused by an antigenically stable organism, such as yellow fever, but where more than one strain can promote infection all must be included in the vaccine, e.g. in the poliomyelitis vaccine there are three antigenic types. The problem becomes most acute when, as in influenza, the organism undergoes frequent variation; the strains responsible for succeeding epidemics are slightly different from each other and it is extremely difficult to produce an entirely satisfactory vaccine before an epidemic arrives.

The incentive to produce effective viral vaccines is particularly strong because there are no reliable chemotherapeutic agents for the majority of virus diseases.

Living and Dead Vaccines

The earliest recorded example of the production of active immunity by artificial means is the ancient practice of variolation which was used to give protection against smallpox (variola). It involved scratching virus from mild cases into the skin, the aim being to produce a harmless form of the disease by employing an unusual route of infection; smallpox virus normally enters the body via the respiratory tract. Enough fatal cases of the disease developed to give clear warning of the serious risk involved in using virulent viruses for immunisation and since the time of Jenner (p. 289) attempts have been made to induce viral immunity by attenuated or inactivated organisms.

Compared with inactivated (dead) vaccines, attenuated (living) vaccines have important advantages—

1. The immunity is stronger and more lasting because the virus multiplies in the tissues.

2. As a result of the multiplication a smaller dose can be given.
3. Satisfactory products can be made from viruses with labile antigens that are destroyed by inactivation processes; e.g. cowpox and yellow fever.
4. Administration by the normal route of infection may be possible. In some cases this makes injections unnecessary. Attenuated poliomyelitis vaccine given by the (natural) oral route can be taken on a sugar lump.

They also have a number of disadvantages—

1. The virus may spread to other individuals and, theoretically at least, could become exalted in virulence as a result of transfer from person to person. On the other hand, if the strain remained stable, this spread could be a useful way of increasing immunity in the population.
2. It is much more difficult to attenuate than to inactivate an organism. The attenuated strain must retain its antigenicity but be free from virulence and incapable of regaining it. However, inactivated vaccines are not entirely free from danger since faulty inactivation could leave fully virulent strains in the preparation.
3. Because there is no inactivation process great care must be taken to prevent contamination with viruses capable of causing other infectious diseases or tumours.

While in some cases the choice between the two methods is straightforward, as with cowpox and yellow fever where inactivation destroys antigenicity, in others it is far less simple and both types are available.

Cultivation of Viruses in Vaccine Production

Since viruses are intracellular parasites they will grow only within other living cells. These can be provided in free-living animals, fertile eggs or tissue cultures.

FREE-LIVING ANIMALS

Nowadays very few vaccines are made from viruses grown in free-living animals. The products are good antigens but the method is inconvenient and costly and adventitious contamination is difficult to prevent. In some parts of the world typhus vaccine is prepared from rickettsiae grown in the lungs of small rodents or the peritoneal cavities of gerbils, and rabies vaccine may be produced from the brains of sheep or rabbits, but in the UK, the most important prophylactic prepared from free-living animals is vaccine lymph (smallpox vaccine). There are alternative sources of this vaccine but the products are less thermostable and no more effective than the material from free-living animals.

FERTILE EGGS

Many viruses can be grown in some part of the chick embryo (Fig. 33.1). The advantages of this method over the use of free-living animals include—

(a) It is much easier to keep the product free from contaminating micro-organisms;
(b) At the age of use the embryo cannot produce antiviral antibodies, which might affect the yield.

Nevertheless, in using eggs a number of precautions must be taken—

(a) Strict aseptic technique must be maintained throughout, to prevent bacterial contamination. The yolk sac is an excellent medium for bacterial growth, and although the amniotic and allantoic fluids are antibacterial they cannot cope with heavy infection.

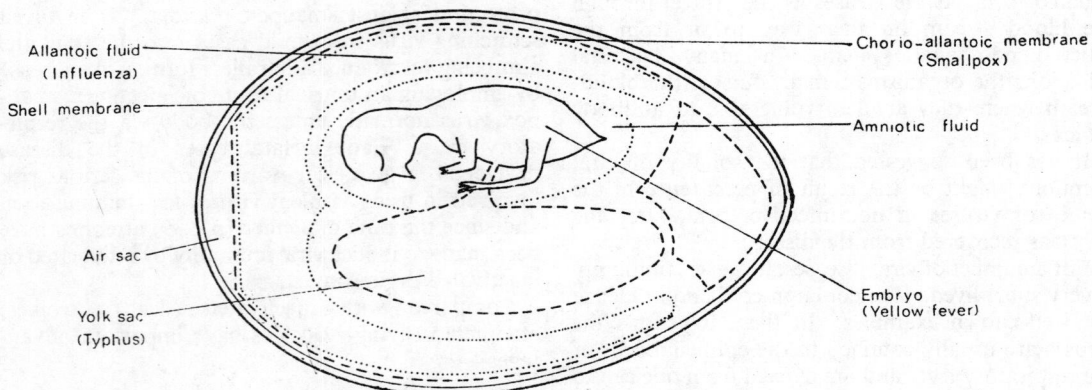

Fig. 33.1   Regions of egg used in production of official vaccines

(b) Repeated passage of virus from egg to egg must be avoided because the virus may become adapted to embryo tissue and less virulent for its natural host. To ensure an adequate supply of virus of satisfactory virulence the vaccine strain is grown in quantity in one batch of eggs and then freeze-dried or stored at a low temperature so that the same virus can be used for many future batches of vaccine.

(c) Viruses grown in the yolk sac or embryo are separated by grinding and, as a result, traces of egg protein get into the vaccine and may cause reactions in the recipient similar to those produced by the injection of serum proteins (p. 402). When either of these two regions is used the egg must not be more than ten to eleven days old at harvesting because before this time its proteins are not sufficiently developed to cause hypersensitivity reactions.

(d) The eggs must be candled to confirm that the embryos are alive. This involves examination in front of a bright light, when spontaneous movement or well-defined blood vessels indicate a living embryo.

TISSUE CULTURE

It has been known for many years that vaccinia virus (see Smallpox vaccine) will grow in certain minced animal tissues kept alive in suitable solutions of salts but the method remained undeveloped as a means of growing viruses because of the success of chick embryo techniques and the difficulty of preventing contamination of the cultures. Eventually, the fertile egg was found unsuitable for the growth of several important viruses, such as those causing chickenpox, german measles, measles and poliomyelitis, and this problem, combined with the discovery of antibiotics, which could be used to control accidental contamination, led to renewed interest in tissue culture. It is now a major method of virus vaccine production. The essential features are—

1. Selection of a Suitable Tissue

A large number of tissues can be successfully cultivated outside the animal body but, because certain viruses will grow only in primate cells, monkey kidney has become the most widely used (e.g. in the manufacture of both poliomyelitis vaccines and one measles vaccine). Chick embryo is more satisfactory in some cases, e.g. for attenuated measles virus and cowpox, and the latter has also been successfully grown in calf embryo skin.

Ideally the tissues should be free from living micro-organisms but while the absence of major bacterial diseases such as tuberculosis in monkeys is comparatively easy to confirm by quarantine of the animals and a post mortem before use of the kidneys, it is far more difficult to ensure freedom from contaminating viruses; for example, it was believed for many years that the chick embryo was not a natural carrier of viruses, but now it is known that avian leucosis may be present. This virus causes tumours in birds and, although there is no evidence of transmission to humans, eggs from leucosis-free flocks are used for measles vaccine. As would be expected, the tissues of free-living animals such as the monkey carry many more viruses, and while most are non-pathogenic to man, constant vigilance, including long quarantine and numerous safety tests, is necessary.

Eventually it may be possible to maintain clean lines of cells by continuous subculture (cf. Maintenance of Bacterial Cultures). This has been done for many years with certain malignant cells (e.g. the HeLa line, from a patient, Helen Langley, with cancer of the cervix) but normal cells usually die after a few subcultures. In the last few years progress has been reported on the development of non-malignant lines one of which, from foetal lung tissue, will propagate for about 50 passages without deleterious cytological changes. If such a line could be established it would be possible to avoid constant use of fresh tissue for each vaccine and to ensure that the cells are free from contamination.

2. Establishment of Growth and/or Maintenance of Metabolism under Artificial Conditions

After the organ or tissue has been removed from the animal under surgically clean conditions, it is cut up or minced and treated, usually with trypsin, to disperse the cells. The result is a suspension of single cells or small aggregates and this is used in one of two types of culture—

(a) Suspended Cell Culture. In this, the cells are merely suspended in a liquid medium. The aim is simply to maintain cell metabolism, and since there is very little or no proliferation, an adequate quantity of cells for virus growth must be included initially.

(b) Fixed Cell (Monolayer) Culture. Fewer cells are added to the medium and these are allowed to settle on to one side of a large flat-sided bottle. During a period of incubation they become attached to the glass and multiply into a uniform layer one cell thick. When this has spread over the lower side of the bottle the medium is changed from one that will support growth to another that is adequate to maintain cell metabolism.

Fixed cell cultures are claimed to give higher yields of virus per cell, possibly because, as is indicated by the fact that multiplication occurs, the viability of the cells is higher. Also, it is easier to change the medium and, as there are fewer floating cell aggregates to protect the virus, to sterilise the suspension when a dead vaccine is required.

Extremely complex media are needed to grow and maintain these cultures. They contain—

(a) A balanced salt solution, to provide the optimum pH and osmotic pressure.

(b) Nutrients. The nutritional needs of tissue culture cells are very exacting and necessitate particularly complicated media. In addition, in vaccine production, complex materials such as serum and proteins must be excluded as far as possible because they may cause reactions when the vaccine is administered. To satisfy these requirements, many ingredients (sixty or more) are included, e.g. essential amino-acids, growth factors, dextrose, purines, pyrimidines and inorganic salts. Growth, as distinct from maintenance, media usually contain more complex ingredients such as protein hydrolysates, tissue extracts and, sometimes, serum, but the latter must be completely absent from the final product to prevent hypersensitivity reactions in recipients. Heavy metals are very toxic to tissue culture cells and their concentration must be extremely low.

(c) A pH indicator, often phenol red, to show the state of cell metabolism and when the pH has fallen to a level that necessitates a change of medium.

(d) Antibiotics, both antibacterial and antifungal, to prevent growth of contaminants. Care is taken largely to inactivate these by the end of processing because sensitisation of a patient, by administration of small amounts in a vaccine, could make dangerous the subsequent administration of urgently needed antibiotic. This problem is so great with penicillin that the *Pharmacopoeia* does not allow its use and although streptomycin may be used in the production of cell cultures it must be absent when the virus is added.

3. *Cultivation of Viruses in the Cells*

After the suspended cells have become adjusted to the medium, or the monolayer has fully developed, the seed virus is added and the culture is returned to the incubator, where it is slowly rocked to prevent accumulation of high concentrations of harmful metabolites on the surfaces of the tissue cells and to ensure free exchange of oxygen and carbon dioxide. The virus invades the cells, multiplies, and is released into the medium which, at the end of incuba-

tion and after suspended cells have been allowed to settle, is siphoned off aseptically.

Official Viral Vaccines

In the following account the vaccines are classified under the method of production commonly used in the United Kingdom.

A. FROM FREE-LIVING ANIMALS

1. *Smallpox Vaccine*

When Jenner introduced vaccination (p. 289) he used living cowpox virus which gave good immunity to smallpox because the viruses of the two diseases are closely related. Since then, smallpox vaccines have not always been made from natural cowpox strains; variola virus attenuated by passage through animals, such as calves or rabbits, and known as vaccinia, has also been used. The origin of the strains used for vaccine production today is by no means certain.

The vaccine is usually obtained from lesions produced on the skin of suitable living mammals, e.g. calves or sheep—

Selection of Animals. Healthy calves or sheep are quarantined and given thorough examinations to exclude communicable diseases.

Inoculation. The flanks and abdomen (only the former in sheep because the abdomen is less easy to keep clean) are scrubbed, disinfected, shaved, rescrubbed, and redisinfected. Then, in special rooms, the shaved areas are—

(a) Scarified, i.e. lightly scratched with a comb-like device, without drawing blood.

(b) Inoculated, by rubbing a seed virus of known potency into the scratches. Sometimes this seed is propagated in rabbits when it is known as lapine.

Incubation. During the next four to five days, vesicles containing the virus develop along the lines of scarification, and throughout this period every precaution is taken to keep the inoculated areas aseptically clean.

Harvesting. The animals are killed, exsanguinated and washed. Then the contents of the vesicles (i.e. the lymph) are removed by curretage, i.e. by scraping with a special (Volkmann's) spoon that has a very sharp edge to the bowl. The pooled material is homogenised. A post mortem is done on the animal's carcase to confirm the absence of infectious diseases.

Purification. Because it is not possible entirely to prevent contamination with extraneous micro-organisms the lymph must be treated to kill pathogens and to reduce the number of residual bacteria to a very low level. For many years this was done by grinding with an equal volume of glycerin and storing for a long time at −10°C. Nowadays a more efficient method is used—

(*a*) The lymph is extracted with a protein solvent, e.g. trichlorofluoroethane. Presence of protein lowers the efficiency of the bactericidal agent (p. 345).

(*b*) Phenol is added to produce a concentration of 0·4 per cent and the material is incubated at 22°C for two days or until the bacterial count is low enough. The viruses are unharmed by this treatment because they are much more resistant than bacteria to phenol.

(*c*) Glycerin and peptone are included to give concentrations of 40 per cent and 1 per cent respectively. The glycerin assists the bactericidal action of the phenol during the subsequent storage at −10°C, which continues until issue. The glycerin also gives the product a viscosity similar to the earlier preparations that were treated with glycerin alone, a viscous preparation being easier to use for vaccination. The peptone helps to preserve the viability of the viruses, particularly if the product is to be freeze-dried.

(*d*) Sometimes brilliant green, or another suitable colouring matter, is added to mark the area of application of the vaccine.

Tests are performed to confirm the absence of *Escherichia coli*, aerobic pathogens, and anaerobic pathogens and to show that the number of living extraneous micro-organisms is not more than 500 per ml.

Alternative Methods of Preparation. Vaccines prepared from virus grown on the chorioallantoic membrane of the fertile hen's egg are used in parts of the USA. The technique is described on page 394. Tissue culture methods using calf embryo skin or chick embryo cells have also been developed and the products appear antigenically equivalent to vaccines from other sources.

A major advantage of these alternative methods is that a sterile preparation can be obtained. When they are used the *Pharmacopoeia* states that the vaccine must comply with the official tests for sterility, a requirement that the product from free-living animals could not meet because of its virtually unavoidable contamination with living bacteria.

For obvious reasons the *Pharmacopoeia* restricts the name Vaccine Lymph, a well-known synonym for smallpox vaccine, to the product obtained from free-living animals.

Freeze-dried Smallpox Vaccine. Liquid smallpox vaccine retains its potency for a year at −10°C but at higher temperatures its stability is much lower, particularly if it is not protected from light. For example, the storage life at 2 to 10°C and 10 to 20°C is only two weeks and one week respectively. The freeze-dried product is far more stable and keeps indefinitely below 10°C, for a year at 22°C and for a month at 37°C; this is an advantage in the tropics and in situations where it is necessary to keep emergency stocks. After reconstitution it keeps its potency for a week if stored below 10°C.

Packaging. Although multi-dose containers may be used, the liquid vaccine is commonly packed in single-dose capillary tubes of glass or plastic. The freeze-dried material is supplied in multi-dose containers together with suitable volumes of reconstituting fluid.

2. Rabies Vaccine

The development of the first rabies vaccine by Louis Pasteur is one of the greatest achievements in the history of immunisation. First, he showed that the virulence of the natural ('street') virus, obtained from the saliva of mad dogs, could be increased by passage through a series of several dozen rabbits until it eventually became stable ('fixed') virus. At this point the incubation time of the virus in the host had been shortened from about 60 to 6 days. Pasteur found next that this stable strain could be attenuated by drying the infected spinal cords of rabbits, the degree of attenuation depending on the length of drying. By starting immunisation with an emulsion of highly attenuated cord (dried for 14 days), and following this on each of the succeeding eleven days with a preparation that had received a day's less drying than that used on the previous day, he was able to prevent the development of rabies in animals and, later, in humans who had been bitten by rabid animals. Protection after infection is possible with this disease because rabies is unique in having a very long incubation period ranging from about 60 days for leg bites to about 30 days for bites in the region of the head. Consequently, there is enough time for *large* doses of vaccine to stimulate an adequate antibody response before the virulent virus is poured out into the bloodstream (p. 389).

Over the years, Pasteur's method has been modified in two respects. Firstly, rabbit spinal cords have been replaced by rabbit brains, which give better yields, and, secondly, attenuation by drying has, in general, been superseded by inactivation with chemicals. In the *Pharmacopoeia* method—

(*a*) Rabbits or sheep are injected intracerebrally with fixed rabies virus.

(*b*) When they have shown typical symptoms for 24 hours and have become completely paralysed, they are killed and the brains are harvested and homogenised in Sodium Chloride Injection.

(*c*) The viruses are inactivated. Phenol is often preferred, but treatment with other chemicals, e.g. formaldehyde or beta-propiolactone, or ultraviolet light has also been successful.

(*d*) The preparation is diluted to contain a suitable amount of brain material.

Alternative Method of Preparation. Vaccines containing nervous tissue may cause an allergic response in the brain, leading to nerve cell deterioration and paralysis. These reactions are rare when vaccines are prepared in fertile hen or duck eggs. The latter are preferred because yields are better. The usual inactivating agent is beta-propiolactone.

B. FROM FERTILE EGGS

Because some viruses grow better in particular parts of the embryo (e.g. vaccinia in the chorioallantoic membrane, influenza in the allantoic fluid, yellow fever in the embryo itself and typhus *rickettsia* in the yolk sac) several methods of inoculation are used—

1. *Inoculation on to the Chorioallantoic Membrane*

Eggs that have been incubated for twelve days are candled, and while they are in front of the lamp the air sac is marked and a triangle (about 10 mm in side) is drawn at a place where the chorioallantoic membrane is well-developed (Fig. 33.2a). The triangle is carefully cut out with the edge of a carborundum disc driven by a dental motor, and at the same time a tiny groove is cut over the air space.

The triangle is then lifted gently to separate it from the shell membrane without damaging the latter, and a drop of sterile saline is pipetted on to the membrane which is then split with a blunt mounted needle.

Gentle suction is next applied to the hole over the air sac and, as the air is removed, the essentially fluid contents of the egg are drawn towards the hole. Consequently, the chorioallantoic membrane falls away from the shell membrane, below the triangular opening, forming a new sac into which the saline is

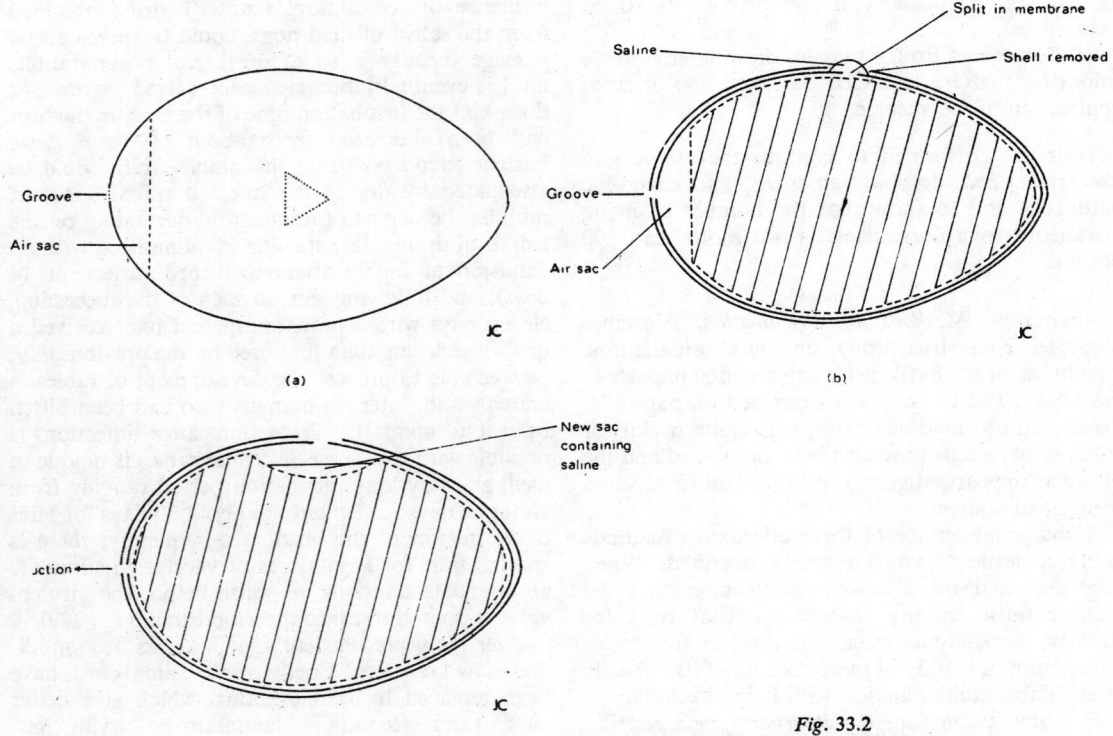

Fig. 33.2
Inoculation of the chorioallantoic membrane

drawn (Fig. 33.2*b* and *c*). The split in the shell membrane is then widened, the virus is inoculated through the opening, and the site is covered. A variety of methods have been used to achieve this, including replacement of the triangular flap and sealing with hard or soft paraffin, and covering the opening with a strip of transparent adhesive tape.

The eggs are incubated, taking care to keep the inoculation site uppermost.

2. *Inoculation into the Embryo*

Eggs that have been incubated for only seven to eight days are used (p. 391). The seed virus is inoculated directly into the embryo through a small hole over the air sac, using a syringe and long needle.

3. *Inoculation into the Yolk Sac*

The method is similar to the embryo technique. To deposit the inoculum in the yolk sac accurately, the needle is inserted along the long axis of the egg to just beyond the centre.

4. *Inoculation into the Allantoic Fluid*

After ten to thirteen days incubation, the eggs are marked to show the air sac and the point of inoculation, which is a small hole made on the side of the egg with a dentist's drill, without damaging the shell membrane. It is positioned to avoid blood vessels. Another hole is drilled over the air sac to relieve any excess pressure when the inoculum is introduced. The virus is injected with a syringe and needle and the inoculation hole is then sealed with melted sterile hard paraffin.

(*a*) SMALLPOX VACCINE

After incubation for three days the shell is removed aseptically and the thickened and infected chorio-allantoic membrane is separated into saline. The material is frozen and in this condition is ground to free the viruses. The suspension is diluted with a diluent similar to that used for the vaccine from free-living animals.

(*b*) YELLOW FEVER VACCINE

This vaccine contains an attenuated strain of yellow fever virus known as the 17D strain, which was produced from the highly virulent Asibi strain (named after a patient) by numerous passages through tissue cultures, first in mouse embryo cells

and then in chick embryo from which the central nervous tissue had been removed. The virulent virus has two properties—

(i) Viscerotropic. This is shown in humans and monkeys by damage to the viscera; e.g. the jaundice that gives the patient the colour from which the disease is named is a result of necrosis of the liver.

(ii) Neurotropic. This leads to encephalitis when the virus is injected intracerebrally into mice.

The 17D strain has entirely lost its viscerotropism but the neurotropism, although diminished, is still evident. These facts are reflected in the official identification tests for the vaccine which show that the preparation is harmless to rhesus monkeys but lethal to mice.

Because the virus is living, a strong, long-lasting immunity is produced, and reaches a satisfactory level about ten days after injection, lasting for at least ten years.

The vaccine is prepared from embryo-inoculated fertile eggs in the following way—

After incubation for three to four days, the tops of the eggs are removed and the embryos are lifted out with forceps, the pooled embryos being ground with sterile water to extract the virus from the cells. The resulting suspension is then centrifuged to remove cell debris, and the supernatant fluid containing the viruses is freeze-dried. After drying, the ampoules are immediately filled with pure dry sterile nitrogen and sealed.

The vaccine undergoes rapid deterioration in the presence of air and this is increased by moisture; consequently, when the preparation has been reconstituted, with Sodium Chloride Injection, it must be administered within half an hour.

(*c*) INFLUENZA VACCINE

The preparation of a satisfactory prophylactic for influenza is complicated by the capacity of the virus for variation. Most influenza outbreaks are caused by one of two types of virus—

Type A, which is responsible for quickly spreading major epidemics that are sometimes worldwide, and type B, which gives rise to small localised outbreaks and only occasionally produces a widespread epidemic.

There is no cross immunity between these types and in addition, variation takes place within the types, particularly in type A which shows considerable lack of stability in antigenic structure. Since 1933 three distinct antigenic classes of A have appeared—

Classical A	1933–1946
A1 (A prime)	1946–1957
A2 (Asian)	1957–

and two classes of B have been recognised.

There is no cross-immunity between any of these five classes, and it follows that, in theory, protection against influenza can be provided in two ways. By

1. *Producing a Polyvalent Vaccine that will give Blanket Coverage.*

This method will be successful only if the antigenic components of the virus are limited. Then, if each is strongly represented by the strains chosen for the vaccine, the product should be effective. In the USA, preparations of this kind, containing one or more strains of each of A, A1, A2, and B, have been used for many years.

2. *Obtaining Information on the Antigenic Composition of the Strain Likely to Cause the Next Outbreak, in Time to Prepare a Specific Vaccine for it.*

The World Health Organisation has an influenza centre to which any outbreak in member countries is reported immediately. The virus is identified as quickly as possible and the strain is made available to vaccine manufacturers. If the latter have adequate warning, this method has the advantage of providing a vaccine specific for the on-coming epidemic. To cover major and local outbreaks, due to types A and B respectively, it is an advantage to include the most recently isolated strains of each in the vaccine. As there is an upper limit to the amount of virus that can be injected without toxic reactions, the quantity of antigen relevant to the next epidemic can be much greater in these uni- or di-valent vaccines than in the polyvalent type. The official vaccine contains the strains currently recommended by the World Health Organisation.

Preparation

After incubation for two to three days the inoculated eggs are chilled in a refrigerator for a day. This kills the embryo and, therefore, prevents haemorrhage into the allantoic fluid during harvesting. The shell is removed from over the air sac, the underlying membranes are cut away, and the allantoic fluid is drawn off into a flask. Pools of the fluid from small batches of eggs are separately tested for sterility. The use of small pools avoids rejection of an unnecessarily large amount of fluid that might have been contaminated by only one or two eggs.

The virus is purified, usually by centrifugation. First a low speed is used to separate a flocculent precipitate of protein and then a change to a very high speed throws out the viruses. They are removed into a suitable vehicle. The resulting concentrated suspension is treated with about 0·01 per cent formaldehyde at 0 to 4°C for two to three days to inactivate the virus which is finally suspended in a neutral buffered saline solution containing thiomersal or other suitable bactericide.

Polyvalent vaccines are made by mixing purified and inactivated suspensions of each strain.

Adjuvant Vaccines

The antigenic effect of influenza vaccine can be potentiated by emulsifying the aqueous suspension in mineral oil using a water-in-oil emulsifying agent. The oil stimulates the formation of a granuloma (a small harmless growth of cells) at the site of injection, and this protects the virus and delays its destruction. The result is an improved level and duration of immunity. The pharmacopoeial vaccine is an aqueous suspension, but commercial oil-adjuvant products are available.

Active immunity to influenza develops quickly—in ten to fourteen days. Only one injection is given as there is no improvement in antibody response from a second. The protection, however, is short-lived and lasts for about six months only.

C. FROM TISSUE CULTURES

1. *Poliomyelitis Vaccines*

Poliomyelitis is a much-feared disease because it can cause paralysis but it more often occurs in latent or mild, non-paralytic forms. Probably about 90 per cent of infections cause no symptoms and only 1 per cent lead to paralysis. The explanation is that the virus first invades the cells of the oropharyngeal and intestinal mucosae and in most individuals remains there until it is eliminated by cell replacement. Meanwhile it stimulates a lasting immunity. In a small percentage of infections, however, it finds its way via the lymphatics and the blood-stream to the central nervous system where it causes the degenerative changes that produce paralysis.

The first successful prophylactic was the inactivated vaccine which is administered parenterally and stimulates the production of antibodies in the blood. This type of vaccine gives protection by neutralising the virus as it passes through the bloodstream on the way from the alimentary canal to the central nervous system. It does not, however, prevent establishment of infective virus in the mucosae and an individual, actively immunised with the inactivated vaccine, could act as a carrier for virulent virus and infect others.

The second type of vaccine contains attenuated organisms which, when the preparation is given orally (e.g. on a sugar lump), invade by the normal route. In the mucosa of the alimentary canal they prevent the establishment of infective virus by stimulating the production of local antibodies and, possibly, through interferon production (p. 313). Antibodies also develop in the bloodstream.

Both types of vaccine are represented in the *Pharmacopoeia* but, in practice, live, oral vaccine is usually preferred.

Preparation

There are three distinct antigenic types of poliomyelitis virus, types I, II, and III, and each has much greater antigenic stability than, for example, the types of influenza virus. This means that, although strains of all three types are known, infection by one gives protection against all other strains of that type. Therefore, by including one important strain of each type in a polyvalent vaccine a satisfactory and long-lasting immunity is produced.

The three types of virus are grown separately in either suspended or fixed cell cultures of monkey kidney tissue. Nerve cells, a more obvious choice, are avoided as they have a short life in tissue culture and because traces of nervous tissue in vaccines sometimes cause an allergic reaction in the brain (p. 394). Rhesus monkeys are used; they are quarantined on arrival and checked for tuberculosis and other communicable diseases, both before and after death.

The monkey kidney cells must not have been propagated in series, i.e. obtained from a continuous line of cells (p. 391). This exclusion is based on fear that, because it has been easier to produce continuous lines of malignant than normal cells, ability to maintain a line of the latter is indicative of a transformation towards malignancy in the cells.

For both types of vaccine, serum is forbidden in the culture media used for maintaining cell growth during virus propagation but it may be included in media used to initiate the growth of tissue cells. This is to prevent serum reactions when the preparations are administered and is more important in the inactivated vaccine, which is given parenterally; for this there is a limit of not more than one part per million of serum in the final product.

(*a*) *Inactivated Vaccine.* This is often called Salk-type vaccine after the American virologist who first developed it.

After the virus suspension has been harvested it is tested to confirm that—

(i) only the correct strain of poliomyelitis virus is present;
(ii) the virus titre is above a minimum level;
(iii) it is free from viral, bacterial and fungal contaminants.

Then it is passed through filters of increasing fineness which remove remnants of tissue cells and, finally, bacteria; the former could protect some of the virus from the inactivating agent.

Inactivation is by 0·01 per cent formaldehyde under accurately controlled conditions of pH and temperature and with magnetic stirring. It is usually complete in six days but at least twice this time is allowed to make sure that no active virus remains. The suspension may be refiltered at the halfway point. The rate at which inactivation is proceeding is followed for several days and then at about the 9th and 12th days large samples are tested for absence of infective virus; the suspension is not used unless both are sterile.

The univalent vaccines are then blended to give the trivalent product and further very large samples are tested for freedom from infective virus.

Finally, the formaldehyde is neutralised with sodium metabisulphite, and thiomersal is added as a bactericide. Disodium edetate is also included to sequester heavy metals that catalyse decomposition of thiomersal to products that are toxic to the virus.

(*b*) *Attenuated (Oral) Vaccine.* This is often called Sabin-type vaccine after the American who developed it. It is manufactured in essentially the same way as Salk-type vaccine except that—

(i) Attenuated strains, prepared by rapid passages through tissue cultures of monkey kidney cells, are used.
(ii) The virus in the final vaccine must not represent more than three subcultures from a strain that laboratory and clinical tests have shown to be satisfactory. This reduces the chance of using a variant that has become more virulent or has lost antigenicity.
(iii) There is no inactivation stage.
(iv) In addition to testing for freedom from extraneous bacteria, moulds and viruses, special tests are necessary, because the virus in the vaccine is living, to confirm the absence of virulent poliomyelitis virus (p. 408).

2. Measles Vaccines

Measles is rarely a fatal disease in Britain but a great deal of childhood misery is caused by complications due to respiratory and middle ear involvement. Mortality is still high in countries where there is malnutrition. The virus was not isolated until 1954, when Enders and Peebles grew it in a tissue culture of human kidney cells. More recently, cell systems applicable to vaccine production, i.e. from monkey kidney or chick embryo cells, have been successfully substituted.

In general, attenuated vaccines with high antigenicity cause severe reactions when administered, while inactivated products, although virtually reaction-free, are very poor immunising agents.

The *Pharmacopoeia* includes a vaccine of each type. The attenuated one, which, like the corresponding poliomyelitis preparation, is given parenterally, includes a strain of virus in which the degree of attenuation provides the best compromise so far between antigenicity and reactivity. Only a minority of patients show side effects (fever, transient rash and irritability). A single injection is considered adequate but it is too early to know how protection compares with the life-long immunity from an attack of the disease.

The official inactivated vaccine is not intended to be used alone. It may be given four to six weeks previously to reduce reactions from the living vaccine.

(a) *Inactivated Vaccine.* This is manufactured by a method similar to that used for inactivated poliomyelitis vaccine. The main differences are—

(i) The vaccine is univalent. Measles virus has high antigenic stability.

(ii) The tissue culture may be of chick embryo or monkey kidney cells.

(iii) The final vaccine represents not more than ten passages from the seed virus.

(iv) Among possible contaminants are avian leucosis viruses (p. 391). Eggs used for chick embryo tissue cultures must come from leucosis-free flocks of birds.

(v) The virus may be adsorbed on to aluminium hydroxide or phosphate. The resulting depot preparations are more efficient antigens (cf. diphtheria vaccine) and satisfactory but short immunity can be obtained with three doses.

(b) *Attenuated Vaccine.* Again, the method of preparation is similar to that used for the corresponding poliomyelitis vaccine, but in addition to points (i), (iii), and (iv) mentioned under measles inactivated virus the following differences apply—

(i) The virus is grown in chick embryo tissue only, because it is to this that the attenuated strain has been adapted.

(ii) In addition to the usual tests for the absence of extraneous bacteria and viruses, the viral suspension must also be free from mycoplasma.

These are frequent contaminants of tissue cultures, often causing cytopathogenic effects similar to those caused by viruses and confusing the interpretation of tests in which tissue cultures are used. In addition, some species of mycoplasma are pathogenic (p. 326).

(ii) The vaccine is freeze-dried after suitable stabilisers have been added.

(iv) The product must be handled with extreme care. The virus is rapidly inactivated by most bactericides, including bactericidal soaps, alcohols and chlorinated water. Absolutely clean equipment (e.g. radiation-sterilised disposable syringes) is essential for reconstitution and administration. Traces of heavy metals catalyse deleterious changes and, therefore, contact with metals must be avoided as far as possible.

RICKETTSIAL SUSPENSIONS

Although rickettsiae are small bacteria they, like viruses, require the environment of living cells for growth and multiplication. In the *Pharmacopoeia* there is only one rickettsial vaccine, typhus, and the organisms for this are usually grown in the yolk sac of the fertile egg.

TYPHUS VACCINE

There are two forms of typhus, epidemic and murine, caused by *Rickettsia prowazeki* and *R. typhi* respectively. Epidemic typhus ('jail fever') is carried from person to person by lice. It has always been associated with war, famine, and overcrowding and, if untreated, the mortality is high. Murine (rat) typhus is a much milder disease transmitted by the rat flea.

Both forms can be treated successfully with wide-spectrum antibiotics but vaccines are useful to protect members of the armed services and medical staff against epidemic typhus in endemic areas. Immunisation against murine typhus is not considered essential except for laboratory workers using the organism. The Pharmacopoeial vaccine contains both species.

Preparation

After the embryos have died or become moribund, the heavily infected yolk sacs are removed and ground to liberate the rickettsiae.

The ground material is suspended in an isotonic solution containing 0·2 to 0·5 per cent of formaldehyde to kill the organisms. Inactivation is necessary because attenuated typhus vaccines cause severe reactions. At this stage the preparation contains 10 to 15 per cent of yolk sac material and, to reduce the hazard to individuals sensitive to egg protein it is treated with ether or trichlorotrifluoroethane.

The aqueous phase is separated and used as the vaccine. Thiomersal may be added as a bactericide.

R. prowazeki liberates soluble antigen into the yolk sac and care is taken to retain this in the preparation.

Alternative Methods of Preparation. Although typhus vaccine is usually made in eggs it can also be obtained from free-living animals, i.e.: (*a*) from the lungs of small rodents (e.g. mice) that have been infected intranasally with massive doses of typhus rickettsiae to give them typhus pneumonia; (*b*) from the intraperitoneal fluid of gerbils (North African rodents) infected by intraperitoneal injections of rickettsiae.

DIAGNOSTIC PREPARATIONS

These are preparations containing bacterial *toxins*. They are used to test individuals for—

A. Susceptibility or immunity to a particular infection.
B. A useful degree of protection after immunisation.
C. The presence of a particular disease.

There are four official preparations—

1. Schick test toxin
2. Schick control
3. Old tuberculin
4. Tuberculin purified protein derivative (Tuberculin PPD)

Schick test and control are used together for applications A and B in connection with immunity to diphtheria. The tuberculins can be used for A, B, and C in investigations of tuberculosis.

The Schick Test

This is based on the following facts—

(*a*) The presence of an adequate level of diphtheria antitoxin in the blood renders an individual immune to diphtheria and, conversely, the absence of this antitoxin makes him susceptible.

(*b*) The introduction of a minute quantity of diphtheria toxin into the skin produces no effect (negative reaction) if antitoxin is present because the toxin is neutralised and made harmless. If antitoxin is absent or its level is too low to give protection, the toxin produces a local inflammation (positive reaction). Hence negative and positive reactions indicate immunity and susceptibility respectively.

SCHICK TEST TOXIN

This is a sterile filtrate prepared from a culture of *Corynebacterium diphtheriae* grown on a suitable nutrient broth. The filtrate contains diphtheria exotoxin; for some time this loses potency, then its toxicity becomes relatively stable and at this point it may be used.

It is diluted so that—

1. The test dose is contained in 0·2 ml. The volume must be small because the preparation is injected intracutaneously.
2. It is isotonic with blood plasma—to prevent false reactions due to paratonicity.
3. Its pH is stabilised. If the toxin is diluted with Sodium Chloride Injection it loses its potency in a few days even at 0°C but when the official diluent, containing a borax-boric acid buffer as well as sodium chloride, is used the preparation is stable for at least two months at a temperature not exceeding 25°C.

The amount of toxin in the test dose is critical; if too small it may give a negative result when antitoxin is absent or insufficient to cause immunity; if too great it may swamp the antitoxin in an immune person and produce a positive result. The *Pharmacopoeia* outlines tests that fix the upper and lower limits of toxin concentration at satisfactory levels.

SCHICK CONTROL

This is Schick test toxin from the same batch as that used for the test which has been heated at not lower than 70°C and not higher than 85°C for at least five minutes to destroy the toxin. It is used to discover if individuals are sensitive to non-specific constituents (i.e. substances other than the toxin) in the broth. If this sensitivity was not detected their pseudo-reactions might be interpreted as lack of immunity.

Application of the Test

On the same occasion, the test dose is injected intracutaneously into the left forearm and an equal volume of the control is given into the right forearm. The arms are first examined one to two days later. The possible results, explanations and inferences are shown in Table 33.3.

Table 33.3

	Left arm (Toxin)	Right arm (Control)	Explanation Toxin is—	Inference Individual is—
1.	Large flushed area	No reaction	not neutralised	not immune
2.	No reaction	No reaction	neutralised	immune
3.	Large flushed area	Smaller flushed area	not neutralised; sensitivity to broth constituents	not immune and a pseudo-reactor
4.	Small flushed area*	Small flushed area (same size as*)	neutralised; sensitivity to broth constituents	immune and a pseudo-reactor

A true positive persists longer than a pseudo-reaction and, therefore, results 3 and 4 (Table 33.3) are re-examined after a week when the false result will have faded.

The Schick test is less often used now that more reliable diphtheria prophylactics are available.

The Tuberculins

Persons suffering from tuberculosis or who have recovered from an active or latent infection are extremely sensitive to a protein constituent of the tubercle bacillus, *Mycobacterium tuberculosis*. The tuberculins contain this protein and, therefore, when they are applied to or injected into the skin of sensitised individuals a local inflammation is set up. Minute doses are sufficient to cause the reaction. In general, only people who have never been infected will give a negative result.

The bacterial protein (tuberculin), which may be regarded as a toxin, acts as an antigen which stimulates the tissues to produce corresponding antibodies. These antibodies react strongly with the antigen when they meet it again, causing inflammation, and even necrosis, of the cells in the area. This hypersensitivity reaction, or allergy, appears to be a defence mechanism designed to limit the spread of infection.

The mechanism of immunity to tuberculosis is uncertain and reference should be made to more specialised textbooks for discussions of the subject. In individuals who are not actually suffering from the disease the presence of tuberculin sensitivity usually indicates immunity. It is the tuberculin negative group, therefore, that can usefully be given BCG vaccine after which, if the immunisation has been successful, the tuberculin reaction should be positive.

OLD TUBERCULIN

Tuberculin was first made by Koch, and as the official preparation is still based on his preparation it is known as *Old* tuberculin. It is the heat-concentrated fluid from a culture of either the human or bovine strain of *Mycobacterium tuberculosis* grown in a fluid medium.

Early products contained large amounts of non-specific, reaction-causing impurities, partly from the meat broth used for growing the organisms and partly from the metabolism and autolysis of the latter. Unwanted broth constituents are now excluded by the use of a synthetic medium containing 5 per cent glycerin, dextrose and, as the only sources of nitrogen, asparagine (an amino acid) and ammonium salts.

After inoculation with the organisms the medium is incubated at 37°C for six weeks or more. *Mycobacterium tuberculosis* has a very long generation time of about a day and, therefore, prolonged incubation is necessary to obtain abundant growth.

The culture is then steamed for an hour. This kills the organisms and destroys the antigenicity of many of the protein impurities but does not harm the tuberculin which is very heat stable.

The preparation is then concentrated to about one-tenth of its original volume, a preservative bactericide is added, and the solution is sterilised by filtration.

TUBERCULIN PURIFIED PROTEIN DERIVATIVE (TUBERCULIN PPD)

The active protein from Old Tuberculin was isolated by Seibert in the 1930s and is now known by the above names or simply as PPD. It is free from broth constituents and metabolic and autolytic products of the bacteria.

Two types are officially recognised, mammalian and avian. The former is prepared from the human or bovine strain of *Mycobacterium tuberculosis*, the latter from the avian type.

After growing the organisms in a synthetic medium, as in the preparation of Old Tuberculin, the culture is filtered through paper pulp, to remove the bacteria, and then subjected to ultra-filtration to remove the glycerin and mineral salts. To this a protein precipitant (e.g. ammonium sulphate or trichloracetic acid) is added. The precipitated protein is separated, purified, and made available as a freeze-dried powder, hypodermic solution tablets, or a concentrated solution.

TUBERCULIN TESTS

1. The Mantoux Test

This is the most precise method. Initially, a very low dose (1 unit) is injected intracutaneously in a volume of 0·1 ml. If the result is negative the dose is increased to 10 units and, if there is still no reaction, to 100 units. Graded dosage is necessary because of the great difference in tuberculin sensitivity between individuals. It is necessary to start with a low dose since very sensitive persons may show severe reactions to the higher concentrations.

To avoid repeated testing, the World Health Organisation has used, in some of its surveys, a single dose of 5 units, which explains why the *Pharmacopoeia* mentions four strengths.

2. The Heaf Test

This has become the most popular method in the UK because the method of inoculation is less painful, simpler, and more reliable than use of a syringe and needle.

A spring-release device makes several intracutaneous punctures of equal depth through a film of tuberculin previously applied to the skin. PPD is preferred for this test.

3. The Tine Test

An ethylene-oxide sterilised, disposable unit consisting of a short plastic handle connected to a stainless-steel disc carrying four tines (teeth) coated with old tuberculin (5 unit strength) is commercially available. The results compare favourably with those from the Mantoux test. The method is painless and quick, and syringes, solutions etc. are unnecessary.

The results of these tests are read after 72 hours. A positive reaction consists of a raised indurated area; erythema without induration is disregarded.

Various percutaneous tests have been tried. They involve application of tuberculin to the surface of the skin in an ointment, jelly, filter paper patch etc., but they are much less reliable than intracutaneous methods.

Table 33.4 compares the results of the Schick test and the tuberculins in immune and non-immune individuals.

Table 33.4

Individual	Schick test	Tuberculins
Immune	Negative	Positive
Non-immune	Positive	Negative

PRECAUTIONS WHEN HANDLING DIAGNOSTIC MATERIALS

False results will be obtained if Schick control becomes contaminated with the test toxin or a dilute solution of a tuberculin with a stronger one. This may happen if glassware or syringes are not kept exclusively for one preparation because traces of diagnostic materials adhere strongly to glass and only by unusually drastic treatments are they entirely removed. Disposable syringes are preferable and it is helpful to colour-code or otherwise mark glassware for tuberculin dilutions. Apparatus contaminated with Schick test toxin or the tuberculins should never be used for any other biological product; diagnostic preparations are potentially dangerous materials (e.g. PPD may cause toxic effects if inhaled) and great care is necessary when handling them.

ANTIBODY-CONTAINING PREPARATIONS
(SERA)

The plasma of an immune person or animal contains a large number of antibodies which, if the blood is withdrawn and allowed to clot, are found in the serum that separates. A serum may contain antitoxic, antibacterial or antiviral antibodies and, accordingly, is called an antitoxic, antibacterial or antiviral serum. Antitoxic sera, however, are more often known as antitoxins.

Most antisera are obtained from animals in which active immunity has been stimulated artificially, but there are a few diseases such as measles and german measles that cannot be reproduced in animals, and for these, human serum or products derived from it, are used.

Antitoxins (antitoxic sera)

The methods of preparation of the official antitoxins are essentially the same. Diphtheria antitoxin, with occasional references to other antitoxins, will be used to illustrate the general principles.

Diphtheria Antitoxin

CHOICE OF THE ANTIGEN FOR IMMUNISING THE ANIMAL

For diphtheria and staphylococcus antitoxins a toxoid is used but, in some cases, by starting with very small doses, it is safe to use the toxin (e.g. for certain gas-gangrene antitoxins). Occasionally, the course begins with a toxoid and, after an interval of a few months, is completed with a toxin. This method is applicable to the immunisation of horses against tetanus, and towards the end of the course their immunity is so strong that they are being injected with many hundred times the lethal dose for a susceptible animal.

The antigens are prepared by methods essentially similar to that described under diphtheria vaccine, except that the clostridia of botulism, gas gangrene and tetanus, used in the corresponding antitoxins, must be grown under anaerobic conditions.

Immunisation of Horses

Horses are preferred, primarily because they are large and, therefore, considerable volumes of blood can be taken without ill-effects. They are easy to handle, which simplifies administering the injections and withdrawing the blood. In addition, their red blood cells settle quickly and pack tightly, which facilitates separation of the serum. Occasionally, other animals (e.g. goats) are used to provide antitoxin for individuals sensitive to horse protein.

First the horses are isolated for seven days while:

(a) They are examined for infectious diseases such as glanders. This is caused by *Actinobacillus mallei* and can be transmitted to man in whom it can be fatal. It is detected by a diagnostic test, similar in principle to a tuberculin test, in which the reagent is called mallein.

(b) They are immunised against tetanus, to which horses are very susceptible.

(c) Their blood is examined for existing antibodies. Horses may have a basal immunity to certain diseases which shortens very significantly the time needed to obtain a satisfactory antibody level.

After isolation, gradually increasing amounts of toxoid are injected into the neck muscles every few days for several months. The first dose is usually not more than 5 ml but as much as 600 ml is reached by the time a satisfactory antitoxin titre has been attained and the course ended. Titre is a term used to express antibody concentration. It is the highest dilution of the serum capable of causing a particular antigen-antibody reaction (e.g. neutralisation of toxin) under specified conditions.

Eight litres of blood are withdrawn aseptically from the jugular vein into bottles containing anti-coagulant solution. The bleeding is repeated twice over the next eight days, after which the horse is given ten days rest. Then another short course of antigen is administered to stimulate further antibody production, and afterwards the three bleedings are repeated. Rest, courses of antigen, and bleedings are continued until the animal stops producing a satisfactory antitoxin titre; this is usually after four to five courses.

The blood is stored in a refrigerator until the cells have settled. Then the plasma is siphoned off and calcium chloride is added to induce clotting. When this is complete the clot is separated from the serum by filtration.

Refinement of the Serum

Horse serum contains high concentrations of several proteins. Although these belong to the same classes as the proteins of human serum the species difference is sufficiently marked for horse proteins to act as antigens when injected into the human body. In some individuals the response is the development of a hypersensitive state that can make injections of preparations containing horse serum a serious risk. There are two main manifestations of this hyper-sensitivity—

(a) *Severe Anaphylactic Shock.* This can occur almost immediately after injection of the serum. The patient becomes faint and pale, has difficulty in breathing, and may collapse and die if treatment is delayed. It occurs more often after the first injection, usually in individuals with a history of an allergy such as asthma or infantile eczema.

(b) *Serum Sickness.* This is a milder response and may take the form of headache, swelling of the face, aching joints, fever, or a rash. It can occur a day or two after injection in individuals who have received horse serum previously, or it may follow the first dose and, in this case, the reaction is usually delayed for a week or more. The latter effect is due to the tissues becoming sensitised before all the serum has been cleared from the body.

The principal proteins in horse serum are albumins, beta-globulins, and gamma-globulins. Antitoxins are largely associated with the beta-globulins, while antibacterial and antiviral antibodies (and to a small extent antitoxins) are connected with gamma globulins. By separation of non-antitoxic from active proteins sera can be produced that, because of their reduced protein content, are much safer to inject.

Two methods are used—

1. *Concentration by Fractional Precipitation*. This depends upon the fact that the components of a mixture of proteins can often be separated by adding suitable concentrations of ammonium sulphate (salt precipitation—p. 12). Sufficient ammonium sulphate is added to the serum to produce a one-third saturated solution. The gamma-globulin fraction precipitates and is separated and discarded. More ammonium sulphate is then added to give half saturation, whereupon the beta-globulin fraction, together with its associated antitoxin, is slowly precipitated.

The liquid portion containing the albumin is separated by a filter press and discarded. The precipitate is removed from the filter cloths to sheets of cellulose film which are made into bags and suspended in tanks of chlorinated running water. Dialysis takes place and the ammonium sulphate passes out through the cellophane and, as it is removed, the antitoxic globulin passes back into solution. The process takes from one to two days and, meantime, the chlorine in the water prevents microbial contaminants from multiplying and producing pyrogen.

Afterwards the solution is adjusted to isotonicity with blood plasma, and a preservative is added if the preparation is to be packed in multi-dose containers. Finally, it is passed through pyrogen-removing and sterilising filters.

The incidence of serum sickness with crude serum was about 50 per cent; the use of sera prepared by fractional precipitation reduced this by about a half.

2. *Concentration by Proteolytic Digestion*. The serum is diluted, pepsin is added and the pH is adjusted to the optimum for this enzyme's activity, i.e. approximately 4. After incubation at 37°C for about two days the following changes have occurred—

(*a*) The albumin is almost completely digested and the products will pass through a dialysing membrane.

(*b*) The gamma-globulin fraction is partly digested to dialysable compounds and partly precipitated by he pH.

(*c*) The beta-globulin is split into two fragments nly one of which has antitoxic activity. Both are colloidal solution and are too large to pass rough a dialysing membrane.

The liquid is filtered to remove the precipitated gamma-globulin and the filtrate is subjected to ultrafiltration during which the dialysable products of the digestion, inorganic salts, and the bulk of the water are removed.

The concentrate is heated at 55°C for one hour after addition of ammonium sulphate. The inactive fragment of the beta-globulin is denatured by this treatment and, in the presence of the inorganic salt, is precipitated. It is filtered off and more ammonium sulphate is added to the filtrate to precipitate the active fragment. This is separated, dialysed, adjusted to isotonicity, and preserved as in the fractional precipitation method. The incidence of serum sickness with this product is low (only 5 per cent).

OTHER OFFICIAL ANTITOXINS

1. Botulinum Antitoxin

Botulism is due to the exotoxin produced by *Clostridium botulinum*. Strictly it is not an infection because the organism does not invade the body. Usually it results from eating foods that have been carelessly canned or bottled, and in which the anaerobe has found oxygen-free conditions suitable for its growth and for toxin production. Commercially preserved foods are not a hazard because they are subjected to heat treatments that are more than adequate to kill the spores of *Clostridium botulinum* and well in excess of the few minutes boiling that will destroy its thermolabile toxin.

As stated earlier (p. 376) the toxin is extremely dangerous and the mortality from botulism is high. Antitoxin is of little use therapeutically but is useful for the protection of other individuals who have eaten the contaminated food, provided it is injected before symptoms appear. Antibacterial drugs are useless because of the absence of living organisms.

Three strains of *Cl. botulinum* are responsible for botulism in man—A, B, and E. The A toxin is the most toxic and the E type is often found in fish products. The pharmacopoeial monograph covers simple antitoxins made from each of the three strains and, also, polyvalent preparations containing any mixture of A, B, and E. Polyvalent antitoxins are preferred and are made by preparing the simple products in separate animals, and mixing in appropriate proportions.

2. Gas-gangrene Antitoxins

The commonest cause of gas gangrene is infection of a deep wound with dirt containing the spores of one or more species of a group of anaerobic exotoxin-producing bacilli the most important members of which are—

Clostridium welchii
Clostridium oedematiens
Clostridium septicum (also known as Vibrion Septique)

The infection spreads quickly because of the wealth of invasive abilities (hyaluronidase, collagenase, lecithinase etc.) possessed by the toxins or their associated enzymes. The characteristic that gives the disease its name is the large amount of foul-smelling gas that collects in the tissues and helps to disintegrate them.

The *Pharmacopoeia* includes simple antitoxins made from each of the three strains listed above, and a mixed product prepared by combining the three simple products.

The most potent toxin produced by each species is known as the alpha-toxin and this must be present in the antigen used for immunising the horse. Sometimes two antitoxins are made in the same animal. The mixed antitoxin is preferred because antitoxin treatment must start as early as possible and there is rarely time for bacteriological identification of the organism responsible for the infection. Best results follow intravenous injection but precautions are essential to prevent serum shock.

Occasionally, the triple product is used to provide prophylaxis after serious road and sports-field injuries but antibiotics are increasingly preferred for both this and therapeutic purposes.

3. Staphylococcus Antitoxin

Acute infections caused by *Staphylococcus aureus* (e.g. boils, carbuncles and osteomyelitis) are treated with antibiotics but because of the increasing emergence of drug-resistant strains it is useful to have the antitoxin available as an adjunct to chemotherapy. It is used when the patient is seriously ill from widespread dissemination of the alpha-toxin in the body.

4. Tetanus Antitoxin

The value of this antitoxin for the treatment of tetanus is greatly diminished if it is not administered before symptoms have fully developed, because once the toxin of *Clostridium tetani* has combined with the nerve cells it cannot be neutralised.

For many years it has been widely and successfully employed, in war and peace, as a prophylactic after deep, penetrating and dirty wounds, particularly if these have not been cleaned promptly. There is a fairly high incidence of serum reactions and, occasionally, when hypersensitivity is suspected, human anti-tetanus gamma globulin (p. 405), collected from fully immune volunteers, is used instead. Now that immunisation of infants and schoolchildren frequently includes tetanus it may be possible eventually to replace the prophylactic injection of antitoxin by a dose of tetanus vaccine, particularly if the immunity of the individual has been maintained by booster doses.

Antibacterial Sera

This type of serum is used to provide passive immunity to diseases caused by endotoxin-producing bacteria. Antisera against a number of such diseases, e.g. pneumonia, meningitis and typhoid, were used in the past but have been displaced by chemotherapy. There are no examples in the *British Pharmacopoeia*, but leptospira antiserum is included in the *British Pharmaceutical Codex*.

They are prepared in essentially the same way as antitoxins, the main differences being—

(*a*) The horse is injected with a dead or living suspension of the organism.
(*b*) The intravenous route is used because reactions often follow the injection of large numbers of bacterial cells by the intramuscular route.

(*c*) The methods of refining the sera are different because antibacterial antibodies are associated with the gamma-globulin fraction. The high degree of purification achieved with antitoxins is not obtained.

Leptospira Antiserum

Occasionally, this preparation is used with chemotherapy in the early treatment of spirochaetal jaundice (Weil's disease). It is not used prophylactically.

Weil's disease is caused by the spirochaete *Leptospira icterohaemorrhagiae*, of which rats are the main reservoir. The infection occurs mainly in individuals who work near to water contaminated with rat urine, e.g. sewer workers, coal miners, and fish cleaners.

Antiviral Sera

Antiviral antibodies are believed to act differently from the types of antibody already considered. Since viruses are intracellular parasites, and antibodies cannot penetrate cells, inactivation must take place in the body fluids or on surfaces at which invasion is occurring. The mode of attack appears to involve blockage of sites on the virus that are used in adsorption on to the host cells prior to penetration.

The main source of the antiviral antibodies used in passive immunisation is human serum (*see* Human Normal Immunoglobulin Injection). This is because the horse is not susceptible to several of the important diseases against which protection may be required, e.g. german measles, measles, and poliomyelitis. However, the official rabies antiserum is prepared in horses.

Rabies Antiserum

The horse is first given a course of dead rabies virus and when a good level of immunity has developed living virus is substituted. The methods of protein purification used to refine the serum are designed to separate the gamma-globulin fraction that contains the antiviral antibodies.

This antiserum, because of its high efficiency in preventing rabies if administered within 24 hours of exposure to infection, is given in conjunction with the vaccine to patients who have been bitten in areas of special danger, such as the head and neck, by animals known or suspected to be rabid. The antibodies in the serum interfere with the antigenic activity of rabies vaccine, and additional doses of the latter are necessary to compensate for this.

Human Normal Immunoglobulin Injection

This preparation, which used to be called human gamma globulin injection or simply gamma globulin, contains almost all of the gamma G globulins of human plasma together with smaller amounts of other plasma proteins.

Gamma globulin is now known to consist of at least three distinct components named immunoglobulins G, A, and M but more often referred to as IgG, IgA, and IgM. IgG antibodies seem to be the most important; they constitute 85 to 90 per cent of the total immunoglobulins and are the type produced by strong and prolonged antigenic stimuli. Hence the relevance of the official statement that almost all of these antibodies must be present.

It is obtained from human plasma by a fractionation process but since other blood products of pharmaceutical interest are separated by similar techniques the method is discussed in Chapter 34.

Its use is based on the fact that adults have been exposed to a variety of virus infections and, therefore, if the plasma from bottles of blood taken from a large number of different donors (the *Pharmacopoeia* requires not fewer than 1500) is pooled the product will contain useful levels of a number of important antiviral antibodies.

Because it is made from human (homologous) and not animal (heterologous) serum it is well tolerated.

Reactions are rare and not serious while excretion is slower (over four to six weeks) and is more even than with heterologous sera.

Since particles, caused by aggregation of denatured globulin, may form on storage it should not be given intravenously. The normal route is by intramuscular injection.

Supplies are limited (p. 414) and, therefore, doctors are encouraged to restrict its use to diseases and circumstances in which it has particular value. The following are examples—

Measles. To prevent or attenuate the disease in children under three. To control outbreaks in hospitals and other institutions. To protect individuals who because of ill-health or poor environment seem unlikely to stand up to the disease.

Rubella (german measles). To protect women exposed to infection in the first four months of pregnancy, because during this period there is a definite risk of serious damage to the foetus.

Infectious Hepatitis. To control outbreaks in institutions.

Small quantities of two special types of gamma globulin are available. One is human anti-tetanus immunoglobulin, the use of which was discussed on page 404. The other is human anti-vaccinia immunoglobulin, prepared from the blood of donors recently immunised against smallpox and used, for example, to treat patients suffering from complications of vaccination such as generalised vaccinia.

Preservatives in Immunological Products

The pharmacopoeial requirement that the bactericide included in a multiple dose container of an injection must not interfere with the efficiency of the medicament has particular relevance in the field of immunological products.

Obviously, preservative bactericides cannot be included in suspensions of living bacteria such as BCG vaccine. In addition, they are not used in most living viral vaccines because, although viruses in general have comparatively high resistance to antibacterial agents (*see* Smallpox Vaccine, where phenol and glycerin are used to kill extraneous bacteria) it is necessary to maintain the antigenicity of the attenuated strains at the highest possible level. In some cases (e.g. attenuated measles vaccine) inclusion of a bactericide could be disastrous.

It is preferable not to include in diagnostic preparations anything that might, by irritation of the intracutaneous tissue, cause a false skin reaction. When bactericides are added (e.g. in the concentrated tuberculin solutions) they are usually well-diluted by the time the preparation is used.

Bactericides can be added to the dead bacterial, rickettsial and viral vaccines, the toxoid-containing preparations and the sera. Phenol and cresol have been popular because the activity of phenols is not seriously affected by the presence of organic matter of which there is often a high concentration in immunological preparations. However, in recent years it has become apparent that phenolic compounds sometimes have an adverse effect on bacterial and viral antigens, including exotoxins, and

where this is the case, thiomersal (0·01 to 0·02 per cent) is often a satisfactory alternative. Unfortunately, thiomersal is not a very stable substance; solutions require protection from light and its decomposition, which is accelerated by traces of heavy metals, results in products that are harmful to certain virus strains (p. 397). The deleterious effect of phenols is very significant in preparations containing adsorbed toxoids, e.g. the APT, PTAP, and PTAH forms of diphtheria vaccine, possibly because of high local concentrations of the preservative on the adsorbent.

THE CONTROL OF IMMUNOLOGICAL PRODUCTS

In the United Kingdom the manufacture of immunological products is controlled by the Medicines Act 1968, under which Regulations are laid down that forbid manufacture except under licence issued by the Ministry of Health. Licences are granted only if the licensing authority is convinced that adequate premises and appropriately qualified staff are available. An indication of what is involved in satisfying these requirements was given under BCG vaccine and the demands are even more stringent for viral vaccines where living tissues are necessary for cultivation. In general, facilities and organisation need to be at least as good as those of a modern operating theatre and it should not be difficult to visualise the problems and expense involved in achieving this aim on a manufacturing scale. In addition, the facilities have to be backed up by an experienced team of bacteriologists, virologists, clinicians, histologists, veterinary surgeons, statisticians, engineers, and others.

One of the most important stipulations, aimed at preventing contamination with pathogens, is that each product must be manufactured in isolation from any other. In some cases (e.g. the preparation

of a live vaccine) a separate building is necessary but in others microbiologically isolated parts of the same building are acceptable. Use of one building or area for the production of two or more vaccines in series is permitted provided the rooms are efficiently cleaned and sterilised between each.

Much of the cost of manufacturing these products is caused by the elaborate system of testing, controlled by the Therapeutic Substances Regulations, which ensures safety and efficiency in use. The *Pharmacopoeia* outlines the tests applicable to each official product in the standards specified in the monograph. These standards fall into four main classes—

1. Identification tests—to establish the identity of the preparation.
2. Toxicity tests—to confirm that the active constituents (organisms, toxoids, or toxins) can be safely administered.
3. Sterility tests—to demonstrate freedom from extraneous micro-organisms.
4. Potency tests—to make sure that the product is a satisfactory immunising or diagnostic agent.

Identification Tests

Often the reason for selecting a particular test is obvious.

Antigen-containing preparations are usually identified by their ability to stimulate production of the corresponding antibodies in the blood of suitable animals. A satisfactory response is confirmed in a variety of ways—

(a) by using the appropriate diagnostic preparation where one is available, e.g. Schick test toxin, to indicate a satisfactory level of immunity to diphtheria;
(b) by challenging the immunity of the animals by

infecting them with virulent organisms of the corresponding disease, e.g. typhus and rabies vaccines;
(c) by determining the antibody titre in the serum of the animals, using an *in vitro* test.

Where the production of more than one type of antibody is expected, as in inactivated poliomyelitis vaccine, each is identified.

Occasionally a more unusual test is used, e.g.—

(a) Live measles and live poliomyelitis vaccines when mixed with the appropriate antisera will not infect tissue cultures.

(b) Influenza vaccine. The ability of influenza virus to agglutinate chicken red blood cells (haemagglutination) is used to identify the vaccine. In addition, when appropriate specific antisera are added the agglutination is inhibited.

(c) Yellow fever vaccine. Intracerebral injection into mice causes encephalitis and death, but injection into rhesus monkeys stimulates antibody production. This test illustrates the fine balance between toxicity and antigenicity in the 17D strain of yellow fever virus; although attenuated for man and higher animals it is still lethal for mice.

When the preparation produces a skin reaction this can be used for identification, e.g. smallpox vaccine and the diagnostic preparations.

Antibody-containing preparations are identified by their ability either to neutralise the toxin produced by the corresponding organism and render it harmless to animals (antitoxins), or to combat the organism itself (rabies antiserum).

Toxicity Tests

Toxicity in immunological preparations may be caused by—

(a) Incomplete conversion of toxin to toxoid.
(b) Incomplete sterilisation of a supposedly dead vaccine.
(c) Increased virulence in an attenuated organism.
(d) Excessive toxicity in the toxin used for a diagnostic preparation.

The principle underlying most of the tests is that administration of a human (i.e. a very large) dose, by the usual or by a variety of routes, to a sensitive and small laboratory animal must not cause, within a specified period, either serious symptoms or death.

When, because of the toxic nature of the preparation itself, injection by any other route would cause adverse symptoms in laboratory animals the preparation is tested intracutaneously. For example, for Schick test toxin, injection of $\frac{1}{25}$ of the test dose into guinea-pigs gives a positive Schick reaction, while $\frac{1}{50}$ of the test dose causes no local effect. White or pale coloured animals are used so that the result can be seen clearly. BCG vaccine is also tested in this way; the lesion must not be necrotic.

As up to 500 living extraneous micro-organisms per ml are permitted in smallpox vaccine from free-living animals a reliable toxicity test cannot be imposed for this preparation.

Sterility Tests

Detection of extraneous micro-organisms is a most complex aspect of the manufacture of immunological preparations. The problems are different for—

1. Preparations (other than inactivated viral and rickettsial vaccines) that should be sterile.
2. Attenuated bacterial vaccines.
3. Inactivated viral and rickettsial vaccines.
4. Attenuated viral vaccines.

1. Sterile Preparations

These include dead bacterial vaccines, diagnostic preparations, and sera. The official sterility tests are used to show, subject to the limitations inherent in the methods (Gunn and Carter, 1965), the absence of living bacteria and moulds. For the dead bacterial vaccines additional tests are performed to show that the specific organisms have been destroyed; these have greater reliability than conventional sterility tests because the media and conditions best suited to the organisms are known although, of course, they may not be ideal for damaged organisms (p. 342).

2. Attenuated Bacterial Vaccines

BCG vaccine illustrates two of the difficulties—

(a) *The detection of contaminating bacteria in the presence of living bacterial cells.* This can be done, using the official sterility test media, because the bacillus of Calmette and Guérin does not grow well in these.

(b) *The vital importance of detecting contamination with the virulent strain.* This test is performed in living animals. Guinea-pigs are given a very large dose of the vaccine intramuscularly and the preparation passes the test if there are no deaths within six weeks. The significance of the long time that elapses before the results are available is discussed on page 388.

3. Inactivated Viral and Rickettsial Vaccines

Tests are necessary to detect—

(a) Contaminating bacteria and moulds.
(b) Specific organisms that might have escaped the inactivation process.

(c) Extraneous organisms derived from the animals, eggs, or tissue cultures used in the preparation of the vaccines.

Bacteria and moulds are detected by the official sterility tests and specific organisms by injection into susceptible animals (rabies and poliomyelitis), by inoculation into tissue cultures (poliomyelitis and measles) or by the use of the appropriate part of the fertile egg (influenza and measles).

The introduction of virus contamination via the tissues used for growth is one of the greatest complications of virus vaccine production. Monkey kidney and chick embryo can carry a number of viruses, including types capable of causing tumours in laboratory animals but not, apparently, in man. The latter are known as oncogenic viruses, examples of which are the avian leucosis viruses, sometimes found in fertile eggs and in chick embryo tissue cultures, and SV (simian virus) 40, carried by certain monkeys. The '40' indicates that this was the fortieth contaminating virus strain isolated from monkey kidney.

The problem is attacked on two fronts. Firstly, and most usefully, at source; by procedures such as: (a) avoiding monkey species known to carry many viruses, (b) keeping animals in prolonged quarantine before taking their tissues, and (c) by breeding in isolation, e.g. to obtain leucosis-free hens. Secondly, by repeated tests for extraneous agents throughout manufacture. A typical series in vaccine production by tissue culture is—

(i) Tests on the medium in which the cells are first incubated, i.e. before virus is added.

(ii) Incubation of 25 per cent of the bottles as negative controls (see 'Sterility Testing' in Gunn and Carter, 1965) at the same time as the remainder are incubated with the virus. At harvesting, both inoculated and non-inoculated bottles are tested, the vaccine virus in the former being neutralised with a type-specific serum first.

(iii) Re-incubation of the negative controls for a further fourteen days followed by retesting.

(iv) Tests on the virus suspension after inactivation.

(v) Tests on the final vaccine. These are performed by the manufacturer and by a national control laboratory.

The extraneous viruses are detected by a variety of methods including addition to suitable tissue cultures (some viruses cause cytopathogenic effects, others, such as fowl leucosis, produce no visible signs but interfere with the establishment of a second virus, page 312) and injection into susceptible laboratory animals.

4. Attenuated Viral Vaccines

In most respects the methods of testing inactivated and attenuated viral vaccines are similar, but two new difficulties occur with the latter—

(a) Since the specific virus is alive it must be neutralised with type-specific antiserum before the tests for extraneous viruses are carried out. Sometimes it is possible to test in the presence of living specific virus by using a living cell system in which only the contaminant of interest will grow.

(b) Tests for absence of virulent forms of the specific virus have to be carried out in the presence of attenuated strains of the same virus. As would be expected, the properties of virulent and attenuated strains are similar, e.g. they will grow on the same types of tissue culture, and the design of distinguishing tests is very difficult. For poliomyelitis use is made of the greater plasticity of the virulent strains, e.g. unlike attenuated strains they will grow at 40°C or in a high concentration of bicarbonate or under conditions of oxygen lack such as are provided when a tissue culture is covered with a layer of agar.

In performing the conventional tests for absence of bacterial and fungal contaminants the viruses, although they are alive, do not interfere because they cannot grow in non-living culture media.

Smallpox vaccine prepared from viruses grown in fertile eggs or tissue cultures must be sterile, and although up to 500 micro-organisms per ml are allowed in vaccine lymph, making a sterility test impracticable, it must be tested for freedom from *Escherichia coli* (an organism found in faeces), aerobic pathogens (e.g. *Bacillus anthracis* and beta-haemolytic streptococci) and anaerobic pathogens (e.g. *Clostridium tetani*).

Potency Tests

1. Bacterial Toxoids

There are few products for which the need for potency tests exceeds that for immunological products. This is well-illustrated by the vaccines. In these the balance between toxicity or virulence and antigenicity is delicate and in attempting to remove the former there is a risk of destroying the latter. Consequently, tests for potency are as vital as sterility or toxicity tests.

Guinea-pigs are given a course of the preparation and after a suitable interval the level of active immunity is checked either by the appropriate diagnostic test (as for diphtheria vaccine FT and TAF, where the Schick test is used) or by determining the antitoxin content of the animals' blood by a biological assay (p. 410), as for staphylococcus toxoid, the forms of tetanus vaccine and the adsorbed types of diphtheria vaccine.

For the diphtheria vaccines an *in vitro* test is also used. It involves determining the number of flocculation equivalents in a dose of the preparation. When diphtheria toxoid and antitoxin are mixed in suitable proportions flocculation occurs (p. 378). If the toxoid is kept constant and the amount of antitoxin is varied, the mixture that flocculates first contains the nearest to equivalent amounts of toxoid and antitoxin. The amount of toxoid corresponding to 1 unit of antitoxin in the most rapidly flocculated mixture is known as 1 flocculation equivalent (Lf). A minimum number of flocculation equivalents per dose is specified for each form of the vaccine.

2. Dead Bacterial Vaccines

For these preparations, apart from pertussis, there are no good potency tests in animals. They are standardised by specifying the number of organisms of each species or type per ml of vaccine. This is based on the argument that their antigenicity depends on the amount of antigen present, which is approximately proportional to the number of bacterial cells. Cholera, plague, TAB, and TABC are standardised in this way.

For pertussis vaccine the dose necessary to protect mice against a lethal dose of *Bordetella pertussis*, administered intracerebrally, is compared with the dose of a standard preparation that gives the same protection.

3. BCG Vaccine (living, bacterial)

The vaccine is administered to guinea-pigs and after an appropriate interval the development of tuberculin hypersensitivity is checked by intracutaneous injection of old tuberculin. It will be recalled that this hypersensitivity is usually associated with a useful degree of immunity to tuberculosis.

4. Typhus Vaccine (dead, rickettsial)

Guinea-pigs are immunised with the vaccine and their serum, which contains typhus antibodies, is separated. The test then determines the minimum volume of this serum necessary to protect mice against lethal doses of a product prepared by growing typhus rickettsia in the yolk sacs of fertile eggs and harvesting in a manner that preserves the maximum amount of the soluble toxic antigen (p. 399).

5. Inactivated Viral Vaccines

(a) Poliomyelitis

A course of injections is given to suitable species of monkeys and, after an appropriate time, the concentration of each of the three antibodies in the serum is estimated by a bio-assay. In this the amount of serum required to protect tissue cultures from infection by poliomyelitis virus is compared with the amount of a standard antiserum that gives the same protection. Each of a series of dilutions of sample and standard is mixed with a highly infective dose of virus, which, after incubation to allow neutralisation to take place, is added to a separate tissue culture that is examined for cytopathic degeneration after about a week.

(b) Measles

The antibody titres produced in guinea-pigs by the vaccine under test and a reference vaccine known to give a satisfactory response in man are compared.

(c) Influenza

In this case, the haemagglutinating activity of the vaccine can be used as an indirect indication of potency.

6. Attenuated Viral Vaccines

For oral poliomyelitis and attenuated measles vaccines the virus titre (p. 312) is estimated. This is a satisfactory indication of the capacity of the preparation to cause infection, which is the way in which living vaccines stimulate immunity.

The titres of poliomyelitis and measles virus suspensions are determined in tissue cultures, but a different technique is preferred for smallpox vaccine. The number of infective units is estimated by inoculating known volumes of suitable dilutions on to the chorioallantoic membranes of fertile eggs and counting the lesions, each of which is assumed to have been caused by one virus unit.

The method for yellow fever virus is unusual and is possible because the 17D strain is not attenuated for mice and, therefore, will kill these when injected intracerebrally. The dose that causes 50 per cent of a group of mice to die of yellow fever encephalitis is determined. This is called the LD50 (p. 313) and there should be a specified number in the vaccine.

7. Diagnostic Preparations

The potency tests for these are based on the local reactions produced after intracutaneous injection.

(a) *Schick Test Toxin*

The test dose gives a positive Schick reaction in a non-immune guinea-pig when mixed with $\frac{1}{1250}$ of a unit or less of diphtheria antitoxin but no reaction when mixed with $\frac{1}{750}$ unit or more.

(b) *The Tuberculins*

The preparation is injected into the depilated skin of guinea-pigs previously sensitised to tuberculin by injection of *Mycobacterium tuberculosis*. The lesion diameters produced by the preparation under test are compared with those produced by a standard preparation of tuberculin.

8. Antitoxins

Many of the methods outlined above are full-scale biological assays requiring careful control of factors such as type and weight of animal and volume, route and temperature of injections in order to reduce sources of error to a minimum. They also involve the use of statistics in the design of tests and the interpretation of results. A better appreciation of the problems inherent in biological methods can be obtained from a more detailed study of one type of assay; the standardisation of antitoxins has been selected for this purpose.

PRINCIPLE OF THE METHOD

The potency of the antitoxin under test is determined by comparing the dose necessary to protect animals from the effects of a fixed dose of exotoxin with the dose of a standard antitoxin required to give the same protection.

THE STANDARD PREPARATION

The standard preparation must be stable so that the results of different manufacturers are comparable. For this reason it is not possible to assay antitoxins directly by finding the dose necessary to neutralise the effects of a fixed amount of standard toxin; toxins are too unstable.

Standard preparations originate from the World Health Organisation; under its auspices an International standard is produced. Using samples of this for comparison, the National Institute for Medical Research in this country prepares a national standard and every six months issues fresh samples of this to manufacturers. The latter then make their own laboratory standards which are used for the assays.

The standard preparation for antitoxin assays usually consists of freeze-dried natural horse serum

containing the appropriate antitoxic antibodies. The activity of the national standard is related to that of the international standard and every sample carries an indication of the weight corresponding to 1 international unit.

These procedures ensure that all antitoxins of a particular type and containing the same number of units per dose are of equal potency if they are produced in member countries of the WHO.

OUTLINE OF THE METHOD

Three preparations are used—

(a) The sample antitoxin, i.e. the antitoxin under test.
(b) The corresponding standard antitoxin.
(c) A suitable toxin to use as the test toxin.

The potency of the test toxin is found in relation to the standard antitoxin by a suitable method and then the potency of the sample antitoxin is found in relation to the test toxin by the *same* method.

SELECTION OF A SUITABLE TEST TOXIN

A toxigenic strain of the appropriate organism is grown on a suitable fluid medium and the sterile filtrate containing the exotoxin is collected.

A suitable toxin is chosen by determining certain doses. These are different for the various assays and depend on the nature of the toxic symptoms produced by the particular toxin. Some examples are given in Table 33.5.

All except the Lh dose refer to effects following administration of the dose by a designated route to specified laboratory animals. The Lh result is obtained from an *in vitro* test.

The *Pharmacopoeia* defines a suitable toxin by either specifying the size of the relevant dose or, more often, by indicating the relationship of one dose to another. An example of the latter is found in the assay for diphtheria antitoxin where the doses used are the Lr/100 and the minimum reacting dose; for the toxin to be suitable there must be at least 200 minimum reacting doses in the Lr/100 dose.

When, as with diphtheria toxin, the toxicity declines for a time after preparation, it must be stored until there is no further loss of activity. It is then kept in the dark at a low temperature and preserved with a bactericide that does not affect its toxicity.

The determination of the potency of diphtheria antitoxin will be used to illustrate the remaining stages of a typical assay.

Table 33.5

Name of dose	Largest or smallest amount ...	that causes ...	when used alone or mixed with 1, 0·1, or 0·01 unit of antitoxin
Lo/10	Largest	No local or general reactions	0·1
L+	Smallest	Death in a specified time	1
Lr/100	Smallest	A skin reaction	0·01
Lh	Smallest	50 per cent haemolysis of 10 per cent rabbit red blood cells	1
LD50	Smallest	Death of half of the animals in a specified time	Alone
Minimum reacting dose	Smallest	A skin reaction	Alone

DETERMINATION OF THE TEST DOSE OF TOXIN

Mixtures are made containing 0·01 unit of standard antitoxin and varying amounts of test toxin.

Each mixture is adjusted to the same volume and kept at room temperature for a specified time.

Then each is injected intracutaneously into the shaven or depilated flanks of guinea-pigs. The animals must be healthy, of a prescribed weight, and must not have been treated previously with anything that might interfere with the test. White or pale coloured animals are used so that the reaction can be detected easily. Several different doses at suitably spaced intervals may be given to each guinea-pig.

The Lr/100 dose of the toxin is the amount in the mixture that after two days causes a small characteristic reaction at the site of injection. Mixtures containing larger and smaller amounts cause necrosis and no reaction respectively.

DETERMINATION OF THE POTENCY OF THE SAMPLE ANTITOXIN

The skin reactions caused by mixtures containing the Lr/100 dose of toxin and varying amounts of sample antitoxin are compared with the reaction caused by a mixture containing the Lr/100 dose of toxin and 0·01 unit of standard antitoxin.

The mixture giving the same degree of skin reaction as that produced by injection into the *same* animal of the mixture containing the standard contains 0·01 unit.

Limit of Solids

The solids content of the antitoxins and rabies antiserum must not exceed 20 per cent. If removal of inactive protein has been inadequate the value will be higher. The amount of non-specific protein is further controlled by the limit on total protein and the requirement that not more than a trace of albumin is detectable by electrophoresis. Foreign proteins are excluded by precipitation tests.

STORAGE OF IMMUNOLOGICAL PRODUCTS

Preservation of the potency of immunological products involves maintaining the viability of living cells or preventing the denaturation of proteins (i.e. antigens or antibodies).

The causes of denaturation and loss of viability are largely chemical and, since the rate of a chemical reaction is influenced by temperature in accordance with the Arrhenius equation (Eqn 6.35), storage at low temperatures is essential.

For most products the optimum storage temperature is just above the freezing point and in the past 2 to 4°C was recommended. However, because it is easy to exceed 4°C in a domestic refrigerator the the upper limit is now 10°C. Storage between 2 and 10°C is directed for most vaccines, all antitoxins and the tuberculins.

There is an important difference between the storage of bacterial vaccines and antitoxins, on the one hand, and viral vaccines, on the other. While a number of viral vaccines (e.g. smallpox and oral poliomyelitis) are more stable at or below their freezing points, serious deterioration results if bacterial vaccines or antitoxins are allowed to freeze. This may be due to mechanical damage by ice crystals or the adverse effects of high local concentrations of inorganic salts and preservative bactericides.

Freeze-dried vaccines, although relatively stable compared with the corresponding liquid forms, also require careful storage. For example, freeze-dried smallpox and yellow fever vaccines must be kept at not more than 10°C and approximately 0°C respectively.

Of the official immunological preparations only one (Schick test toxin) may be stored at above 10°C, which underlines the importance of keeping these preparations refrigerated. Failure to do so invalidates the enormous care, illustrated in the preceding sections of this chapter, taken by manufacturers to ensure the reliability of this complex class of pharmaceutical preparations.

Light usually accelerates decomposition and immunological products must be protected from it. Light-resistant glass is not often used because it obscures the contents and makes difficult the detection of slight colour changes or faint precipitates. Storage in a carton is satisfactory provided the container is kept in it except when in use.

The selected examples in Table 33.6 illustrate the need for correct storage.

Table 33.6

Vaccine	Storage temperature (Protected from light)	Life
Poliomyelitis (oral)	Frozen 20°C	2 years Less than 7 days
Smallpox (liquid)	−10°C 2 to 10°C	1 year 14 days
Yellow fever	0°C Room temperature	1 year Few days

Good stock control is particularly important for biological preparations. Expiry dates, which are required on the packages by law, must be watched carefully and items of stock must be sold in chronological order. Sometimes the expiry date on a multidose container is much earlier than on an ampoule. This is related to problems connected with the use of rubber as a closure material for parenteral solutions and these are discussed in detail in Gunn and Carter (1965).

Dilution and the choice of diluent may also influence stability. The diagnostic preparations provide good illustrations of this; e.g. undiluted Old Tuberculin is stable for 8 years but when diluted its stability depends on the degree of dilution and the nature of the diluent.

ABBREVIATED TITLES

To discourage prescribers, frustrated by the long names of many immunological preparations, such as Diphtheria, Tetanus, Pertussis, and Poliomyelitis Vaccine, from using confusing abbreviations the *Pharmacopoeia* gives official abbreviated titles that must also be used on the labels of the container and package of the product.

Each abbreviation is in two or more parts—

The first part is usually a shortened version of the name of the disease or causal organism. Where only one disease or organism is relevant, three letters (usually the first three of the word) are used, thus:

Dip for diphtheria, but
Flu for influenza, and
Typhus is unabbreviated.

Where more than one disease or organism is relevant each is designated by a single letter if the meaning cannot be in doubt; when this is not possible the first three letters of the name are used. Examples—

TAB for Typhoid, paratyphoid A, paratyphoid B, but
TABCho for Typhoid, paratyphoid A, paratyphoid B and Cholera.

The second part, separated from the first by a diagonal line, is a three-letter abbreviation indicating the type of product. Examples—

For vaccines—Vac
For antisera—Ser
But for Staphylococcus toxoid—Sta/Tox

Where there are several forms of a product, as in the diphtheria vaccines, an approved abbreviation for the form follows another diagonal line, e.g.—

Dip/Vac/FT

Some further examples of full abbreviations are given below—

Tet/Ser — Tetanus antitoxin
Plague/Vac — Plague vaccine
Var/Vac — Smallpox vaccine
DTPerPol/Vac — Diphtheria, tetanus, pertussis, poliomyelitis vaccine
Tub/Vac/BCG(Perc) — Percutaneous Bacillus Calmette Guérin vaccine.

BIBLIOGRAPHY

BEVERIDGE, W. I. B. and BURNET, F. M. (1946) *The Cultivation of Viruses and Rickettsiae in the Chick Embryo. Medical Research Council Special Report Series No. 256.* Her Majesty's Stationery Office, London.

BOYD, W. C. (1946) *Fundamentals of Immunology,* 4th ed. Interscience, New York.

BURDON, K. L. and WILLIAMS, R. P. (1964) *Microbiology*, 5th ed. Collier-Macmillan, London.

BURNET, F. M. (1962) *The Natural History of Infectious Disease*, 3rd ed. University Press, Cambridge.

COHEN, A. (1969) *Textbook of Medical Virology*. Blackwell, Oxford.

DAWSON, M. and MILNE, G. R. (1967) *Immunological and Blood Products*. Heinemann, London.

GENERAL MEDICAL COUNCIL (1968) *British Pharmacopoeia*. Pharmaceutical Press, London.

GUNN, C. and CARTER, S. J. (1965) *Dispensing for Pharmaceutical Students*, 11th ed. Pitman Medical, London.

FISHER, P. J. (1967) *The Polio Story*. Heinemann, London.

HARRIS, M. (1964) *Pharmaceutical Microbiology*. Baillière, Tindall and Cox, London.

PARISH, H. J. (1965) *A History of Immunization*. Livingstone, Edinburgh.

PARISH, H. J. (1968) *Victory with Vaccines*. Livingstone, Edinburgh.

PARISH, H. J. and CANNON, D. A. (1961) *Antisera, Toxoids, Vaccines, and Tuberculins in Prophylaxis and Treatment*, 6th ed. Livingstone, Edinburgh.

PAUL, J. (1960) *Cell and Tissue Culture*, 2nd ed. Livingstone, Edinburgh.

PENSO, C. and BALDUCCI, D. (1963) *Tissue Cultures in Biological Research*. Elsevier, Amsterdam and London.

PHARMACEUTICAL SOCIETY (1968) *British Pharmaceutical Codex*. Pharmaceutical Press, London.

STANDFAST, A. F. B., EVANS, D. C., and WEITZ, G. F. (1962) *Proceedings of the 7th International Congress for Microbiological Standardization, London, 1961* Livingstone, Edinburgh.

STEWART, F. S. (1968) *Bacteriology and Immunology for Students of Medicine*, 9th ed. Baillière, Tindall and Cassell, London.

VAN HEYNINGEN, W. E. (1950) *Bacterial Toxins*, Blackwell, Oxford.

WILSON, G. S. and MILES, A. A. (1964) *Topley and Wilson's Principles of Bacteriology and Immunity*, 5th ed. Arnold, London.

WORLD HEALTH ORGANIZATION (1960) *Wld. Hlth. Org. tech. Rep. Ser. 1960, 200. Requirements for Biological Substances b. General Requirements for the Sterility of Biological Substances. Report of a Study Group.* Her Majesty's Stationery Office, London.

SELECTED PAPERS

ANDERSON, T. (1968) Virus infection—prevention and treatment. *Pharm. J.*, 200, 175-177.

HARTLEY, P. (1949) Materials used in Great Britain for the active immunization of man against diphtheria. *J. Pharm. Pharmac.*, 1, 425-433.

ISAACS, A. (1952) Influenza vaccines. *Chemist Drugg.*, 157, 879-883.

ISAACS, A. (1961) Interferon, a round unvarnished tale. *J. Pharm. Pharmac.*, 13, 57T-61T.

PARISH, H. J. (1966) Immunizing agents. *Pharm. J.*, 197, 41-45.

PERKINS, F. T. (1967) The control of viral vaccines. *Pharm. J.*, 198, 29-32.

34

Blood and Related Products

THE importance of blood in health and disease has been appreciated since ancient times but blood transfusion was not practised on a large scale until early this century. Previous attempts were often frustrated by clotting and ignorance of the existence of blood groups; therefore, for centuries blood-letting rather than transfusion remained a pillar of medical therapy.

The discoveries of blood groups by Landsteiner in 1900, and the non-toxic anticoagulant sodium citrate by Hustin in 1915 paved the way for rapid advances. The demands of the army for blood in the First World War provided a further stimulus. Steady progress was made in the aseptic handling and storage of blood, and at the beginning of the Second World War a blood transfusion service was set up under the Ministry of Health. This has continued, and now Regional Blood Transfusion Centres collect, examine, process and store blood and transport it to hospitals as required.

Human blood and the products obtained from it are not available commercially in the United Kingdom. In England and Wales immunoglobulin is obtained from the Public Health Laboratory Service, fibrin foam and thrombin from the Blood Products Laboratory at the Lister Institute, and other products from the Regional Blood Transfusion Centres. There are also special supply centres in Scotland and Northern Ireland.

The relationship of the official preparations is shown in Table 34.1.

Whole Human Blood

This is human blood that has been mixed with a suitable anticoagulant.

Any person in good health is accepted as a donor provided that he or she—

1. Is not suffering from any disease that can be transmitted by transfusion. This includes syphilis, malaria, and serum jaundice.

2. Is not anaemic. The haemoglobin content of the blood should not be less than 12·5 and 13·3 per cent for female and male donors respectively. This can be checked on the spot by allowing a drop of blood to fall into a copper sulphate solution of specific gravity 1·053 (female) or 1·055 (male). If the drop sinks the sample is satisfactory.

COLLECTION

The blood is collected aseptically from the median cubital vein, in front of the elbow, into a sterile container containing an anticoagulant solution. During collection the bottle is gently shaken to ensure that blood and anticoagulant are well mixed, thus preventing the formation of small fibrin clots. Not more than 420 ml is taken at one attendance. Immediately afterwards the container is sealed and cooled to 4–6°C.

The equipment used for taking blood is made from plastics, and is disposable. The container is most often the Medical Research Council blood bottle but plastic bags have been used in America for some years and are likely to be the containers of the future (*see* Gunn and Carter, 1965).

BLOOD CLOTTING

According to classical theory blood clotting takes place in two phases—

1. Prothrombin $\xrightarrow{\text{Thromboplastin + ionised calcium}}$ Thrombin

2. Fibrinogen $\xrightarrow{\text{Thrombin}}$ Fibrin

Although it is now known that several other factors enter into the clotting reaction the above scheme is adequate for an understanding of the aspects of blood products discussed in this chapter.

In response to injury, the tissues and blood platelets free substances that activate the clot-promoting enzyme thromboplastin. This, with the assistance of ionised calcium and other factors, converts prothrombin into the active clotting enzyme thrombin which acts on fibrinogen, converting it into insoluble fibrin, the matrix of the clot.

Table 34.1
Blood Products

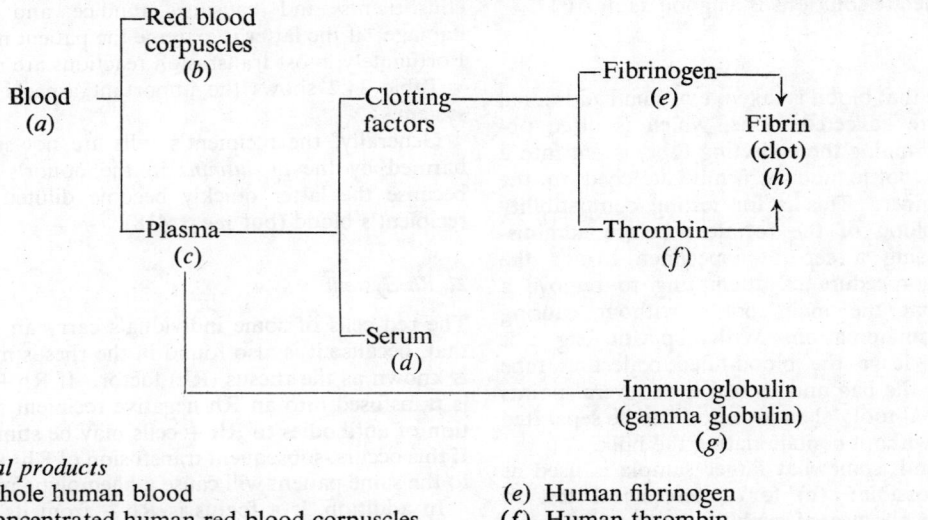

Official products

(*a*) Whole human blood
(*b*) Concentrated human red blood corpuscles
(*c*) Dried human plasma
    Human plasma protein fraction
    Dried human plasma protein fraction
(*d*) Dried human serum

(*e*) Human fibrinogen
(*f*) Human thrombin
(*g*) Human normal immunoglobulin injection

(*h*) Human fibrin foam.

ANTICOAGULANTS

1. *Citrates*

The solution most often used as a blood anti-coagulant is known as Acid–citrate–dextrose (ACD) and has the composition—

Sodium acid citrate	2·0 to 2·5 G
Dextrose	3·0 G
Water for Injections	to 120 ml

The citrate prevents clotting by binding the calcium ions as unionised calcium citrate.

At one time the normal (trisodium) citrate was used but it has a very alkaline pH in solution which causes considerable caramelisation (darkening) of the dextrose during sterilisation and the two solutions have to be autoclaved separately. The acid citrate produces a pH of about 5 and causes little or no caramelisation. In addition, it is less likely to induce flaking of the glass of the container. The higher concentration (2·5 G/120 ml) is often preferred because it more effectively reduces the formation of small clots.

The dextrose delays haemolysis of the erythrocytes *in vitro* and prolongs their life after transfusion. Its function may be connected with the synthesis of compounds, such as adenosine tri-phosphate (ATP) that are important in making energy available to living cells.

2. *Heparin*

This is a naturally occurring anticoagulant made by the mast cells of the connective tissue surrounding blood vessels. It inhibits clotting in the circulatory system. Occasionally it is used in blood for transfusion when large volumes must be given to one patient and the corresponding amounts of citrate would be harmful, e.g. in cardiac surgery.

It quickly loses activity in blood *in vitro* and normal quantities are effective for about a day. ADC, on the other hand, prolongs the storage life to three weeks. Heparin is expensive and may continue its action after transfusion, necessitating the administration of neutralising substances such as protamine sulphate.

3. *Disodium Edetate*

This is a chelating agent which, because it has a strong affinity for divalent metals, will bind calcium firmly. It is sometimes preferred when preservation of blood platelets is essential, although the stability of these seems to depend much more on preventing contact with glass surfaces; if plastic bags or silicone-treated bottles are used, ACD is almost as effective for this purpose. The survival of red cells in dextrose-edetate solutions is as good as in ACD.

TESTING

At the time that blood is taken, two small additional amounts are collected. One, which is often obtained by draining the collecting tube, is put into a small 5 ml bottle and is firmly attached to the main container. This is for testing compatibility with the blood of the recipient before administration; using a separate specimen avoids the dangerous procedure of attempting to remove a sample from the main bottle without causing bacterial contamination. With a plastic bag it is possible to leave the blood-filled collecting tube attached to the bag and to seal it at several points with a special tool; then a section can be separated for testing without contaminating the bulk.

The second, somewhat larger sample is used as soon as possible: (a) for a serological test to confirm the absence of syphilis, and (b) to determine the ABO grouping of the cells and plasma and the Rh grouping of the cells.

BLOOD GROUPS

Fundamentally, the aim of blood grouping is to prevent an antigen-antibody reaction. Red cells carry an antigen that reacts with the corresponding antibody in the plasma of individuals of certain other groups. If the cells are transfused into an individual with the equivalent antibody in his plasma they are rapidly destroyed, with serious consequences.

Although some nine blood group systems are known, only the ABO and Rh are of major importance as causes of haemolytic transfusion reactions.

1. ABO System

The first sign of the haemolytic antigen-antibody reaction is agglutination and, therefore, red-cell

antigens and plasma antibodies are called agglutinogens and agglutinins respectively. The agglutinated cells haemolyse, freeing haemoglobin and other constituents and causing jaundice and kidney damage; if the latter is extreme the patient may die. Fortunately, most transfusion reactions are mild.

Table 34.2 shows the important aspects of this system.

Generally, the recipient's cells are not seriously harmed by the *agglutinins* in the donor's *plasma* because the latter quickly become diluted in the recipient's blood (but see p. 418).

2. Rh System

The red cells of some individuals carry an antigen that, because it is also found in the rhesus monkey, is known as the rhesus (Rh) factor. If Rh+ blood is transfused into an Rh negative recipient production of antibodies to Rh+ cells may be stimulated. If this occurs, subsequent transfusion of Rh+ blood to the same patient will cause a haemolytic reaction.

In addition, if a foetus is Rh+ from its father, and the mother is Rh negative and has the Rh+ antibody in her blood, either from a previous transfusion of Rh+ blood or as a result of stimulation by antigens of the foetus, the mother's antibodies may cross the placenta and destroy the foetal erythrocytes. This haemolytic reaction may kill the foetus or cause the infant to be severely anaemic.

STORAGE

Apart from short periods for transport and examination, which must not exceed thirty minutes, blood must be kept at 4 to 6°C until required for use. Even at this temperature deleterious changes take place. The leucocytes disintegrate in a few hours and the platelets in a few days. The red cells show a fall in ATP and other organic phosphates, a reduction in oxygen-carrying capacity and, due partly to loss of lipid from their membranes,

Table 34.2

Group	Red cell antigen (agglutinogen)	Plasma antibody (agglutinin)	Can donate to:	Can receive from:
A	A	anti-B	A or AB	A or O
B	B	anti-A	B or AB	B or O
AB	A and B	None	AB only	All groups. Universal recipient.
O	O	anti-A and anti-B	All groups. Universal donor	O only

increased fragility. Storage at room temperature, even for only a day, seriously reduces post-transfusion survival of the erythrocytes.

The fitness of blood for transfusion is based on its appearance. On standing, the cells sediment, leaving a layer of yellow supernatant plasma. If the blood has been taken shortly after a heavy fatty meal the plasma may be turbid and show a white layer of fat on its surface. On top of the red cells there may be a complete or partial greyish layer of leucocytes. The most important feature, however, is the line of demarcation between cells and plasma, which must be sharp; if it is obscured by a diffuse red colouration, indicating haemolysis, the blood is unfit for use. Complete haemolysis, especially if it occurs rapidly, is usually a sign of bacterial infection but its absence is not confirmation of sterility since certain psychrophilic bacteria, predominantly pseudomonads and members of the coli-aerogenes group, can grow in blood at refrigerator temperatures without causing haemolysis. Many of the organisms isolated from contaminated blood have been capable of using citrate as their sole source of carbon and, as would be expected, this has led to clot formation.

USES

The volume of the blood in the body can be reduced to a dangerously low level by haemorrhage, shock, burns, and uncontrollable diarrhoea and vomiting. Haemorrhage and certain diseases may result in deficiency or absence of vital blood constituents such as red cells, platelets, or clotting factors. The transfusion of whole blood can be of great value in all these circumstances but often, because of the risk of transfusion reactions, it is not used where the need is solely to make up blood volume but is restricted to haemorrhage and certain diseases where there is deficiency of the vital oxygen-carrying erythrocytes.

Normally whole blood is not administered unless the ABO and Rh groups of donor and recipient are known and a sample of the donor's blood has been tested for compatibility with that of the recipient. In an emergency, group O, Rh negative blood may be given while the above precautions are being taken.

Concentrated Human Red Blood Corpuscles

This product is made by removing most of the citrated plasma from whole blood that is not more than a fortnight old and has been allowed to stand or has been centrifuged to deposit the cells. Not less than 40 per cent of the supernatant fluid is siphoned off through sterile tubes, taking strict aseptic precautions throughout, but, since there is a risk of bacterial contamination, the product must be used within 12 hours. The cells are matched with the recipient's plasma and may then be mixed with matched cells from other bottles. The haemoglobin content must not be less than 15·5 per cent.

USES

This product is used when administration of whole blood might overtax the circulation, i.e. in treatment of diseases, such as chronic anaemia, rather than haemorrhage. Another application is in exchange transfusions in infants; a toxic amount of citrate might be given if whole blood was used.

Dried Human Plasma

Whole blood has several serious disadvantages—

1. It has poor keeping properties necessitating use within three weeks.
2. It requires refrigerated storage.
3. It must be compatible with the blood of the recipient.

Dried plasma, on the other hand, has the following advantages—

1. Properly stored it keeps well for at least five years.
2. If protected from light it can be stored at room temperature provided this is below 20°C.
3. It can be given to patients of any blood group.

Consequently, in suitable circumstances, dried plasma is used as a substitute for whole blood.

PREPARATION

Two major problems have to be overcome—

(a) *Transmission of Viral Jaundice.* Viral jaundice is one of the most serious ill-effects of transfusion. There are two types: infective hepatitis and homologous serum jaundice, distinguished by their incubation times, approximately five and twenty weeks respectively, and their mortality rates, approximately 0·3 and 12 per cent respectively. However, most infections following transfusion are mild.

Control is partly effected by refusing to accept donors with a history of jaundice, but not all cases are recognised and since at present there is no reliable test by which carriers can be detected, an occasional infected bottle is inevitable. Attempts have been made to kill the causative viruses by treatment with ultra-violet light but the method is technically difficult.

If the preparation of a blood product involves pooling material from a large number of donors, infection in one or two bottles will be distributed throughout the pool and appear in each of the units made from it. Nowadays the pools used for making dried plasma and serum are limited to not more than ten donations, and the incidence of jaundice is only slightly greater than when whole blood is transfused. In the past, when pools of 300 or more bottles were made the incidence was 7 to 12 per cent.

(b) *Neutralisation of Plasma Agglutinins.* Earlier it was stated that the agglutinins in the donor's plasma usually do not damage the recipient's red cells. Occasionally, however, the plasma agglutinins are very powerful and can cause serious haemolysis of the cells of the recipient. This means that incompatibility problems are not entirely eliminated by using products such as plasma and serum, that contain no cells.

The problem has been overcome since the discovery that red cell agglutinogens also occur as water soluble forms in plasma, saliva and other body fluids. Consequently, by mixing plasma from different groups in suitable proportions the powerful agglutinins can be cross-neutralised by soluble agglutinogens, producing a preparation that is safe to transfuse to all groups. The most satisfactory ratio for mixing is 9 of A: 9 of O: 2 of B or AB.

Dried plasma is usually prepared from time-expired citrated blood. The supernatant fluid is separated, as described under concentrated red blood corpuscles. Batches of not more than ten bottles are pooled, choosing the correct ratio of blood groups to neutralise powerful agglutinins. The pools are kept at 4 to 6°C while samples are tested for sterility and no pool is used unless it passes. Then 400 ml quantities are dispensed into MRC bottles and subjected to freeze-drying. The general aspects of freeze-drying are discussed on pages 279–280. The following are special features of the plasma process—

Preliminary Freezing

The bottles are sealed with bacteriologically efficient fabric pads covered by ring-type closures and then centrifuged at −18°C. The liquid snap-freezes and becomes distributed around the inside of the bottle in the manner shown in Fig. 24.12.

Primary Drying

The bottles of frozen material are mounted horizontally in the drying chamber and a high vacuum is applied. The ice sublimes on to a condensing coil kept at −50°C and a small heater provides the latent heat required for evaporation. This stage takes about two days, after which the residual moisture content is about 2 per cent.

Secondary Drying

This is done in another chamber by vacuum desiccation over phosphorus pentoxide. It takes about a day, and the product is left with about 0·5 per cent of moisture.

Each fabric seal is then replaced by an MRC type closure (Gunn and Carter, 1965) perforated by a plugged hypodermic needle. The bottles are returned to the secondary drying chamber, re-evacuated, and then the vacuum is broken with dry sterile nitrogen. Finally, the needles are removed and the closure is protected with a sterile viscose cap.

STORAGE

Dried plasma, kept below 20°C and protected from light, moisture, and oxygen, remains usable almost indefinitely, although it is customary to impose an arbitrary expiry date of about five years.

Its fitness for use is shown by its solubility when reconstituted in a volume of Water for Injections, Sodium Chloride Injection or a solution containing 2·5 per cent dextrose and 0·45 per cent sodium chloride, equivalent to the original volume of plasma. It must dissolve completely within ten minutes at room temperature. Gel formation or incomplete solution indicates deterioration. After reconstitution it must be used immediately.

USES

Reconstituted plasma is a satisfactory alternative to whole blood in conditions where there is no loss of red cells. It is of particular value in the treatment of severe burns and scalds where, because of extensive fluid and protein loss, there is considerable haemo-concentration. It may also be given when blood is more appropriate; either because whole blood is unavailable or, in emergency, until the results of matching tests are known.

Because of its long storage life at a convenient temperature dried plasma is more suitable than blood as a reserve stock in a small hospital or a remote community.

Dried Human Serum

This is prepared in the same way as dried plasma except that the blood is collected into dry bottles and allowed to clot, the supernatant serum being separated after the clot has retracted.

Plasma is usually obtained from blood that is out-of-date, i.e. has been available as whole blood for 21 days. By converting blood into serum this period in reserve is lost and, therefore, much less blood is used for serum production.

Its storage and use are the same as for dried plasma.

Liquid Plasma and Serum

The only official liquid blood product is human plasma protein fraction and it is instructive to consider briefly why unmodified liquid plasma and serum are no longer recognised.

Plasma and serum, like blood, are excellent media for bacterial growth and, therefore, the user must be able to detect contamination. Unfortunately, these products are often opalescent due to suspended fat. Further, turbidity and deposits develop during storage and as a result of movement during transport, thus making infection very difficult to identify.

Attempts to remove the fat by filtration were not very successful because it blocked the filter, but centrifugation proved more satisfactory. With serum it was then possible, by passing the product through a sterilising pad, to obtain a clear preparation that would store reasonably well. It has passed out of use because blood is more economically used for dried plasma production.

With plasma there are additional difficulties because, unlike serum, it contains the clotting factors, which can be activated fairly easily. For example, if plasma is filtered through fibrous pads magnesium ions from the asbestos can, like calcium ions *in vivo*, activate prothrombin and cause clots in the filter and, later, in the filtrate. Methods were devised for removing some of the clotting factors and an unstable lipoid-globulin complex by adsorption on to kaolin or fractionation with an organic solvent at low temperatures. Complex aseptic manipulations were involved and, to confirm freedom from contamination, it was necessary, before issue, to store the products for several weeks at a temperature conducive to bacterial growth.

Further progress was made less urgent by the success of dried plasma but investigations continued and have contributed to the development of the product known as human plasma protein fraction.

The Fractionation of Plasma

During the early part of the Second World War the need for a transfusion material with a long life (unlike whole blood) and stability during storage (unlike liquid plasma) led E. J. Cohn and his colleagues in the United States of America to investigate the separation of albumin from plasma. About 60 per cent of the plasma protein is albumin and, therefore, it plays a major part in maintaining the high osmotic pressure necessary to retain fluid in the blood vessels. A very successful solvent precipitation technique was developed by which other proteins, as well as albumin, were separated. Some of these, i.e. fibrinogen, prothrombin, and gamma globulin, proved so valuable that protein fractionation of plasma quickly became an established procedure.

The process selected must not alter the biological properties of the fractions nor affect their solubilities. It must be possible to carry it out aseptically and, ideally, the conditions should discourage bacterial growth. Any additive must be harmless or easily removed after use.

One of the oldest methods of protein separation is salting-out (*see* 'Purification of Antitoxins') but this is unsuitable for plasma fractionation because high concentrations of salt are needed and these are not selective enough. Also, dialysis, a technique that is difficult to perform aseptically, is necessary to remove the salt after the precipitation.

Cohn's technique was based on the use of an organic solvent (ethyl alcohol) to reduce the solubilities of the proteins, and was given flexibility by alterations of pH, ionic strength (an expression of salt concentration), and protein. The use of an organic solvent, instead of salt, as the main precipitant confers a number of incidental advantages—

1. Because of its volatility it can be removed easily during the freeze-drying of the final product.
2. Salt can be used in low concentrations to improve resolution.
3. It helps to control contaminants because of its bacteriostatic activity.
4. Being a liquid, it is easy to add aseptically.

On the other hand, it is necessary to keep the temperature very low (0 to $-5°C$) to prevent solvent denaturation of the proteins.

In the UK ether is preferred to alcohol. It is claimed to cause less protein denaturation. A scheme indicating the preparation of products by ether fractionation is given in Table 34.3.

Human Plasma Protein Fraction

This is a solution of some of the proteins from liquid plasma. It contains albumin and certain globulins that retain their solubility on heating. It is prepared by fractionating pooled citrated plasma and is similar to the fraction shown as crude albumin in Table 34.3.

Table 34.3
Ether Fractionation of Plasma
(For full information *see* Kekwick and Mackay, 1954)

---

1. Plasma $\xrightarrow[\substack{0°C \\ pH\ 7·7}]{\text{Ether 11\%}}$ ↓ Fibrinogen

2. Supernatant 1 $\xrightarrow[\substack{0°C \\ pH\ 5·35}]{\text{Ether 10\%}}$ ↓ Prothrombin

3. Supernatant 2 $\xrightarrow[\substack{-3·5°C \\ pH\ 5·5 \\ \text{ionic concn } 0·035}]{\text{Ether 18·5\%}}$ ↓ Globulins $\xrightarrow[\text{fractionation}]{\text{further}}$ ↓ Gamma globulin

4. Supernatant 3 $\xrightarrow[\substack{-5°C \\ pH\ 5}]{\text{Ether 12\%; Ethanol 16·5\%}}$ ↓ Crude albumin $\xrightarrow[\text{fractionation}]{\text{further}}$ ↓ Albumin

---

A stabiliser, such as sodium caprylate or acetyl-tryptophan, is added. This allows the preparation to be heated for several hours at a low temperature without significant denaturation of the proteins.

Sodium chloride is added to make the preparation approximately isotonic. The solution is sterilised by filtration, aseptically distributed into MRC blood bottles and then heated at $60 \pm 0·5°C$ for ten hours to destroy the viruses of infective hepatitis and homologous serum jaundice.

Although the use of a bactericide or antibiotic would help to control contamination, neither is allowed. A bactericide would be undesirable on toxicity grounds in a preparation given intravenously in large volumes. With an antibiotic there would be a risk of sensitisation.

The fractionation process involves concentration of the albumin fraction. To ensure that, as a result, the amount of sodium citrate is not raised to a harmful level the concentration in the final preparation is limited to 0·4 per cent.

The protein content is not less than 4·3 per cent w/v and the product exerts a colloidal osmotic pressure approximately equivalent to that of pooled liquid plasma containing 5·2 per cent w/v of protein. It must be stored between 5 and 20°C and protected from light. Because the fibrinogen has been removed the preparation remains clear.

Dried human plasma protein fraction is prepared by freeze-drying human plasma protein fraction. Both are used for the same purposes as dried plasma.

Human Fibrinogen

Fibrinogen is the soluble constituent of plasma that, on the addition of thrombin, is converted to fibrin. After separation from plasma by fractionation, the precipitate is collected by centrifugation, dissolved in citrate-saline, and freeze-dried. The air in the containers is displaced by nitrogen.

The citrate prevents spontaneous clotting when the material is reconstituted. Fibrinogen dissolves slowly but since, like many protein solutions, it froths badly if shaken and the solid-stabilised foam is very slow to disperse, agitation should be limited to rocking. The solution should be used as soon as possible and not later than three hours after preparation.

USES

Occasionally, fibrinogen is administered alone to treat fibrinogen deficiency but more often it is used in conjunction with thrombin (see below).

Human Thrombin

This is the enzyme that converts fibrinogen to fibrin. The prothrombin obtained from the fractionation of plasma is washed with distilled water and dissolved in citrate saline. It is converted to thrombin by adjustment to pH 7 and adding thromboplastin and calcium ions. The solution is filtered and freeze-dried, and the air in the containers is replaced with nitrogen. It is reconstituted with saline when required.

USES

The fibrin clot produced when thrombin is mixed with fibrinogen is used in surgery to suture severed nerves and to assist adhesion of skin grafts. The mixture clots at a rate that depends on the amount of thrombin present and, therefore, if necessary, it can be kept fluid long enough for adjustments, e.g. of skin grafts, to be made. The clot also acts as a haemostat (see 'Fibrin Foam'). Since the fibrin is human it is well-tolerated by the body, and new cells penetrate it rapidly.

Human Fibrin Foam

This is a sponge-like mass of human fibrin. It is prepared by whipping a solution of fibrinogen into a froth by mechanical means and then adding thrombin. The product is poured into trays and freeze-dried, then cut into pieces of convenient size and sterilised by dry heat at 130°C for three hours.

The storage conditions for fibrin foam, fibrinogen and thrombin are the same as for dried serum except that fibrin foam need not be kept under nitrogen.

USES

It is used with thrombin as a haemostat in surgery, when other methods used to arrest bleeding have been unsuccessful. A piece is dipped into thrombin solution and applied to the bleeding area. The combination of thrombin and the large rough surface provided by the sponge causes the blood to clot. The foam can be left in situ, where it will be absorbed because it is entirely of human origin.

Human Normal Immunoglobulin Injection

Immuno- or gamma globulin is obtained from the globulins fraction separated in stage 3 of the fractionation of plasma (see Table 34.3).

Globulins (beta and gamma) $\xrightarrow[\substack{0°C \\ pH5 \\ \text{ionic strength } 0.01}]{\text{Ether } 9\%}$ Beta globulins

Supernatant $\xrightarrow[\substack{-3.5°C \\ pH 6.75 \\ \text{ionic strength } 0.025}]{\text{Ether } 18.5\%}$ Gamma globulins

The ionic strengths are critical.

The immunoglobulins are dissolved in a suitable solvent, usually 0·8 per cent sodium chloride solution, and a preservative, e.g. 0·01 per cent thiomersal, is added. The solution is sterilised by filtration, packed in single-dose containers and stored at 4 to 6°C with protection from light.

Normally, pools of not less than 1500 donations are used to ensure a satisfactory representation of the various types of adult antibodies, but when, as in the preparation of antivaccinia and antitetanus immunoglobulins, it is obtained from the blood of recently immunised donors the pools can be smaller.

Its uses are discussed in Chapter 33.

Control of Blood Products

Although all the blood products can save life, many are dangerous. If, for example, blood, plasma, or serum become heavily contaminated with micro-organisms, or the container or solvent is not pyrogen-free, or a bactericide is added to a preparation given in large volumes intravenously the risk to the patient is considerable. The official standards and labelling are designed to reduce the hazards to a minimum.

STANDARDS

Identification

As all blood products contain proteins, the standard methods used in protein identification are often applicable.

Precipitation tests with specific antisera are used to show that only human serum proteins are present in dried serum, dried plasma, the plasma protein fractions, fibrinogen, thrombin, and immunoglobulin.

The characteristic mobilities of blood proteins in an electrophoretic field are a sensitive means of identifying fibrinogen, immunoglobulin, and the plasma protein fraction. In the last-named, for example, there must not be less than 85 per cent of the protein having the mobility of albumin and not more than 1 per cent of gamma globulin.

Proteins can also be identified by their sedimentation rate in an ultra-centrifuge, which method is suitable for identifying and quantifying the different types of gamma globulin (p. 405).

Differences in clotting behaviour are simpler but useful characteristics. Plasma clots when calcium chloride is added, but serum does not. Fibrinogen is identified by the clotting that occurs when thrombin is added, and thrombin by the same result when it is mixed with plasma.

The determination of the blood groups, ABO of plasma and cells and Rh of cells, is an identification test for whole blood, while the descriptions of the latter and of concentrated red blood corpuscles are aids to identity and safeguards against the use of an unsafe product.

Sterility and Pyrogens

All blood products must comply with the official tests for sterility, and those preparations (i.e. immunoglobulins and the plasma protein fractions) that are exposed to special risk of contamination with pyrogens due to lengthy processing must also pass the pyrogen test.

Solubility

Complete solubility in an appropriate volume of the usual solvent, sometimes in a specified time, is required for all solid preparations except fibrin foam. This indicates that the protein constituents have not deteriorated.

Assays

For whole blood and concentrated red cells the assay is a determination of the haemoglobin value. For the remaining products, except fibrin foam (no assay) and thrombin, the protein content is determined chemically. In thrombin there must be a minimum number of clotting doses per mg, a clotting dose being the amount of thrombin required to clot 1 ml of 0·1 per cent fibrinogen in saline buffered at 7·2 to 7·3 in 15 seconds at 37°C.

Determinations of K and Na ions in plasma protein fraction ensure that the levels are not high enough to disturb the electrolyte balance of the recipient. An assay for sodium citrate in the same product prevents toxic effects from excess of this salt.

LABELLING

Probably there is no better group of examples than the blood products for illustrating the care necessary in labelling modern medicaments. Two examples (Table 34.4) will be sufficient to underline this point and to indicate the types of official specification.

Plasma Substitutes

The limited supplies of plasma, the cost of producing the dried form and the risk of transmitting serum hepatitis stimulated attempts to find substitutes of non-human origin that could be used to restore the blood volume temporarily while the recipient replaced the lost protein.

(Table 34.4)

Whole blood	Dried plasma protein fraction
Name of preparation	Name of preparation
ABO group.	Volume of Water for Injections necessary for reconstitution
Rh group and nature of antisera used for testing	Total amount of protein in reconstituted solution
Total volume; proportion of blood; nature and percentage of anticoagulant and any other material introduced	Concentrations of potassium, sodium and citrate ions
Date of donation	Names and concentrations of stabilising agents or other added substances
Expiry date	Expiry date
Storage conditions	Storage conditions
A statement that the contents must not be used if there is any sign of deterioration	A statement that the contents must not be used if, after adding water, a gel forms or solution is incomplete
An indication by which the history of the preparation can be traced	An indication by which the history of the preparation can be traced
	An instruction to discard the reconstituted solution if not used within three hours.

PROPERTIES OF AN IDEAL PLASMA SUBSTITUTE

1. The same colloidal osmotic pressure as whole blood.
2. A viscosity similar to that of plasma.
3. A molecular weight such that the molecules do not easily diffuse through the capillary walls.
4. A fairly low rate of excretion or destruction by the body.
5. Eventual and complete elimination from the body.
6. Freedom from toxicity, e.g. no impairment of renal function.
7. Freedom from antigenicity, pyrogenicity, and confusing effects on important tests such as blood grouping and the erythrocyte sedimentation rate.
8. Isotonicity, in solution, equal to that of blood plasma.
9. High stability in liquid form at normal and sterilising temperatures and during transport and storage.
10. Ease of preparation, ready availability and low cost.

GUM SALINE

This is a synonym for Injection of Sodium Chloride and Acacia, which was official in the 1932 *British Pharmacopoeia.*

In the First World War Bayliss experimented with soluble starch, dextrin, and gelatin as plasma substitutes and finally used 6 per cent acacia in 0·9 per cent sodium chloride solution. It was transfused extensively until signs of liver dysfunction disclosed that the gum was not metabolised but stored in various organs.

POLYVINYLPYRROLIDONE

In the Second World War the Germans introduced a synthetic colloid, polyvinylpyrrolidone, for the treatment of shock. It was marketed in this country in the 1950s but was later withdrawn because of suspected carcinogenicity.

DEXTRAN

To date this is the most satisfactory plasma substitute. It is a polysaccharide produced when the bacterium *Leuconostoc mesenteroides* is grown in a sucrose-containing medium. In the sugar industry it occurs as a slime that clogs pipes and filters and interferes with crystallisation.

The organism secretes an enzyme that converts sucrose to dextran according to the following equation—

$$n \text{ sucrose} \xrightarrow{\text{dextran-sucrase}} n(\text{glucose} - H_2O) + n \text{ fructose}$$

$$\underbrace{}_{\text{dextran}} \qquad \underbrace{}_{\substack{\text{used by} \\ \text{organism}}}$$

Different strains produce dextrans of two main groups—

1. Long, practically unbranched chains of glucose units joined by 1:6 glucosidic linkages.
2. Highly branched polymers consisting of short chains of 1:6 units joined by 1:4 and 1:3 linkages to branches.

Branched chains are more likely to give rise to allergic reactions when injected, and in dextrans used for plasma substitutes the linkages should be almost entirely of the 1:6 type. This is achieved by choosing a suitable specially developed strain of the organism that produces dextran in which about 95 per cent of the linkages are 1:6.

Production

The manufacture of dextran is similar in many respects to the production of an antibiotic (p. 366) and involves laboratory culture followed, in the factory, by growth in seed tanks and then in 4500 dm³ fermenters. Because synthesis of the enzyme and its action on the sucrose are rapid, the high degree of asepsis maintained in antibiotic fermentations is unnecessary. Also, as the process is inhibited by aeration, there is no need for a costly supply of sterile air. Another special feature is the need to prevent the hydrolysis of the sucrose to glucose and fructose during sterilisation of the culture media. If this occurs dextran will not be produced because in nature the conversion does not involve inversion but is a straight transglycosidation. Preventative measures include adjustment of the media to neutral pH before sterilisation, and the avoidance of overheating.

When maximum conversion to dextran has been obtained it is precipitated by adding a suitable organic solvent.

Natural dextran consists of chains of approximately 200 000 glucose units with molecular weights up to about 50 million. Very large molecules, i.e. those with molecular weights above about 250 000 have serious drawbacks—

1. They yield very viscous solutions that are difficult to administer.
2. They may cause renal damage and allergic reactions.
3. They interfere with blood matching and sedimentation tests by causing rouleaux formation.

Rouleaux are aggregates of red cells that resemble piles of plates.

4. They produce colloidal osmotic pressures that are lower than those of small molecules.

Therefore, to produce a material suitable for medical use it is necessary to reduce the size of the natural molecules. This may be done in several ways—

(a) *Acid Hydrolysis.* The dextran is adjusted to a pH of 2 and is heated at 90°C. As hydrolysis proceeds, the preparation becomes less viscous and the reaction is stopped at the required viscosity.

(b) *Thermal Degradation.* A solution of dextran is heated under pressure at 160°C in the presence of sodium sulphite, to prevent oxidative deterioration, and calcium carbonate, to neutralise acidity. The method is slower than acid hydrolysis but the yield of preferred molecules is better and fewer reducing groups are produced.

(c) *Ultrasonic Disintegration.* Bombardment with ultrasonic waves splits the molecules into fragments of approximately the same size and the product is clinically acceptable, unlike the material from the previously mentioned methods, which requires considerable fractionation. Unfortunately, this technique is much more expensive to use.

(d) *Seeding the Fermenter.* If a low molecular weight dextran is included in the culture medium before fermentation the organism will use it as a template on which to build more glucose molecules. The average molecular weight of the product is much lower than if no template dextran is provided.

Acid hydrolysis seems to be the method most often used. The hydrolysed product contains molecules ranging from 10 000 to 1 million in molecular weight.

The very small molecules, i.e. those of below a molecular weight of about 60 000, also have disadvantages—

1. They are rapidly excreted in the urine.
2. They pass into the tissue fluids causing an adverse osmotic pressure.

Therefore, the product should contain the minimum of molecules of molecular weight less than 60 000.

Molecules with molecular weights between approximately 60 000 and 100 000 are not excreted in the urine but they diffuse fairly rapidly into the tissues.

To summarise—

This suggests that the ideal fraction should have a majority of molecules within the range 100 000 to 250 000 with a bias towards the lower end.

However, the American type of dextran has an average molecular weight of about 75 000. The aims are to restore the colloidal osmotic pressure quickly and to ensure fairly rapid elimination of the foreign colloid from the body. The latter advantage. combined with a reduction in rouleaux formation is considered to outweigh the disadvantage of the high dosage necessary to compensate for excretion losses.

The British dextran of the 1963 *British Pharmacopoeia* (Dextran 150 Injection) had an average molecular weight of about 150 000 and produced a more prolonged effect due to the preponderance of larger molecules that are not lost from the blood vessels. This preparation caused rouleaux formation, a condition known as sludging because it slows the flow of blood in the capillaries and post-capillary veins. To overcome the problem, which is less evident with lower molecular weight fractions, the 1968 *British Pharmacopoeia* has replaced Dextran 150 with Dextran 110, which has an average molecular weight of 110 000.

To obtain the clinical ranges of molecular weight, the neutralised hydrolysate is subjected to a long process of fractional precipitation. A water-miscible organic solvent, in which the polysaccharide is insoluble (e.g. acetone or alcohol) is added under very carefully controlled conditions and the required fraction is gradually separated by repeated retreatment of either precipitate or supernatant fluid. Cost decides the narrowness of the fraction finally accepted. In all samples, because of entrainment of one fraction with another, there are small proportions of very large and very small molecules.

The selected fraction still requires considerable purification to remove—

(a) Reducing sugars—by further solvent precipitation. The main contaminant is fructose, the by-product of the fermentation.

(b) Fractionation solvents—by evaporation under reduced pressure.

(c) Inorganic salts—by demineralisation in a mixed bed ion exchanger. It is particularly important to remove phosphates because they cause precipitation during sterilisation and storage.

(d) Colour—by adsorption on to activated charcoal.

(e) Pyrogens—by adsorption on to asbestos, or cellulose derivatives.

◄──────── 60 000 ◄────────► 100 000 ◄────────► 250 000 ──────────►			
Rapidly excreted in urine	Lost into tissue fluids	Acceptable range	Cause allergy and renal damage
Lost into tissue fluids			Interfere with tests

— -

(f) Micro-organisms—by filtration. Between each treatment the preparation is passed through a fibrous pad and just before bottling a membrane filter is used.

The solution is diluted to a concentration of 5 per cent in either 5 per cent Dextrose Injection or Sodium Chloride Injection, packed in sulphur-treated soda-lime bottles (Gunn and Carter, 1965) and closed with lacquered rubber plugs. Finally, it is sterilised, usually by heating in an autoclave.

Control

The following tests from the official specification for Dextran 110 Injection illustrate the precautions taken to confirm that the product is suitable as a plasma substitute.

Chemical techniques limit the amounts of lead, acetone and alcohol, reducing sugars, nitrogen (from the culture medium), and, acid and alkali.

Biological methods show that the preparation is not pyrogenic, is sterile, and is free from proteins that could cause anaphylaxis.

The dextran content is determined by polarimetry and there are limit tests for small and large molecules. The former involves injection into rabbits; the urine collected throughout the succeeding 48 hours must not contain more than 30 per cent of the injected dose. The latter necessitates precipitation of the top 10 per cent of the fraction with alcohol and determining its intrinsic viscosity; this must not be greater than 0·4 which is equivalent to an average molecular weight of about 240 000. The intrinsic viscosity of the fraction as a whole is also found and must indicate an average molecular weight of about 110 000.

Dextran 40 Injection

A number of conditions, including severe burns, crush injuries and acute peritonitis, are accompanied by a severe degree of sludging in the blood. This can be reduced by the administration of Dextran 40 injection which, because it contains polymers of low molecular weight, lowers plasma viscosity and improves capillary flow. Both changes reduce cell aggregation and this, in turn, further improves the flow.

A crude dextran of low molecular weight is manufactured by including very small template molecules in the fermentation medium. Then fractionation is used to produce the clinical material which has an average molecular weight of 40 000.

Absorbable Haemostats

These materials are used to control bleeding when it cannot be checked by more conventional means. They are gradually absorbed by the tissues and, therefore, if used during surgery can be left in the body when the incision is closed, and if applied to a surface wound need not be removed when the dressing is changed.

There are four important types: human fibrin foam (p. 421), gelatin sponge, oxidised cellulose, and calcium alginate. Fibrin foam is the most acceptable because it is of human origin and is particularly well tolerated by the tissues, but supplies are limited.

ABSORBABLE GELATIN SPONGE

This is prepared by adding a small percentage of formaldehyde to a warm solution of good quality gelatin which is then whisked into a foam and freeze-dried. The porous product is cut into pieces of suitable size and sterilised by dry heat at 140°C. It is marketed as white or near-white, rectangular, very porous pieces that are extremely light and have a papery feel.

It absorbs many times its own weight of blood and the official standard for absorbency requires absorption of not less than thirty times its weight of water. When pressed tightly on to a bleeding area blood is taken up and clotting is encouraged by the large rough surface which causes platelet disintegration. The sponge also acts as a plug by sticking to the underlying tissues and mechanically supporting the clot over the oozing vessels. Sometimes it is previously soaked in a saline, antibiotic or thrombin solution, when it must be pressed to remove air and excess liquid before application.

Since some organisms liquefy gelatin it should not be used in septic wounds; nor is it suitable for arresting haemorrhage from large vessels.

Absorption occurs in four to six weeks. The sponge is non-antigenic and tissue reactions have been mild.

The standards include a test for digestibility in acid pepsin solution.

Unless aseptic handling has been perfect it is advisable to discard any unused part of the contents of a container. Resterilisation should not be attempted.

OXIDISED CELLULOSE

Cellulose can be converted into polyanhydro-glucuronic acid, an absorbable haemostatic material, by oxidation with nitrogen dioxide. Early products were made from cotton in the form of wool, lint and, particularly, gauze. More recently a knitted material, in which cotton is replaced by regenerated cellulose (viscose rayon) has been introduced. Fibres of the latter are of uniform diameter and the size distribution of the polymers is less wide and more constant than in cotton. As a result the oxidation can be carried out in a more reproducible manner and the product is claimed to show less variation in absorption time, haemostatic efficiency, and tissue reactivity.

Oxidation is carried out on the fabricated dressing and involves conversion of about 20 per cent of the primary alcohol groups to carboxyls. Gaseous sterilisation, often by formaldehyde, is used because heat causes serious deterioration.

The material has the appearance of the original dressing except that it may be less white in colour. It has a faint odour and acid taste.

In contact with blood it turns dark brown and swells to a gelatinous coagulum. Its haemostatic activity may be partly due to chemical reaction between the polyuronic acid and haemoglobin or other blood proteins but the fabric also acts as a scaffolding for clot formation and a plug at cut ends of the vessels. It is more effective if used dry.

Small pieces are absorbed in two to seven days but very large amounts may take several weeks.

It inactivates thrombin, unless previously neutralised with sodium bicarbonate injection, and is incompatible with penicillin. It should not be used in bone surgery because callus formation is inhibited. Unused pieces from an opened container should be discarded.

CALCIUM ALGINATE

This is derived from alginic acid, a colloidal substance obtained from the seaweeds *Laminaria digitata* and *Laminaria cloustoni* which grow off the Scottish and Irish coasts.

Alginic acid is a polyuronide built up from d-mannuronic acid units. Its carboxyl groups react with metallic ions to form alginates and, since the parent acid is unstable, the water-soluble sodium salt is used as the source of other alginates.

If an ionised calcium salt is added to sodium alginate solution instantaneous precipitation of calcium alginate occurs, a sensitive reaction that can be used for preparing foams, fabrics and other physical forms. These can be sterilised by autoclaving or dry heat.

$$2 \text{ Na alginate} + Ca^{++} \rightleftarrows \text{Ca alginate} + 2 \text{ Na}^+$$

Calcium alginate dressings have a marked haemostatic effect that is probably due mainly to mechanical pressure. As long as twelve weeks may be necessary for complete absorption and, although it is possible to make products that are absorbed in about ten days, by including a small proportion of sodium alginate, the tendency is to restrict the use of alginates to the arrest of external bleeding, e.g. from surgical incisions, tooth sockets, and sites from which grafts have been taken.

A transparent protective film can be made *in situ* over a burn, wound or incision by applying a solution of sodium alginate and then spraying with calcium chloride solution. This film is impervious to water but permeable to water vapour.

Alginate dressings can be removed, if necessary, by washing with a solution of a sodium salt, e.g. 5 per cent sodium citrate, which reverses the reaction shown in the equation above. They are compatible with penicillin and can be resterilised if necessary.

BIBLIOGRAPHY

DAWSON, M. and MILNE, G. R. (1967) *Immunological and Blood Products.* Heinemann, London.

GUNN, C. and CARTER, S. J. (1965) *Cooper and Gunn's Dispensing for Pharmaceutical Students* 11th ed. Pitman Medical, London.

HURN, B. A. L. (1968) *Storage of Blood.* Academic Press, London and New York.

KEKWICK, R. A. and MACKAY, M. E. (1954) *The Separation of Protein Fractions from Human Plasma with Ether. Medical Research Council Special Report Series No. 286.* H.M.S.O., London.

MOLLISON, P. L. (1967) *Blood Transfusion in Clinical Medicine,* 4th ed. Blackwell, Oxford.

SELECTED PAPERS

BLAINE, G. (1949) Alginate dressings. *Chemist Drugg.,* **151,** 214–215.

BETTS, T. J. and WHITTET, T. D. (1962) A new absorbable haemostatic—its use and identification. *Pharm. J.,* **188,** 269–270.

FAIRBURN, J. W. and WHITTET, T. D. (1948) Absorbable haemostatics; their uses and identification. *Pharm. J.,* **160,** 149–150.

FISH, F. (1959) Newer surgical materials. *Pharm. J.,* **183,** 49–53.

FOSTER, F. H. (1968) Dextran—Manufacture and use. *Process Biochem.,* 3 (2), 15–19; 3 (3), 55–57, 62.

HUGO, W. B. (1954) Blood products of the British Pharmacopoeia. *Alchemist, Leeds.* **18,** 336–342; 389–391; 432–434.

HURWITT, E. S., HENDERSON, J., LORD, G. H., GITLITZ, G. F., and LEBENDIGER, A. (1960) A new surgical absorbable haemostatic agent. *Amer. J. Surg.,* **100,** 439–446.

JORPES, J. E. (1956) The blood clotting mechanism. *J. Pharm. Pharmac.,* **8,** 73–83.

MACINTOSH, F. C. (1949) Anticoagulants. *J. Pharm. Pharmac.,* **1,** 353–367.

NANCE, M. (1950) Blood and blood products. *J. Pharm. Pharmac.,* **2,** 273–285.

REVOL, L. A. (1956) Products of human blood. *J. Pharm. Pharmac.,* **8,** 84–92.

PART FOUR

Ligatures and Sutures

35

Surgical Ligatures and Sutures

SURGICAL ligatures and sutures are threads or strings specially prepared and sterilised for use in surgery, the former for tying blood vessels and other tissues, the latter for sewing tissues together.

Numerous materials have been used for these purposes, including intestinal tissues and tendons of a large assortment of animals and birds, various kinds of thread spun from vegetable fibres, human hair, horse and camel hair, synthetic threads and metallic wire. Some are absorbed or digested in the tissues of the body after their ligaturing or suturing function has been performed and, provided the material is non-irritant and sterile, may be left in the body with confidence. These include animal intestine and other tissues. The others are insoluble in the body and their use will depend, among other things, on their non-irritant properties. They may disintegrate after a long period but commonly become encysted and cause no trouble. Surface stitches of non-absorbable material, used to bind the edges of a wound, are removed after healing has taken place.

Among the most essential properties of ligatures and sutures are the following—

1. They must be sterile.
2. Their strength must be adequate for the purpose for which they are used.
3. They must cause as little irritation as possible.
4. Their gauge should be as fine as possible.
5. If absorbable the approximate time of absorption should be known.

Catgut

This is the most widely used absorbable suture and ligature material. The following outline of its preparation for surgical use will give some idea of the extreme care necessary in the production of a suitable thread—

Catgut or violin gut is prepared from the intestine of the sheep. The name is said to be derived from the word 'kitgut' (a 'kit' being a small violin used in olden times), and has, of course, nothing to do with

the cat. Gut sutures have been used for hundreds of years and it is said that Rhazes of Baghdad used harp strings for surgical suturing over a thousand years ago. The unsatisfactory nature of these early materials will be realised when it is remembered that sheep gut is normally infected with sporing pathogenic bacteria, unknown until a much later date. Pasteur's discovery of the bacterial cause of many diseases was followed up by Lister, the surgeon who introduced the use of sterile materials into surgery, including catgut sterilised with phenol. Today, catgut is a carefully standardised material.

Raw Materials

When the sheep are slaughtered the intestines are roughly deprived of their contents and placed in cold storage or packed in brine for transport. About the first 7·5 m of the intestine is selected for surgical gut preparation.

Selection and Washing

The first process at the catgut works is to clean the intestines, or casings as they are called, by alternately drawing them through the hands and soaking them in water. This is done repeatedly until the casings are as clean as possible. At the same time the opportunity is taken to inspect the gut for abnormalities and poor samples, which are rejected.

Splitting the Casings

The end of the intestinal tube is fitted over the end of a flat curved peg and pulled against two sharp knives. The curved peg fits the natural curve of the intestine so that it 'feeds' to the knives in such a way that it is split into a 'rough' and a 'smooth' ribbon, corresponding to the mesenteric and antimesenteric parts of the intestine. The smooth ribbon is the one chosen for surgical gut.

Removal of Unwanted Layers

The gut consists of four layers—outer mesenteric, muscular, submucous and mucous layers. All but the submucous layer or submucosa are scraped away mechanically by blunt knives, the process being aided by soaking in alkaline solutions.

Orientation of Fibres

During the above scraping process the constituent fibres of the gut become arranged in a more parallel way. This greatly increases tensile strength.

Hardening

At this stage the ribbons may be tanned or hardened by soaking in solutions of chromic salts. This causes delay in the absorption of the gut in the body, the time of absorption depending on the strength of solutions used. At one time, surgical gut was labelled 'ten day', 'twenty day', or 'forty day', but since time of absorption will depend on various factors such as the tissue in which it is implanted, such precise terms are not favoured to-day. The terms, 'plain', 'chromic', and 'extra chromic' compare with the terms mentioned above.

Spinning

The ribbons are next tied at the ends in groups of two, three or more, depending on the gauge of thread to be prepared, pulled to an even tension and spun. The number of twists used in spinning the thread must be carefully controlled to ensure a uniform product of good tensile strength. Hardening or chromicising may be done at this stage rather than at the ribbon stage, but here it produces a case-hardening effect, the centre of the string being unaffected by the chromic solution.

Drying

This is done in an atmosphere conditioned with regard to temperature and humidity, the strings being kept under a suitable tension.

Finishing

The dried strings are 'polished' by mechanical means. This is really a smoothing process, in which the strings are rubbed against an abrasive surface to produce a smooth, uniform string of circular section. This is a highly important part of the manufacture of good quality surgical gut.

Gauging

The gauge of the strings is carefully checked at this stage and should show uniformity between strings of the same batch and, also, along the length of each string.

Sterilisation

The gut may be sterilised by heat, chemicals, or ionising radiations. The chemical process involves the use of iodine. The disadvantages of this process are the long period of immersion in the iodine solution and, more important, the variable increase in absorption time in the body. Heat processes, in spite of the problems involved, produce a more satisfactory product. In 1961 a start was made to develop the process of sterilisation by gamma irradiation, a method that has the great advantage of being carried out on the finally sealed containers.

Difficulties

Sheep intestine is normally infected with bacteria and is likely to contain pathogenic organisms such as the sporing anaerobic bacteria responsible for tetanus and gas gangrene. The sterilisation process must, therefore, be a thorough one and rigorously checked by sterility tests. In addition, catgut consists of collagen, which is converted into gelatin if heated in presence of moisture, thus ruining it as a suture material. Heat sterilisation must, therefore, be carried out in absence of moisture.

The Heat Process

Tubing. Suitable lengths of gut are coiled on heat-resisting fibre card and placed in glass tubes along with a label of heat-resisting material, printed with heat-resisting ink.

Drying. The tubes are placed in baskets and dried in a drying oven in which the temperature is raised slowly to avoid damaging the gut. When thoroughly dried it is ready for the sterilisation process which may be done in one of two ways.

1. The baskets of tubes are placed in an autoclave containing an anhydrous fluid such as toluene or xylol. A temperature of 160°C is maintained for several hours.

2. Alternatively, the heating may be done in a non-pressure vessel using an anhydrous liquid of high boiling point so that a temperature of 160°C may be readily maintained.

The tubes are then filled with a sterile tubing fluid and sealed by fusion of the glass. This part of the process must be done under stringent aseptic conditions.

The Irradiation Process

In this process the prepared gut is packed in aluminium foil envelopes containing 90 per cent isopropyl alcohol as a preservative. The envelopes are then passed through an irradiation area on a conveyor system. Thus the catgut is sterilised when sealed in its final container and, since the process is a rapid one, there is no lengthy hold up of material as in other processes. The irradiation to which the gut is subjected is considered to be 40 per cent greater than that necessary to destroy the most resistant organisms, each suture receiving a minimum dose of 2·5 megarads.

The exterior of the packets is sterilised before opening by immersion in a solution of 1 per cent formaldehyde in 90 per cent isopropyl alcohol.

'Boilable' and 'Non-boilable' Catgut

If the tubing fluid contains any water the tubes of catgut are labelled 'Non-boilable'. This is a warning to avoid the use of heat in sterilising the outside of the tube prior to opening it for use. If the tubing fluid is anhydrous the tubes may be boiled before opening. Non-boilable gut is more popular because the water in the tube keeps it pliable and immediately ready for use. In this case the outside is sterilised by washing in soapy water and steeping in a germicidal solution before opening.

The non-boilable tubes are filled with alcohol containing a small quantity of water. Gut from boilable tubes must be conditioned before use. This is done by soaking for a few minutes in sterile industrial methylated spirit or for a few seconds in sterile saline solution.

Official catgut is of the non-boilable variety.

Standards

All catgut for surgical use in the UK is subject to sterility tests under the Therapeutic Substances Act. The following tests are indicated or described in the *British Pharmaceutical Codex*.

1. *Sterility tests.* Such tests must take into account the fact that bactericides are likely to be present in the tubing fluid.
2. *Gauge.* This is measured by means of a dial reading micrometer at several points along the strand, and after the gut has been conditioned as described above.
3. *Tensile strength.* This is done by means of a machine in which the load necessary to rupture the gut is measured, the test being performed on 'straight' and 'knotted' samples.

Gauge limits and minimum tensile strength figures are given in tabular form for the various gauges. No standards are given for absorption time. The problem has been investigated by several workers, notably by Holder who used both *in vitro* and *in vivo* methods, the latter giving more satisfactory results.

The student is referred to this work, which is indicated at the end of this chapter.

Other Materials

The following are used to a lesser extent than catgut—

ABSORBABLE

Kangaroo tendons are obtained from the tails of kangaroos and are processed and sterilised in a manner similar to that for catgut. The strings are prepared in three gauge sizes and are used to a limited extent. It is absorbed slowly in the body and is chiefly used in hernia and in bone repair.

Brocafil. This is a suture material introduced by Dutch research workers. It is prepared from animal sinew by maceration, in a special acid solution to disintegrate the tissue, and homogenisation. This does not damage the constituent fibrils of the tissue, however, and the product is a viscous fluid containing these fibrils in suspension. This fluid is squirted continuously into a basic liquid where it solidifies as a ribbon. The ribbons are then polished and sterilised. Certain advantages are claimed for this suture, e.g.

1. Little original contamination.
2. Exact and uniform gauging.
3. Threads may be as long as required.
4. Good tensile strength.
5. Ease of sterilisation.
6. Good absorption qualities.

A reference to this material is given below.

NON-ABSORBABLE

Silk, linen, cotton, and synthetic threads have their advocates and special uses. All are readily obtainable and easily sterilised by autoclaving. Unless specially treated, spun yarns have wick-like capillary properties that may allow contamination to be conveyed through the threads. Synthetic monofilament threads are free from this defect. The technique necessary for their use requires longer operational time than that for catgut.

Synthetic. The BPC describes nylon and polyester sutures. These may be monofilaments or plaited threads.

Silkworm 'gut' is prepared from the sacs of viscous material in the silkworm, which the insect would have spun into silk if allowed to mature. The sacs are pulled out into a thread and after drying, grading, polishing, etc, are used as sutures or ligatures. It has several disadvantages, such as lack of uniformity in gauge, brittleness, and limited length. It is, however, strong and has a smooth surface.

Horsehair, from the tail hairs of the horse, is of fine gauge and is non-capillary and non-irritant. It is, however, uneven in gauge and has low tensile strength. Original contamination is almost certain, but it may be readily sterilised by means of the autoclave.

Metals and Alloys are considered to have special advantages, as for example in hernia. The BPC describes monofilament, plaited and twisted stainless steel sutures. They are non-irritant, have high tensile strength in fine gauge, and have been found useful in plastic and orthopaedic surgery. They are of course, readily sterilised.

BIBLIOGRAPHY

GROSS, M. Z. *The Ethicon Book of Sutures*. Ethicon Suture Laboratories, Edinburgh.

HOLDER, E. J. (1939) *Surgical Sutures and Ligatures*. Livingstone, Edinburgh.

HOLDER, E. J. (1946) *Desirable Factors in Surgical Sutures*. Blackwood, Edinburgh.

REFERENCES

DAWSON, J. O. (1962) Ligatures and sutures. *Chemist Drugg.*, **160**, 177–179.

LAWRIE, P. (1959) A survey of the absorbability of surgical catgut. *Br. J. Surg.*, **46**, 634–637.

LAWRIE, P., ANGUS, G. E., and REESE, A. J. M. (1959) The absorption of surgical catgut. *Br. J. Surg.*, **46**, 638–642.

OS, D. VAN. (1946) A new surgical suture. *Pharm. J.*, **103**, 164.

PART FIVE

Radioactive Isotopes

36

Radioactive Isotopes

In medical fields, radioisotopes are used—

1. As Sources of Radiation

(a) As alternatives to radium and X-ray machines for treatment of disease, particularly cancer.

(b) For radiation sterilisation (see Gunn and Carter, 1965).

2. For Tracer Techniques

These are of value in diagnosis and research. Radioactive and normal atoms of the same element behave chemically in exactly the same way. The fate of a substance in the body can be followed by administering a small amount in a radioactive form and tracing its course by observing the radiations emitted.

Radioactive isotopes are dispensed and used in larger hospitals, and pharmacists should be able to deal with the pharmaceutical aspects.

This chapter will be particularly concerned with the formulation and dispensing of radioactive substances but to assist the understanding of these subjects some of the fundamental aspects of radioactivity will be summarised first.

Aspects of Nuclear Physics

Atomic Structure

The atom consists of a small heavy nucleus, containing most of the mass, surrounded by planetary electrons that determine its chemical nature.

The nucleus contains two fundamental particles—

1. Protons (hydrogen nuclei)—which carry a single positive charge.
2. Neutrons—which are uncharged.

The *Atomic number* (Z) is the number of protons in the nucleus. It is always constant for and characteristic of a particular element, e.g. C–6, P–15, Na–11, and is conventionally indicated in the following way—

$$_6C \qquad _{15}P \qquad _{11}Na$$

The *Mass number* (A) is the total number of particles (protons and neutrons) in the nucleus. The atoms of a particular element can have different mass numbers because the number of neutrons can vary.

Nuclide

A nuclide is a particular nuclear species characterised by its atomic number and mass number, e.g. $^{12}_6C$ and $^{23}_{11}Na$ are nuclides. (Note the method of indicating the mass number.)

Isotopes

These are nuclides with the same atomic number but different mass numbers, i.e. different numbers of neutrons in the nucleus, e.g. ^1_1H, ^2_1H, and ^3_1H are isotopes of hydrogen.

Isotopes may be stable or unstable; if the latter, they undergo radioactive decay and are known as radioactive isotopes or radionuclides. Carbon has five isotopes—

Two are stable: $^{12}_6C$ and $^{13}_6C$

Three are radioactive: $^{10}_6C$, $^{11}_6C$, and $^{14}_6C$.

Since the atomic number is characteristic of all isotopes of one element and is indicated by the symbol, C, H, P, etc, it is convenient to omit the subscripts. Consequently, the radioactive isotopes of carbon are usually written as ^{10}C, ^{11}C, and ^{14}C.

Isomers

These are atomic species with the same mass and atomic numbers but differing in energy content. They are not common and when they occur, one is usually metastable (m is the symbol) and decays to the other—

$$^{87\,m}Sr \text{ and } ^{87}Sr \qquad ^{99\,m}Tc \text{ and } ^{99}Tc$$

Stable and Unstable Nuclei

The nuclei of elements of low atomic number are most stable if the number of neutrons is equal to or slightly greater (1 more) than the number of protons. If the neutron number is less or significantly greater (2 or more) than the number of protons, the nucleus is unstable, e.g. for carbon—

Protons	Neutrons	
6	4	unstable
6	5	unstable
6	6	stable
6	7	stable
6	8	unstable

For elements of higher atomic number the most stable neutron:proton ratio approximates to 1·5:1.

Unstable nuclei have excess energy, and by discharging this in the form of particles or radiation they achieve a stable structure.

The Electron Volt

The energy of radiations is measured in electron volts (eV) or millions of electron volts (MeV). An electron volt is the energy acquired by an electron in falling through a potential difference of 1 volt.

$$1 \text{ eV} = 10^{-19} \text{ joules.}$$

Types of Radiation

The radiation emitted from radioactive isotopes is in the form of charged particles of matter (alpha- or beta-particles). Sometimes, after the emission of a particle, the nucleus still has too much energy; this is dissipated in the form of gamma rays, a type of electromagnetic radiation.

1. ALPHA PARTICLES

These have the following characteristics—

(a) They are equivalent to the nuclei of helium atoms, i.e. ^4_2He.
(b) They are heavy and positively charged.
(c) Their range is—
    a few cm in air,
    a fraction of a mm in body tissues.
(d) They have discrete energies, typically 4 MeV; e.g.

$$^{226}\text{Ra} \dashrightarrow {}^{222}\text{Ra} + {}^4\text{He}$$

Alpha-emitters are not used in pharmaceutical preparations.

2. BETA PARTICLES

(a) Have the same mass as an electron (approximately 1/1800 of a mass unit; an alpha particle has a mass of 4 mass units; one atomic mass unit, amu, is 1/16 of the mass of the oxygen-16 atom).
(b) May be charged negatively (negatron or electron) or positively (positron); the former is most common.
(c) Their range is—
    a few metres in air,
    about a cm in body tissues.
(d) The particles from a particular nuclear change have a continuous spectrum of energies. Typically, the maximum energy (E^{max}) is 1·5 MeV and the mean energy ($\overline{E}$) is 0·6 MeV; e.g.

$$^{24}_{11}\text{Na} \dashrightarrow {}^{24}_{12}\text{Mg} + \beta^-$$

3. GAMMA RADIATION

This is similar to X-radiation but while gamma radiation is emitted from the nucleus, X-radiation is produced from the planetary electrons.

(a) When it reacts with matter it behaves as if composed of discrete packets (quanta) of energy. These are sometimes called photons.
(b) Since it is an electromagnetic radiation it has no mass or charge and travels with the speed of light.
(c) It is very penetrating; high-energy rays can pass through several feet of solid matter.
(d) Gamma quanta have discrete energies, typically 2 MeV.

Types of Disintegration

Alpha emission will not be discussed because of its lack of importance in the field in which we are interested.

BETA EMISSION

Emission of negatively charged beta particles is usually called, simply, beta emission. It occurs if the number of neutrons in the nucleus is too high for stability, e.g. ^{14}C. A more stable structure is achieved by the conversion of a neutron into a proton. The positive charge on the latter is balanced by the formation of an electron which is emitted as beta radiation.

$$n \rightarrow p + \beta^-$$

Any residual excess nuclear energy is discharged as gamma-radiation.

POSITRON EMISSION

This takes place if the nucleus is deficient in neutrons, e.g. ^{11}C. A proton changes to a neutron and a positron is emitted—

$$p \rightarrow n + \beta^+$$

Positrons have only a brief existence; each combines with an electron to yield two gamma rays in opposite directions (annihilation radiation). Each ray has an energy of 0·51 MeV.

ELECTRON CAPTURE

This occurs when a neutron-deficient nucleus has insufficient energy for positron emission. A planetary electron is captured by the nucleus producing the same result as in positron emission—

$$p + \beta^- \dashrightarrow n$$

Often the electron is taken from the inner (K) shell of orbital electrons; hence the alternative name of K-capture. The gap in the K shell (which contains relatively low-energy electrons) may be filled by an electron of higher energy from an outer orbit and this leads to the emission of X-rays. No particle is emitted and the X-ray is usually the only sign that a change has occurred, although occasionally the capture leaves the nucleus with excess energy which it dissipates as gamma radiation.

INTERNAL CONVERSION

This happens when the excess energy of an excited nucleus, instead of being emitted as gamma radiation, is given to one of the planetary electrons, resulting in the ejection of the electron from the atom. Conversion electrons are always accompanied by X-radiation and, unlike normal beta particles, all have the same energy.

Most of the radioactive isotopes that are used in medicine emit either beta radiation or beta and gamma radiation.

Decay Schemes

The changes that occur during disintegration can be shown diagrammatically (Fig. 36.1). These diagrams, which are known as decay schemes, are interpreted as follows—

Horizontal lines represent energy levels.

Vertical lines represent energy changes without change in atomic number, e.g. gamma emission.

Left and right sloping lines indicate energy changes associated with a change in atomic number. A left slope represents positron emission and a right slope beta particle (negatron) emission.

The schemes show that in certain radionuclides some of the atoms disintegrate in a different manner from the others. However, the proportion that changes by a particular route is always constant. These proportions are usually shown on the decay scheme.

Disintegration Rate

The rate at which the atoms of a particular radioisotope disintegrate depends on the degree of instability of their nuclei. The moment of disintegration of a particular atom is unpredictable but the rate of disintegration of the whole population of atoms in any radioisotope obeys the exponential law—

$$\frac{dN}{dt} = -\lambda N \qquad (36.1)$$

where dN/dt represents the rate of change in the number of radioactive nuclei with time, λ is the probability of disintegration in unit time, for a particular radionuclide, and is known as the decay constant, and N is the number of radioactive nuclei present at a particular time.

When Eqn (36.1) is integrated for a period of time between $t = 0$ and $t = t$ hours the result is:

$$\ln N_t - \ln N_0 = -\lambda t$$

or

$$\frac{N_t}{N_0} = e^{-\lambda t}$$

or

$$N_t = N_0 e^{-\lambda t} \qquad (36.2)$$

where N_0 = initial number of radioactive nuclei;

N_t = number of radioactive nuclei at time t.

If the logarithm of the activity is plotted against time a straight line is obtained.

HALF-LIFE

The time taken for half of the radioactive nuclei to disintegrate (i.e. for the activity to fall to half of its original value) is known as the half-life ($t_{\frac{1}{2}}$). After two half-lives half of the remainder will have changed (25 per cent remain); after three half-lives 12·5 per cent remain, etc.

After one half-life:

$$N_t = \tfrac{1}{2}N_0 \quad \text{and} \quad t = t_{\frac{1}{2}}$$

Substituting these values in Eqn (36.2)

$$\tfrac{1}{2}N_0 = N_0 e^{-\lambda t_{\frac{1}{2}}}$$

or

$$\tfrac{1}{2} = e^{-\lambda t_{\frac{1}{2}}}$$

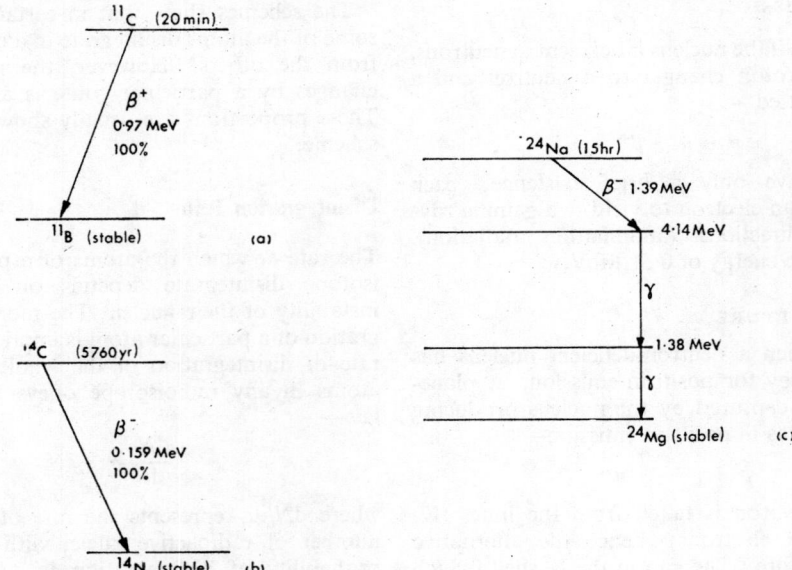

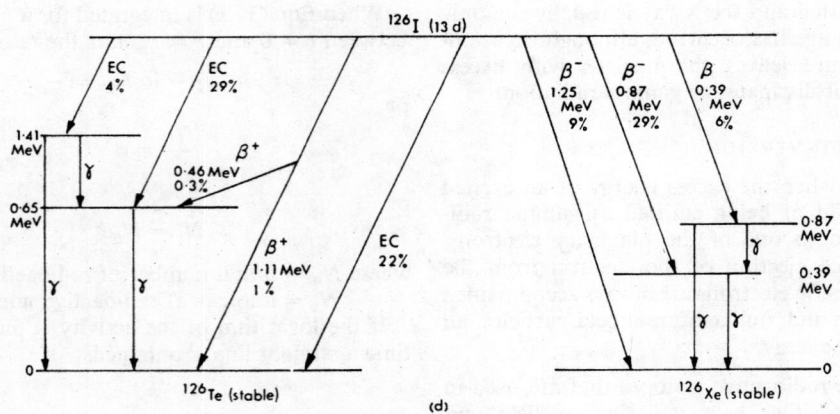

Fig. 36.1   Decay schemes

Hence

$$\ln \tfrac{1}{2} = -\lambda t_{\frac{1}{2}}$$

Multiplying by -1,

$$-\ln \tfrac{1}{2} = \lambda t_{\frac{1}{2}}$$

and

$$-(\ln 1 - \ln 2) = \lambda t_{\frac{1}{2}}$$

i.e.

$$\ln 2 - \ln 1 = \lambda t_{\frac{1}{2}}$$

and

$$\ln \frac{2}{1} = \lambda t_{\frac{1}{2}}$$

i.e. the decay constant, λ, is given by—

$$\lambda = \frac{\ln 2}{t_{\frac{1}{2}}}$$

$$\lambda = \frac{0 \cdot 693}{t_{\frac{1}{2}}} \qquad (36.3)$$

Knowledge of the half-life of a radionuclide is important in some of the calculations involved in the dispensing of radioactive isotopes.

Units of Radioactivity

The fundamental unit of radioactivity is the curie (Ci). It is defined as the amount of radioactive material in which the number of disintegrations per second is $3 \cdot 7 \times 10^{10}$. Consequently a millicurie (mCi) and a microcurie (μCi) are the amounts of radioactive material in which the numbers of disintegrations per second are $3 \cdot 7 \times 10^7$ and $3 \cdot 7 \times 10^4$ respectively.

SPECIFIC ACTIVITY

Essentially this is the ratio of active atoms to inactive atoms in a sample. In practice it is commonly expressed in such units as mCi per mg, mCi per mEq, and μCi per ml.

Effects of Radiations

1. Ionisation

All nuclear disintegrations result directly or indirectly in the production of fast-moving, charged particles. As these pass through matter they collide with atoms in their path and share their energies with the planetary electrons. Some of the latter may acquire sufficient energy to tear themselves away from the atom. Thus, a track of negative electrons and positively charged molecules is produced. Each positively charged molecule together with its separated electron is called an ion pair and the 'tearing-away' process is known as ionisation.

2. Excitation

Sometimes, when radiations react with matter, ionisation does not take place. Instead, the atoms simply acquire extra energy from the particles and assume an excited state, a process known as excitation. This excess energy may be discharged in several ways, one of which is the emission of light.

Alpha and beta particles cause ionisation and excitation directly. Gamma radiation, because it is without mass or charge, reacts much less strongly with matter. However, it does interact with some of the planetary electrons and these escape, often with high energy, causing the above effects.

Factors Influencing Magnitude of Ionisation

1. The velocity of the ionising radiation—this determines the length of the collision time.
2. The charge on the ionising particle—this determines the magnitude of the forces acting during the collision.

Consequently, the amount of ionisation produced is directly proportional to the charge and inversely proportional to the velocity of the particle.

Linear Energy Transfer

This is the energy lost per unit length of path of an ionising particle. A similar term is *specific ionisation* which is the number of ionisations per unit length of track. In air about $32 \cdot 5$ eV is required to produce one ion pair.

Alpha particles—double charge.
    —heavy and, therefore, of low velocity.
    —consequently, the linear energy transfer (LET) and specific ionisation are high.

Beta particles—single charge.
    —light and, therefore, of high
    —velocity. consequently, the LET and specific ionisation are low.

Gamma rays—no charge.
    —no mass; very high velocity.
    —consequently, the LET and specific ionisation are very low.

METHODS OF MEASUREMENT AND DETECTION

The following properties of radiation are used:

1. Ionisation of gases.
2. Production of scintillations in phosphors.
3. Blackening of photographic paper.

In the first two types of method the particle or photon is caused to produce a pulse of electricity. These pulses are amplified and counted electronically. Alternatively, the charges may be integrated and measured as an electric current.

Ionisation Methods

(a) IONISATION CHAMBER

The ionisation produced in a gas by radiation can be collected on electrically charged plates. If the voltage is low the ions move to the plates slowly and many recombine; consequently the current is not a measure of particle emission. However, as the voltage is increased the current (number of ions collected) gradually increases until a point is reached where the ions are swept so rapidly to the electrodes that practically none is lost and the current remains constant. Considerable further increase in voltage is possible without altering this, so-called, saturation current.

Because the current is very small, especially with beta and gamma radiations, which do not produce dense ionisation, very sensitive current-measuring devices are needed to detect it.

Ionisation chambers are operated under these conditions. They have high stability and are used for very accurate work.

(b) PROPORTIONAL COUNTER

If the voltage is increased to well above the range necessary to produce a saturation current the light negative ions are accelerated so much that they become capable of causing ionisation themselves. Hence, the ionisation is multiplied several hundred or thousand times (depending on the gas used in the counter) and the amplified pulses are more easily detected.

Proportional counters are used in this region of voltage. They get their name from the fact that the total number of ions collected is proportional to the number of primary ions formed. Since the latter depends on the energy of the radiation these counters can be used to determine particle energy. They are sometimes suitable for measuring low energy (soft) beta emitters.

(c) GEIGER-MÜLLER COUNTER

If the voltage gradient is increased even further, the amplification of the ionisation becomes so great that, even if the initial occurrence is only a single ionisation, an avalanche of secondary ionisation is produced. This results in a very large pulse that requires very little amplification to make it operate a counting device.

Scintillation Counters

This type of counter depends on the fact that radiation causes the emission of flashes of light (scintillations) from certain materials known as phosphors as a result of excitation of their atoms. The phosphor is coupled to a photomultiplier, i.e. a photoelectrode in the same envelope as an electron multiplier.

The scintillations stimulate the emission of electrons from the photocathode and these are accelerated to the first electrode (dynode) of the multiplier. From this dynode 3 to 4 electrons are emitted for each incident electron and are accelerated to the next dynode where the same multiplication takes place. Since a typical photomultiplier contains about eleven dynodes the overall gain by the time the electrons arrive at the final anode is considerable (about 10^6) and the resultant pulses require only low amplification for detection in a counting unit.

Geiger-Müller and scintillation counters are the main types used for routine work. The former count beta particles with very high efficiency, and gamma particles with very low efficiency. Scintillation counters have very high efficiency for particles, and high efficiency for gamma radiation. Low energy (soft or weak) beta emitters cannot be detected satisfactorily with a Geiger counter because their particles are unable to penetrate the wall of the instrument. A suitable method is to dissolve them in, or mix them with, a liquid phosphor and use scintillation counting.

For details of these counters a textbook on radioisotope techniques should be consulted.

Photographic Film

This is widely used to measure the amounts of radiation to which individuals working with radioactive isotopes have been subjected (p. 443).

HARMFUL EFFECTS OF RADIATION

Before this subject can be discussed some additional units must be defined—

RAD

This is the unit of absorbed dose. It is that quantity of radiation from any source that delivers 100×10^{-7} joules of energy per gramme of tissue or other specified medium.

ROENTGEN

This is the unit of exposure dose. Unlike the rad it can be measured directly. It is the quantity of X- or gamma radiation that produces in 1 cm³ of air ions carrying 1 esu of charge of either sign.

One roentgen (r) is equivalent to about 84×10^{-7} joules per gramme in air and about 93×10^{-7} joules per gramme in water or soft tissue.

REM

It might be expected that a particular absorbed dose would produce the same biological response regardless of the type of radiation from which it was delivered. This is not so. The pattern of energy release depends on the nature and energy of the incident radiation and, therefore, particles (e.g.

alpha) that produce tracks of intense ionisation produce a different biological response from that caused by, for example, beta particles, which give sparser ionisations along a much longer and less direct path (*see* Linear Energy Transfer).

To allow for these differences a modifying factor known as the Relative Biological Effectiveness (RBE) is introduced. For gamma and X-rays and beta particles this is 1, while for alpha particles, protons and fast neutrons it is 10. It follows that the biological effectiveness of an absorbed dose can be indicated by multiplying the latter by the RBE.

The unit of biological effectiveness is the rem (Roentgen Equivalent Man) which is equal to the dose in rads multiplied by the appropriate RBE factor, i.e.—

$$\text{dose in rems} = \text{dose in rads} \times \text{RBE}$$

For the radiations of interest in medicine (beta particles and gamma radiation) the rem and the rad are identical because their RBE is one.

Biological Effects

Ionisation and excitation of molecules in the body cause abnormal chemical reactions. For example, essential enzymes are inactivated, proteins are coagulated, nucleic acids in the genetic apparatus are damaged, and histamine-like substances are produced. These primary effects lead to the recognisable signs of radiation damage.

Damage to only a small fraction of the molecules in a living cell is sufficient to produce serious effects, as is illustrated by the following calculation.

A dose of 500 rads received over the whole body is approximately the LD 50 (p. 313) for man.

Since 1 rad = 100×10^{-7} joules, the energy produced by the above radiation = $500 \times 100 \times 10^{-7}$ joules per gramme.

If it is assumed that the energy required to produce 1 ion pair in tissue is the same as in air, i.e. 34 eV, the number of ion pairs produced (since 1 eV = $1 \cdot 6 \times 10^{-19}$ joules) =

$$\frac{500 \times 100 \times 10^{-7}}{34 \times 1 \cdot 6 \times 10^{-19}} = 0 \cdot 92 \times 10^{15}$$

But 1 gramme of tissue contains about 8×10^{22} atoms; therefore, fraction of atoms ionised

$$= \frac{0 \cdot 92 \times 10^{15}}{8 \times 10^{22}}$$

$$= 1 \cdot 15 \times 10^{-8}$$

i.e. the dose that causes ionisation of only one molecule in 10^8 may destroy a cell.

Some of the damage caused by radiations is due to an indirect effect. Action on water molecules leads to the production of free radicals—

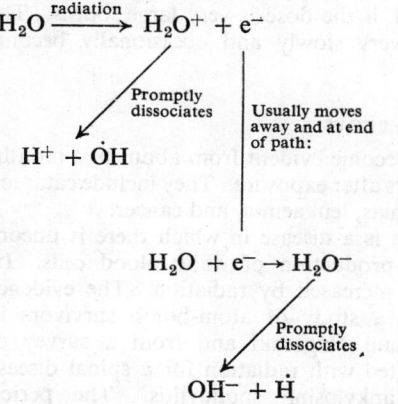

The free radicals $\dot{O}H$ and $\dot{H}$ may react—

$$\dot{O}H + \dot{O}H \rightarrow H_2O_2$$
$$\dot{H} + \dot{H} \rightarrow H_2$$

If atmospheric oxygen is present—

$$\dot{H} + O_2 \rightarrow H\dot{O}_2$$
$$2H\dot{O}_2 \rightarrow H_2O_2 + O_2$$

The powerful oxidising activity of the hydrogen peroxide and the $\dot{O}H$ and $H\dot{O}_2$ free radicals is thought to be responsible for some of the destructive effects of radiations. Support for this theory is provided by the fact that in the absence of oxygen or in the presence of certain reducing agents, e.g. cysteine, the extent of radiation damage is reduced.

The degree of damage is influenced by the radiation intensity and the exposure time. In general, if the dose is insufficient to damage the tissue irretrievably, healing modifies the effects. Hence, a number of small doses spread over several weeks does less damage than the same amount of radiation in one dose. However, this does not apply to the reproductive cells of the testes and ovaries, the effect on which is cumulative.

Actively dividing cells are the most radiation sensitive (e.g. the cells of the reproductive organs, blood forming tissues, skin, hair roots, and the lining of the alimentary canal). This suggests that harmful effects may be due to interference with nucleic acid synthesis; abnormal chromosomes can often be seen microscopically after radiation damage.

SKIN DAMAGE

This was observed in early workers with X-rays who received very large doses over a prolonged period.

A short exposure to intense radiation produces erythema. Longer exposure can cause brittleness and dryness (due to destruction of the sebaceous glands), loss of hair (due to damage to the hair follicles) and, if the dose is very large, burns. The latter heal very slowly and occasionally become malignant.

SOMATIC EFFECTS

These may become evident from about two months to many years after exposure. They include cataract, severe anaemias, leukaemia, and cancer.

Leukaemia is a disease in which there is uncontrolled over-production of white blood cells. Its incidence is increased by radiation. The evidence comes from a study of atom-bomb survivors in Hiroshima and Nagasaki and from a survey of patients treated with radiation for a spinal disease known as ankylosing spondylitis. The period between exposure and symptoms of leukaemia was about six years.

Cancer tends to occur in tissues severely damaged by radiation. The latent period is very long and often exceeds twenty years. The evidence for a relationship between radiation and cancer comes from several sources, e.g. the pitchblende miners of Schneeberg and Joachimsthal, who developed lung cancer through inhalation of radon gas; the occurrence of bone cancer in painters of the luminous dials of watches who used to 'point' the tips of their brushes in their mouths and thus ingested the radium-containing paint; and the early radiologists (see Skin damage).

GENETIC EFFECTS

Radiation has two effects on reproductive cells. It can damage the chromosomes and increase the frequency of gene mutation. The former is not very important because it is caused only by long exposure to low intensity X- and gamma-rays.

Because damage to genetic material is cumulative and irreparable, long exposure at low intensity affects the mutation rate as much as an equivalent dose of high intensity, i.e. there appears to be no safe threshold dose. The mutations will be inherited by future generations and most are believed to be harmful. Consequently, it is not the exposed person who is at special risk but, rather, future generations and, through these, the whole population. For this reason it is particularly important that radiation exposure should be minimised during the early years (i.e. the first 30) of life.

For additional information on biological effects of radiation see Lea (1947) and the MRC Report (1960).

Exposure to Radiation

RADIATION FROM NATURAL SOURCES

Man is continually exposed to external and internal radiations of natural origin (background radiation), e.g.—

(a) The earth's crust contains radioactive minerals and, therefore, man-made structures of brick and concrete emanate measurable amounts of radiation.
(b) Cosmic rays from outer space.
(c) The atmosphere contains minute amounts of radon and thoron, gaseous decay products of radium and thorium.
(d) Radioactive constituents of the human body, e.g. ^{40}K, ^{14}C, and ^{226}Ra.

The total dose to the gonads from these sources is shown in Table 36.1.

Table 36.1

Source	Dose (mrads/wk)
Earth's crust	1–3
Cosmic radiation	0·5
Atmosphere	0·05
Body constituents	0·5
	2–4

i.e. the yearly dose is 0·1–0·2 rads

RADIATION FROM OTHER SOURCES

Man also receives radiation from the appurtenances of civilisation. The approximate doses to the population of Great Britain as a whole are given below. They are expressed as percentages of the natural background.

Source	Dose to gonads (%)
Natural background	100
X-ray examinations	22
Fall-out from test explosions	1
Luminous watches and clocks	1
Occupational exposure	3

i.e. the total dose due to man-made sources of radiation is about 25 per cent of that received from the natural background. Clearly, certain types of X-ray examination should not be repeated too often; e.g. a gastro-intestinal series averages 13·7 r. On the other hand, it should be mentioned that a chest X-ray contributes only 0·03 r.

Maximum Permissible Doses

These are the doses of radiation that, in the light of present knowledge, are not expected to cause appreciable body harm to an individual at any time during his life. They are based on the recommendations of the International Committee on Radiation Protection (1959, 1966).

Their main object is to prevent harmful effects on the gonads and the blood-forming organs. The maximum permissible accumulated dose to these at any age over 18 years is $5(N - 18)$ rems, where N is the age in years. This works out to an average of 5 rems per year and ensures that the dose to the gonads is not more than 60 rems by the age of 30.

To prevent dangerously uneven accumulation of the maximum dose, not more than 3 rems may be received during any 13 consecutive weeks (or one calendar quarter).

Organs and parts of the body in which radiation damage is less critical may receive somewhat higher doses—

	Maximum permissible doses (rems)	
	Quarterly	Yearly
Hands, forearms, feet, and ankles	20	75
Skin, except as above	8	30

In addition, the maximum body burdens of various isotopes are laid down.

The above doses apply to occupationally exposed (designated) persons and are extra to the natural background and medical exposures. For the general population the maximum level is much lower, i.e. only 0·1 rems per year, excluding medical exposures. The concentration of isotopes in drinking water is also limited.

To ensure that exposures are kept well below the maximum permissible levels it is important to check, for each operation, e.g. dispensing procedure—

1. The dose rate from the isotope being used.
2. The dose received by the operator.

1. DOSE RATE

This is the rate of delivery of energy from a radionuclide. It is best measured under working conditions, using suitable radiation detectors, but for selecting a procedure and deciding the appropriate type of shielding it is convenient to use formulae—

(a) For Beta-emitters

Dose rate at 100 mm = 3100 × Ci rads per hour in tissue, where Ci = the source strength in curies.

For other distances the inverse square law can be applied. The results, although not accurate, are on the safe side because air absorption of the radiation will reduce the dose delivered.

It is also useful to know the dose rate at the surface of a solution. This is $s \times E$ rads per hour, where s is the specific activity of the isotope in microcuries per ml and E is the mean energy (see p. 436) per disintegration.

(b) For Gamma-emitters

Dose rate $D = \dfrac{0·5\ Ci\ E}{d^2}$

where D = dose rate in rads per hour; Ci = source strength in curies; E = total energy of the gamma radiation in MeV per transformation; d = distance from the source in metres.

This formula is applicable only if the distance is large compared with the size of the source (because the inverse square law refers to point sources). This is often the case, but in other circumstances reference books, such as the Radiochemical Manual (1966), should be consulted.

2. DOSE RECEIVED

The methods used to measure the doses of radiation received by workers with radionuclides are—

(a) Film Badges

These are clipped on to the breast pocket and contain a small strip of a suitable photographic paper, such as Ilford Industrial X-ray film, in a dental packing. The degree of blackening of the film depends on the amount of energy absorbed by the emulsion. They are used to measure the dose over a fairly long period, e.g. a week or a month. The film is then developed and the results compared with films exposed to standard doses of radiation and, to ensure uniformity of treatment, developed at the same time. Part of the film is covered with a thin sheet of metal such as tin or lead which absorbs the beta particles. Consequently, the uncovered part indicates the beta plus gamma dose and the covered part the gamma dose.

However, it can be extremely difficult to discover exactly when a serious exposure took place. Also, the film indicates no more than the dose received where the badge is pinned to the body; to obtain information about dosage to other parts (e.g. the hands) which usually will have received much greater doses, it is necessary to attach film packs to the appropriate area.

15

(b) Pocket Ionisation Chambers (dosimeters)

These instruments give immediate indication of the dose received during a particularly hazardous operation. Essentially they are quartz fibre electroscopes; before use they are charged, which makes the fibre move away from its support. Ionisation caused by the radiation causes the charge to leak away, and the fibre gradually moves back. Its image is viewed against a scale by lenses. A variation is to fit an audible alarm which sounds when the dose rate exceeds a preset value.

Dosimeters do not indicate the magnitude of gross over-exposure, which is a disadvantage.

Every designated person must have an annual medical examination, which usually includes an examination of the blood for signs of radiation damage.

Hazards from Handling Isotopes Used in Medicine

Radionuclides are a health hazard to the user in two ways—

1. External radiation of the body.
2. Internal radiation of the body; due to ingestion, inhalation, or absorption through the skin or abrasions.

Gamma emitters present external hazards because of the penetrating power of gamma rays.

Because it is easy to shield against beta radiation, beta-emitters provide no appreciable external hazard but, within the body, they are more dangerous than gamma-emitters because their linear energy transfer is higher.

The safest radioisotopes to use and handle are those in which—

(a) The particles or rays have relatively low energy.
(b) The physical half-life is short, e.g. ^{132}I (2·3 h); ^{99}Tc (Technetium) (6 h).
(c) The biological half-life is short.

The biological half-life is a term used to describe the rate of elimination of a radionuclide from the body. It is the time taken for 50 per cent of the radioactive nuclei to be eliminated. ^{14}C has a very long physical half-life (5760 years) but provided it is administered in the form of carbonate, i.e. not in an organic compound, it is quickly expelled in the expired air.

A further term, the effective half-life, is sometimes used in connection with the duration of radioactivity in the body following intake of an isotope. It describes the decrease in activity due to both physical and biological half-lives.

TOXICITY OF RADIOACTIVE ISOTOPES

Radionuclides have been classified according to their toxicity (International Atomic Energy Authority, 1963)—

Class 1 Radionuclides (high toxicity)

This includes alpha-emitters. Because of the high linear energy transfer from alpha particles considerable damage is produced in tissues near to the site of the ingested isotope. Radium and plutonium are examples.

Class 2 Radionuclides (medium toxicity-upper sub-group A)

This includes—

(a) Isotopes with a relatively long effective half-life, e.g. ^{22}Na, ^{60}Co, and ^{36}Cl.
(b) Isotopes that concentrate in a particular organ or tissue and therefore irradiate it heavily, e.g.:
(i) ^{131}I, which concentrates in the thyroid gland.
(ii) ^{45}Ca and ^{90}Sr, which are deposited in bone and, because they have a low rate of excretion, cause damage to erythropoietic tissue in the marrow over a long period.

Class 3 Radionuclides (medium toxicity—lower sub-group B)

This includes most of the radioactive isotopes used in medicine, e.g. ^{14}C, ^{24}Na, ^{32}P, ^{35}S, ^{42}K, ^{55}Fe, ^{59}Fe, ^{58}Co, ^{51}Cr, ^{74}As, ^{132}I, ^{198}Au.

Class 4 Radionuclides (low toxicity)

This includes isotopes with very weak emissions or a short effective half-life. Medical examples include ^{3}H, ^{91m}Y, ^{99m}Te.

The position of an isotope in this classification is a guide to the amount that can be safely handled, which is also determined by the type of laboratory and the circumstances in which the isotope is being handled (i.e. a simple or complex operation in which the nuclide is in solution or a manipulation of dry material; the latter is particularly hazardous because of the risk of inhaling radioactive dust).

SHIELDING

For many simple operations there is no significant hazard from working without shielding provided the work is performed quickly and at an adequate distance from the active material. Nevertheless, before this it is essential to confirm with a suitable monitor that the consequent exposure is acceptable.

Beta-emitters

Although the range of beta-particles in air is a few metres, it is much shorter in denser materials. Beta-particles lose energy in matter by interaction with the electrons of atoms and, therefore, their absorption depends largely on the number of electrons in their path. For materials of low atomic number this is nearly proportional to the weight per unit area and, consequently, absorbing power for beta-particles is expressed in mg/cm^2, i.e. the weight of material behind 1 cm^2 of surface.

The amount of material necessary to stop a beta-particle entirely is known as the range of the particle, e.g. the range for a 2 MeV particle in aluminium is 1000 mg/cm^2.

Provided the energy is less than 1 MeV, glass containers give satisfactory protection from their contents. If the isotope is in solution the solvent provides some shielding. The shielding material should be of low atomic number (e.g. aluminium, perspex, and thick rubber). In materials of high atomic number some of the beta energy is converted into a highly penetrating form of X-ray known as braking radiation (bremsstrahlung). However, the danger from this is not significant unless large sources of about 1 Ci or more are involved.

Perspex of 6 mm thickness absorbs beta-particles of energy up to 1 MeV, and adequate protection is given by a perspex asepsis screen made from sheet 5 mm thick.

Gamma-emitters

Shielding against gamma radiation is much more difficult because gamma rays are never completely absorbed however great the thickness of the absorber. The intensity of the transmitted radiation decreases exponentially with absorber thickness, and the degree of attenuation depends on the energy of the rays and the geometry of the source. Calculations are complicated, and reference must be made to more specialised sources of information for details. However, in general, the heavier (i.e. the greater the atomic number) the shielding material the greater the attenuation; therefore, lead is often used. For example, 1 MeV rays are 90 per cent attenuated by 45 mm of lead or 250 mm of concrete. The lead bricks used in dispensing radiopharmaceuticals interlock in a way that prevents radiation passing between the bricks.

Laboratory Design

Work with isotopes should be segregated into special rooms. A good suite for dispensing would include a dispensary, a counting room, a hot laboratory, a store, and an annexe.

DISPENSARY

As the preparation of radionuclides for medical use often involves aseptic technique, a well-designed asepsis laboratory is essential.

COUNTING ROOM

This should be well away from the hot laboratory. Nearby sources of high activity increase the background radiation in the counting room. A low background is necessary for accurate use of radiation measuring equipment. Sources taken to the room for counting should not exceed a few microcuries so that the effect on equipment adjacent to that being used is minimal. It should be appreciated also that, although tracer levels of isotopes present no health hazard to the dispenser, spread of contamination may greatly upset counting (e.g. 1% of 1 μCi $\equiv$ 370 disintegrations per second).

HOT LABORATORY

A separate room is desirable for handling materials above the tracer level. It should have a strengthened fume cupboard with an air flow rate, away from the operator, of 0·5 to 1 m/s. There must be no risk of back draughts carrying contamination into other rooms.

STORE

Additional safety is provided by a separate store. Entrance from outside, as well as from inside, the building avoids transport of supplies through the suite. A steel locker provided with lead containers or bricks, particularly for gamma-emitters, is suitable for storage.

ANNEXE

This is an inactive area leading into the dispensary. It includes changing, washing, and monitoring facilities.

Constructional Materials

The problem is contamination control and is similar to that faced by a pharmacist when

asepsis suite. Many of the solutions are the same.

A detailed discussion of the design of asepsis laboratories will be found in *Dispensing for Pharmaceutical Students* but the following points are of special importance in connection with laboratories for dispensing isotopes.

All surfaces should be smooth, non-porous, non-wetting, and heat-resistant. The flooring should be removable and replaceable easily should it become badly contaminated. Well-laid and heavily waxed linoleum is popular because usually it is possible to clean up a spillage by just removing the wax.

Wall finishes should be hard and smooth for ease of decontamination. High gloss paint is preferable to tiles because it is easier to remove if necessary.

The amount of wood should be minimal; benches and cupboards can be plastic-faced and wood surrounds treated with a sealer. Junctions, e.g. where a bench joins a wall, can be closed with a waterproof sealing compound and covered with a sealed beading. Benches that have to carry lead bricks must be strengthened; this applies particularly to the fume cupboard in the hot laboratory.

OTHER ASPECTS

Wastes from sinks should be easily accessible, preferably of glass and provided with a trap to prevent active material, accidentally discarded, from reaching the main system immediately. Ideally, sinks should not have overflows because they are difficult to clean.

Each worker should be allocated adequate floor space to minimise receipt of radiation from adjacent workers; 18 square metres is a suitable area.

Equipment

Surgical Rubber Gloves

These are worn when open sources are being handled. They must be removed or well washed before counting equipment, taps etc. are handled.

Trays

A tray is necessary as a working surface. It must be flat-bottomed and large enough to contain the whole volume of any liquid being handled, should spillage occur. Its internal surface should be covered, first with bitumen-interleaved paper or plastic sheeting and then with a layer of blotting paper. It is useful to cover the whole bench in the same way. Stainless-steel trays are ideal but costly. A compromise is to use one of reasonable size within a much larger plastic tray, the latter covering most of the working area.

Pipettes

These must be of the safety type of which many kinds are available. The most convenient are piston-operated. Alternatively, a suitable attachment, e.g. a safety bulb or tubing to a remote syringe, may be used. Wash bottles, also, must not be mouth-operated; the plastic squeeze-type is satisfactory.

Paper Tissues

Tissues are of great value for mopping-up small volumes of spillage, resting the tips of used pipettes etc.

Long Forceps

Even 75 mm forceps reduce the dose to the hands to $\frac{1}{100}$th because of the reduction of radiation intensity with distance, according to the inverse square law. Remote handling tools may be required for gamma-emitters.

Beakers

These are useful for containing bottles of active material for extra safety. If required, the space between the bottle and beaker may be filled with lead shot to reduce the dose rate.

Waste Containers

For solid waste, a foot-operated bin lined with a tough paper bag is suitable. For liquid waste, bottles or carboys made from thick plastic are necessary.

Container Carriers

Containers of active material should not be carried in the hands or pockets. A tin lined with cotton wool and fitted with a handle is usually adequate but special lead containers are available for strong gamma sources.

Shielding

A plastic asepsis screen with a closed front is satisfactory for most beta-emitters, provided the perspex sheet is of adequate thickness, but many types of totally enclosed glove boxes, with special air control systems and gauntlets in the arm holes are available commercially.

When lead bricks are necessary for gamma-emitters it may be possible to give adequate protection by a screen around the source rather than by a more bulky and inconvenient wall directly in front of the worker. A large, suitably tilted mirror may be necessary. Since gamma-rays are not significantly attenuated by a wooden bench the lower parts of the body must be protected by, for example, a layer of lead bricks on the bench surface.

Laboratory Discipline

Laboratory coats must always be worn.

Non-essential items should not be taken into active laboratories.

Drinking, eating, smoking, and application of cosmetics are forbidden.

No mouth operations are allowed.

Paper, not normal handkerchiefs, should be used and treated as active waste.

All waste must be retained in special receptacles.

The working area, hands, and clothing must be carefully monitored after use.

In every active room a monitor, giving audible signals, should be in constant use to provide warning of excessive build-up of background radiation.

A personal monitor, usually a film badge, must be carried.

Radiopharmaceuticals

The importance of radionuclides in medicine is reflected in the Pharmacopoeia which includes several monographs on radioactive products (*see* list at end of chapter). These and similar preparations are called radiopharmaceuticals.

The main source of supply in the UK is the Radiochemical Centre at Amersham. The isotope is sent to the user in one of the following forms—

1. A solution for parenteral use.
2. A solution for oral use.
3. A stock solution to be diluted and, if appropriate, sterilised before parenteral or oral use.
4. Nuclide generators.

The first three are self-explanatory apart from the fact that the oral preparations include isotopes in oil solution and packed in gelatin capsules. Each capsule provides a single dose of defined activity at a particular time; the use of this form also eliminates the need for a flavouring agent.

Nuclide Generators

The hazard to a patient during a diagnostic investigation is reduced by using an isotope with a very short physical half-life but it is difficult to distribute such isotopes to users directly. A solution sometimes possible is to supply it in the form of a long-lived parent that decays to the isotope required. The parent is prepared in the form of a suitable ion which is adsorbed on to a column, usually of alumina; the whole is known as a generator or cow (Richards, 1966). The user elutes (milks) the daughter with a suitable solution.

An important example is the technetium 99^m generator. This isotope is used for brain, liver, and thyroid scanning because, as well as having a short half-life (6 h), it does not emit beta radiation, which makes it safer to use in the body. Also, the one gamma photon it produces has an energy of 0·14

MeV which is very suitable for scanning techniques because it is low enough for the detector to be shielded fairly easily from radiation from parts of the organ at which it is not looking immediately; at the same time the energy is not so low that loss by absorption and scattering in the tissues is significant.

The parent, in this case, is molybdenum-99, which has a half-life of 67 hours and is prepared as ammonium molybdate before adsorption of the molybdate ion on to the alumina. The technetium is removed as pertechnate ion by elution with isotonic saline—

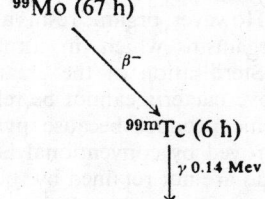

When the daughter has been removed, more parent decays and further milking can be done. After a week a new column is required. Figure 36.2 shows a growth-decay scheme for this system.

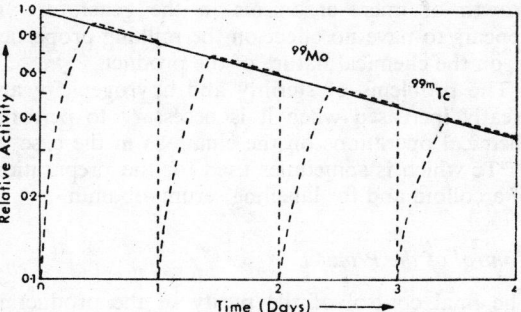

Fig. 36.2 Growth-decay curve for ^{99}Mo – ^{99m}Tc system

Table 36.2
Parent-daughter Systems

	System		Half-lives Parent	Daughter	Applications
^{132}Te	$\xrightarrow{\beta^-}$	^{132}I	78 h	2·3 h	Thyroid studies
^{87}Y	$\xrightarrow{EC}$	^{87m}Sr	80 h	2·8 h	Bone scanning
^{68}Ge	$\xrightarrow{EC}$	^{68}Ga	280 d	68 min	Bone studies
^{90}Sr	$\xrightarrow{\beta^-}$	^{90}Y	28 yr	64 h	Cancer therapy
^{113}Sn	$\xrightarrow{\beta^-}$	^{113m}In	118 d	1·7 h	Kidney function

Other examples of parent-daughter systems are shown in Table 36.2.

PRACTICAL ASPECTS

Shielding

The columns contain considerable activity (e.g. for ^{99}Mo, 25 to 200 millicuries) and adequate lead shielding must be set up around them.

Bacterial Contamination

The method of choice for separating a parent and daughter system is ion exchange because of its simplicity. However, organic resins allow the growth of micro-organisms which, in turn, may produce pyrogens. Sterilisation of the eluate while it will kill or remove bacteria cannot be relied on to yield an apyrogenic product because pyrogens are not always destroyed by conventional heat sterilisation processes and are not retained by the usual types of bacteria-proof filters. If possible, inorganic adsorbents are chosen because they are less likely to support microbial growth; also, they are more resistant to radiation damage.

Charlton (1966) has suggested the addition of 0·5 per cent phenol to the eluent to prevent the growth of micro-organisms in the generator; it appears to have no effect on the milking properties or on the chemical nature of the product.

The problems of sterility and apyrogenicity are greatly increased when it is necessary to perform chemical operations on the eluate as in the case of ^{99m}Tc which is sometimes used for the preparation of a colloid and for labelling serum albumin.

Control of the Product

The final control of the purity of the product is not in the hands of the manufacturer of the generator. The user must be aware of the appropriate control procedures and should analyse samples for radionuclidic purity between milkings of diagnostic doses.

A self-explanatory drawing of a unit for collecting a daughter product from a generator is shown in Fig. 36.3, but considerable variation in design is possible (Hutchinson and McLeod, 1965).

Stability

Apart from decomposition due to decay of the radionuclide itself which, inevitably, adds impurity to the preparation, the purity of the product may be

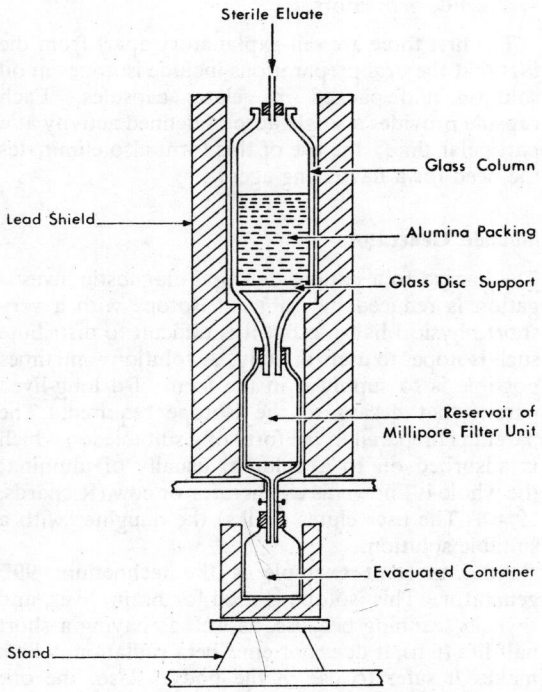

Fig. 36.3   A typical generator unit

affected by damage to the labelled compound or the adjuncts as a result of—

1. Direct action of the radiations from the radionuclide.
2. Indirect action, due to free radicals and other species produced, from the solvent or impurities, by the radiations.
3. Chemical action unconnected with the radiations.

1. DIRECT ACTION

This can be reduced by lowering the specific activity, or by dilution. Dilution leads to absorption of much of the radiation by the diluent (e.g. solvent) instead of by the active ingredient; it is a useful technique but it may be accompanied by an increase in the indirect effect.

Occasionally it may be possible to use a less energetic isotope of the same element. An example is the replacement of ^{131}I by ^{125}I for labelling insulin and triiodothyronine.

2. INDIRECT ACTION

This can be reduced by—

(a) Storage at a low temperature, which reduces the mobility of the free radicals.
(b) Changing to a non-aqueous solvent.
(c) Lowering the specific activity.
(d) Adding a reducing agent.
(e) Adding a radical scavenger.

The last-named is a substance that is preferentially attacked by the free radicals; e.g. benzyl alcohol 0·9 per cent improves the stability of high specific activity cyanocobalamin ^{57}Co from 47 per cent loss of activity in six months to less than 2 per cent in three months.

3. CHEMICAL ACTION

This is controlled by conventional means such as the addition of buffers, antioxidants, sequestering agents; use of scrupulously clean containers; and protection from light (by storage in the dark), moisture (by freeze-drying or packaging in a hermetically-sealed container) and oxygen (by using evacuated or nitrogen-filled ampoules).

Formulation of Parenteral Products

Apart from the aspects mentioned in the previous section this closely follows the formulation of other injections, but some special features are considered below—

1. SOLVENT

All the radioactive injections in the Pharmacopoeia are aqueous, i.e. the solvent is Water for Injections. Occasionally propylene glycol is included, e.g. 50 per cent in Water for Injections for iodinated thyroxine.

Oily solutions are uncommon but a solution of iodinated (^{131}I) triolein in iodised oil injection is used for investigations of the lymphatic system.

2. OSMOTIC PRESSURE

When an injection or solution is required for a haematological investigation isotonicity with blood plasma is desirable. For example, Ferric Citrate (^{59}Fe) Injection and Sodium Chromate (^{51}Cr) Solution are made isotonic with sodium chloride.

3. BACTERICIDES

Usually, parenteral solutions of radionuclides are supplied in multi-dose containers, because of the constantly changing dose of the preparation due to decay. Also, a multi-dose container is less expensive to shield for transport than the equivalent number of single dose units.

The choice of a suitable bactericide is complicated by the instability of many of them under the influence of radiations. One of the most suitable is benzyl alcohol 0·9 per cent. This is mentioned in the Pharmacopoeia as a satisfactory bactericide for Iodinated (^{131}I) Human Serum Albumin Injection. However, it has two disadvantages—

(a) It is a vasodilator and, therefore, is not universally suitable, e.g. it cannot be used in injections used to investigate the circulatory system.
(b) It decomposes in solutions of high radioactivity; e.g. in $Na_2H^{32}PO_4$ injection of strength 10 mCi/ml a heavy white precipitate is produced after several weeks storage. (This precipitate may be due to oxidation to benzoic acid.) The esters of parahydroxybenzoic acid behave similarly.

Sometimes, as with sodium chromate (^{51}Cr), the medicament is an oxidising agent. Oxidation of the bactericide might render it inactive while the accompanying reduction of the chromate could make it unsuitable for its purpose, the labelling of red blood cells.

Mercurial compounds are used as bactericides in such low concentrations that a small amount of radiation-induced change might render them ineffective.

When a suitable bactericide cannot be found the Pharmacopoeia permits omission provided the container is labelled to indicate this. The physician must then decide whether or not to use the container more than once.

For further information see Charlton (1965), Cohen (1966), Peng (1961), and Wolf and Tubis (1967).

4. ANTIOXIDANTS

These may be used to maintain a radionuclide in the correct valency state (e.g. Ferrous Citrate ^{59}Fe) or to prevent other oxidative changes (e.g. Sodium Iodide Injection (^{131}I), which contains thiosulphate to prevent volatilisation of iodine produced by atmospheric oxidation and by secondary radiation effects). For further information see Briner (1963, 1966) and Wolf and Tubis (1967).

5. OTHER ADDITIVES

Special stabilisers are used in certain cases. Iodinated (^{131}I) human serum albumin that has been partially coagulated by heat treatment is sometimes used for lung scanning. The particles are temporarily trapped in the lungs. To prevent excessive heat denaturation of the albumin, sodium caprylate or acetyltryptophanate is added (p. 420).

^{198}Au in colloidal suspension is used to treat malignant serous effusions in the pleural or peritoneal cavities. The gold colloid is prepared by reducing a salt of gold-198 by dextrose in alkaline solution in the presence of gelatin as a stabiliser. The latter acts as a protective colloid (p. 61).

Calculation of the Activity of a Radiopharmaceutical

In dispensing radiopharmaceuticals it is often necessary to calculate the activity of a preparation at some future time. This can be done in two ways;

1. FROM EQUATIONS (36.2) AND (36.3)

Example

The activity of a sample of ^{131}I was 500 microcuries per millilitre at noon on Monday. Calculate its activity at 4·0 p.m. on Thursday (Half-life of ^{131}I = 8 days). From Eqn (36.3)—

$$\lambda = \frac{0.693}{t_{\frac{1}{2}}}$$

Since $t_{\frac{1}{2}}$ for ^{131}I = 8 days (8 × 24 hours):

$$\lambda = \frac{0.693}{8 \times 24}$$

From Eqn (36.2)—

$$\ln N_t - \ln N_0 = -\lambda t$$

$$N_0 = 500 \ \mu\text{Ci/ml}$$

t = the time from noon Monday to 4 p.m. Thursday = 76 h

$$\therefore \ \ln N_t - \ln 500 = -\frac{0.693}{8 \times 24} \times 76$$

i.e.

$$\ln N_t = 6.218 - 0.2743$$
$$= 5.944$$

Hence, N_t = 381·1 microcuries per millilitre.

Any units may be used for N_0 and N_t provided they are the same for both, e.g. microcuries per ml or disintegrations per minute per unit volume. The time is usually expressed in hours.

2. GRAPHICALLY

Using the preceding example—

At time 0 the activity   = 500 μCi/ml
After exactly eight days
    the activity = 250 μCi/ml because the
half-life is 8 days.

The appropriate points are plotted on semi-log paper as shown in Fig. 36.4, and because the relationship between the logarithm of the activity of a radionuclide and time is linear, a straight line can be drawn between these points. From extrapolation of this line the activity at 4 p.m. Thursday can be read off. It is 381 μCi/ml.

Any error in obtaining the activity from the graph is much less than that involved in measuring the aliquot of the radioactive solution.

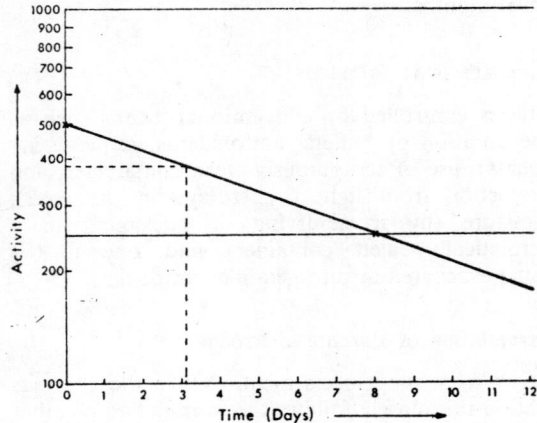

Fig. 36.4 Logarithm of activity plotted against time for ^{131}I

Dispensing

Most of the principles relevant to the safe dispensing of radiopharmaceuticals have been outlined earlier. Adaptation of aseptic technique (*see Dispensing for Pharmaceutical Students*) to allow for these should permit most problems to be faced with confidence.

Nevertheless, a dummy run should always be done before any new procedure is attempted, because this will disclose any special difficulties and provide the opportunity to work out quicker manipulations, possibly at a greater distance, so that when the isotope is used the time of exposure and dose rate will be minimal. In this preliminary work it is valuable to use highly coloured dye solutions to show that spillage has either not occurred or has been satisfactorily contained. During the first active manipulation the dose rate should be most carefully monitored.

Sterilisation

When the preparation is stable to autoclaving sterilisation presents no special problems except that small portable autoclaves should be used to avoid the inconvenience that a breakage in a large hospital steriliser would cause.

For isotopes, such as ^{132}I and ^{99m}Tc, with very short half-lives there is insufficient time for autoclaving, and sterilisation by filtration is necessary. Solutions of radiopharmaceuticals are very dilute, and adsorptive filters such as fibrous pads are unsuitable. The best media are cellulose ester membranes (e.g. Millipore filters). A 13 mm size is available that can be used in a hypodermic syringe adaptor. The membrane with a pore size of 0.22 μm is most satisfactory. A polypropylene disposable adaptor is also available. The method can be used, with a 0.45 μm membrane, for filtration of oily solutions. Strict aseptic technique is essential during the subsequent transfer to the final container which, in some cases, can conveniently be a disposable syringe.

When the product is thermolabile and a suspension, the entire preparation must be carried out aseptically.

Sterility Testing

Sterility testing of radiopharmaceuticals presents three problems—

1. The long incubation time of the tests (normally seven days in the UK) often precludes testing before issue, either because the preparation has a very short half-life or because it is unstable. An example of the latter is the colloidal solution of chromium phosphate (^{32}P).

This is not a serious difficulty with injections sterilised by autoclaving because it is common practice to rely mainly on process controls for this method.

For other injections, where sterilisation by filtration or preparation by aseptic technique is used, reliance should be put on good asepsis and, where possible, a 48-hour sterility test. In any case a retrospective test is desirable to confirm the reliability of the method of preparation.

2. The culture media are subjected to intense radiation and there is some evidence that this may slightly affect their constituents and, therefore, their sensitivities. It is possible, also, that high activities may prevent the recovery of damaged organisms. The dose received by 10 ml of broth containing 1 ml of Sodium Phosphate (^{32}P) Injection of specific activity 5 mCi/ml is 170 000 rads over 14 days (Burianek, 1965).

Use of the filtration method of sterility testing would considerably reduce this problem.

3. The additional difficulties of manipulation imposed by the radioactivity.

Pyrogen Testing

As with sterility testing, radiopharmaceuticals present special problems.

1. TIME TAKEN FOR TEST

For a conventional test it is advisable to allow a day in case repeat tests are necessary. This, added to transport time, means that short-lived isotopes cannot be tested before despatch. The problem is made worse by the preference of most users for delivery of short-lived isotopes at the beginning of the week.

2. PYRETIC EFFECTS OF THE RADIATIONS

There is little information on this aspect, but for the high activity preparations used in cancer treatment it is advisable to allow a period of decay before test, if this is practicable. The Pharmacopoeia specifies use of a volume of colloidal ^{198}Au, corresponding to 10 mCi, that has been allowed to decay to 100 μCi before testing. This kind of requirement makes testing before issue impracticable.

For diagnostic preparations pyretic effects due to radiation are unlikely to be significant.

Because of these two problems it is suggested that, as for other injections, pyrogen tests should be obligatory only if the preparation—

(a) is administered in large volume, e.g. ^{198}Au, or

(b) is a good medium for bacterial growth, e.g. iodinated (^{131}I) human serum albumin, or

(c) contains medicaments prone to contamination with pyrogens.

In addition, the solvent and any ingredients likely to be pyrogenic, e.g. gelatin in ^{198}Au colloid, should be tested before use, and occasional tests should be performed on all products to confirm that regular testing is not necessary.

In carrying out pyrogen tests on gamma-emitters it may be necessary to use either (a) a syringe encased in lead, with the consequent disadvantages of weight and difficulty of viewing the contents, or (b) a remote syringe to which is attached a long capillary tube that is passed through the bore of a needle previously inserted into the vein of the animal.

.For general aspects of sterility and pyrogen testing see Gunn and Carter (1965) and for aspects of the testing of radiopharmaceuticals see Charlton (1965a and b).

Adsorption

Adsorption of radioactive substances from solution on to the surfaces of containers and on to materials in suspension can be a serious problem, partly because desorption is difficult and partly because the amount of radioactive material in solution is often very small and, therefore, loss can be serious.

It can be minimised by—

(a) using silicone-coated glassware;

(b) maintaining an acid pH, since in glass containers adsorption is greatest from neutral or alkaline solutions;

(c) very carefully clarifying the solution to remove suspended impurities that might act as adsorbents.

Waste Disposal

Management of waste is one of the most important problems for workers with radionuclides. It must not be allowed to accumulate in working laboratories, because it will increase the background radiation, nor must its disposal become a danger to the general public. Useful precautions include—

(a) Separation of liquid and solid waste.

(b) Storage of the waste for each isotope separately or mixed only with waste from other isotopes of about the same half-life. Admixture of short and long-lived waste would delay disposal of the former.

(c) Labelling of waste containers with contents, date, and radiation level.

(d) Storage in a special area, e.g. a separate room or in an appropriately shielded part of the isotope store.

(e) Waste is not poured down the sink, incinerated, or put into the public health service refuse bin until its activity is no more than background or is not in excess of the level allowed for disposal by the local authority.

Isotopes of long half-life may require concentration by suitable techniques such as precipitation, evaporation, adsorption, and incineration to reduce bulk and, therefore, storage space. Sometimes it is possible by dilution or addition of a stable isotope in an appropriate chemical form to reduce the specific activity to a point at which earlier disposal is permissible.

The possibility of atmospheric pollution by the air from fume cupboards is slight when no more than a few curies of medical isotopes are being handled. Air filtration of the effluent is unlikely to be needed unless liquids of very great activity or powders are being handled. The air should be vented high above the roof.

Carcases of laboratory animals are preserved before storage, e.g. by covering with bleaching powder and Vermiculite and heat-sealing into a plastic bag. They must be kept cool. For further information on this subject see Code of Practice (1964).

Decontamination

Areas contaminated by spillage must be immediately and clearly marked and decontaminated promptly.

Spilt liquid can be absorbed by paper tissues or, if the amount is large, by Vermiculite.

Subsequent stages involve the use of swabs dampened with water or a detergent containing one or more complexing agents, such as EDTA or citric acid. In stubborn cases a gentle abrasive cleaner may be necessary. For spillage on linoleum an organic solvent may be required to take off the wax.

Powders should be 'fixed' immediately to prevent dispersal. A good method is to spray on a strippable coating which, on removal, will bring away the powder.

Glassware is cleaned before the isotope becomes firmly attached to the surfaces. Usually, water or a detergent plus a complexing agent is adequate. Success should be confirmed by monitoring both the glassware and the last rinsing. If the activity of the washing fluids is greater than 1 μCi they should be stored.

For detailed information on decontaminating laboratories see Code of Practice (1964, 1968).

Official Preparations

Preparation	Half-life (days)	Type of decay	Radiations	Dose range (approx.) μCi	mCi	Use Diagnostic	Therapeutic
Injections							
Chlormerodrin (^{197}Hg)	2.7	EC	γ X	20		Brain tumour localisation.	
Ferric citrate (^{59}Fe)	45	β^-	$\beta^-\gamma$	5–30		Iron metabolism	
Gold (^{198}Au)	2.7	β^-	$\beta^-\gamma$		50–200		Malignant effusions
Iodinated (^{125}I) human serum albumin	60	EC	γ X	2–5		Various, particularly blood volume determinations	
Iodinated (^{131}I) human serum albumin	8.04	β^-	$\beta^-\gamma$	5–50		Plasma volume. Circulation time	
Sodium iodide (^{131}I)	8.04	β^-	$\beta^-\gamma$	2–50	100–150	Thyroid function	Thyroid carcinoma
Sodium hippurate (^{131}I)	8.04	β^-	$\beta^-\gamma$	20		Renography	
Sodium phosphate (^{32}P)	14.3	β^-	β^-		5	Tumour localisation	Polycythæmia vera Leukaemia
Solutions							
Sodium chromate (^{51}Cr)	27.8	EC	γ X	20–100		Labelling of red blood cells	
Sodium iodide (^{125}I)						◄------- See Injection -------	
Sodium iodide (^{131}I)						◄------- See Injection -------►	
Solution and capsules (oral use): Injection							
Cyanocobalamin (^{57}Co)	270	EC	γ		1	Cyanocobalamin metabolism	
Cyanocobalamin (^{58}Co)	71	β^- EC	$\beta^-\gamma$		1	Cyanocobalamin metabolism	

Labelling

The Pharmacopoeia requires the following information on both package and container labels of radiopharmaceutical injections.

1. The name of the injection.
2. The strength, stated in either microcuries or millicuries per millilitre, at a given time and date.
3. An indication that the injection is radioactive.
4. The name and percentage of any added bactericide or, if appropriate, a statement that the injection does not contain one.
5. A mark or number whereby the history of the injection may be traced.

In addition the package label must state—

1. The total volume of the injection.
2. The total content of active and inactive elements, in certain instances.

REFERENCES

BRINER, W. H. (1963) The preparation of radioactive chemicals for clinical use. *Am. J. Hosp. Pharm.*, **20**, 553–561.

BRINER, W. H. (1966) *Radioactive Pharmaceuticals* (Edited by Andrews, G. A. *et al.*) U.S Atomic Energy Commission, Oak Ridge. 93–111.

BURIANEK, J. (1965) *Radiopharmaceuticals, Specifications. I. Sterility tests, II. Pyrogen tests.* W.H.O./Pharm./Fd. Sec./122.65.

CHARLTON, J. C. (1965a) *Radiopharmaceuticals. Specifications I. Pyrogen tests, II. Addition of bactericides to multi-dose bottles.* W.H.O./Pharm./ Ed. Sec./123.65.

CHARLTON, J. C. (1965b) Radioactive pharmaceuticals *Pharm. J.*, **195**, 37–41.

CHARLTON, J. C. (1966) *Radioactive Pharmaceuticals* (Edited by Andrews, G. A. *et al.*) U.S. Atomic Energy Commission, Oak Ridge. 33–50.

CHRISTIAN, J. E. (1961) Radioisotopes in the pharmaceutical sciences and industry. *J. pharm. Sci.*, **50**, 1–13.

CODE OF PRACTICE (1964, 1968) *Code of Practice for the Protection of Persons Exposed to Ionising Radiations in Research and Teaching.* 1st and 2nd ed. Her Majesty's Stationery Office, London.

COHEN, Y. (1966) *Radioactive Pharmaceuticals* (Edited by Andrews, G. A. *et al.*) U.S. Atomic Energy Commission, Oak Ridge. 165–175.

GUNN, C. and CARTER, S. J. (1965) *Dispensing for Pharmaceutical Students.* 11th ed. Pitman Medical, London. 529–534.

HUTCHINSON, F. and MACLEOD, T. M. (1965) Radiopharmaceutics. *Pharm. J.*, **195**, 461–462.

INTERNATIONAL ATOMIC ENERGY AUTHORITY (1963) *Classification of Radionuclides. Technical Report Series No. 15.*

LEA, D. E. (1947) *Action of Radiations on Living Cells.* Macmillan, New York.

M.R.C. REPORT (1960) *The Hazards to Man of Nuclear and Allied Radiations. Medical Research Council Report.* Her Majesty's Stationery Office, London.

PENG, C. T. (1961) Radioactive drugs in the United States Pharmacopoeia. *J. pharm. Sci.*, **50**, 88–90.

RADIOCHEMICAL MANUAL (1966) Ed. by Wilson, B. J. 2nd ed. The Radiochemical Centre, Amersham.

RECOMMENDATIONS OF THE INTERNATIONAL COMMISSION ON RADIOLOGICAL PROTECTION (1959, 1966) Pergamon, London.

RICHARDS, P. (1966) *Radioactive Pharmaceuticals.* (Edited by Andrews, G. A. *et al.*) U.S. Atomic Energy Commission, Oak Ridge.

WOLF, W. and TUBIS, M. (1967) Radiopharmaceuticals. *J. pharm. Sci.*, **56**, 1–17.

Appendix

Forces between Molecules, Ions and Atoms

When molecules, ions, or atoms are near enough to influence each other then forces of attraction and repulsion operate. Attractive forces are necessary to produce the coherence between molecules that is responsible for the liquid and solid states. However, if repulsive forces did not operate there would be nothing to prevent the attractive forces from causing interpenetration and mutual destruction of molecules.

REPULSIVE FORCES

Two types of repulsive force exist.

(*a*) A general repulsion, which arises if any two atoms are brought too close together, since there is a reluctance for their electron clouds to overlap. This effect is only important for distances of the order of atomic dimensions because it decreases extremely rapidly with distance of separation between atoms. In fact, this repulsive force is approximately proportional to the inverse twelfth power of the interatomic distance, r; i.e. repulsion α $1/r^{12}$.

(*b*) Coulombic repulsion between two similarly charged ions. The force, F, of this repulsive effect between two ions with net charges Q_1 and Q_2 respectively, separated by a distance r in a vacuum, is given by Eqn (A.1), where ε_0 is known as the permittivity of the vacuum.

$$F = \frac{Q_1 Q_2}{4\pi\varepsilon_0 r^2} \qquad (A.1)$$

When the ions are separated by a uniform dielectric medium the force exerted between them is less than when they are in a vacuum. This effect is taken into account by Eqn (A.2), where ε_r is the permittivity of the medium relative to that of a vacuum.

$$F = \frac{Q_1 Q_2}{4\pi\varepsilon_r r^2} \qquad (A.2)$$

ATTRACTIVE FORCES

These are classified on the basis of the natures of the two components, between which attraction occurs.

There are three types of component: i.e. ions permanent dipoles, and induced dipoles.

1. Ions arise from the transfer of electrons from one atom to another.

2. In covalent bonds complete transfer of electrons between one atom and another does not occur, and these bonds involve shared electrons. However, if the bond is formed between two different atoms the shared electrons will be closer to the more electronegative atom. Thus, the positive and negative centres do not coincide. This separation of charge gives rise to a permanent dipole moment associated with that bond. This dipole moment will possess a particular value and will act in a particular direction. The various bond moments that may arise in a compound, which contains several bonds, contribute to an overall value for the dipole moment of that compound. If this value is finite (i.e. >0) the molecule is said to possess a permanent dipole moment, whereas a molecule with a dipole moment of zero is said to be non-polar. (It should be borne in mind that a non-polar molecule may still contain polar bonds, since its dipole moment of zero may result from opposing bond moments within the molecule; e.g. bond moments with equal values acting in opposite directions.)

3. In completely covalent bonds the electrons are shared equally by the two atoms involved in the bond. The latter does not therefore possess a dipole moment. However, if an ion is brought up to one end of this bond the shared electrons may be displaced towards one or other of the involved atoms and so give rise to an induced dipole moment in the bond. For example, a negatively charged ion will repel the bonding electrons as shown in Fig. A.1a. This effect will disappear when the inducing ion is removed. A similar effect can arise when a molecule with a permanent dipole moment approaches the non-polar molecule. This is illustrated by Fig. A.1b.

Since there are three different types of component between which attraction can occur, then six types of attraction may arise. These are summarised in Table A.1. In addition, the forces of these various attractions differ in their dependence on the distance of separation of the components. The relationship

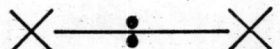

Covalent bond between two
similar atoms. Bonding
electrons are equally shared
and molecule is non-polar.

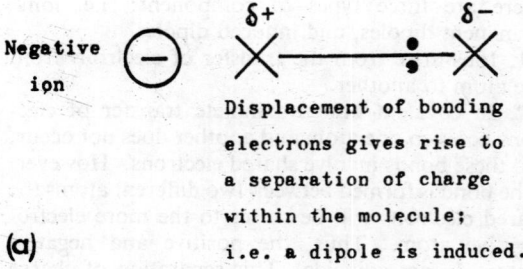

Displacement of bonding
electrons gives rise to
a separation of charge
within the molecule;
i.e. a dipole is induced.

Molecule with a
permanent dipole.

Molecule with
an induced
dipole arising
from displacement
of bonding electrons.

(b)

Fig. A.1

(a) Ion-induced dipole interaction

(b) Permanent dipole-induced dipole interaction

between these forces and distance is also given in Table A.1.

The potential energy of attraction may be regarded as the work required to overcome the attraction and separate the components from a distance of closest approach to infinity. Since work is equal to force × distance, then the potential energies of the various attractions listed in Table A.1 are inversely proportional to one less power of the distance of separation than the corresponding forces of attraction.

The last three types of attraction listed in the table are known collectively as van der Waals forces. It can be seen that their effects are much more dependent on the distance of separation than the electrostatic forces between ions or ions and dipoles. The attractive forces that are exerted between non-polar molecules are known as London or dispersion forces. These arise from the fact that the vibrations of electrons produces a mutual induction of dipoles within the molecules.

Finally, a special type of attraction that involves the sharing of a hydrogen atom between two electronegative atoms, such as oxygen, nitrogen or fluorine, may occur. This interaction is known as hydrogen bonding. The electronegative atoms may be contained in different molecules so that intermolecular association results from the hydrogen bonding, or they may be in the same molecule, so that intramolecular hydrogen bond formation occurs. The energy of a hydrogen bond is about one tenth that of a covalent bond. This energy is therefore appreciable, and hydrogen bonding is of particular importance in intermolecular complex formation and solvation.

Table A1
Types of Attraction and the Relationship of their Forces and Potential Energies to Distance of Separation, *r*

Type of attraction	Potential energy proportional to	Force proportional to
Ion—ion	$1/r$	$1/r^2$
Ion—permanent dipole	$1/r^3$	$1/r^4$
Ion—induced dipole	$1/r^4$	$1/r^5$
Permanent dipole—permanent dipole	$1/r^6$	$1/r^7$
Permanent dipole—induced dipole	$1/r^6$	$1/r^7$
Induced dipole—induced dipole	$1/r^6$	$1/r^7$

Index

Note. Where one of a series of references is of particular importance it is printed in **bold type**.

Autoclave 294, 304, 331
Autoradiography 306
Autotroph 303
Autoxidation 99, 100
Azeotropic mixture **23**, 24, 267

BACILLUS sp. **299**, 308, 320, **324**, 332, 354, 363
Bacillus anthracis, in vaccine lymph 408
Bacitracin 372
Bacteria
  biochemical tests for 322
  capsules 298, 307, 321, 325, 335, 385
  classification 303, 323, 324, 331, 332
  counting **326**, 342, 347
  cultural characters **323**, 335
  cultural conditions 344
  cultural techniques 317, 321, 366
  morphology 307, 323, 324, 335
  motility 299, 307, 318, 320, 324, 325, 326
  nutrition 303, 342
  reproduction 305, 306, 342
  toxins 376
  vegetative 304, 308, 335, 350, 353, 255, 358
Bactericides **333**, 341, 342, 354, 363, 368
  biochemical effects 337, 342, 373
Bacteriolysins 378
Bacteriophages 306, **314**, 323, 366
Bacteriophrenic 341
Bacteriostat 341, 343, **347**, 352, 362
Ball mill 187
Bar 4, 5
BCG Vaccine, *see* Vaccines
Behring, E. A. 292
Benethamine penicillin 369
Bentonite 80, 126
  gel 68, 69, 118
Benzalkonium chloride 360, 364
Benzathine penicillin 369
Benzocaine 99
Benzoic acid and salts 353, 364
Benzoyl peroxide 99
Benzyl alcohol 359, 364, 365
Benzyl penicillin 296, 366, 368, 369
Bergey's Manual 323, 331
Berry and Bean's method of testing disinfectants 346
BET adsorption isotherm 45
Beta-haemolytic streptococci in vaccine lymph 408
Beta particles 436
Bile salts 110, 320, 321
Bimolecular layer 105, 106
Binary fission 305, 326
Binder, in tablets 217
Bingham bodies 117
Bingham equation 117
Biological half-life 111
Biological Oxygen Demand (BOD) 337
Biological response to radiations 441
Biotransformation 105, 110, 111, 113
Bisphenols 357, 358

Bithionol 358
Black fluid 358
Bleach 294
Blood:
  anticoagulants 415
  brain barrier 109
  clotting 69, **414**, 418
  Concentrated Human Red Corpuscles 417
  concentrations of drugs 111
  Dried Plasma 417
  Dried Serum 418
  groups 416
  Liquid Plasma 419
  Liquid Serum 419
  Whole Human 414
  products 414
    control 421
    labelling 421
Boiling point 18
  composition diagram 26
  diagram 25, 26
  effect of pressure 19
  elevation of 15
Bonding of tablet granules 232
Bordetella sp. 320, 325
  Bordetella pertussis 325, 376, 387, 409
Boric acid 353
Born repulsion 56
Botulinum Antitoxin 381, **403**
Boundary layers 148
Braking effect 64
Breaking of emulsions 80
Bredig's method 57
Brilliant green, *see* Dyes
Bronchial mucus 67
Brown's tubes 328, 386
Brownian movement 54, 59, 118
Brucella sp. 325
Bubble cap plates 266
Buffer(s) 337, 350, 354, 366, 368, 369, 371
Bulk density of powder beds 226
n-Butyl gallate 101
Butyl hydroxyanisole (BHA) 101

CAFFEINE 99, 113
Calamine lotion 79
Calandria 167
Calcium acetate solubility curve 9
Calcium alginate 426
Capillary condensation:
  in xerogels 70
  theory 46
Capillary rise:
  mechanism 35
  method 36
Capping, of tablets 218, 232
Caps, screw 137
Capsules, bacterial, *see* Bacteria
Capsules, as a dose form 71, 77, 112
Carbenicillin 369
Carbohydrates 303, 307, 322, 324, 367
Carbolic acid, *see* Phenol
Carbon dioxide 30, 87
Carrell flask 317

Carriers of disease 289, 292
Casein 79
Catalysis:
  heterogeneous 96
  homogeneous 96
Catgut 429
  boilable and non-boilable 431
  chromic 430
Cation 295, 360, 361
  exchanger 94, 95
Cationic agents 360, 362
Cationic dyes 295, 361, 362
Cell membrane 104, 106
  transport across 15, 104, **105**, 106
Cell wall, bacterial 276, 298, 308, 355, 368, 371
Cellulose acetate 72
  phthalate 113
Centrifugal effect 245, 246
Centrifugation 245
  principles 245
Centrifuges **246**, 328
  conical disc 248
  continuous 250
  perforated basket 246
  tubular bowl 247
Cephaloridine 372
Cetomacrogol 41, 80
  Emulsifying Ointment **68**
Cetostearyl alcohol 83
Cetrimide 41, 83, 360, 364
  Emulsifying Ointment **68**
  Emulsifying Wax 83
Cetylpyridinium salts 360
Cetyl trimethyl ammonium bromide 41
Chain inhibitor 100
Chain initiation 99, 100
  suppressors 100, 101
Chain propagation 99
Chain reactions 93, 103
Chain termination 99
  agents of 100
Charcoal 48, 49
  activated 48, 50
Chemical kinetics 89
Chemical potential 335
Chemical reactions in gels **70**
Chemical standards 346
Chemisorption **43**, 96
Chemotherapy 289, 294, 295, 364, 366, 373
Chi-squared test 327, 331, 347
Chick-Martin Test **344**, 352
Chloramines 354
Chloramphenicol 30, 113, 296, 366, 370, 373
  palmitate 20, 78, 113
Chlorbutol 359, 363, 364
Chlorhexidine 345, 362, 364
Chlorine 353, 355
Chlorocresol 364
Chloroform 49, 67, 364
Chlorothiazide 99
Chloroxylenol 67, 348, 357, 358
Chlorpromazine 110
Chlortetracycline 296, 370
Cholera 291, 292, 324, 376, 386
  vaccine, *see* Vaccines
Cholesterol 105

DISPENSING FOR PHARMACEUTICAL STUDENTS

Contents